MULTIPLE SCLEROSIS

MULTIPLE SCLEROSIS

Editors

DONALD W. PATY, MD, FRCPC
Professor, Department of Medicine
Division of Neurology
University of British Columbia
Vancouver Hospital and Health Sciences Center
Vancouver, British Columbia, Canada

GEORGE C. EBERS, MD, FRCPC
Professor, Department of Clinical Neurological
    Sciences
University of Western Ontario
University Campus–London Health
    Sciences Centre
London, Ontario, Canada

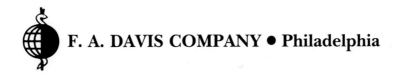 F. A. DAVIS COMPANY • Philadelphia

F.A. Davis Company
1915 Arch Street
Philadelphia, PA 19103

Printed in the United States of America

Last digit indicates print number: 10 9 8 7 6 5 4 3 2 1

Medical Editor: Robert W. Reinhardt
Medical Developmental Editor: Bernice M. Wissler
Cover Designer: Louis Forgione

As new scientific information becomes available through basic and clinical research, recommended treatments and drug therapies undergo changes. The author(s) and publisher have done everything possible to make this book accurate, up to date, and in accord with accepted standards at the time of publication. The authors, editors, and publisher are not responsible for errors or omissions or for consequences from application of the book, and make no warranty, expressed or implied, in regard to the contents of the book. Any practice described in this book should be applied by the reader in accordance with professional standards of care used in regard to the unique circumstances that may apply in each situation. The reader is advised always to check product information (package inserts) for changes and new information regarding dose and contraindications before administering any drug. Caution is especially urged when using new or infrequently ordered drugs.

Library of Congress Cataloging-in-Publication Data
Multiple sclerosis/editors, Donald W. Paty, George C. Ebers.
    p.   cm.—(Contemporary neurology series; 50)
  Includes bibliographical references and index.
  ISBN 0-8036-6784-1
  1. Multiple sclerosis I. Paty, Donald W. II. Ebers, George C.
III. Series.
  [DNLM: 1. Multiple Sclerosis. W1 CO769N v. 50 1997 / WL 360 M9556 1997]
RC377.M839 1997
616.8'34—dc21
DNLM/DLC
for Library of Congress   97-3052

We dedicate this book to our many patients with multiple sclerosis, who over the years have taught us so much about the disease, about themselves, about ourselves, and about courage and the unsinkable nature of the human spirit.

FOREWORD

About 20 years ago I gave a talk on multiple sclerosis treatment to the neurology department at the University of Western Ontario. Dr. Donald Paty had started his academic career there five years previously, and Dr. George Ebers had just arrived. Numerous research projects were underway. During my visit, one of the patients with MS in the hospital died. Within minutes after obtaining permission for autopsy, Drs. Paty and Ebers were in the morgue, with a well-organized team of technicians to collect specimens for their research. This type of enthusiasm for multiple sclerosis research has continued, both in Western Ontario and in Dr. Paty's new location at the University of British Columbia (UBC), where he assumed the post of Head of the Division of Neurology in 1980.

George Ebers, trained in both neurology and clinical immunology, has made signal contributions in the study of spinal fluid abnormalities and in clinical natural history studies, and has become an authority in the difficult field of MS genetics. Donald Paty, soon after arriving at UBC, became a lead investigator in the study of the natural history of MS as revealed by serial MRI scans, work that paralleled similar studies at the National Institute, Queen Square, London, by David Miller, Ian McDonald, and their colleagues. The MRI has provided a measuring tool that has revolutionized MS research in the past 12 years. All research involves measurement, and neurologists had only the CSF and cumbersome clinical scales to work with prior to its introduction.

The current volume reflects knowledge obtained from hundreds of well-studied cases of MS, most of whom have had complete CSF and imaging studies, and tissue typing. It also reflects the excellent teaching abilities of both authors: They are good at it, and like to do it. Some of their students and colleagues have participated in writing sections of this work.

Thanks in large measure to the prodigious efforts of Paty and Ebers, the development of new treatments for MS accelerated and culminated in the demonstration of effectiveness of new therapies. New therapies continue to be evaluated against the background of the natural history information which they, and their colleagues, have patiently accumulated. While the specifics of treatment will change rapidly in the next decade, this book will remain a valuable source of MS clinical and natural history data for many years to come.

William A. Sibley, MD
Tucson, Arizona

PREFACE

Why have we written this book? On reflection, we felt that our collective experience in clinical research and clinical management of MS justified putting some of our thoughts down on paper. We have seen or been involved in the management of over 6,000 patients with multiple sclerosis over the last 25 years. Therefore, we feel that it is appropriate at this time of flux and excitement in the multiple sclerosis world to organize our own thoughts on many day-to-day aspects of the disease.

The explosion of interest in and knowledge about multiple sclerosis has carried us well past the preoccupation with diagnosis that characterized our early years in the field. We are encouraged that finally the problem of MS is ripe for solution. Several things have simultaneously converged to engender this kind of optimism. Major developments include improvements in imaging, neurobiology, and the understanding of MS genetics. A better understanding of the natural history of the disease also has provided a major impetus for clinical trials. Improvements in the design and execution of such studies have led to confidence that patients are well-served by their participation. In contrast to studies in the past, modern trials have a high likelihood of being definitive, and increased potential to show meaningful therapeutic benefit. Nevertheless, as for most chronic disease, the most important outcome (long-term protection from disability) still remains an elusive target.

We wish to make a few apologies to the prospective reader. The book is primarily oriented toward the clinical practitioner in neurology, but we believe that it will also be useful to other physicians and allied health professionals. Some chapters may be helpful to patients and their families. Those who are interested in a basic understanding of immunology, the biology of myelin, or neurophysiology, however, will need to look elsewhere. Although we have made some effort to catalogue and tabulate a variety of topics that lend themselves well to such an approach, we recognize that in many cases we have opted to give our own opinions and interpretations of what are often complex data. Consensus in MS has not been easy, and we are certain that some of our interpretations will find disfavor. We therefore caution the reader to accept this book as our best effort, but to challenge all undocumented statements. We take full responsibility for errors of fact and emphasis.

Because the book covers many disciplines, we have attempted to write most chapters so that each can be read somewhat independently of the others. This method of organization is intended to save the reader from having to refer to other chapters via the index for a full understanding of the concepts being presented. This way of writing has caused some redundancy. However, we feel that the book expresses our point of view. We hope that it also provides enough raw data to help readers make up their own minds about controversial topics. We welcome comments so that we can better understand our readers' needs.

D.W. Paty, MD, FRCPC
G.C. Ebers, MD, FRCPC
May 1997

ACKNOWLEDGMENTS

This book owes its successful completion to many present and former colleagues from the MS Clinic at University Hospital, London, Ontario, and the MS Clinic at the Vancouver Hospital, Vancouver, B.C. These people include Holly Armstrong, Brenda Bass, Cathy-Lee Benbow, Kathy Eisen, Marg Elliott, Rochelle Farquhar, Eunice Gorman, Erin Johnston, Jane LeSaux, Lynn McEwan, Wendy Morrison, Jill Nelson, Ken Redekop, Peggy Vandervoort, and Sharon Vitali. Numerous physicians have played a key role in helping run the clinics and in stimulating us to address questions, some of which they have raised about MS. These physicians include M.B. D'Hooghe, Michael Farrell, Stan Hashimoto, John Hooge, Lorne Kastrukoff, Bill McGinnis, Michael Nicolle, John Noseworthy, Joël Oger, Beth Pringle, George Rice, Galina Vorobeychik, Lee Voulters, and Brian Weinshenker.

Funding from the MS Society of Canada, MS Foundation of Canada, the BC Health Research Foundation, the Jack Cohen Family, the Selena Aitken Fund, and the Medical Research Council of Canada have been instrumental in putting together many of the studies highlighted in this book. A special thanks is due to Bob Kibler and Jerome Posner for having shown us how clinical experience can be translated into deeper understanding of a disease.

Outstanding secretarial and data assistance has been provided by Vilma Brandjes, Lynn Dyck, Christain Guillou, Lynne Hannay, Cheryl Johnson, Debra King, Marion Lawson, Monique Schareck, and Marian Young.

We are very grateful for the editorial help of Bernice Wissler and Linda Weinerman from FA Davis. Special thanks is also due to our research colleagues Dennis Bulman, Keith Cover, David Li, Rob Koopmans, Brenda Rhodes, Andrew Riddehough, and Guojun Zhao.

CONTRIBUTORS

Duncan P. Anderson, MD, FRCSC
Associate Professor of Ophthalmology
University of British Columbia
Head, Department of Ophthalmology
St. Paul's Hospital
Vancouver, British Columbia, Canada

Terry A. Cox, MD
Duke University Eye Center
Durham, North Carolina

George C. Ebers, MD, FRCPC
Professor
Department of Clinical Neurological
  Sciences
University of Western Ontario
London Health Sciences Centre–
  University Campus
London, Ontario, Canada

Stanley A. Hashimoto, MD, FRCPC
Clinical Professor
Department of Medicine
Division of Neurology
University of British Columbia
Vancouver Hospital & Health Sciences
  Center
Vancouver, British Columbia, Canada

Lorne F. Kastrukoff, MD, FRCPC
Department of Medicine
Division of Neurology
University of British Columbia
Vancouver Hospital & Health Sciences
  Center
Vancouver, British Columbia, Canada

G.R. Wayne Moore, MD, CM, FRCPC
Clinical Professor of Pathology and
  Laboratory Medicine
Neuropathologist, Multiple Sclerosis Clinic
University of British Columbia
Vancouver Hospital & Health Sciences Center
Vancouver, British Columbia, Canada

John H. Noseworthy, MD, FRCPC
Professor and Chair
Division of Neuroimmunology
Department of Neurology
Mayo Clinic
Rochester, Minnesota

Donald W. Paty, MD, FRCPC
Professor
Department of Medicine
Division of Neurology
University of British Columbia
Vancouver Hospital & Health Sciences Center
Vancouver, British Columbia, Canada

George P. A. Rice, MD, FRCPC
Professor
Department of Clinical Neurological Sciences
University of Western Ontario
London Health Sciences Centre–University
  Campus
London, Ontario, Canada

A. Dessa Sadovnick, PhD
Associate Professor
Department of Medical Genetics and
  Medicine (Associate Member)
University of British Columbia
Vancouver, British Columbia, Canada

CONTENTS

CHAPTER 1

INTRODUCTION: A HISTORICAL OVERVIEW

George C. Ebers, MD

EARLY INVESTIGATORS
MORE RECENT HISTORY
SOME NOTES ON TERMINOLOGY

Any physician fortunate enough to have been familiar with or participated in the identification of a new disorder will appreciate the difference between recognizing an already established pattern and delimiting the boundaries of a new one. In this context, we can best appreciate the problems encountered by early investigators presented with a condition as pleomorphic as MS. The historical development of MS as a specific disease entity spans the golden age of neurology, includes many of its major figures as central players, is controversial, and is still in the process of modification.

EARLY INVESTIGATORS

The first reported case in the medical literature that represents an unmistakable example of relapsing-remitting MS appears to be that found in *Maladies de la moelle epinière* by Charles Prosper Ollivier.[19] This first clinical monograph on disorders of the spinal cord was published in 1824 in Paris. The description, first pointed out by Spillane,[23] is unaltered in the first three editions of Ollivier's monograph. The patient was a 20-year-old man who, in 1808, developed transient weakness of his right foot. At age 29 years he had considerable paraplegia, but again, this was followed by improvement, which allowed him to walk with a cane. At age 30 years he found that hot spa waters aggravated his disability (the first recorded hot tub test?), and he experienced an acute loss of feeling in the right leg, accompanied by numbness and clumsiness of both hands. Urinary retention developed, and evacuation was aided by pressure on the abdomen. His intellect remained preserved, although his motor function and speech deteriorated. When last seen, he was said to have lost none of the "gaiety of his character" despite advanced disability. This description is included in Ollivier's chapter on "myelitis," although we do not know who was responsible for the application of this rather apt term to the patient's disorder. Presumably, no pathology became available to Ollivier, nor do later editions of his book (the last in 1837) further clarify this disorder. Ollivier listed several possible causes of myelitis, which included the extension of erysipelas or an exanthem, thereby anticipating Pierre Marie's similar suggestions.[15] To treat the disorder, he advised general

1

bleedings and plenty of leeches over the thoracic area.

Other early investigators include Richard Bright,[3] who, in 1831, described a case suggestive of MS, and Robert Carswell,[4] whose celebrated atlas of anatomical pathology, which appeared in 1838, demonstrates in plate 4 a "peculiar disease state of the cord and pons varolii," which is unmistakably that of MS. This appears to be the first pathological representation of the lesions of MS, but it provides no clinical description. It appears that Carswell's seed fell on fallow ground in the British Isles, and it was not until more than three decades later that clinical descriptions of the disease in England were given by Moxon.[18]

Controversy still exists over who were among the earliest investigators to describe MS. Although priority for having published illustrated lesions of MS may go to Carswell, Cruveilhier,[9] whose clinical descriptions as well as pathological plates date to a slightly later period,[8] provided one of the earliest clearly recorded attempts to understand the disease process. Furthermore, his observations led to the classic studies of Charcot, Vulpian, and their students.

In the mid-nineteenth century, several authors from Germany described cases of multiple sclerosis both clinically and pathologically. Notable among these was Frerichs,[12] who was probably the first to diagnose "spinal sclerosis" in a living subject, if we choose to overlook Ollivier's approximation. This case was documented by his student Valentiner,[24] who despite grouping tabes, MS, and combined sclerosis together, did point out the existence of remissions in some cases. Additional contributions were made by Turck, Rokitansky, and Rindfleisch, among others.

In 1866, Vulpian[25] coined the term "sclerose en plaque disseminé" in print. He presented three cases of MS before the Societé Médical of the Paris hospitals. One of these, Mademoiselle V., was presented at Charcot's famous clinical lessons in 1868, having been "bequeathed" (along with Vulpian's careful and detailed notes on her) to Charcot when Vulpian left the Salpêtrière in 1865.

Although Charcot did not describe the first cases clinically or pathologically, nor was he the first to diagnose MS in life, he played a major role in establishing the disease as a clinical pathological entity through his widely read lectures.[5–7] Charcot published relatively little on MS himself, but there is every indication that the writings of his pupils Bourneville and Guerard[1] and Ordenstein[20] were direct extensions of his own thoughts and views and probably his words.

There is no doubt about the importance of Charcot's contribution in shaping the clinical features of MS into a reasonably discrete and diagnosable entity. Although it was tremor that originally directed Charcot's attention to this disorder, with the evident contrast between the resting tremor of Parkinson's disease and the intention tremor of MS, he soon pursued other aspects of this strange new malady. He defined the clinical features of the disease, including the recognition of atypical and incomplete forms. He emphasized the importance of a probing history to uncover fleeting early episodes and was thus aware of temporary complete remission. He recognized the pure spinal forms and enumerated atypical features such as amyotrophy. He first described the microscopic pathology in such a definite way that the woodcuts from his classic 1868 paper[5] served, in the words of Putnam, as "the textbooks of a generation." As late as 1938, Putnam[21] commented that the modern development of new and specific staining methods had added almost nothing to Charcot's descriptions achieved with his carmine stain.

The first monograph on MS was actually the aggregation thesis of Ordenstein,[20] Charcot's pupil at the Salpêtrière, which was published in 1867. This volume, which is roughly half devoted to Parkinson's disease and the other half to MS, is most notable for the first appearance of the famous chromolithograph of the drawing of gross MS plaques by Charcot.[7] However, the text is repetitious and spare on critical analysis, contains numerous errors of fact, and gives the previous writers on MS less than their due. Not surprisingly, Ordenstein gives credit for elucidating the clinical features of MS to Charcot.

The monograph by Bourneville and Guerard,[1] in contrast to that by Ordenstein, contains much more information and describes many more cases of MS. It contains the woodcuts from the 1868 Gazette Hô-pitaux article and contains extensive, careful clinical notes and analyses. The discussion of previous contributions is also much more satisfactory. Two of the clinical descriptions recorded in great detail appear to come from two of the patients in Cruveilhier's atlas and accordingly have special historical significance.

In North America, investigators included Morris,[17] who reported the first case of MS in North America by autopsy; Hammond,[13] who in his textbook of nervous diseases, stated that he had collected 11 cases of cerebrospinal MS; and finally, Osler.[11] Sir William Osler's experiences with the pathology of MS at the Montreal General Hospital in the latter part of the nineteenth century include one definite case and two possible cases out of a total of almost 800 autopsies. This remarkable series may represent the best available data for estimating the prevalence of MS in Canada a century ago. The data are severely limited in numbers but suggest a prevalence of the disease that is not much different than it is today.

William Moxon[18] reported on eight cases of "insular sclerosis," a term that he used in 1875. Some authors believe this to be the first authoritative description of MS in the English literature. The etiology of the disease drew few more thoughtful comments than those by Pierre Marie in 1884.[15] Based on personal observations, he suggested that MS was the complication of a large number of infective diseases, including typhoid, smallpox, erysipelas, pneumonia, measles, scarlatina, whooping cough, dysentery, cholera, and others. This concept has its attractions and adherents even today.

MORE RECENT HISTORY

In the latter part of the nineteenth century, MS became well recognized in neurological clinics, although evidence that it caused considerable diagnostic difficulty has continued to accumulate until most recently. However by 1930, Brain[2] estimated a prevalence rate of 16 per 100,000 population in England, even though he assumed a mean duration of disease of only 8 years. Davenport[10] had already noted the pre-dilection of the disease for certain ethnic groups.

The early history of MS is somewhat easier to put into context and perspective than that of the last 50 years. Certainly, many of the early observations have been extended. In 1935, Rivers and Schwentker[22] produced experimental allergic encephalitis (EAE) in monkeys, and the relevance of EAE animal models has grown steadily. Relapsing and progressive forms of EAE appear to have close parallels to the human disease. The mediation of demyelination by T cells (and myelin-specific T-cell lines), which, when activated, have no difficulty crossing the blood-brain barrier, has important implications for the understanding of MS. In addition, several viral models of central nervous system demyelination exist with and without a conjoined immune-mediated component. Advances in diagnoses have occurred pari passu, notably including cerebrospinal fluid (CSF) electrophoresis,[14] evoked potential studies,[16] and finally, magnetic resonance imaging (MRI).[26] These developments will be covered in subsequent chapters.

SOME NOTES ON TERMINOLOGY

Although Carswell may have published the first drawings to illustrate the pathology of MS, his label of a "peculiar disease state" might be criticized as being economical with the imagination. Cruveilhier, on the other hand, termed the pathology "gray degeneration of the cord." This term necessarily lacked precision at the time, and we have found it applied to other disorders with grayish spinal discoloration. The term remained in use until at least the 1880s, when we find Osler in one of his Montreal General Hospital cases employing it. "Disseminated sclerosis" was the term used in England after Moxon.[18] The term *multiple sclerosis* derives from the German usage and is a direct translation of "multiple sklerose."

REFERENCES

1. Bourneville DM, and Guerard I: De la Sclerose en Plaques Disseminees. A Delahaye, Paris, 1867.

2. Brain WR: Critical review: Disseminated sclerosis. QJM 23:343–391, 1930.

3. Bright R: Report of Clinical Cases. Longmans, London, 1831.

4. Carswell R: Pathologic Anatomy: Illustrations of the Elementary Forms of Disease. Longman, Orme, Brown, Green and Longman, London, 1838.

5. Charcot JM: Histologie de la sclerose en plaques. Gazette Hôpitaux (Paris) 41:554–555, 557–558, 566, 1868.

6. Charcot JM: Lectures on Disease of the Nervous System. New Sydenham Society Series, London, 1887.

7. Charcot JM: Seance du 14 mars. Cr Soc Biol (Paris) 20:13–14, 1868.

8. Compston A: Priorities in the history of multiple sclerosis. Ital J Neurol Sci (in press).

9. Cruveilhier J: Anatomie pathologique du corps humain. JB Bailliere, Paris, 1829–1842.

10. Davenport CB: Multiple sclerosis from the standpoint of geographic distribution and race. Archives of Neurology and Psychiatry 8:51, 1922.

11. Ebers GC: Osler and neurology. Can J Neurol Sci 12:236–242, 1985.

12. Frerichs FT: Ueber hirnsklerose. Arch Ges Med 10:334–337, 1849.

13. Hammond A: A Treatise on Disease of the Nervous System. D Appleton & Co, New York, 1871.

14. Lowenthal AM, Vansande M, and Karcher D: The differential diagnosis of neurological disease by fractionating electrophoretically, the CSF–globulins. J Neurochem 6:51, 1960.

15. Marie P: Sclerose en plaques et maladies infecteuses. Prog Med (Paris) 12:287–289, 305–307, 349–351, 365–366, 1884.

16. Matthews WB, Wattam–Bell JRB, and Pountney E: Evoked potentials in the diagnosis of multiple sclerosis: A follow–up study. J Neurol Neurosurg Psychiatry 45:303–307, 1982.

17. Morris JC: Case of the late Dr. DW Pennock. Am J Med Sci 56:138, 1868.

18. Moxon W: Eight cases of insular sclerosis of the brain and spinal cord. Journal of Neurology, Neurosurgery and Psychiatry 20:437–478, 1875.

19. Ollivier CP: De la moelle epinière et de ses maladies. Crevot, Paris, 1824.

20. Ordenstein M: Sur la Paralysie Agitante et la Sclerose en Plaques Generalisee. A Delahaye, Paris, 1867.

21. Putnam TJ: The centenary of multiple sclerosis. Archives of Neurology and Psychiatry 40:806–813, 1938.

22. Rivers TM, and Schwentker F: Encephalomyelitis accompanied by myelin destruction experimentally produced in monkeys. J Exp Med 61:698–702, 1935.

23. Spillane JD: The Doctrine of the Nerves. Oxford University Press, Oxford, New York, 1981.

24. Valentiner W: Ueber die sklerose des Gehirns und Ruckenmarks. Deutsche Kliniks 8:147, 158, 167, 1856.

25. Vulpian E: Note sur la sclerosie en plaques de la moelle epiniere. Union Médicale Pratique Français 30:459–465, 475–482, 541–548, 1866.

26. Young IR, Hall AS, Pallis CA, et al: Nuclear magnetic resonance imaging of the brain in multiple sclerosis. Lancet 2:1063–1066, 1981.

CHAPTER 2

EPIDEMIOLOGY

George C. Ebers, MD
A. Dessa Sadovnick, PhD

The nonrandom geographic distribution of MS has provided considerable allure for epidemiological study, because the patterns are believed to relate to underlying causes. Charcot[23] was the first to comment on the geographic distribution of MS, noting that while prevalent in France, the disease was not well recognized in Germany or England. Subsequent study has shown that both these countries actually surpass France in prevalence and incidence and perhaps have always done so.

Epidemiological studies have traditionally focused on the geographic distribution (comparing prevalence data) or on case-control studies, which seek to establish correlations with putative environmental causes. Few other diseases of unknown cause have such detailed information available about worldwide prevalence and incidence. Yet despite this wealth of data (over 300 community-based epidemiological studies on MS to date), the results have often led to ambiguous interpretation rather than to definitive correlations supporting specific environmental hypotheses. More consensus has been reached on demographic and clinical features than on concepts of pathogenesis derived from the epidemiological approach.

Key factors for successful epidemiological studies include accurate diagnosis and unbiased case ascertainment, both difficult to attain in MS. Certain diagnosis (and exclusion of diagnosis) of MS is not always possible in the living patient, even given modern advances in laboratory diagnosis.[109] One obstacle in identifying actual cases and control cases for epidemiological studies is the acknowledged lag time from the clinical onset of MS to diagnosis, which averages 4 years. Complete case ascertainment in a defined geographic region lessens the chance that observations result from subtle or unrecognized selection bias.

5

Repeated surveys often appear to increase prevalence figures. Comparison of prevalence rates, however, is not without hazard, because the methodology employed is rarely identical.

In an attempt to explain the geographic distribution of MS, considerable effort has been focused on traditional environmental factors. Numerous investigators have supported a purely environmental cause of MS. The attractiveness of this notion comes from the possibility that a relatively simple act of omission (or commission) could prevent the disease. The intensive study of MS prevalence in the 1950s and 1960s coincided with research on paralytic poliomyelitis, which culminated in the elucidation of the cause and the subsequent development of an effective vaccine. Not surprisingly, a number of investigators sought parallels between the epidemiology of the two diseases. Prevailing concepts of the geographic distribution, age specificity of a putative precipitating infection, and socioeconomic predilection in MS have owed some of their vitality to reasoning by analogy. Specifically, Poskanzer and colleagues[113] proposed that the geographic distribution of MS was analogous to that of poliomyelitis, which has a critical age of exposure and is more common in northern latitudes, temperate climates, and developed regions than in southern latitudes and underdeveloped regions.

Contemporaneously, the notion of a common viral infection of long latency in which only a relatively small proportion of those affected by the virus actually develop the disease in question became a popular notion. For MS, a critical age for susceptibility was suggested by data from migration studies. The identification of "slow viruses" provided evidence by both precedent and analogy to support the long-latency concept.

To test the latent virus theory, sanitation practices in regions where the MS prevalence varies have been studied, but a connection has not been found. For example, studies in Australia and Israel could not explain differences in prevalence within the country on the basis of sanitation.[9,95]

The influential studies of migration to South Africa by Geoffrey Dean[29] and Alter and colleagues in Israel[5,6] again implicated some crucial childhood event related to the later development of MS. The demonstration that a number of infections of the central nervous system (CNS) could be followed by a long-delayed expression of symptoms and signs (e.g., subacute sclerosing panencephalitis, kuru) refocused attention on events of early life, but the mechanism by which observed epidemiological facts were explained by inferences drawn from these possible analogies was neither crystallized nor well defined.

INCIDENCE AND PREVALENCE OF MULTIPLE SCLEROSIS

To understand the epidemiology of multiple sclerosis, it is necessary to define the terms *incidence* and *prevalence*. Incidence is the number of new cases developing (i.e., with symptom onset) per unit of time and population.[74] In general, accurate incidence rates (as for some readily identifiable birth defects in a monitored population) are difficult to obtain. In MS, the calculation of incidence is further complicated by uncertainty about the date of disease onset (initial symptoms are often subtle and only recognized in retrospect), lag time, and diagnostic uncertainty in the early stages. For these reasons, most epidemiological studies on MS either have made deductions about incidence from prevalence or mortality data, or both, or have been limited to prevalence data.

Prevalence is the number of cases present (alive) at one time (prevalence day) within a circumscribed population.[74] The ratio of cases per population is the *point prevalence rate*, or *prevalence ratio*. Prevalence is easier to calculate than incidence, because all cases are included regardless of disease duration. Nevertheless, accurate assessment of prevalence is still difficult; a major problem is that prevalence data rely on diagnostic accuracy, which has changed over time, as well as on completeness of case ascertainment. Even within North America, comparisons between Canada and the United States are influenced by differences in health-care systems. Because Canadians have essentially equal financial access to diagnostic procedures and medical care, the MS population attending Canadian medical centers may potentially be more representative of the overall MS population for disability distribution (benign or mild to severe) as well as of ethnicity and socio-economic distribution. Given the relative homogeneity of Canadian health care, prevalence comparisons within this country may have more than average validity. Finally, major changes in birth rates over the period evaluated can influence crude prevalence rates, thus emphasizing the value of age-specific prevalence rates.

Geographic Distribution

In reviewing the massive literature on MS prevalence, it is important to assess the methodology of each study critically and to compare data from different regions only after carefully determining whether such comparisons are in fact valid. This point and its application are clearly demonstrated in the thorough analyses of prevalence by Kurtzke,[74] who classified MS prevalence rates into "high-," "medium-," and "low-"risk groups. Rates greater than 30 per 100,000 population (now mostly 50 to 120) characterize *high-risk* areas, such as northern and central Europe, Italy, northern United States, Canada, southeastern Australia, parts of the former Soviet Union, and New Zealand. *Medium-risk* areas (prevalence between 5 and 29 per 100,000 population) include southern Europe, southern United States, northern Australia, northernmost Scandinavia, much of the north Mediterranean basin, parts of the former Soviet Union, white South Africa, and possibly central South America. *Low-risk* areas (prevalence less than 5 per 100,000 population) include other known areas of Africa and Asia, the Caribbean, Mexico, and possibly northern South America. However, even within a general geographic region, there can be considerable variation. The marked difference in prevalence between Sicily and Malta serves as an outstanding example of this variation for two areas in close proximity (Fig. 2–1).[31,150] Such varia-

tion may be explained by environmental factors, genetic factors, or a combination of the two.

As early as the 1920s, it was recognized that the distribution of MS was not uniform across geographic regions.[11,28,74] In general, all types of epidemiological surveys (prevalence, incidence, mortality) find that among regions with temperate climates, many economically developed occidental countries tend to have a higher rate of MS. In the Northern Hemisphere, a diminishing north-south gradient for MS prevalence has been well described.[73,75] The reverse, a south-north gradient, has been reported in the Southern Hemisphere.[57,58] These geographic patterns have been postulated to result from environmental factors, such as climate, diet (e.g., consumption of saturated or unsaturated fats), or the differential presence of an infective agent that is in some way climate dependent.[83] Two main lines of evidence, migration studies and geographic trends, support the role of environmental factors in the geographic distribution.

Migration Studies

At least in theory, migration studies should be decisive in distinguishing between environmental and genetic factors. It has been oft-stated that a crucial environmental event that determines subsequent MS susceptibility occurs at age 15 years or earlier. However, the numbers on which this statement rests are relatively small and it cannot be considered yet to have been established that a discrete or age-specific event at or before age 15 years is decisive.

It has been demonstrated that when age at migration is controlled, immigrants tend to adopt the epidemiological patterns seen in the indigenous population.[5,6,29] This trend has been reported for migration to and from both high- and low-risk prevalence regions. However, interpretation of these studies can be ambiguous, because genetic and environmental explanations of observed results are not mutually exclusive.

Studies of migration are much easier in concept than in execution. In principle,

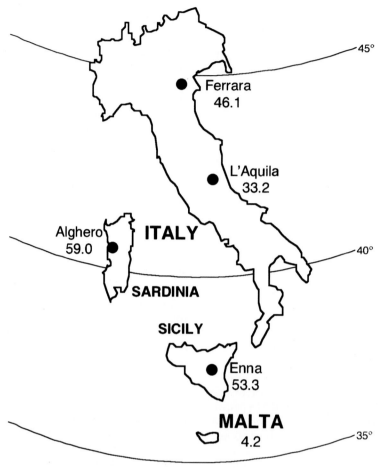

Figure 2–1. Comparison of MS prevalence (per 10[5]) in Malta[150] and in four Italian centers (Alghero, Sardinia[48]; Enna, Sicily[31]; L'Aquila, Italy[47]; Ferrara, Italy[49]).

studies focus on migrants who move from an area of high risk to an area of low risk for MS (or vice versa). If migrants adopt the risk of their new area of residence, an environmental cause is believed to be operative. However, these studies often assume that migrants are representative of the country from which they come. They also assume that these migrants, on settling in their new homeland, distribute themselves randomly. It is doubtful if either of these assumptions is ever true. The greatest migrations in history invariably have been prompted by religious persecution, wars, and other upheavals; and migrants are commonly selected for economic, social, religious, health-related, and even personality and anthropological characteristics. The most striking

example in which these considerations were ignored may have been the study of Vietnamese migrating to France, whose MS risk on migration was found to increase. These migrants all had a French parent, the factor which enabled them to emigrate from Vietnam. This was presumably not true of the population who opted to remain in Vietnam. However, this obvious genetic difference was ignored as the population in Vietnam was used to estimate the expected prevalence of MS in Vietnamese migrants to France.[78]

The frequency of MS has been shown to differ among populations of the same ethnic origin, some of whom have remained in the region of origin and others who migrated to areas where MS occurs at a different rate from the region of origin. Dean[29] showed in South Africa that immigrants tend to adopt the low-MS frequency patterns seen in the indigenous population. This trend has been reported for migration to and from both high- and low-risk prevalence regions.

Geographic Gradients in Ethnically Stable Populations

The second line of evidence that supports the role of environmental factors in the geographic distribution of MS comes from studies of the geographic gradients observed in smaller areas where MS has been surveyed serially. Studies in both 1961 and 1987 showed that in continental Australia, there is a gradient in the frequency of MS. MS is less common in Queensland compared with western Australia, New South Wales, and Tasmania.[58] Similar data are available for New Zealand, where the prevalence and incidence of MS are higher in the South Island than the North Island.[135] It is not possible to conclude from these important and careful studies that environmental factors alone are responsible for the geographic distribution. No formal genetic analyses were carried out, but relative genetic homogeneity among whites is well recognized in the Antipodes at least up to a generation ago.

The influential case-control data of Kurtzke and coworkers[77] deserve special mention. As Davenport[28] had done previously, Kurtzke and coworkers' work has made use of the remarkable record keeping of the US armed forces. In addition, they had the special advantage that MS was considered a service-related disease and therefore compensable on this ground. The implication is that case ascertainment was uniquely high because of potential financial benefits. Furthermore, the availability of extensive demographic data enabled the study of migration within this data set. This work showed that a geographic gradient for a decreasing rate of MS exists in the United States from north to south and, to a lesser extent, west to east.[77] In addition, data on migration within the United

States for this population suggest that the risks for MS changed according to age at migration. However, at the time of the study, it was impossible to control for genetic factors. As a result, the possibility that some of the north-south gradient reflected the distribution of genetic susceptibility alleles was not entertained. These data were recently reanalyzed, and some of the distribution may be influenced by ethnic or genetic factors, because north-south and west-east gradients also exist for specific subpopulations of northern European origin (Fig. 2–2).[77]

However, north-south gradients have also been well documented in New Zealand, France, and Japan (see later), as well as for Australia and the United States. These observations, taken together, seem to overwhelmingly favor an environmentally based latitude effect.

Multiple sclerosis incidence, prevalence, and mortality have been higher in northeast Scotland and in the Orkney Islands over a prolonged period than in any other part of the world. Less well-documented regional trends have also been observed elsewhere in the United Kingdom, but these distribution figures are not all based on recent data. More up-to-date studies have found that, at least in the southern part of England and Wales, the prevalence of MS is uniformly more than 100 per 100,000 population.[143] Nevertheless, a roughly linear relationship may exist between regional variations in the prevalence of MS and the frequency of HLA-DR2 in the unaffected population in the United Kingdom.[142] Sutherland[139] suggested that the parts of Scotland with the highest prevalence of MS were regions whose population was of Nordic origin. This hypothesis is consistent with a more recent report[135] that counted surnames starting with "Mac" or "Mc" in the telephone directory and concluded that the distribution of MS in the south and north of New Zealand showed some correlation with the pattern of immigration from Scotland. Although none of these approaches is methodologically robust, together they support some role of genetic factors in the geographic distribution of MS.

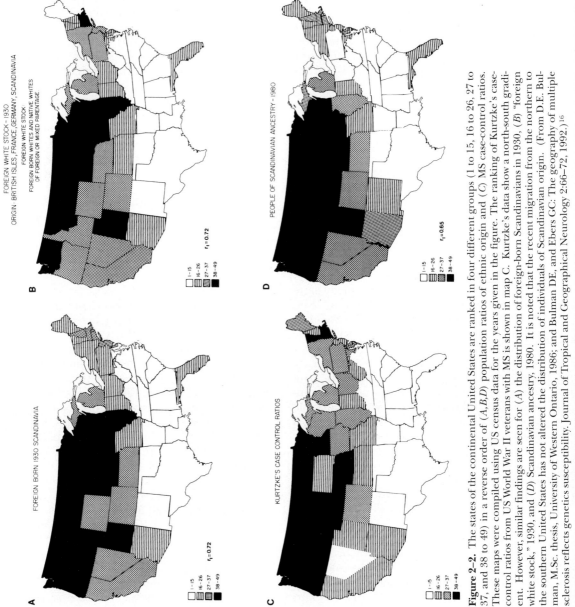

Figure 2–2. The states of the continental United States are ranked in four different groups (1 to 15, 16 to 26, 27 to 37, and 38 to 49) in a reverse order of (A,B,D) population ratios of ethnic origin and (C) MS case-control ratios. These maps were compiled using US census data for the years given in the figure. The ranking of Kurtzke's case-control ratios from US World War II veterans with MS is shown in map C. Kurtzke's data show a north-south gradient. However, similar findings are seen for (A) the distribution of foreign-born Scandinavians in 1930, (B) "foreign white stock," 1930, and (D) Scandinavian ancestry, 1980. It is noted that the recent migration from the northern to the southern United States has not altered the distribution of individuals of Scandinavian origin. (From D.E. Bulman, M.Sc. thesis, University of Western Ontario, 1986; and Bulman DE, and Ebers GC: The geography of multiple sclerosis reflects genetics susceptibility. Journal of Tropical and Geographical Neurology 2:66–72, 1992.)[16]

Racial Distribution

Racial susceptibility and resistance to MS have repeatedly been demonstrated. MS is virtually unknown among black Africans,[29] with only one or two cases reported to date. In a number of previously suspected cases, other diagnoses were confirmed at autopsy.[65] Today, infection by HTLV-1 has to be excluded. The observation that African Americans develop MS could be explained by an admixture of white genes,[34] a change in environment, or both. Similarly, the majority of Native Americans with MS have a white ancestor, although this admixture may have occurred in a grandparental generation.[56]

Asians appear to be relatively resistant to MS, regardless of where they live.[32,73,167] It is of special interest that in Japan, despite the low overall prevalence, a north-south gradient also exists. In Japan and the Orient in general, the clinical manifestations of MS (an optico-spinal form)[72] differ somewhat from that seen in most European populations. Genetically and culturally restricted communities that seem to remain relatively or entirely free from MS despite living in an otherwise high-prevalence area include Hutterites,[38] Lapps,[50] Inuit,[38] Native Americans,[56,77] Saudis,[166] Hispanics,[40] American blacks,[77] Asians,[77] Maoris,[135] and Yakutes.[106] Notably, to date, in all the studies cited on MS in different racial groups, no effort has been made to take into account the evolutionary distance between populations, as recently outlined in a study combining genetic, archeological, and linguistic data.[21]

Geographic Clusters

There are numerous reports of "clusters" (excess of disease occurrence) where several cases of MS have occurred at a similar point, or in individuals who grew up together or were exposed to a specific locale over the same period, or as a result of some combination of these factors. Examples of regions where clusters have been reported include Key West (Florida),[131] Henribourg (Saskatchewan),[64] Colchester County (Nova Scotia),[100] Vaasa (Finland),[68] Hordaland (Norway),[85] Los Alamos County (New Mexico),[60] and Mansfield (Massachusetts).[37] (A cluster has also been reported among workers in a zinc-related manufacturing plant.[138]) Analysis of such clusters is not straightforward for several reasons; for example, the denominator (the number of groups from which the identified high-risk subgroup has been selected) is often unknown.

Extremely high prevalence rates for MS occur in the Orkney (309 per 100,000 population) and Shetland Islands (184 per 100,000 population).[112] Within the Orkney Islands, clustering of cases in time and space has been noted.[114] Lifetime data showed temporal or spatial clustering of patients with MS at least 21 years before disease onset and just before onset. Each of the two-time clusters appeared on three separate islands. No clustering could be demonstrated in the Shetland Islands.

It has not yet been possible to explain clusters; indeed, there is no consensus that true clusters have occurred. None is entirely clear-cut in interpretation. Familial clusters must also be considered. It is, however, important to consider such reports as thoroughly as possible both to continue to identify causal agents and to confirm the veracity of a reported cluster.

Epidemics

Two MS "epidemics" have been identified since World War II. The first and most dramatic has been in the Faroe Islands, whose population is largely of Scandinavian ancestry. Before World War II, there were no reported cases of MS in the Faroe Islands; however, 46 cases were identified from 1943 to 1982,[80,81] and an additional four cases had onsets between 1986 and 1989.[82] The point prevalence rate was reported as 41 in 1950, 64 in 1961, 38 in 1972, and 34 in 1977. These data have been interpreted to indicate a point-source epidemic temporally related to the stationing of approximately 8000 British troops on the islands during World War II. Although the investigators in these studies made impeccable use of available methodology, their interpretation has been open to criticism. In particular, questions have been raised about the completeness of case ascertainment before World War II, when medical services were less readily available. Further questions concern the possibility that the date of clinical onset may bear no relationship to the probable date of acquisition, which could occur as early as age 5 years, and the lack of good objective case-control data with respect to the degree of exposure to British troops.[107,108] These issues have been repeatedly addressed by the authors,[82] who concluded that none of these criticisms are substantiated. They maintain that the primary MS affection (PMSA) was introduced to the Faroe Islands by British troops and that four consecutive and decreasing epidemics of MS occurred (the fourth epidemic consisting of seven patients with symptom onset between 1984 and 1989). They further contend that PMSA is a single, widespread, specific systemic infectious disease whose acquisition in virgin (with respect to MS) populations follows 2 years of exposure starting between ages 11 and 45 years. Clinical MS is said to occur in only a small proportion of those infected and this only after a 6-year incubation period. The agent was deemed to be transmissible only during part or all of this systemic PMSA phase, which is said to end before the usual onset age for clinical MS.

A second but less convincing epidemic reportedly occurred in Iceland, also in relation to the stationing of British troops during World War II.[79] The annual average incidence of MS during the period 1945 to 1954 was 3.2 per 100,000 population, compared with incidence rates of 1.6 per 100,000 population for 1923 to 1944 and 1.9 per 100,000 population for 1955 to 1974. Kurtzke and colleagues conclude that the incidence of MS during the period 1945 to 1954 meets the criteria for a point-source epidemic whose tail thereafter merges with the baseline for Iceland. However, the situation in Iceland differs from that in the Faroe Islands in that MS was known to exist before the occupation by British troops. In addition, one of the authors of the report was the first neurologist in Iceland, arriving in 1942. Therefore, it is conceivable that his arrival may have influenced the apparent increase in MS over the next few years, particularly among younger Icelanders, probably due

to the detection of more relatively benign cases.

Despite these reported epidemics, the identity of any putative infectious agents remains unknown. Many observers remain unconvinced that these tantalizing data have proved transmissibility. Finally, the action of one transmissible agent is only one possible explanation for the observed findings. It is also conceivable that the introduction of a large number of common viruses into a virgin susceptible population could serve to trigger an apparent epidemic without the implication of a specific transmissible agent. Kurtzke[76] has recently published an exhaustively referenced and thoughtful review that emphasizes his interpretation of the existing data as supporting an infectious etiology for MS.

Two recent studies (also mentioned in Chapter 3) have an important bearing on the notion of epidemics. The Canadian Adoptee Study[124a] collected 238 MS patients adopted at or near birth. Among 1201 first degree non-biological relatives, only 1 developed MS; some 25 would have been expected if the parents, sibs and children had been blood relatives. It is to be emphasized that the rate of MS ($\frac{1}{1201}$) is very like that in the Canadian population. Accordingly, living and/or growing up with someone destined to get MS produces no detectable change in one's risk of getting MS. This represents a difficult hurdle for the many avid adherents of infectious theories to overcome. In a different study which addresses the same question, it was found that among almost 2000 half-siblings of MS patients, no difference in risk of growing up together vs. growing up apart could be found.[39a] These results strongly imply that familial aggregation is determined by genes and that population risk is strongly influenced by environment.

Lessons from Animal Models of Autoimmune Disease

All models of spontaneous autoimmune disease in mice show oliogenic or polygenic inheritance of susceptibility, and some demonstrate fascinating epidemiological lessons (see Chapter 3 for a discussion of the genetics of spontaneous autoimmune disease in mice). The best understood of these models is the nonobese diabetic mouse (NOD) developed by Makano in Japan.[87] When colonies of these inbred mice were shipped around the world, a most surprising and initially puzzling fact emerged. Despite documented purity of breeding stocks and approximate genetic homogeneity ensured by generations of inbreeding, the penetrance of diabetes was remarkably variable. Mice reared in Auckland, New Zealand, did not develop diabetes, whereas those mice reared in Edmonton, Canada, developed diabetes without exception. Initial suspicions about genetic contamination proved unfounded, and subsequent examination of these phenomena established several intriguing facts. Despite the presence of the appropriate background of genetic susceptibility, the penetrance proved to be very strongly influenced by diet and cleanliness of environment in early life and by viral contamination of breeding colonies. It must be emphasized, however, that penetrance rose with age and that even in low-penetrance conditions, the clinical penetrance of glycosuria was greatly exceeded by histological penetrance of islet cell inflammation. A germ-free environment in early life resulted in full penetrance of glycosuric diabetes. It is too early to know if these observations are relevant to the epidemiology of MS, but they serve to emphasize several relatively unexplored avenues in MS and to provide a fascinating example of the interaction of genes and the microenvironment in early life.

Temporal Changes

The epidemiological literature contains numerous examples of changes in incidence and prevalence for specific disorders over time. However, these follow-up studies must be critically assessed to determine whether observed changes are real or reflect changes in diagnostic custom, environment, or other factors.

Several large prevalence studies have been conducted in Canada.* Re-evaluation of the same population was first done in

---

*References 4, 13, 54, 55, 116, 137, 141, 158, 159.

Winnipeg, Manitoba. The initial survey used data from patient records and death certificates for the years 1939 to 1948 and found a prevalence rate of 39.6 per 100,000 population.[158] A follow-up study in 1961[137] diagnostically re-evaluated 144 of the patients from the earlier survey. Diagnoses agreed among the two studies for 103 (71.5 percent) of the original 144 patients.[137] Of the 109 patients diagnosed as "probable MS" in the first study, re-evaluation confirmed this diagnosis in 85 cases (78 percent). Of the remaining 24 cases, 7 (6.4 percent) were reclassified as "possible MS," and the remaining were diagnosed as either "unlikely MS" (14 of 109, or 12.8 percent) or "not MS" (3 of 109, or 2.8 percent). In part because of more stringent diagnostic criteria, the prevalence rate in the follow-up study was 35.4 per 100,000 population, slightly lower than that in the earlier work. In western Poland, as shown on Table 2–1, a resurvey similarly found a lower prevalence rate in the more recent study,[22,157] but this change may reflect an increase in population figures due to a higher birth rate rather than a true fall in MS frequency. Yet despite the examples from Manitoba and western Poland, repeated surveys on the same population generally result in a higher prevalence on the second survey (see Table 2–1).

Prevalence rates in Canada as documented in published reports have increased in more recent times. This was most dramatically noted in Saskatoon, Saskatchewan, with a reported prevalence rate of 134 per 100,000 population.[54] Initially, the consensus was that MS research should focus on Saskatoon to determine why the prevalence was so high. However, it soon became evident that this high rate probably reflected the timing of the survey rather than specific risk factors for MS being higher in the region. At the time of publication, the Saskatoon study was the only one in recent years designed specifically to determine prevalence. Furthermore, improved survival, the availability of various diagnostic tests to assist in the diagnosis of MS,[109] and the institution of the universal coverage medical insurance program in Canada all contributed to the apparent rise in prevalence. Subsequent studies[54,55,141] also reported comparable

Table 2–1. TEMPORAL CHANGES IN THE PREVALENCE OF MULTIPLE SCLEROSIS

Location	Prevalence Date or Period	Prevalence per 100,000 Population	Senior Author
Canada			
Winnipeg, Manitoba	1939–1948	39.6	Westlund[158]
Winnipeg, Manitoba	Jan 1, 1960	35.4	Stazio[137]
Rochester, Minnesota	1915	46	Percy[104]
	1978	108	Kranz[70]
	Jan 1, 1985	173	Wynn[164]
Australia			
Perth	Jun 30, 1961	19.6	McCall[95]
Perth	Jun 30, 1981	29.9	Hammond[58]
Newcastle	Jun 30, 1961	19.3	McCall[95]
Newcastle	Jun 30, 1981	36.5	Hammond[58]
Hobart	Jun 30, 1961	33	McCall[95]
Hobart	Jun 30, 1981	75.6	Hammond[58]
Hordaland, Western Norway	Jan 1, 1963	20	Presthus[115]
	Jan 1, 1983	59.8	Larsen[84]
Barbagia, Sardinia	Dec 31, 1975	40.7	Granieri[48]
	Oct 24, 1981	65.3	Granieri[47]
Western Poland	Jan 1, 1965	51.19	Cendrowski[22]
	Dec 31, 1981	42.87	Wender[157]

prevalence rates (Fig. 2–3), with the notable exception of Newfoundland.[116]

Incidence and prevalence rates for MS have been repeatedly reassessed for Rochester and Olmsted County, Minnesota, largely because of the excellent data base at the Mayo Clinic. The reported prevalence rate in Rochester has increased from approximately 46 per 100,000 in 1915[104] to 108 per 100,000 in 1978[70] to 173 per 100,000 in 1985[164] (see Table 2–1). Of interest, the incidence rate for Rochester remained stable at approximately 3.6 per 100,000 from 1905 to 1974.[70, 104] However, re-evaluation of all possible MS cases for the period 1905 to 1984[165] found an increased crude incidence rate of approximately 3.4 and 7.7 per 100,000 population for males and females respectively. It remains uncertain whether this increase in incidence is real or reflects less rigid application of diagnostic criteria or improved case ascertainment, study design, and diagnostic capabilities, or some combination of these factors.[164] Similar findings are reported from western Norway. In Hordaland County, the incidence for clinically definite and clinically probable MS appears to have increased from 1.12 per 100,000 in 1953 to 1957 to 3.5 per 100,000 for 1973 to 1977.[84] The incidence for 1978 to 1982 was lower than for the previous 5-year period, but these data must be interpreted with care because of the acknowledged interval from

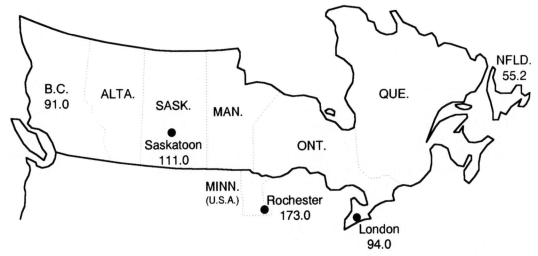

Figure 2–3. Comparison of MS prevalence (per 10^5) in four Canadian locations: British Columbia (1982)[141]; Saskatoon, Saskatchewan (1977)[54]; London, Ontario (1984)[55]; and Newfoundland (1985),[116] and in one American location: Rochester, Minnesota (1985).[164] These prevalence rates include probable MS only. Rates may thus differ from those in Tables 2–1 and 2–3, which may include possible cases also.

MS onset to diagnosis. In More and Romsdal counties, the average annual incidence increased from 1.94 per 100,000 during the period 1950 to 1954 to 3.78 per 100,000 for 1975 to 1979.[96]

Reports of increased prevalence rates over time have been made elsewhere in both the Northern and Southern Hemispheres (see Table 2–1).[44,47,48,58,95,115] The question of an apparent increase in MS prevalence has dashed the hopes of those who may have thought that they had heard the last of MS prevalence studies. In fact, the lack of understanding of the nature of the environmental effect demands an open mind. Implications of an increasing incidence and prevalence are too important to ignore.

SEX RATIO

Multiple sclerosis susceptibility has long been known to vary according to sex. Females are more susceptible by a factor that approaches 2:1 in population studies, but this varies among surveys.[55,141] Males are more likely to have progressive disease from onset.[154,155] A review of the literature[36,39,154,155] suggests that this female preponderance is further increased in early-onset cases, and possibly in familial cases,

in twins, and in individuals who are HLA-DR2-positive. The explanation for the sex-related skew in age-of-onset distribution is unclear, but differences in immune responsiveness may be influenced by neuroendocrine interactions with the immune system. In one recent study,[156] a review of the literature found that relatives (siblings, second-degree, first-degree cousins) concordant for MS were more often of the same sex, but this observation does not necessarily imply a genetic or hormonal mechanism among siblings, because such pairs may in fact have more environmental sharing compared with different-sex siblings. However, a more recent prospective study[123] did not confirm this finding. Different-sex siblings of patients with MS also have a significantly higher risk to develop MS compared with the general population.[121,122] There is evidence that gender may interact with the major histocompatibility complex (MHC), because the frequency of HLA-DR2 is reported to be significantly higher in females than in males.[39,149] Curiously, postmenopausal onset did not appear to alter the sex ratio in our population, based on a study of MS with onset after age 50 years.[62,101] These data provide evidence for a possible interaction among genetic susceptibility, hormonal factors, and environmental sharing.[51,52] It is likely that gender and associated hormonal differences influence disease susceptibility on more than one level, as is seen in several animal models of spontaneous autoimmune disease.[136]

AGE OF ONSET

Multiple sclerosis is primarily a disease of young adults. Diagnostic criteria[109] define the age-of-onset range as 10 to 59 years, extending the previous upper limit from age 50 years.[128] However, childhood MS is a recognized entity and approximately 2.7 percent of cases have their onset before age 16 years.[35] A recent study[35] based on a white population with an onset before age 16 years found that childhood MS is more frequent in females (75.2 percent) and often follows a relapsing-remitting course (80 percent were relapsing-remitting or relapsing progressive). In these patients, the initial attack, from which there is usually complete recovery, tended to involve afferent structures of the CNS, and the progress was usually slow.

The onset of MS is also known to occur after age 59 years,[93,101] even into the eighth decade. The differential diagnosis is usually less straightforward in older patients. They tend to have a chronic progressive course from onset, similar to that characteristic of many degenerative diseases seen in older age, such as system degenerations, which can occasionally mimic MS.

Two recent studies[17,123] found a correlation in age of onset among sibling pairs concordant for MS. In addition, a stronger correlation was observed when concordant monozygotic twin pairs were compared with nontwin MS sibling pairs,[17] suggesting that age of onset in MS may be partly under genetic control.

PRECIPITATING FACTORS (SEE CHAPTERS 5 AND 6)

A number of factors including diet[140] and heavy metals,[19,94] as well as emotional stress, lumbar puncture, surgery and anesthesia, pregnancy, exertion, fatigue, and heat,[94] have been proposed as influencing the onset of symptoms or worsening of MS. The role of trauma (exposure to cold, falling, illness, or stress) as a possible precipitating factor in MS was first raised by Charcot,[23] but any causal relationship has yet to be demonstrated. In reporting MS relapses in relation to trauma, recall bias is always a concern. Often the trauma, such as a fall, has been symptomatic rather than causal.

Despite the various proposals, a universal precipitating factor has not been identified. Many data are supported only by methodologically weak or unconfirmed studies, often anecdotal in nature, yet receiving considerable attention from patients.

Infection

The role of infectious agents as triggering factors in MS has frequently been proposed. Identification of clusters and epidemics has often been interpreted as support for the role of infectious agents as causal factors in the onset of MS. Canine distemper virus was a leading candidate in the 1970s,[25] but subsequent case-control studies have failed to support this.[18,111,118] Nevertheless, surveys of antibodies to different viruses in various MS populations worldwide have shown that on average, patients with MS have high antibody levels to many viruses, including measles. Therefore, existing data give little support to the theory that MS results from exposure to a single, relatively rare virus. Most studies of viral antibodies have not included other autoimmune diseases as controls. When titers in MS are compared to lupus or chronic hepatitis, the values are not at all impressive.

The role of infectious agents in precipitating the clinical onset or relapses of MS remains unresolved. Most research in this area has been based on retrospective data, so that recall bias becomes a problem. Estimates show that the onset of MS was preceded by a reported infective disease in approximately 10 percent of cases.[96] Sibley and colleagues[132] found that minor respiratory tract infections preceded 27 percent of MS relapses. Chronic sinus infection has been reported to be associated with the timing of MS relapses, as well as with the age and season when these occurred.[45] Sibley and Foley[134] reported a seasonal increase in MS relapses in Ohio during the months when respiratory infections are common, and subsequent work in London, Ontario,[33] confirmed this observation. It is unclear, however, whether these seasonal influences are related to viral infection or to some other concomitant event. Do the same factors influencing seasonal variation also account for some of the geographic gradient? Although the relationship between infectious agents and MS remains unclear, it is conceivable that infection in general may act as a nonspecific trigger for the immune system, initiating the onset of a relapse.

Pregnancy

The original and classic study on the association between pregnancy, delivery, and MS relapses was done by Millar and colleagues.[97] Using retrospective data, they found that the average relapse rate per pregnancy year (9 months' gestation plus 3 months after delivery) was 0.265, an elevated rate compared with the rate of 0.10 relapses per year experienced by women who did not have pregnancies. It is troublesome that neither of these rates approached the 0.5 to 1.4 attack per year found in prospective studies.[69,161] The majority of pregnancy-related relapses reported by Millar occurred after delivery. The issue of whether these relapses were physiologically related to labor, delivery, or both or were a result of the stress and fatigue associated with having a newborn in the house remained unresolved. Subsequent retrospective studies continued to confirm the observation that the period after delivery posed the highest risk for a MS relapse, but that gestation itself was relatively quiescent with respect to disease activity.[97] As with other studies on MS, the major methodological problem with research on the relationship between MS and pregnancy has been the use of retrospective data with their inherent recall bias. The definition of an attack has often been imprecise and not clearly separable from nonspecific phenomena associated with the

postpartum period. The unusually low relapse rates in the paper by Millar and colleagues[97] serve to emphasize this drawback.

Birk and colleagues[15] followed eight women *prospectively* for the course of their pregnancies. However, these cases were first ascertained after the onset of pregnancy, and no information was given about pregestational relapse rates. They found that although the MS did not worsen significantly during gestation in any patient, six of the eight women experienced relapses within 7 weeks of delivery.

In a recent study,[126] women were assessed *before the onset of pregnancy* and followed up throughout successful pregnancies and for up to 6 months after delivery. The study concluded that neither pregnancy nor the 6-month period after delivery is a risk factor for MS relapse. Our own experience suggests a modest decrease of exacerbations during pregnancy but this has little impact on clinical practice.

DISEASES ASSOCIATED WITH MULTIPLE SCLEROSIS

Diseases such as systemic lupus erythematosus,[61] myasthenia gravis,[1,91,130] ankylosing spondylitis,[92,145] inflammatory bowel disease,[127] and scleroderma[147] have been reported to be associated with MS. However, none of these reports has yet been confirmed by appropriate and careful case-control population-based surveys. The most that can be said is that MS does not protect individuals from these conditions, nor does it make them more likely to occur.

Every large MS center can identify cases in which a variety of autoimmune diseases have occurred in patients with MS. Some evidence suggests that certain families have a genetic predisposition to autoimmune diseases.[14] For example, in the Vancouver MS Clinic, where all patients have detailed family histories documented by the geneticist, several such families have been clearly identified. In one instance, the mother has MS, her son has juvenile diabetes mellitus, and her daughter has juvenile rheumatoid arthritis. However, such families are rare. In Olmsted County, Minnesota, a detailed survey calculated the relative risk (RR) for 17

Table 2–2. **MS PREVALENCE: ALPHABETICAL LISTING BY COUNTRY**[*][†]

Country	Prevalence Date or Period	Prevalence per 100,000 Population	Senior Author
Albania	Mar 1, 1988	10.3	Kruja[71]
Australia			
Perth	Jun 30, 1981	29.9	Hammond[58]
Newcastle	Jun 30, 1981	36.5	
Hobart	Jun 30, 1981	75.6	
Austria			
Vienna		41.6	Bauer[11]
Upper Austria		29.4	
Lower Austria		21.7	
Belgium	1983	80–100	Bauer[11]
Bulgaria			
Plovdiv areas	Dec 31, 1992	18.3	Trendafilova[146]
Sofia	1983	30	Georgiev[46]
Canada			
British Columbia	Jul 1, 1982	117.2	Sweeney[141]
Saskatoon, Saskatchewan	Jan 1, 1977	134	Hader[54]
Newfoundland	Mar 31, 1985	55.2	Pryse-Phillips[116]
London, Ontario	Jan 1984	94	Hader[55]
Croatia	Jun 30, 1986	143.5	Sepcic[129]
Czechoslovakia (Western)			Bauer[11]
Prague		67	
Northern Bohemia		108	
Denmark	1965	101	Bauer[11]
Finland			Bauer[11]
Uusima (South)	1979	54	
Vaasa (West)	1979	91	
France			
Brittany	1976–1978	25	Gallou[43]
Chalon-sur-Saone		58	Bauer[11]
Avignon		49	Bauer[11]
Haute Pyrenees	Jan 1, 1988	38	Roth[120]
Germany			
Hesse	Dec 31, 1980	58.3	Bauer[11]
Southern Lower Saxony		131	Poser[110]
Rostock		69.1	Bauer[11]
Halle		42.6	Bauer[11]
Northwest Germany	Jun 1990	95	Haupts[59]
Greece			
Macedonia and Thrace	Dec 31, 1984	29.5	Milonas[98]

Continued on following page

Table 2–2.—*continued*

Country	Prevalence Date or Period	Prevalence per 100,000 Population	Senior Author
Hong Kong	Dec 31, 1987	0.88	Yu[167]
Hungary			
Fejer County, West Hungary (Hungarians)	Dec 1992	78.7	Guseo[53]
Gypsies	Dec 1992	98	Guseo[53]
Baranya County (gypsies)	Jan 1, 1993	5	Pàlffy[102]
India			
Zoroastrians (Parsis)	Mar 1, 1988		Wadia[152]
Bombay		26	
Poona		58	
Israel			
Immigrants	Jan 1, 1966		Leibowitz[86]
Europeans		31.3	
Afro-Asians		6.8	
Native-born Israelis	Jan 1, 1965		Leibowitz[86]
Europeans		8.8	
Afro-Asians		2.7	
Italy			
Barbagia, Sardinia	Oct 24, 1981	65.3	Granieri[48]
Enna, Sicily	Jan 1, 1975	53	Dean[31]
Valle d'Aosta	Dec 31, 1985	39	Granieri[49]
Japan		1–4	Kuroiwa[73]
Korea			
Busan	1971–1981	1.8	Kim and Kim[67]
Seoul	1958–1966	2.4	Park[103]
Kuwait			
Kuwaitis	Dec 31, 1988	9.5	Al-Din[2]
Palestinians	Dec 31, 1988	23.8	Al-Din[2]
Libya	Jul 1, 1984	5.9	Radharkrishnan[117]
Macedonia	Jun 30, 1991	15.5	Ljapcher[89]
Malaysia	1968–1986	2	Tan[144]
Malta		4	Vassallo[150]
Mexico			
(Government workers and their families)		1.5	Alter[8]
Netherlands			
Groningen	1992	76.3	Minderhoud[99]

Continued on following page

Table 2–2—*continued*

Country	Prevalence Date or Period	Prevalence per 100,000 Population	Senior Author
New Zealand			Skegg[135]
Waikato (North Island)	1981	27.9	
Otago and Southland (South Island)	1981	79.4	
Norway			
Hordaland	Jan 1, 1983	59.8	Larsen[84]
More and Romsdal Counties	Jan 1, 1985	75.4	Midgard[96]
Poland (Western)	Dec 31, 1981	42.87	Wender[157]
Portugal		15	Bauer[11]
Romania			Bauer[11]
Brasov, Transylvania		43	
Cluj, Transylvania		43	
Bucharest		79.4	
Danube (Southern Regions)		<6	
Saudi Arabia	Jan 1983–Dec 1986	8	Yaquib[166]
South Africa			Dean[29]
White South Africans			
(English-speaking)	1960	12.7	
(Afrikaans-speaking)	1960	3.6	
Spain			
Asturias, Northern Spain		45	Uria[148]
Lanzarote (Canary Islands)	Dec 21, 1987	15	Garcia[44]
Malaga	Mar 1, 1984	53	Fernàndez[41]
Barcelona	Dec 1, 1991	57	Fernàndez[41]
Sweden		130	Bauer[11]
Switzerland			
Bern	Jan 1, 1986	110	Kesselring[66]
Valais		25	Bartschi-Rochaix[10]

Continued on following page

autoimmune diseases, including rheumatoid arthritis (RR = 1.8) and autoimmune thyroid disease (RR = 3.3), for patients with MS compared to control subjects.[42,88,162] The only statistically significant result was for autoimmune thyroid disease (Hashimoto's thyroiditis and Graves' disease). Similar data were collected in London, Ontario, for relatives of 194 patients with MS and spousal control subjects. An increased frequency of poliomyelitis and thyroid disease and a mild reduction of cancer were found in the families with MS compared with control subjects (A. Rudd and G.C. Ebers, 1986). This area does not appear to represent a promising avenue of exploration. The data serve more to underscore the remarkable organ specificity of MS than to support the hypothesis of some general autoimmune diathesis. It should be noted

Table 2–2.—*continued*

Country	Prevalence Date or Period	Prevalence per 100,000 Population	Senior Author
Taiwan	May 1975	0.95	Hung[63]
Tunisia		10	Ben Hamida[12]
United Kingdom			
England: London, Borough of Sutton	Jan 1, 1985	115	Williams[160]
Southeast Wales (South Glamorgan)	Jan 1, 1985	117	Swingler[143]
Northeast Scotland (Grampian region)	Dec 1, 1980	144	Phadke[105]
Shetland Islands	Apr 30, 1984	170	Cook[24]
Orkney Islands	Sept 21, 1983	224	Cook[26]
Outer Hebrides	Jul 1, 1979	97.3	Dean[30]
United States			
Hawaii			Alter[7]
Asians	Jan 1, 1969	8.8	
Whites	Jan 1, 1969	10.5	
California			
Spanish-surnamed (California-born)		0.42	Enstrom[40]
Foreign (mostly Mexican-born)		0.07	
Los Angeles (whites, Los Angeles-born)	Apr 1, 1970	22	Visscher[151]
Washington (whites born in King and Pierce Counties)	Apr 1, 1970	69	
Minnesota, Rochester	Jan 1, 1985	173	Wynn[165]

Source: Adapted from Sadovnick AD, and Ebers GC: Epidemiology of multiple sclerosis: A critical overview. Can J Neurol Sci 20:17–29, 1993.[124]

*The reader is referred to the appropriate references. These rates are not necessarily comparable with each other but should provide the most up-to-date information known for the country. Studies vary on the diagnostic criteria, ascertainment, and year of study.

†This table is not meant to be a comprehensive list of every prevalence survey ever conducted in a given country.

that both poliomyelitis and thyroid disease have MHC associations present in MS (DR2 and DR3, respectively). This chapter discusses a selected few possible disease associations with MS.

Diabetes Mellitus

A study in Olmsted County, Minnesota,[162] reported an RR for diabetes mellitus of 2.5 in patients with MS, but this was not statistically significant. Warren and Warren[153] re-

ported a higher association of diabetes mellitus in both patients with MS and their relatives compared with control subjects.

Neoplasia

The study in Olmsted County[163] reported an RR for neoplasia of 1.4 in patients with MS, but this was not statistically significant. Some investigators[133] have reported that neoplasia occurs in patients with MS at the same rate as in control subjects, whereas

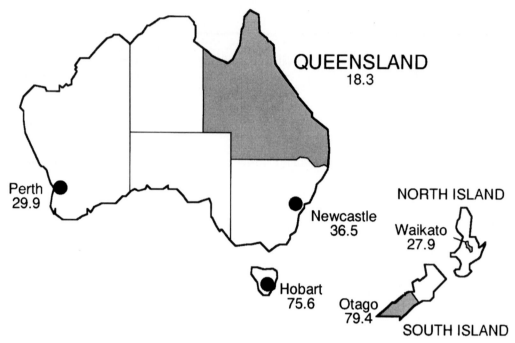

Figure 2–4. Comparison of MS prevalence (per 10[5]) and illustration of north-south gradient in Australia[57, 58]: State of Queensland (1987), Perth (1988), Newcastle (1988), Hobart (1988), and in New Zealand[135]: North Island, Waikato (1987); and South Island, Otago (1987).

others have found an increased rate. Zimmerman and Netsky[168] reported a 20 percent incidence of malignant tumors in 50 autopsied cases of MS, including two brain tumors. Others have also reported concurrent MS and primary brain tumors.[20,27,90,119] An autopsy series of 120 cases found neither an increase in the rate of neoplasia among patients with MS compared with general control subjects nor any cases with brain tumors.[3] A recent study[125] found that neoplasia was identified as an underlying cause of death significantly less often than expected among patients with MS. Although it is conceivable that changes in the immune system may protect patients with MS from neoplasia, it is more likely that neoplasia is less readily diagnosed in patients with MS not having autopsies because the symptoms of neoplasia may either be attributed to MS or else not be investigated in severely disabled patients. Even if neoplasia were slightly increased, the role of the MS could be indirect, such as its being associated with the use of cytotoxic drugs. In any event, these studies provide important bases for comparison now that cytotoxic

agents have achieved relatively widespread usage.

Uveitis

Uveitis in different forms has been reported in association with various infectious and autoimmune diseases, including Behçet's disease, toxoplasmosis, ankylosing spondylitis, sarcoidosis, syphilis, and MS.[94] Uveitis has been reported in up to 5 percent of patients in studied series, and an even higher rate is found for retinal perivenous sheathing. The main implication is the association of uveitis with infectious and autoimmune disorders. It should be remembered that the uveal tract, although not myelinated, does participate in the inflammatory process in a substantial proportion of patients.

SUMMARY

In a review of the epidemiology of MS, it is tempting to visually represent the worldwide prevalence of MS in a single, comprehensive map. However, the reader may find such a map more misleading than meaningful. Existing prevalence and incidence studies for most countries are not comparable. Data are influenced by temporal differences as well as by differences in healthcare systems, neurological expertise, and even cultural practices. For these reasons, we have listed prevalence data alphabetically by country in Table 2–2; in this way, it is retrievable for reference without the implication that these studies can be directly compared. The main conclusions drawn from worldwide prevalence studies using contemporaneous data from the most informative comparative studies are as follows:

1. A north-south gradient exists independent from genetic or racial factors. Several countries exhibiting relative racial homogeneity show a north-south gradient (e.g., Australia, New Zealand; Fig. 2–4). A west-east gradient is also seen in the United States.

2. Major differences in prevalence occur in the absence of difference in latitude. There are a number of exceptions to the north-south gradient when regions of different ethnic derivation are included. Two examples illustrate this observation. Sicily and Malta were simultaneously subjected to a prevalence study[31,150] by the same investigator (see Fig. 2–1). The prevalence in Sicily was 10-fold that in Malta. The second example is in North America, where five recent prevalence studies using similar methods demonstrate an almost four-fold difference in prevalence (see Fig. 2–3). The rate for Rochester, Minnesota, closely approximates rates for northeast Scotland and the Shetland and Orkney islands.

3. Individuals from the same ethnic derivation either have similar prevalence rates or have different prevalence rates in widely separated geographic areas. The former is illustrated by Minnesota and Scandinavia, and the latter by the United Kingdom, northern Australia, and South Africa.

4. Specific resistant isolates are shown to exist regardless of latitude. The sum of the prevalence information leads to the almost inescapable conclusion that the geography of MS cannot be explained by any single known environmental factor in isolation. Similarly, it seems very unlikely that the distribution of any genetic factors, singly or in combination, could account for the observed worldwide distribution of MS.

Future research should refrain from further attempts to force an exclusively genetic or environmental explanation on an abundant collection of facts that simply will not accommodate such an interpretation. Further epidemiological studies should examine populations in which control of genetic factors is optimized (see Chapter 3). Re-examination of a number of individual environmental factors may then prove informative.

REFERENCES

1. Aita JF, Snyder DH, and Reichl W: Myasthenia gravis and multiple sclerosis: A usual combination of diseases. Neurology 24:72–75, 1974.
2. Al-Din AS: Multiple sclerosis in Kuwait: Clinical and epidemiological study. J Neurol Neurosurg Psychiatry 49:928–931, 1986.
3. Allen IV, Millar JH, and Hutchinson MJ: General disease in 120 necropsy-proven cases of multiple sclerosis. Neuropathol Appl Neurobiol 4:279–284, 1978.
4. Alter M, Allison RS, Talbert OR, Godden JO, and Kurland LT: The geographic distribution of multiple sclerosis: A comparison of prevalence in Charleston County, South Carolina and Halifax County, Nova Scotia. NS Med Bull 39:203–210, 1960.
5. Alter M, Hapern L, Kurland LT, Bornstein B, Leibowitz U, and Silberstein J: Prevalence among migrants and native inhabitants. Arch Neurol 7:253–263, 1962.
6. Alter M, Leibowitz U, and Speer J: Risk of multiple sclerosis related to age of immigration to Israel. Arch Neurol 15:234–237, 1966.
7. Alter M, Okihiro M, Rowley W, and Morris T: Multiple sclerosis among orientals and caucasians in Hawaii. Neurology 21:122–130, 1971.
8. Alter M, and Olivares L: Multiple sclerosis in Mexico. Arch Neurol 23:451–459, 1970.
9. Antonovsky A, Leibowitz U, Medalie JM, Halpern L, Smith AH, and Alter M: Reappraisal of possible aetological factors in multiple sclerosis. Am J Public Health 58:836–848, 1968.
10. Bartschi-Rochaiz W: MS in Switzerland Canton Wallis. In Bauer HJ, Poser S, and Ritter G (eds): Progress in Multiple Sclerosis Research. Springer, New York, 1980, pp 535–538.
11. Bauer HJ: Multiple sclerosis in Europe. Symposium Report. J Neurol 234:195–206, 1987.
12. Ben Hamida M: La sclerose en plaques en

Tunisie: Etude clinique de 100 observations. Rev Neurol (Paris) 33:109–117, 1977.

13. Bennett L, Hamilton R, Neutel CI, Pearson JC, and Talbot B: Survey of persons with multiple sclerosis in Ottawa, 1974–1975. Can J Public Health 68:141–147, 1977.

14. Bias WB, Reveille JD, Beaty TH, Meyers DA, and Arnett FC: Evidence that autoimmunity in man is a Mendelian dominant trait. Am J Hum Genet 39:584–602, 1986.

15. Birk K, Ford C, Smeltzer S, Ryan D, Miller R, and Rudick RA: The clinical course of multiple sclerosis during pregnancy and the puerperium. Arch Neurol 47:738–742, 1990.

16. Bulman DE, and Ebers GC: The geography of multiple sclerosis reflects genetics susceptability. Journal of Tropical and Geographical Neurology 2:66–72, 1992.

17. Bulman DE, Sadovnick AD, and Ebers GC: Age of onset in siblings concordant for multiple sclerosis. Brain 114:937–950, 1991.

18. Bunnell DH, Visscher BR, and Detels R: Multiple sclerosis and house dogs: A case control study. Neurology 29:1027–1029, 1979.

19. Butler EJ: Chronic neurological disease as a possible form of lead poisoning. J Neurol Neurosurg Psychiatry 15:119–128, 1952.

20. Castaigne P, Escourelle R, and Brunet P: Reticulosarcome cerebral primitif associe a des lesions de sclerose en plaques. Revue Neurologique 130:181–188, 1974.

21. Cavalli-Sforza LL, Piazza A, Menozzi P, and Mountain J: Reconstruction of human evolution: Bringing together genetic, archaelogical and linguistic data. Proc Natl Acad Sci USA 85:6002–6006, 1988.

22. Cendrowski W, Wender M, Dominik W, Flejsierowicz Z, Owsianowski M, and Popiel M: Epidemiological study of multiple sclerosis in Western Poland. Eur Neurol 2:90–103, 1968.

23. Charcot JM: Lectures on the Diseases of the Nervous System (translated by G. Siegerson). New Sydenham Society, London, 1877, pp 157–222.

24. Cook SD, Cromarty JI, Tapp W, Poskanzer D, Walker J, and Dowling PC: Declining incidence of multiple sclerosis in the Orkney Islands. Neurology 35:545–551, 1985.

25. Cook SD, and Dowling PC: A possible association between housepets and multiple sclerosis. Lancet 1:980–982, 1977.

26. Cook SD, MacDonald J, Tapp W, Poskanzer D, and Dowling PC: Multiple sclerosis in the Shetland Islands: An update. Acta Neurol Scand 77:148–151, 1988.

27. Currie S, and Urich H: Concurrence of multiple sclerosis and glioma. J Neurol Neurosurg Psychiatry 37:598–605, 1974.

28. Davenport CB: Multiple sclerosis from the standpoint of geographic distribution and race. Arch Neurol 8:51–58, 1922.

29. Dean G: Annual incidence, prevalence and mortality of MS in white South African–born and in white immigrants to South Africa. BMJ 2:724–730, 1967.

30. Dean G, Goodall J, and Downie A: The prevalence of multiple sclerosis in the Outer Hebrides compared with northeast Scotland and the Orkney and Shetland Islands. J Epidemiol Community Health 35:110–113, 1981.

31. Dean G, Grimaldi G, Kelly R, and Karhausen L: Multiple sclerosis in southern Europe. I. Prevalence in Sicily in 1975. J Epidemiol Community Health 33:107–110, 1979.

32. Detels R, Visscher BR, Malmgren RM, Coulson AH, Lucia MV, and Dudley JP: Evidence for lower susceptibility to multiple sclerosis in Japanese Americans. Am J Epidemiol 105:303–310, 1977.

33. D'Hooghe MB, and Ebers GC: A population-based study of seasonal onset of multiple sclerosis in London, Ontario (abstract). Neurology 39:284, 1989.

34. Dupont B, Lisak RP, and Jersild C: HLA antigens in black American patients with multiple sclerosis. Transplant Proc 91:181–185, 1976.

35. Duquette P, Murray TJ, Pleines J, et al: Multiple sclerosis in childhood: Clinical profile in 125 patients. J Pediat 111:359–363, 1987.

36. Duquette P, Pleines J, Girard M, Charest L, Senecal-Quevillon M, and Massé C: The increased susceptability of women to multiple sclerosis. Can J Neurol Sci 19:466–471, 1992.

37. Eastman R, Sheridan J, and Poskanzer DC: Multiple sclerosis clustering in a small Massachusetts community, with possible common exposure 23 years before onset. N Engl J Med 289:793–794, 1973.

38. Ebers GC: Genetic factors in multiple sclerosis. Neurol Clin 1:645–654, 1983.

39. Ebers GC: Multiple sclerosis and other demyelinating diseases. In Asbury A, McKhann G, and McDonald I (eds): Diseases of the Nervous System. WB Saunders, Philadelphia, 1986, pp 1268–1281.

39a. Ebers GC, Sadovnick AD, Risch NJ: A genetic basis for familial aggregation in Multiple Sclerosis. Nature 377:150–151, 1995.

40. Enstrom JE, and Operskalski EA: Multiple sclerosis among Spanish surnamed Californians. Neurology 28:434–438, 1978.

41. Fernàndez O, and Bufill E: Prevalence of multiple sclerosis in Spain: Validation of an epidemiological protocol in two geographically separated areas. In Firnhaber W, and Lauer K (eds): Multiple Sclerosis in Europe. An Epidemiological Update. Leuchtturrn-Verlag/LTV Press, Darmstadt, Germany 1994, pp 184–189.

42. Furszyfer J, Kurland LT, McConahey WM, Wollner LB, and Elveback LR: Epidemiologic aspects of Hashimoto's thyroiditis and Graves disease in Rochester, Minnesota (1935-1967) with special reference to temporal trends. Metabolism 3:197–204, 1972.

43. Gallou M, Madigand M, Masse L, Morel G, Oger J, and Sabouraud O: Epidemiologie de la sclerose en plaques en Bretagne. Presse Med 12:995–999, 1983.

44. Garcia JR, Rodriguez S, Henriquez MS, et al: Prevalence of multiple sclerosis in Lanzarote (Canary Islands). Neurology 39:265–267, 1989.

45. Gay D, Dick G, and Upton G: Multiple sclerosis associated with sinusitis: Case-controlled study in general practice. Lancet 1:815–819, 1986.

46. Georgiev D, Milanov I, Tzonev V, and Kalafatova O: The epidemiology of multiple sclerosis in Sofia. In Firnhaber W, and Lauer K (eds): Multiple Sclerosis in Europe. An Epidemiological Update. Leuchtturrn-Verlag/LTV Press, Darmstadt, Germany 1994, pp 322–325.

47. Granieri E, Casetta I, Tola MR, et al: Multiple sclerosis: Does epidemiology contribute to providing etiological clues? J Neurol Sci 115 (suppl):16–23, 1993.

48. Granieri E, and Rosati G: Italy: A medium or high-risk area for multiple sclerosis? An epidemiologic study in Barbagia, Sardinia, southern Italy. Neurology 32:466–472, 1982.

49. Granieri E, Tola R, Paolino E, Rosati G, Carreras M, and Monetti VC: The frequency of multiple sclerosis in Italy: A descriptive study in Ferrara. Ann Neurol 17:80–84, 1985.

50. Gronning M, and Mellgren SI: Multiple sclerosis in the two northernmost counties of Norway. Acta Neurol Scand 72:321–327, 1985.

51. Grufferman S, Barton JW, and Eby NL: Increased sex concordance of sibling pairs with Behcet's disease, Hodgkin's disease, multiple sclerosis and sarcoidosis. Am J Epidemiol 126:365–369, 1987.

52. Grufferman S, Cole P, and Lukes RJ: Hodgkin's disease in siblings. N Engl J Med 296:248–250, 1977.

53. Guseo A, Jofejü E, and Kocsis A: Epidemiology of multiple sclerosis in Western Hungary 1957-1992. In Firnhaber W, Lauer K (eds): Multiple Sclerosis in Europe. An Epidemiological Update. Leuchtturrn-Verlag/LTV Press, Germany 1994, pp 279–286.

54. Hader WJ: Prevalence of multiple sclerosis in Saskatoon. Can Med Assoc J 127:295–297, 1982.

55. Hader WJ, Elliot M, and Ebers GC: Epidemiology of multiple sclerosis in London and Middlesex County, Ontario, Canada. Neurology 38:617–621, 1988.

56. Hader WJ, Feasby TE, Noseworthy JH, Rice GP, and Ebers GC: Multiple sclerosis in Canadian Native People. Neurology 35:300, 1985.

57. Hammond SR, de Wytt C, Maxwell LC, et al: The epidemiology of multiple sclerosis in Queensland, Australia. J Neurol Sci 80:185–204, 1987.

58. Hammond SR, McLeod JG, Millingen KS, et al: The epidemiology of multiple sclerosis in three Australian cities: Perth, Newcastle and Hobart. Brain 111:1–25, 1988.

59. Haupts M, Schejbal P, Pöhlau D, Malin J, Przuntek H, and Gehlen W: Epidemiological data on multiple sclerosis from an industrial area in North-West Germany. In Firnhaber W, Lauer K (eds): Multiple Sclerosis in Europe: An Epidemiological Update. Leuchtturrn-Verlag/LTV Press, Darmstadt, Germany 1994, pp 143–146.

60. Hoffman RE, Zack MM, Davis LE, and Burchfiel CM: Increased incidence and prevalence of multiple sclerosis in Los Alamos County, New Mexico. Neurology 31:1489–1492, 1981.

61. Holmes FF, Stubbs DW, and Larsen WE: Systemic lupus erythematosus and multiple sclerosis in identical twins. Arch Intern Med 119:302, 1967.

62. Hooge JP, and Redekop WK: Multiple sclerosis with very late onset. Neurology 42:1907–1910, 1992.

63. Hung TP: Multiple sclerosis in Taiwan: A reappraisal. In Kuroiwa Y, and Kurland LT (eds): Multiple Sclerosis: East and West. Kyushu University Press, Kyushu, Japan, 1982, pp 83–96.

64. Irvine DG, and Schiefer HB: Geotoxicology of multiple sclerosis: The Henribourg, Saskatchewan, Cluster Focus. II. The soil. Sci Total Environ 77:175–188, 1988.

65. Kaufmann JC, and Lipschitz R: Trigeminal neurofibroma: Review and follow-up report of a case in a Bantu mimicking disseminated sclerosis. S Afr Med J 36:872–881, 1962.

66. Kesselring J, and Beer S: Epidemiology of multiple sclerosis in Switzerland. In Firnhaber W, and Lauer K (eds): Multiple Sclerosis in Europe: An Epidemiological Update. Leuchtturrn-Verlag/LTV Press, Darmstadt, Germany 1994, pp 166–167.

67. Kim SW, and Kim SY: Multiple sclerosis in Busan, Korea. Clinical features and prevalence. In Kuroiwa Y, and Kurland LT (eds): Multiple sclerosis: East and West. Kyushu University Press, Kyushu, Japan, 1982, pp 57–69.

68. Kinnunen E: Multiple sclerosis in Finland: Evidence of increasing frequency and uneven geographic distribution. Neurology 34:457–461, 1984.

69. Koopmans RA, Li DKB, and Oger JJ: The lesion of multiple sclerosis: Imaging of acute and chronic stages. Neurology 39:959–963, 1990.

70. Kranz JM, Kurland LT, Schuman LM, and Layton D: Multiple sclerosis in Olmsted and Mower Counties, Minnesota. Neuroepidemiology 2:206–218, 1983.

71. Kruja J: Multiple sclerosis in Albania. In Firnhaber W, and Lauer K (eds): Multiple Sclerosis in Europe. An Epidemiological Update. Leuchtturrn-Verlag/LTV Press, Darmstadt, Germany 1994, pp 309–315.

72. Kuroiwa Y, Igata A, Itahara K, et al: Nationwide survey of multiple sclerosis in Japan. Clinical analysis of 1084 cases. Neurology 25:845–851, 1975.

73. Kuroiwa Y, Shibasaki H, and Ikeda M: Prevalence of multiple sclerosis and its north-south gradient in Japan. Neuroepidemiology 2:62–69, 1983.

74. Kurtzke JF: A reassessment of the distribution of multiple sclerosis: Pts I and II. Acta Neurol Scand 51:110–136, 137–157, 1975.

75. Kurtzke JF: Geography in multiple sclerosis. J Neurol 215:1–26, 1977.

76. Kurtzke JF: Epidemiological evidence for multiple sclerosis as an infection. Clin Microbiol Rev 6:382–427, 1993.

77. Kurtzke JF, Beebe GW, and Norman JE: Epidemiology of multiple sclerosis in U.S. veterans. I. Race, sex and geographic distribution. Neurology 29:1228–1235, 1979.

78. Kurtzke JF, and Bui QH: Multiple sclerosis in a migrant population. II. Half-orientals immigrating in childhood. Ann Neurol 8:256–260, 1980.

79. Kurtzke JF, Gudmundsson KR, and Bergmann S: Multiple sclerosis in Iceland. I. Evidence of a postwar epidemic. Neurology 32:143–150, 1982.

80. Kurtzke JF, and Hyllested K: Multiple sclerosis in

the Faroe Islands. I. Clinical and epidemiological features. Ann Neurol 5:6–21, 1979.

81. Kurtzke JF, and Hyllested K: Multiple sclerosis in the Faroe Islands. II. Clinical update, transmission and the nature of multiple sclerosis. Neurology 36:307–328, 1986.

82. Kurtzke JF, and Hyllested K: Validity of the epidemics of multiple sclerosis in the Faroe Islands. Neuroepidemiol 7:190–227, 1988.

83. Laborde JM, Dando WA, and Teetzel ML: Climate, diffuse solar radiation and multiple sclerosis. Soc Sci Med 27:231–238, 1988.

84. Larsen JP, Aarli JA, and Riise T: Western Norway, a high risk area for multiple sclerosis: A prevalence incidence study in the county of Hordaland. Neurology 34:1202–1207, 1984.

85. Larsen JP, Riise T, Nyland H, Kvale G, and Aarli JA: Clustering of multiple sclerosis in the county of Hordaland, Western Norway. Acta Neurol Scand 71:390–395, 1985.

86. Leibowitz U, Kahana E, and Alter M: Multiple sclerosis in immigrant and native populations of Israel. Lancet 1:1323–1325, 1970.

87. Leiter EH, Serreze DV, and Prochazka M: The genetics and epidemiology of diabetes in NOD mice. Immunol Today 11:147–149, 1990.

88. Linos A, Worthington JW, O'Fallon WM, and Kurland LT: The epidemiology of rheumatoid arthritis in Rochester, Minnesota: A study of incidence, prevalence and mortality. Am J Epidemiol 111:87–98, 1980.

89. Ljapchev R, and Daskalovaska V: Epidemiological studies of multiple sclerosis in the republic of Macedonia. In Firnhaber W, and Lauer K (eds): Multiple Sclerosis in Europe: An Epidemiological Update. Leuchtturrn-Verlag/LTV Press, Darmstadt, Germany 1994, pp 301–308.

90. Lynch PG: Multiple sclerosis and malignant glioma. BMJ 3:577, 1974.

91. Margolis LN, and Graves RW: The occurrence of myasthenia gravis in a patient with multiple sclerosis. North Carolina Medical Journal 24:243–244, 1945.

92. Matthews WB: The neurological complications of ankylosing spondylitis. J Neurol Sci 5:561–573, 1968.

93. Matthews WB: Course and prognosis. In Matthews WB, Acheson ED, Batchelor JR, and Weller RO (eds): McAlpine's Multiple Sclerosis. Churchill Livingstone, New York, 1985, pp 49–52.

94. Matthews WB: Some aspects of the natural history. In Matthews WB, Acheson ED, Batchelor JR, and Weller RO (eds): McAlpine's Multiple Sclerosis. Churchill Livingstone, New York, 1985, pp 73–95.

95. McCall MG, Brereton TLG, Dawson A, Millingen K, Sutherland JM, and Acheson ED: Frequency of multiple sclerosis in three Australian centres, Perth, Newcastle and Hobart. J Neurol Neurosurg Psychiatry 31:1–9, 1968.

96. Midgard R, Riise T, and Nyland H: Epidemiologic trends in multiple sclerosis in More and Romsdal, Norway: A prevalence/incidence study in a stable population. Neurology 41:887–892, 1991.

97. Millar JH, Allison RS, Cheesman EA, and Merrett JD: Pregnancy as a factor influencing relapse in disseminated sclerosis. Brain 82:417–426, 1959.

98. Milonas I, Tsounis MI, and Logothetis S: Epidemiology of multiple sclerosis in northern Greece. Acta Neurol Scand 81:43–47, 1990.

99. Minderhoud JM, and Zwanikken CP: Increasing prevalence and incidence of multiple sclerosis: An epidemiological study in the province of Groningen, the Netherlands. In Firnhaber W, and Lauer K (eds): Multiple Sclerosis in Europe: An Epidemiological Update. Leuchtturrn-Verlag/LTV Press, Darmstadt, Germany 1994, pp 113–121.

100. Murray TJ: An unusual occurrence of multiple sclerosis in a small rural community. Can J Neurol Sci 3:163–166, 1976.

101. Noseworthy J, Paty DW, Wonnacott T, Feasby T, and Ebers G: Multiple sclerosis after age 50. Neurology 33:1537–1544, 1983.

102. Pàlffy G, Czopf J, Kuntàr L, and Gyodi E: Multiple sclerosis in Baranya County in Hungarians and in gipsies. In Firnhaber W, and Lauer K (eds): Multiple Sclerosis in Europe. An Epidemiological Update. Leuchtturrn-Verlag/LTV Press, Darmstadt, Germany 1994, pp 274–278.

103. Park CS: Multiple sclerosis in Korea. Neurology 16:919–926, 1966.

104. Percy AK, Nobrega FT, Okazaki H, Glattre E, and Kurland LT: Multiple sclerosis in Rochester, Minn: A 60-year appraisal. Arch Neurol 25:105–111, 1971.

105. Phadke JG, and Downie AW: Epidemiology of multiple sclerosis in the northeast (Grampian Region) of Scotland: An update. J Epidemiol Community Health 41:5–13, 1987.

106. Popov VS: Clinical picture and epidemiology of disseminated sclerosis. Zh Nevropatol Psikhiatr IM S S Korsakova 83:1330–1334, 1983.

107. Poser CM, and Hibberd PL: Analysis of the "epidemic" of multiple sclerosis in the Faroe Islands. I. Biostatistical aspects. Neuroepidemiol 7:181–189, 1988.

108. Poser CM, Hibberd PL, Benedikz J, Gudmundsson G: Analysis of the "epidemic" of multiple sclerosis in the Faroe Islands. I. Clinical and epidemiological aspects. Neuroepidemiology 7:168–180, 1988.

109. Poser CM, Paty DW, Scheinberg L, et al: New diagnostic criteria for multiple sclerosis: Guidelines for research protocols. Ann Neurol 13:227–231, 1983.

110. Poser S: The epidemiology of multiple sclerosis in Southern Lower Saxony. In Firnhaber W, and Lauer K (eds): Multiple Sclerosis in Europe: An Epidemiological Update. Leuchtturrn-Verlag/LTV Press, Darmstadt, Germany 1994, pp 130–133.

111. Poskanzer DC, Prenney LB, and Sheridan JL: Housepets and multiple sclerosis. The Lancet 1:1204, 1977.

112. Poskanzer DC, Prenney LB, Sheridan JL, and Kondy JY: Multiple sclerosis in the Orkney and Shetland Islands. I. Epidemiology, clinical factors and methodology. J Epidemiol Community Health 34:229–239, 1980.

113. Poskanzer DC, Schapira K, and Miller H: Multi-

ple sclerosis and poliomyelitis. The Lancet 2: 917–921, 1963.

114. Poskanzer DC, Walker AM, Prenney LB, and Sheridan JL: The etiology of multiple sclerosis: Temporal-spatial clustering indicating two environmental exposures before onset. Neurology 31:708–713, 1981.

115. Presthus J: Report on the multiple sclerosis investigations in West-Norway. Acta Psychiatr Neurol Scand 35:88–92, 1960.

116. Pryse-Phillips WE: The incidence and prevalence of multiple sclerosis in Newfoundland and Labrador, 1960–1984. Ann Neurol 20:323–328, 1986.

117. Radhakrishnan K, Ashok PP, Sridharan R, and Mousa ME: Prevalence and pattern of multiple sclerosis in Benghazi, North-Eastern Libya. J Neurol Sci 70:39–46, 1985.

118. Read D, Nassim D, Smith P, Patterson C, and Warlow C: Multiple sclerosis and dog ownership: A case-control investigation. J Neurol Sci 55:359–365, 1982.

119. Reagan TJ, and Frieman IS: Multiple cerebral gliomas in multiple sclerosis. J Neurol Neurosurg Psychiatr 36:523–528, 1973.

120. Roth MP, Ballivet S, Descoins P, Ruidavets JB, Clanet M, and Cambon-Thomsen A: Multiple sclerosis in the Pyrénées-Atlantiques: A case-control study conducted in the Southwest of France. In Firnhaber W, and Lauer K (eds): Multiple Sclerosis in Europe. An Epidemiological Update. Leuchtturrn-Verlag/LTV Press, Darmstadt, Germany 1994, pp 177–178.

121. Sadovnick AD, and Baird PA: The familial nature of multiple sclerosis: Age-corrected empiric recurrence risks or children and siblings of patients. Neurology 38:990–991, 1988.

122. Sadovnick AD, Baird PA, and Ward RH: Multiple Sclerosis: Updated risks for relatives. Am J Med Genet 29:533–541, 1988.

123. Sadovnick AD, Bulman DE, and Ebers GC: Influence of gender on the susceptibility to multiple sclerosis in siblings. Arch Neurol 48:586–588, 1991.

124. Sadovnick AD, and Ebers GC: Epidemiology of multiple sclerosis: A critical overview. Can J Neurol Sci 20:17–29, 1993.

124a. Sadovnick AD, Ebers GC, Dyment D, Risch N and the Canadian Collaborative Study Group. Evidence for the genetic basis of Multiple Sclerosis. The Lancet 347:1728–1730, 1996.

125. Sadovnick AD, Ebers GC, Eisen K, and Paty DW: Cause of death in patients attending multiple sclerosis clinics. Neurology 41:1193–1196, 1991.

126. Sadovnick AD, Eisen K, Hashimoto SA, et al: Multiple sclerosis and pregnancy: A prospective study. Arch Neurol 51:1120–1124, 1994.

127. Sadovnick AD, Paty DW, and Yannakoulias G: Concurrence of multiple sclerosis and inflammatory bowel disease. N Engl J Med 321:762–763, 1989.

128. Schumacher GA, Beebe G, Kibler RF, et al: Problems of experimental trials of therapy in multiple sclerosis: Report by the panel on the evaluation of experimental trials of therapy in multiple sclerosis. Ann NY Acad Sci 122:552–568, 1965.

129. Sepcic J, Antonelli L, Materljan E, and Sepic-Grahovac D: Multiple sclerosis cluster in Gorski Kotar, Croatia, Yugoslavia. In Battaglia MA (ed): Multiple Sclerosis Research. Elsevier, Amsterdam, 1989, pp 165–169.

130. Shakir RA, Hussuen MM, and Trontelj JV: Myasthenia gravis and multiple sclerosis. J Neuroimmunol 4:161–165, 1983.

131. Sheremata WA, Poskanzer DC, Withum DG, MacLeod CL, and Whiteside ME: Unusual occurrence on a tropical island of multiple sclerosis. Lancet 2:618, 1985.

132. Sibley WA, Bamford CR, and Clark K: Clinical viral infections and multiple sclerosis. Lancet 1 (8441):1313–1315, 1985.

133. Sibley WA, Bamford CR, and Laguna JF: Anamnestic studies in multiple sclerosis: A relationship between familial multiple sclerosis and neoplasia. Neurology 28:125–128, 1978.

134. Sibley WA, and Foley JM: Infection and immunization in multiple sclerosis. Ann NY Acad Sci 122: 457–468, 1965.

135. Skegg DC, Corwin PA, Craven RS, Malloch JA, and Pollock M: Occurrence of multiple sclerosis in the north and south of New Zealand. J Neurol Neurosurg Psychiatry 50:134–139, 1987.

136. Smith HR, and Steinberg AD: Autoimmunity: A perspective review. Annu Rev Immunol 1:175–210, 1983.

137. Stazio A, Kurland LT, Bell GL, Saunders MG, and Robot E: Multiple sclerosis in Winnipeg, Manitoba. Methodological consideration of epidemiologic survey: Ten-year follow-up of a community-wide study and population re-survey. Journal of Chronic Diseases 17:415–438, 1964.

138. Stein EC, Schiffer RB, Hall J, and Young Y: Multiple sclerosis and the workplace: Report of an industry-based cluster. Neurology 37:1672–1677, 1987.

139. Sutherland JM: Observations on the prevalence of multiple sclerosis in northern Scotland. Brain 79:635–654, 1956.

140. Swank RL: Multiple sclerosis: Correlation of its incidence with dietary fat. Am J Med Sci 220:421–430, 1951.

141. Sweeney VP, Sadovnick AD, and Brandejs V: Prevalance of multiple sclerosis in British Columbia. Can J Neurol Sci 13:47–51, 1986.

142. Swingler RJ, and Compston DA: The distribution of multiple sclerosis in the United Kingdom. J Neurol Neurosurg Psychiatry 49:1115–1124, 1986.

143. Swingler RJ, and Compston DA: The prevalence of multiple sclerosis in southeast Wales. J Neurol Neurosurg Psychiatry 51:1520–1524, 1988.

144. Tan CT: Multiple sclerosis in Malaysia. Arch Neurol 45:624–627, 1988.

145. Thomas DJ, Kendall MJ, and Whitfield AG: Nervous system involvement in ankylosing spondylitis. BMJ 1:148–150, 1974.

146. Trendafilova L, Manova M, and Hadjipetrova K: Multiple sclerosis in the Plovdiv area, Bulgari. In Firnhaber W, and Lauer K (eds): Multiple Sclerosis in Europe: An Epidemiological Update. Leuchtturrn-Verlag/LTV Press, Darmstadt, Germany 1994, pp 326–331.

147. Trostle DC, Helfrich D, and Medsger TAJ: Systemic sclerosis (scleroderma) and multiple sclerosis. Arthritis Rheum 29:124–127, 1986.

148. Uria DF, Abad P, Virgala P, and Calatayud MT: Prevalence and incidence of multiple sclerosis in Gijon (Northern Spain). In Firnhaber W, and Lauer K (eds): Multiple Sclerosis in Europe: An Epidemiological Update. Leuchtturrn-Verlag/LTV Press, Darmstadt, Germany 1994, pp 179–183.

149. Van Lambalgen R, Sanders EA, and D'Amaro J: Sex distribution, age of onset and HLA profiles in two types of multiple sclerosis: A role for sex hormones and microbial infections in the development of autoimmunity? J Neurol Sci 76:13–21, 1986.

150. Vassallo L, Elian M, and Dean G: Multiple sclerosis in southern Europe. II. Prevalence in Malta in 1978. J Epidemiol Comm Health 33:111–113, 1979.

151. Visscher BR, Detels R, Coulson AH: Latitude, migration and the prevalence of multiple sclerosis. Am J Epidemiol 106:470–475, 1977.

152. Wadia NH, and Bhatia K: Multiple sclerosis is prevalent in the Zoroastrians (Parsis) of India. Ann Neurol 28:177–179, 1990.

153. Warren S, and Warren KG: Multiple sclerosis and associated diseases: A relationship to diabetes mellitus. Can J Neurol Sci 8:35–39, 1981.

154. Weinshenker B, Bass B, Rice GP, and Ebers GC: The natural history of multiple sclerosis: A geographically-based study. I. Clinical course and disability. Brain 112:133–146, 1989.

155. Weinshenker B, Bass B, Rice GP, and Ebers GC: The natural history of multiple sclerosis: A geographically-based study. II. The predictive value of the early clinical course. Brain 112:1419–1428, 1989.

156. Weitkamp LR: Multiple sclerosis susceptibility: Interaction between sex and HLA. Arch Neurol 40:399–401, 1983.

157. Wender M, Pruchnik-Grabowska D, Hertmanowska H, et al: Epidemiology of multiple sclerosis in Western Poland. Acta Neurol Scand 72:210–217, 1985.

158. Westlund KB, and Kurland LT: Studies on multiple sclerosis in Winnipeg, Manitoba and New Orleans, Louisiana. I. Prevalence: Comparison between the patient groups in Winnipeg and New Orleans. American Journal of Hygiene 57:380–396, 1953.

159. White DN, and Wheelan L: Disseminated sclerosis. A survey of patients in the Kingston, Ontario area. Neurology 9:256–272, 1959.

160. Williams ES, and McKeran RO: Prevalence of multiple sclerosis in a south London borough. Br Med J 293:237–239, 1986.

161. Willoughby EW, Grochowski E, and Li DKB: Serial magnetic resonance scanning in multiple sclerosis: A second prospective study in relapsing patients. Ann Neurol 25:43–49, 1989.

162. Wynn DR, Codd MB, Kurland LT, and Rodriguez M: Multiple sclerosis: A population–based investigation of the association with possible autoimmune diseases and diabetes mellitus (abstract). Neurology 37:272, 1987.

163. Wynn DR, Codd MB, Kurland LT, and Rodriguez M: Multiple sclerosis: A population-based investigation of the association with neoplastic disorders (abstract). Neurology 37:151, 1987.

164. Wynn DR, Kurland LT, O'Fallon WM, and Rodriguez M: A reappraisal of the epidemiology of multiple sclerosis in Olmsted County, Minnesota. Neurology 40:780–786, 1990.

165. Wynn DR, Rodriguez M, O'Fallon WM, and Kurland LT: Update on the epidemiology of multiple sclerosis. Mayo Clinic Proc 64:808–817, 1989.

166. Yaquib BA, and Daif AK: Multiple sclerosis in Saudi Arabia. Neurology 38:621–623, 1988.

167. Yu YL, Woo E, Hawkins BR, Ho HC, and Huang CY: Multiple sclerosis amongst Chinese in Hong Kong. Brain 112:1445–1467, 1989.

168. Zimmerman HM, and Netsky MG: The pathology of multiple sclerosis. Res Publ Assoc Res Nerv Ment Dis 28:271–312, 1950.

CHAPTER 3

SUSCEPTIBILITY: GENETICS IN MULTIPLE SCLEROSIS

George C. Ebers, MD
A. Dessa Sadovnick, PhD

The most common and important human diseases are complex traits that result from genetic/environmental interactions. Among these are the autoimmune disorders, a group that may include MS. The possible role of inherited factors influencing the development of MS has intrigued neurologists for almost a century. Eichhorst[20] labeled MS an "inherited, transmissible" disease. By 1950, 85 families in which there were at least two family members with MS were reported in the literature.[64] Genetic analysis of such families led to limited speculation about the nature of susceptibility to MS. It was clear, however, that the data were inconsistent with fully penetrant mendelian patterns of inheritance. Concepts of genetic or environmental interactions have been relatively recent developments. The early literature indicates that most early investigators concluded that "nurture" was much more important than "nature" in the etiology of MS.

Although few imaginable hypotheses have not been at one time proposed to explain MS susceptibility, early systematic studies[13,64] stand out as providing special insights. Davenport,[13] using data from the US armed services, suggested that the distribution of MS matched the geographic distribution for immigration to the United States from Scandinavia. He concluded that "there are internal conditions that inhibit and those that facilitate the development of the disease or the factors on which it depends." Pratt and colleagues[64] believed that susceptibility to MS arose from the presence of two or more independently segregating genes, thus suggesting the concept of oligogenic or polygenic inheritance.

29

Table 3–1. **EVIDENCE AGAINST A PURELY TRANSMISSIBLE ETIOLOGY IN MULTIPLE SCLEROSIS**

Table 3–1. **EVIDENCE AGAINST A PURELY TRANSMISSIBLE ETIOLOGY IN MULTIPLE SCLEROSIS**

1. Low rate in dizygotic twins[4,16,39,44,57,74]
2. Low rate in conjugal pairs[22,43,82]
3. Negative birth-order studies[29]
4. High rate of MS in second- and third-degree relatives of patients[75,76]
5. Groups resistant to MS in high-risk areas
   Native Americans (North America)[35,46]
   Inuit (northern Canada, Alaska)[15]
   Hutterites (western Canada)[15]
   Hispanics (California)[21]
   Asians, such as Chinese and Japanese (North America)[14,46]
   American blacks (North America)[46]
   Lapps (Scandinavia)[33]
   Maoris (New Zealand)[89]
   Yakutes (Far North, Russia)[64]
6. Reported association/linkage with candidate loci[20]

In 1972, the report of an association between certain alleles of the human leukocyte antigen (HLA) system and MS provided the first direct evidence supporting a genetic contribution.[42] Because the major histocompatibility complex (MHC) was found to encode immune response genes in mice, it was plausibly advanced that individuals develop MS because they inherit genes that influence immune response (possibly viral), leading to a chain of immunologic events resulting in myelin injury. Although nothing has been discovered since 1972 to discount the role played by the MHC in restricting and regulating immune response in mice and humans, it has become clear that genes outside the MHC are also important.[80]

The search for loci influencing MS susceptibility has largely been confined to specific candidate genes influencing immune response. In addition to the MHC, these include the T-cell receptor *(TcR)*, immunoglobulin constant *(C)* and variable *(V)* regions, several complement loci and several structural genes of myelin.

It remains undetermined whether any particular genes are truly necessary for the development of MS. Existing data suggest that, at the very least, two genes (and almost certainly several genes) will be found to be influential and to interact in undetermined ways. Taken together, data to date (vide infra) provide evidence against a purely transmissible etiology in MS (Table 3–1).

DISTRIBUTION OF MULTIPLE SCLEROSIS

Geographic distribution, including migration studies, has been discussed in Chapter 2. The contribution of genetic factors to the geographic distribution of MS, however, is discussed in this chapter.

Multiple Sclerosis Susceptibility

Some evidence suggests that in persons who are innately susceptible to MS, the conditions leading to widespread multifocal myelin injury are established during a fairly short period of susceptibility in childhood. Although the studies are retrospective and thus subject to recall bias, the age in childhood at which individuals are affected by the common exanthematous illnesses appears to associate with the risk of subsequently developing MS. This concept applies especially to HLA-DR2–positive children exposed to measles, mumps, and rubella at a relatively older age.[11] If this association is in fact true, it remains unclear whether it is causal or represents a secondary phenomenon. For example, later age of childhood exanthems may be associated with higher socioeconomic status, which may itself be associated with MS and susceptibility without any implication of causality.

The epidemiological approach has clear limits for understanding the geographic distribution of MS. Without clear information on the distribution of susceptibility alleles (some of which are presumably yet to be identified), it is difficult to interpret the entire body of MS geographic data. If MS susceptibility is determined by oligogenes (a small number of interacting genes), it is likely that each locus presumably differs in its effect on susceptibility. The distribution of these loci may not be evenly distributed in an "at-risk" population. There is room for daunting complexity, because the effects of susceptibility genes, singly or in combination, could be overridden by resistance genes. Indeed, multiple alleles at a given locus may determine a hierarchy of risks. Where a given factor is common, MS prevalence would also be expected to be high. The probability would then increase that the other risk factors would occur in the individual. However, the primary factor determining susceptibility in an at-risk population may not itself appear to be strongly associated. This explanation has been advanced for the lack of association with HLA-DR2 in the Orkney Islands. While HLA-DR2 is present in 50 percent of the unaffected population, the distribution of HLA-DR2 among patients with MS is similar to that found elsewhere in northern Europe.[10,65] In contrast, factors that do not have a high frequency in the unaffected population and may only in fact be making a small contribution to heritability may appear to be most strongly associated with the disease in these populations. In the situation where all risk factors for the disease are uncommon, the local frequency of MS will also be low, and the factors that are biologically most significant will then most easily emerge in disease association studies. More detailed surveys involving larger numbers of subjects are needed to identify the subsidiary associations. It must be remembered that many populations may not yet have reached equilibrium (panmixia) and that population associations with genetic markers may reflect this lack of equilibrium rather than being an indication of the pattern of susceptibility.

TWIN STUDIES

The classic method for distinguishing between the relative importance of genetic and environmental factors in disease has been the study of twins. This method is straightforward in concept but, like migration studies, difficult in execution. Simply stated, twin studies allow comparison of concordance in monozygotic (MZ) twins, who are genetically identical, with that in dizygotic (DZ) twins, who are no more genetically alike than nontwin siblings, but who would be expected to share a more common environment than nontwin siblings. Comparison of concordance rates between MZ and DZ pairs measures the influence of genetic factors. Comparison of concordance rates between DZ pairs and nontwin siblings measures the influence of environment (perhaps better called non-genetic factors).

The major problem in twin studies, including some of those in MS, is ascertainment.[74] Twins occur in approximately 1 per 80 births with an expected monozygotic (MZ):dizygotic (DZ) ratio of 1:2.[92] One measure of ascertainment bias is therefore to determine whether the MZ:DZ ratio in a study sample approaches 1:2. For example, the large twin study conducted by MacKay and Myrianthopoulos[53] consisted of substantially more MZ pairs than expected. This study exemplifies some of the practical problems associated with twin studies. Because there are few available patient populations with a sufficiently large number of twins in which to conduct such a study, most investigators have relied on the solicitation of volunteers by public appeal. This method tends to result in overrepresentation of females, MZ pairs, and concordant pairs. The excess of females has been seen in many studies for different diseases in which volunteers are solicited. The excess of MZ pairs is probably because the twin status of MZ pairs is more likely to be known to friends, more distant relatives, and physicians than it is for DZ pairs. For example, at the Vancouver MS Clinic, all patients who were MZ twins were identified as such by the referring physician, but this was not the case for the majority of patients who were DZ twins. The excess of concordant pairs is probably (and understandably) because such pairs would have more motivation to participate in a genetic study than would discordant pairs, when only one member of the twin pair is affected with the disease in question. In addition, the likelihood of ascertainment of the same pair is apparently doubled when both members of the pair are affected.

To minimize ascertainment bias, several studies have identified twin pairs from large populations either of patients with MS or of twins.[4,16,39,44,58,74] The combined results of the population-based studies[4,39,44,58,74] (Table 3–2) demonstrate a concordance rate of approximately 26 percent for MZ pairs compared with only 2.4 percent for same-sex DZ pairs, a figure close to the rate derived for nontwin siblings of patients with MS (not corrected for sex). The risk for concordance among same-sex sibling pairs appears to be increased from empirical risk data.[75,76] These data give the same-sex concordance rate for MS as 4.14 ± 1.28 percent for male-male pairs and 5.65 ± 1.10 percent for female-female pairs (see Table 3–4).

Twin data from France[25] seem not to agree with the population-based data from other centers, including the most recent work from the British Isles. The French study was not population based, and among 116 twin pairs identified, over half could not be fully evaluated. The zygosity status of more than 20 pairs could not be determined. It is suggested that a difference exists in the importance of genetic influence between France and other geographic regions studied but the confidence intervals of concordance for MZ twins in the French, Canadian, and British studies are overlapping.[18]

A number of inferences can be drawn from the data in Table 3–2:

- The genetic component to susceptibility appears substantial (although one must consider the possible increased environmental sharing in MZ compared with DZ twins).
- Genetic susceptibility is unlikely to be accounted for by a single dominant or even a single recessive gene, because the difference in concordance rates suggests the operation of at least two or more genes. The large difference in concordance rates between MZ and DZ twins recalls the difference between F1 (50 percent) and F2 (2 percent) generations in graft acceptance that led Little[48] to conclude that some 15 different loci determined the acceptance or rejection of allografts.
- A modest tendency for concordant pairs to be female (data not shown), even controlling for the expected female-to-male excess in MS, shows that gender is an independent factor influencing susceptibility (see also the discussion on the influence of gender on susceptibility in Chapter 2).
- Twin data also have implications for the nature of the environmental effect, because most MZ twins are discordant even after age correction and magnetic resonance imaging (MRI) scans (which can show clinically asympto-

Table 3–2. **RESULTS FROM POPULATION-BASED TWIN STUDIES**

Senior Author	Monozygotic Concordance	Dizygotic Concordance	Sibling Concordance
Heltberg[37]	4/19 (21.1%)	1/28 (3.6%)*	Not Available
Bobowick[4]	2/5 (40.0%)	0/4*	Not Available
Kinnunen[42]	2/7 (28.6%)	0/6*	Not Available
Sadovnick[69]	8/26 (30.8%)†	2/43 (4.7%)	5.1%‡
Mumford[54]	11/44 (25.0%)	2/61 (3.3%)	Not Available
Totals (excluding ref 25)	27/101 (26.7%)	5/142 (3.5%)	1.5%‡
French Research Group on MS[23]	1/17 (5.9%)§	1/37 (2.7%)§	Not Available

*Sample is comprised of same sex-pairs.
†Sample includes one pair with MS in one twin and isolated optic neuritis in the co-twin.
‡Figures are derived from refs 16 and 74.
§Study was not population-based.

matic white matter lesions in some clinically unaffected co-twins).

These factors suggest that a substantial environmental effect is required. It must be acknowledged that the number of DZ twins reported in the cited studies is still small, with wide confidence intervals. However, the similar concordance rate for DZ twins and siblings suggests a more global environmental effect such as climate, diet, or the operation of ubiquitous infectious agents. This notion is supported by the finding that sibling pairs tend more toward the same age of onset than year of onset,[9,77] and that affected sibling pairs are randomly ordered in birth sequence.[29] These observations do not rule out the long-held speculation that a specific infectious agent triggers MS, but they make it seem less attractive.

It is important, however, to interpret the results of twin studies in MS in the context of classic infectious diseases, such as polio and tuberculosis, in which similar twin studies have been carried out. In polio, data from a twin study that was methodologically very similar to the Canadian MS twin study[16,74] found concordance rates of 35.7 percent for MZ pairs and 6 percent for DZ pairs.[92] In one large study of tuberculosis, the MZ concordance rate was 51 percent, compared with 26 percent for DZ pairs and a similar figure for nontwin siblings.[34] The high rate of MZ discordance does not necessarily imply the operation of an environmental agent. It is worth mentioning the possibility of other reasons for discordance such as translocations, deletions, somatic mutations, and other random or chance processes, such as differential X-inactivation. It is recognized that reported MS concordance rates in twins (and in families in general) are probably underestimates. Subclinical disease in clinically asymptomatic individuals,[31] including co-twins of patients with MS, has been reported when diagnostic procedures have included cerebrospinal fluid (CSF) examination,[74,96] evoked potentials,[59] and MRI scans.[52,74] In the Canadian twin study, MRI was done on 21 clinically unaffected co-twins (14 MZ, 7 DZ).[74] MRIs for only 2 of the 14 MZ co-twins and 1 of the 7 DZ co-twins showed MRI abnormalities consistent with MS.[74] Of those with no lesions on MRI, four MZ co-twins underwent CSF electrophoresis, and none showed oligoclonal banding or any other central nervous system (CNS) abnormality.[74]

Thus from twin studies, we can conclude that genetic factors are important in MS susceptibility and that at least two genes are involved. For a single dominant or recessive susceptibility locus, the MZ:DZ concordance ratio should approximate 2:1 and 4:1, respectively, if nonheritable factors are equally important for MZ and DZ twins. The combined population-based studies (see Table 3–2) have an MZ:DZ concordance ratio of 7.7:1. In part because the environmental factors have been inscrutable and in part because investigators have exhausted many standard epidemiological approaches in trying to identify environmental stimuli that lead to MS, much research has turned to what may be a less intractable problem, the identification of specific genetic susceptibility loci.

ADOPTEE AND HALF-SIBLING STUDIES

This approach has been stimulated and to some extent validated by two studies indicating that familial aggregation is determined by genes and that singly or multiply affected pedigrees represent the segregation of gene loci interacting with factors influencing penetrance. The first of these was our study of adoptees.[19] Among 1,201 first degree nonbiological relatives of MS patients adopted at or near birth, only one case of MS was found. In contrast, 25 cases would have been expected in biological relatives.

The second study focused on the half-siblings of MS patients. No difference in recurrence risk between half-siblings reared apart versus those raised together was identified.[80] This study conveniently addressed several other issues including in utero effects, breast-feeding, genomic imprinting, vertical transmission, and mitochondrial inheritance. No significant difference was found between maternal and paternal half-sibling rates, casting doubt on some previously viable concepts such as maternal retroviral transmission. The future role of case-control studies in MS research should be considered in the context of the adoptee and half-sibling results.

SUSCEPTIBILITY LOCI IN MULTIPLE SCLEROSIS

Animal Models of Autoimmunity

Studies of animal models of autoimmunity have had a large impact on the thinking of clinical investigators researching genes that make humans susceptible to a number of known or suspected autoimmune disorders. Unfortunately, there is no *spontaneous* experimental animal model for MS. It remains unclear whether the induction of the various forms of experimental allergic encephalitis (EAE) has direct relevance because the immunologic stimulus given to induce disease may not be "physiological." Injection of myelin basic protein (MBP) or an extract of crude white matter can, in the presence of adjuvant, lead to paralysis in a wide range of experimental animals. Nevertheless, susceptibility to EAE appears to be related to the genetic strain of animal used[2] and further study seems relevant (see Chapter 11).

It is beyond the scope of this chapter to deal with the genetics of spontaneous autoimmunity in any detail. However, a few general lessons may be learned from these animal models:

- In virtually all cases, the inheritance of susceptibility is polygenic.

Table 3–3. SPONTANEOUS AUTOIMMUNE ANIMAL MODELS

INSULIN DEPENDENT DIABETES		
	NOD Mice	**BB Rat**
Genes (gene complexes)	>3	≥2
MHC	NOD H-2-C17 (Idd-1)	+
Other gene loci	D9Nds5-C9 (Idd-2)	—
	D3Nds1-C3 (Idd-3)	—
	D11Nds1-C11 (Idd-4)	—
	D6MIT14-C6	—
	D15Nds1-C15	—
	D1MIT5-C1	—
	D13Nds1-C13	—
	D7Nds6-C7	—
	D14Nds1-C14	—
Sex	Female: male ratio >2:1	Female: male ratio >2:1
	Enhanced by estrogen	Enhanced by estrogen
	Decreased by androgen	Decreased by androgen
Known environmental factors	Diet, cleanliness of cages, viruses infecting the colony	Not known
Neonatal thymectomy effect	Abrogates	None
Organ specificities	Pancreas	Pancreas
	Other glands	
	+T-cell hyperplasia	

LUPUS			
	NZB	**(NZB × NZW) F$_1$** **MRL/lpr/lpr**	**BXSB**
Genes (gene complexes)	≥6	NZB + 1NZW (dominant) ≥3	—
MHC	+	+ +	+
Other gene loci	Not known	— —	Y-linked accelerator epistatic (?) to autosomal gene

Continued on following page

- The number of genes interacting may be quite large.
- Genes conferring susceptibility appear to interact at different steps in the initiation of the autoimmune process. This finding is not surprising because there are many steps during the induction of an immune response in which genetic regulation might be expected.

Table 3–3 details spontaneous autoimmune animal models. Perhaps the most informative autoimmune animal model has been the nonobese diabetic (NOD) mouse. Susceptibility to diabetes in this strain appears to be determined by at least 10 genes,* and the role of the MHC has been dissected at a molecular level. The pres-

*References 12, 28, 30, 47, 49, 56, 67, 71, 91.

ence or absence of aspartic acid at position 57 on the MHC class II DQ β chain confers susceptibility or resistance in both the NOD mouse and in human type I juvenile diabetes. Clearly other as yet unidentified genes are also involved, some of which have been linked. The lupus models seem similarly complex, with at least six genes determining the NZB murine lupus. Crosses with the nonsusceptible NZW yield surprisingly severe glomerulonephritis that is not present in either parental strain, demonstrating the important role of background genes and their reactions. The MRL/lpr and BXSB models are probably no less complex.

This discussion has focused on spontaneous models of autoimmunity. However, in the context of genetic susceptibility, it needs

Table 3–3.—*continued*

	NZB	(NZB X NZW) F$_1$	MRL/lpr/lpr	BXSB
Sex	—	Enhanced by estrogen Decreased by androgen	Enhanced by estrogen Decreased by androgen	Enhanced in males (nonhormonal)
Known environmental factors	Stress, diet, virus can all influence NZB	—	—	—
Neonatal thymectomy effect	Enhanced	Enhanced	Abrogates	Enhanced
Organ specificities	Hemolytic anemia	Sjögren's GN	Arthritis GN	Arteritis GN

THYROIDITIS			
	Obese Chicken (OS)	Buffalo Rat (BR)	Experimental Allergic Thyroiditis
Genes (gene complexes)	≥3	≥3	≥2
MHC	+	+	+
Other gene loci	Not known	—	—
Sex	—	—	—
Known environmental factors	—	—	—
Neonatal thymectomy effect	Enhanced	Enhanced	Abrogates
Organ specificities	—	—	—

Source: Modified with permission from Smith HR, and Steinberg AD: A perspective. Ann Rev Immunol 1:175–210, 1983.

GN = glomerulonephritis.

to be emphasized that the processes associated with viral infection tend to be heavily regulated by genes. For example, in the carefully studied model (largely by Frank Lilly and associates) of leukemia caused by the Friend virus, more than 12 loci influence the development of leukemia.[3]

Human Autoimmune Disease

The breeding experiments that have enabled mouse geneticists to determine the individual contribution of susceptibility genes are, of course, impossible in human autoimmune disease. Empirically, however, it has been possible to carry out studies on the frequency of MS among family members of affected index cases. The most exhaustive and systematic studies have been those carried out at the Vancouver MS Clinic,[75,76] where all consecutive, unrelated patients' index cases have detailed genetic histories documented by the clinic's geneticist A. D. Sadovnick. These family histories are updated annually. The familial rate for MS in this population approaches 20 percent (combined rate for first-, second- and third-degree relatives of index cases). The data indicate, for example, that the risk for the offspring, given an otherwise negative family history with respect to MS, may be as high as 5 percent (compared with a point prevalence of 0.1 percent and an estimated lifetime prevalence for clinical MS in Canada that approaches 1 of 500 persons, or 0.2 percent). Although this risk seems low in absolute terms, it is consistent with the predictions of a polygenic model. Details on lifetime risks for MS for various categories of relatives of patients with MS are given in Table 3–4. Table 3–5 gives age-specific risks for MS.

The Canadian family study data[16,74-76] clearly exclude simple mendelian (autosomal dominant, autosomal recessive) inheritance. Autosomal recessive inheritance, postulated by Mackay and Myrianthopoulos[53] (although nothing in their data suggested it), is readily rejected because the frequency of parent-child concordance is similar to that for siblings.[78] A recessive locus with a dominant modifier is less easily excluded. Autosomal dominant inheritance would require *extremely low* penetrance and does not explain either the altered sex ratio among affected individuals or the observed differential parent-child concordance rates.[79] X-linked recessive inheritance is completely incompatible with both the sex ratio of affected cases and with

Table 3–4. **AGE-ADJUSTED EMPIRIC RISKS FOR MS**

Relationship to Index Case	MALE INDEX CASES		FEMALE INDEX CASES	
	Proportion Affected	% Risk ± 95% Confidence Intervals	Proportion Affected	% Risk ± 95% Confidence Intervals
Mother	7/184	3.84 ± 1.42%	14/383	3.71 ± 0.97%
Father	1/128	0.79 ± 0.79%	6/303	2.00 ± 0.18%
Parents	8/312	2.56 ± 0.90%	20/686	2.95 ± 0.65%
Daughter	2/223	5.13 ± 3.53%	5/386	4.96 ± 2.17%
Son	0/248	0.00 ± 1.49%	0/411	0.00 ± 0.90%
Children	2/471	2.47 ± 1.72%	5/797	2.58 ± 1.14%
Sister	9/340	3.46 ± 1.14%	25/608	5.65 ± 1.10%
Brother	10/326	4.15 ± 1.28%	10/612	2.27 ± 0.71%
Siblings	19/666	3.81 ± 0.86%	35/1220	3.97 ± 0.66%
Aunt/uncle	15/560	2.68 ± 0.68%	23/1491	1.59 ± 0.33%
Niece/nephew	3/1000	1.47 ± 0.84%	7/1789	1.83 ± 0.69%
First cousins	7/795	1.53 ± 0.57%	34/2347	2.37 ± 0.40%

Source: From Sadovnick AD, Baird PA, and Ward RH: Multiple Sclerosis: Updated risks for relatives. Am J Med Genet 29:553–541, 1988. Reprinted by permission of Wiley-Liss, Inc. a subsidiary of John Wiley & Sons, Inc.

Table 3–5. **AGES AT WHICH MULTIPLE SCLEROSIS BIRTH (LIFETIME) RISK DECREASES (2.5% to 0.5%)**

Relationship to Index Case	% Risk at Birth (Lifetime Risk)	Age (yr) at Which Risk Decreased to 2.5%	Age (yr) at Which Risk Decreased to 1.5%	Age (yr) at Which Risk Decreased to 0.5%
Male Index Cases				
Daughter	5.13	28	33	43
Son	—	—	—	—
Sister	3.46	23	29	39
Brother	4.15	26	33	42
Niece	3.06	20	28	39
Nephew	—	—	—	—
Maternal first cousin	0.89	N/A*	N/A†	36
Female Index Cases				
Daughter	4.96	28	33	43
Son	—	—	—	—
Sister	5.65	28	33	42
Brother	2.27	N/A	25	38
Niece	2.70	17	26	37
Nephew	1.02	N/A*	N/A†	29
Maternal first cousin	1.93	N/A*	23	36
Paternal first cousin	2.89	23	30	40

Source: Sadovnick AD, Baird PA, and Ward RH: Multiple Sclerosis: Updated risks for relatives. Am J Med Genet 29:533–541, 1988. Reprinted by permission of Wiley-Liss, Inc. a subsidiary of John Wiley & Sons, Inc.
*Birth (lifetime) risk for MS is lower than 2.5%.
†Birth (lifetime) risk for MS is lower than 1.5%.

the parental concordance pattern. X-linked dominant inheritance would account for the almost 2:1 sex ratio among affected cases and the paucity of paternal concordance. However, in multiplex pedigrees, apparent concordance is no less frequent through the unaffected father than the mother; that is, paternal and maternal uncles have almost equal risks[78]. For male and female index cases, the proportion of affected paternal ($\chi^2 = 0.04$) and maternal ($\chi^2 = 0.96$) uncles does not differ significantly ($df = 1$; $P > .05$). In addition, the frequency of concordant father-daughter pairs is as expected when adjusted for the sex ratio, excluding vertical (mitochondrial or placental) transmission.

Although a Y-linked resistance gene (or genes) could be postulated to explain the altered sex ratio in the MS population, this postulation would not easily explain the observed lack of concordant father-son

pairs.[79] By selecting for fathers with MS in that study, we in fact selected for men who did not have resistance genes. Therefore, male offspring would not be expected to be resistant to MS. The recent demonstration of parental imprinting may be of some relevance. This phenomenon results from a differential degree of methylation of at least some genes, depending on which parent (mother or father) transmits the gene. Such an effect might be expected to produce different risks to offspring of affected fathers and mothers. While family data[75,76,79] show a difference in that there is a modest excess of affected offspring of mothers with MS (N = 53) compared to fathers with MS (N = 21), this effect is not as strong as the overall excess of affected daughters (N = 61) compared with affected sons (N = 14), regardless of parental sex. This finding, however, still does not account for the difference between sons and daughters of affected fathers. Parental imprinting would also have to differ by sex of offspring to explain the data. It is therefore likely for these and other reasons that the inheritance of MS susceptibility is polygenic (involving more than one locus).

Specific Susceptibility Loci

Excepting those for MHC, association studies have provided little useful information to date in understanding MS susceptibility. Many of the reported studies have been methodologically suboptimal and non-MHC loci have not been conclusively demonstrated. Nevertheless, there will continue to be a role for association data in demonstrating linkage disequilibrium once linkage has been found. This will be done by saturation of the implicated chromosomal region with flanking markers and will require the identification of polymorphisms very close to the responsible gene. Nevertheless, the coincidental co-association of mendelian genetic diseases and MS could provide a clue for gene localization. Association studies are more sensitive than linkage studies, even those having very large numbers of families. This was recently quantitated by Risch and Merikangas[72], who have raised the sobering spectre of the potential necessity for whole genome association studies.

The likelihood of finding linkage in MS will depend on (1) the number of loci involved in MS susceptibility; (2) the magnitude of their individual effects; (3) the population frequencies of high-risk alleles; (4) the relationship of genotypes at multiple loci to risk (encompassing concepts of genetic heterogeneity, epistasis, or both where genes at different loci may or may not interact in producing risk); (5) the density (map distance) of the dinucleotide (tri-tetra) repeat map (and other restriction fragment length polymorphisms, RFLPs); (6) the polymorphism information content of the markers involved; and finally (7) the number and type of multicase families available for study.

The types of multicase families and their individual value for linkage detection in complex traits have been considered in great detail by Risch.[69,70] He calculated the power and efficiency of readily accessible "pair" methods designed for several specific relationships (i.e., first cousins, half-siblings, grandparents, aunt-uncle, or niece-nephew). These considerations are most appropriate for designing a strategy in MS where by far the most common type of multicase family has but two affected individuals.

It remains to be proven that families with three or more affected siblings are the most informative for linkage studies in complex traits. It is possible that for MS, such families will consist of several individuals who are homozygous at putative dominant or semidominant susceptibility loci (i.e., decreasing the probability of parental heterozygosity), thus making such families less informative than it might appear. It is a reasonable expectation that individual susceptibility alleles in MS will be common. Index maps are being constructed for every chromosome by several laboratories. Preliminary versions of index-type maps are already available, and the average distance between highly polymorphic markers is less than a centimorgan.

Candidate Loci

Table 3–6 outlines processes and gene loci that are candidates for genetic regulation of

Table 3–6. SOME POSSIBLE LEVELS OF GENETIC CONTROL OF AUTOIMMUNITY

Disease initiation
Disease severity
T-cell regulation
T-cell receptors
MHC class I and class II
MHC expression
Vascular permeability
Macrophage presentation
Control of inflammatory mediators
Repair mechanisms

Table 3–7. **PUTATIVE GENETIC SUSCEPTIBILITY LOCI IN MULTIPLE SCLEROSIS**

Complex	Chromosome	Gene Product	Allelic Association	Confirmation	Family Study
MHC	6	Class II DR, DQ	DR2, DQW1[24]	C	D
T-cell receptor	7	*Beta chain* Vβ8 (Bam HI) Vβ11 (Bam HI) Cβ (BglII)	*Haplotype* Vβ8 23b/Vβ11 20Kb/Cβ 9Kb	NC	Increased[94] or not increased[50] haplotype sharing in siblings[1,60,83]
T-cell receptor	14	*Alpha chain* Valpha12 Calpha	6.3Kb (Pss1)[26,60] 2Kb[56]	NC[87]	No increased haplotype sharing[36,51]
Immunoglobulin variable region	14	Immunoglobulin heavy chain variable region VH2	VH2-5 3.4Kb (Bgl 11)[93]	ND	Increased VH2-5 genotype sharing in siblings[37]
Immunoglobulin constant region	14	Immunoglobulin heavy chain constant region	Gm 1-, 17-, 21-kb gamma 3 polymorphisms[28,93]	NC	D
MBP	18	Myelin basic protein		C-NC	Increased haplotype sharing;[6,90] no increased haplotype sharing[32]
Complement	19	Third component of complement	C3F7	NC	ND
Alpha-1 antitrypsin	14	Alpha-1	M allele[55]	C-NC	ND

Source: Adapted from Ebers GC, and Sadovnick AD: The role of genetic factors in multiple sclerosis susceptibility: A critical review. J Neuroimmunol 54:117–122, 1994, with kind permission of Elswier Science-NL, Sara Burgerhart-Straat 25, 1055 KV Amsterdam, The Netherlands.
C = confirmed; D = done; NC = not confirmed; ND = not done.

MS susceptibility. Existing genetic data in MS are summarized in Table 3–7.

MAJOR HISTOCOMPATIBILITY COMPLEX

The role of MHC in MS susceptibility has been recently reviewed in detail by Olerup and Hillert.[61] Despite highly reproducible evidence for a strong association between MS and the HLA-A3, B7, DR2/DQw1 haplotype, studies of haplotype sharing have provided modest if any evidence for linkage.

Canadian data on MHC haplotype sharing in 51 sibling pairs, in which unequivocal haplotypes were derived by typing parents, affected siblings, and unaffected siblings were published some 15 years ago.[77] In this study, 16 individuals shared two haplotypes, 21 shared one haplotype, and 14 shared none. This does not differ from chance expectation. These results are interpreted to mean that the overall contribution of MHC to MS susceptibility is likely to be small. This can be more definitively assessed by determining the risk of MS in MHC haplo-identical siblings compared with siblings sharing no haplotypes. Further studies are warranted to more accurately define the MHC contribution. We have addressed this by examining sibling pairs in which *one* MHC haplotype is shared and, if DR2 is present, asking whether it is the haplotype shared. For 14 such pairs, in 50 percent the non-DR2 haplotype is shared, the chance expectation (G.C. Ebers, unpublished data 1985). There is weak evidence for linkage if very large numbers of affected relative pairs are used. The recent British and American genome searches [57,81] found elevated lod scores using microsatellite markers in 6p21. However since this area had been already implicated by association study it cannot be compared to the many other "anonymous" polymorphic microsatellite markers used in the genome searches to conclude that this is a "major" effect. In summary, data to date indicate that although class II MHC alleles increase the liability for MS, no specific allele (or sequence common to several alleles) has yet been identified as necessary for the development of the disease.

T-CELL RECEPTOR POLYMORPHISMS

The second part of the trimolecular complex involved in T-cell activation (MHC class II antigen, T-cell receptors) is the T-cell receptor itself, formed in part by the association of the alpha chain coded on chromosome 14 with the beta chain on chromosome 7. Accordingly, these have been considered plausible susceptibility loci for autoimmune disorders.

A number of studies have reported associations between alleles at the $V\alpha$ *(TcR)*[50,51,60] and $V\beta$ *(TcR)* loci.[1,83] However, most recent work concludes that it is unlikely that germline polymorphism in the *TcRBV* locus makes a major contribution to MS susceptibility.[36,94]

IMMUNOGLOBULIN VARIABLE REGION

V-region genes for immunoglobulins are responsible for antibody specificity, and accordingly represent candidate loci for MS susceptibility. Some evidence exists for the use of specific *V* genes in the production of autoantibodies.[93] An association has been reported between a VH2–5 polymorphism and MS. We have recently examined haplotype sharing in affected sibling pairs and have found no alteration from that expected.[37] This should be confirmed in another population, but if the *V* region plays a role in MS susceptibility, the effect appears to be weak.

IMMUNOGLOBULIN CONSTANT REGION

An association between MS and alleles at several immunoglobulin constant region loci has not been clearly demonstrated.[93] An association was suggested between MS and Gm allotypes, coded on chromosome 14,[68] but again, this has not been confirmed on either a population or family level.[8,24] This highly polymorphic family of loci is located in the constant region of the human immunoglobulin complex and shows considerable ethnic variation. These studies have illustrated one of the major problems in identifying population associations with human disease. Because the frequency of the Gm allotype alleles is highly ethnic specific, it is imperative in comparing MS cases to control cases that they be matched for racial and ethnic background.

The use of DNA polymorphisms has supplanted Gm typing. One study using constant region DNA probes that showed an association with MS employed the extraordinary design of comparing patients from one continent with control subjects from another.[27]

TUMOR NECROSIS FACTOR-α

Considerable accumulated evidence supports a role for tumor necrosis factor-α (TNF-α) in the pathogenesis of the MS lesion. Although the evidence is circumstantial, it has been demonstrated that TNF-α is present in MS lesions pathologically.[40,84] T-cell clones from the CSF of patients with MS have been found to produce more interferon gamma and TNF-α than control T-cell clones. More recently, Sharief and colleagues[86] found increased levels of TNF in both serum and CSF, and found that these correlate with disease activity and with other evidence of blood-brain barrier disturbance. These studies have been extended to demonstrate that TNF-α levels correlate with disease progression and severity.[84,85] Hauser and associates[38] found elevated levels of both TNF and interleukin-1 (IL-1), with the latter being more elevated. Some earlier work did not demonstrate TNF-α, but this could have been due to methodological problems.[23]

Little information is available on the role of TNF polymorphism as it might relate to genetic susceptibility. One study using a relatively uninformative RFLP, examined allele distribution in patients with MS and control subjects and found no difference.[26] Recently, a number of highly polymorphic markers have become available for this locus. These have taken the form of dinucleotide repeat polymorphisms. Three of these are microsatellite markers, two of which are 3.5 kb upstream of the *TNF*β gene and have 13 and 7 alleles, respectively. Size variants at *TNF* microsatellite loci in

the mouse have clear functional (level of secretion) correlates.[41] Furthermore, recent data have indicated that one of the alleles at the 13-allele human microsatellite locus (*TNF*β) (*A*2) is strongly associated with hypersecretion of TNF-α in response to standard stimuli (J. Todd et al., personal communication, 1993). This functional correlation with polymorphism makes this locus a candidate region for MS susceptibility at the germ-line level. Furthermore, it may also be a candidate for influencing the severity of the disease and its progression.

MYELIN BASIC PROTEIN

Autoimmunity to MBP has been considered a factor in MS pathogenesis based on studies of experimental allergic encephalomyelitis (EAE). A number of studies have suggested that patients with MS have abnormal immunity to MBP. Studies using single-cell T-cell assays have demonstrated high frequencies of T cells specifically reactive with MBP in peripheral blood and in the spinal fluid of patients with MS.[63] Evidence exists that humoral immunity to MBP is also present both in serum and CSF, as reviewed by Olsson.[62] Accordingly, MBP as the major protein component of myelin and the best studied precipitant of EAE has been a candidate gene for MS susceptibility.

The MBP gene is located on the long arm of chromosome 18, and a high degree of polymorphism has been identified in repetitive DNA sequences 1.5 kb 5' to the first exon of this gene.[6] An association has been demonstrated in patients with MS compared with control subjects with other neurological disorders characterized by alleles in the "2.14 to 2.15-kb range" at this locus.[5] Family studies using this polymorphism not only have indicated confirmation of the association but also have provided evidence for linkage at this locus using a polymerase chain reaction-based allele system.[90] We have recalculated the lod scores for these studies and find them to be considerably less than reported. Furthermore, we find no association in the pedigrees if "married-ins" are used as control subjects (G.C. Ebers and N. Risch, 1993). Re-evaluation of this locus using a highly informative tandem tetranucleotide repeat polymorphism has resulted in the finding that MS susceptibility is not linked to the MBP gene.[32,73,95]

NRAMP 1 LOCUS

The importance of this locus in determining susceptibility to a wide variety of intracellular mycobacteria and other pathogens has been demonstrated.[54,87] The *NRAMP 1 LOCUS* gene directly regulates the process of T-cell independent macrophage activation for antimycobacterial function and indirectly regulates the magnitude and quality of specific immune responses to mycobacterial antigens. Its possible role in autoimmune disease has had little study, but recent findings in the NOD mouse indicate that this locus may be a major susceptibility gene that influences the degree of severity of diabetes in this murine autoimmune model.[12]

COMPLEMENT LOCI

The association of complement alleles at the *C2, C3,* and *C4* loci has been studied, but results have not found either a primary association *(C3)* or a secondary association *(C2* and *C4)* attributable to the primary association with DR2.[7]

GENETIC CONTRIBUTION TO MULTIPLE SCLEROSIS: IS IT RESOLVABLE?

The conclusion that MS susceptibility is determined by polygenes must remain tentative until specific loci are identified. However, consideration of possible models of susceptibility may be more than a sterile exercise. It has an important bearing on how the problem is to be approached, particularly with respect to the type of family data that are likely to be most informative.

In no polygenic disorder, including spontaneous animal models of autoimmunity, is the genetic control fully (or even largely) understood. Nevertheless, the scientific problem has considerable allure, not only as a novel avenue of exploration but also because susceptibility to many of the major causes of human mortality and morbidity is, in fact, determined by polygenes. This category of disorders would appear to include atherosclerosis, hypertension, and diabetes, among others. Nevertheless, formidable obstacles could exist to understanding genetic susceptibility in disorders where polygenic control is suspected. Even for single-gene disorders, a number of independent influences on phenotype are known, such as epistatic interactions, parental imprinting, and genetic heterogeneity. A priori genetic heterogeneity or better termed, genetic complexity, should be proportional to the number of operative loci and is to be anticipated in a condition as complex as MS. Although clinical or demographic heterogeneity between familial and sporadic cases, with the possible exception of sex ratio, has not yet been found, this by no means excludes heterogeneity. It is reasonable and warranted to exclude a single major dominant or recessive influence as a first step.

Individual Loci

Because single-gene disorders are the most familiar to the majority of clinicians, we are accustomed to thinking in terms of the presence or absence of a disease phenotype being absolutely dependent on an allele at a particular locus. Nevertheless, some loci are highly polymorphic, and a more complex relationship may exist. This phenomenon may be true for the role of MHC in MS where, despite two decades of study, its role is still incompletely understood. Given the high concentration of different loci within this complex that control immune responsiveness, at least two levels of complexity seem plausible. First, more than one locus in MHC could influence susceptibility. Second, individual class II alleles may influence susceptibility in a type of hierarchy, such that more than alleles may be graded from susceptibility to neutral to resistant.

Interaction of Loci

Possibly the action or effect of individual loci may be altered or nullified by yet other loci. Several orders of interaction are possible, making one observer suggest that the entire human genome could be sequenced, and we could still be no wiser (D. Weatherall, personal communication, 1987). Potential interactions may need to be specifically and systematically sought. Similarly, it is possible that susceptibility for some disorders reflects the additive effects of a number of loci, none of which is individually necessary or sufficient.

Table 3–8. **STUDIES SEARCHING FOR MULTIPLE SCLEROSIS GENES CHROMOSOMAL REGIONS SHOWING POSITIVE RESULTS (MLS>0.5)**[*†]

GENOME SCREENS			STUDY OF EAE LOCI
AMERICAN[38]	BRITISH[81]	CANADIAN[17]	FINNISH[45]
	1p36-p33 1p21	1p36-p33	
2p23	2p23-p21	2p23-p21 2q33-q36	
		3p25	
	3p14-p13	3p14-p13	
3q22-q24		3q22-q24	
		3q26	
4q31-qter	4q31-qter		
5p15			5p14-p12
5q13-q23	5q12-q13	5q12-q13	
6p21	6p21	6p21	
6q27	6q22-q27		
	7p15		
7q11-q22		7q21-q22	
7q32-q34			
9pter-p22			
9q34.3			
10q21-q22		10q24-q26	
		11q14-q22	
	12p13-p12		
12q23-qter			
13q33-q34			
	14q32		
16p13-cen			
	17pter-q11 17q22		
		18pter	
18p11		18p11	
		18q21.2	
19q13	19q12-q13	19q13	
	22q12.3-q13		
		Xp22.1-p21	
	Xcen-q27		

[*]MLS range between ~0.5 and ~3
[†]Positive scores found in at least 1 dataset studied; these were not always reproduced in all datasets.

Prognosis Genes Versus Susceptibility Genes

Because subclinical forms of MS exist and may be common, the presence of genes that serve to lower detection threshold (symptoms and disability) could be manifested by population associations for such a locus in the absence of an effect on susceptibility. This is one possible, although unattractive, explanation for the finding of an association at a population level with no linkage in families.

Preliminary Genome Search Results

The lack of success of the candidate gene approach and the development of technology that allows for rapid, large-scale genotyping using highly informative PCR-based polymorphisms has led several groups studying complex traits to collect large numbers of families and "screen" the genome. Table 3–8 gives results from three screens and one candidate region recently published. These regions must all be regarded as tentative and will be the subject of much activity in the near future.

SUMMARY

The degree of complexity of genetic control in MS may be large and not easily defined. In some models, the understanding of susceptibility would be intractable because of the complexities of interactions and heterogeneity.

Three recent major advances now make possible a focused effort to advance our understanding of MS in a significant way:
- The collection of large numbers of MS patients and families in several countries that provide a suitably large data base of well-documented and compliant patients.
- The development of statistical methods to explore inheritance in complex disorders efficiently.
- The ongoing construction of a human linkage map based on highly informative markers. These now carry sufficient power to localize genes exerting even small effects, provided that the pool of families with several affected members ("multicase families") is sufficiently large.

REFERENCES

1. Beall SS, Concannon P, Charmley P, et al: The germline repertoire of T cell receptor β chain genes in patients with chronic progressive multiple sclerosis. J Neuroimmunol 21:59–66, 1989.
2. Bernard CC: Experimental autoimmune encephalomyelitis in mice: Genetic control of susceptibility. Journal of Immunogenetics 3:263–274, 1976.
3. Blank KJ, and Klyczek KK: Host genetic control of retrovirus-induced leukemogenesis in the mouse. J Leuko Biol 140:479–490, 1986.
4. Bobowick AR, Kurtzke JF, Brody JA, Hrubec Z, and Gillespie M: Twin study of multiple sclerosis: An epidemiologic inquiry. Neurology 28: 978–987, 1978.
5. Boylan KB, Aryes TM, Popko B, Takahashi N, Hood LE, and Prusiner SB: Repetitive DNA (TGGA)n5' to the human myelin basic protein gene: A new form of oligonucleotide repetitive sequence showing length polymorphism. Genomics 6:16–22, 1990B.
6. Boylan KB, Takahashi N, Paty DW, et al: DNA length polymorphism 5' to the myelin basic protein gene is associated with multiple sclerosis. Ann Neurol 27:291–297, 1990.
7. Bulman DE, Armstrong H, and Ebers GC: Allele frequencies of the third component of complement (C3) in MS patients. J Neurol Neurosurg Psychiatry 54:554–555, 1991.
8. Bulman DE, Pandey JP, and Ebers GC: Gm allotypes in multiple sclerosis. In Lowenthal A, and Raus J (eds): Components of Cerebrospinal Fluid in Multiple Sclerosis. Plenum, New York, 1992, pp 81–86.
9. Bulman DE, Sadovnick AD, Cripps J, and Ebers GC: Age of onset in siblings concordant for multiple sclerosis. Brain 114:937–950, 1991.
10. Compston DA: Multiple sclerosis in the Orkneys. Lancet 2:98, 1981.
11. Compston DA, Vakarelis BM, Paul E, McDonald WI, Batchelor JR, and Mims CA: Viral infection in patients with multiple sclerosis and HLA DR matched controls. Brain 109:325–344, 1986.
12. Cornall RJ, Rins BS, Todd JA, et al: Type 1 diabetes in mice is linked to the interleukin-1 receptor and Lsh/Ity/Bcg genes on chromosome 1. Nature 353:262–265, 1991.
13. Davenport CB: Multiple sclerosis from the standpoint of geographic distribution and race. Arch Neurol 8:51–58, 1922.
14. Detels R, Visscher BR, Malmgren RM, Coulson AH, Lucia MV, and Dudley JP: Evidence for lower susceptibility to multiple sclerosis in Japanese Americans. Am J Epidemiol 105:303– 310, 1977.

15. Ebers GC, Kukay K, Bulman DE, et al. A full genome search in multiple sclerosis. Nature Genetics 13:472–476, 1996.

16. Ebers GC: Genetic factors in multiple sclerosis. Neurol Clin 1:645–654, 1983.

17. Ebers GC, Bulman DE, Sadovnick AD, et al: A population-based twin study in multiple sclerosis. N Engl J Med 315:1638–1642, 1986.

18. Ebers GC, and Sadovnick AD: The role of genetic factors in multiple sclerosis susceptibility: A critical review. J Neuroimmunol 54:117–122, 1994.

19. Ebers GC, Sadovnick AD, Risch NJ. A genetic basis for familial aggregation in multiple sclerosis. Nature (1995) 377:150–151.

20. Eichhorst H: Cited by Schapira. Virchows Arch 146:173–192, 1963.

21. Enstrom JE, and Operskalski EA: Multiple sclerosis among Spanish-surnamed Californians. Neurology 28:434–438, 1978.

22. Finelli PF: Conjugal multiple sclerosis: A clinical and laboratory study. Neurology 41:1320–1321, 1991.

23. Franciotti DM, Grimaldi LM, and Martino GV: Tumor necrosis factor in serum and cerebrospinal fluid of patients with multiple sclerosis. Ann Neurol 26:1989.

24. Francis D, Brazier DM, Batchelor JR, McDonald WI, Downie AW, and Hern JE: Gm allotypes in multiple sclerosis influence susceptibility in HLA-DQw1-positive patients from the North-East of Scotland. Immunology and Immunopathology 41:409–416, 1986.

25. French Research Group on Multiple Sclerosis: Multiple sclerosis in 54 twinships: Concordance rate is independent of zygosity. Ann Neurol 32:724–727, 1992.

26. Fugger LM, Morling N, Sandberg-Wollheim M, Ryder LP, and Svejgaard A: Tumour necrosis factor α gene polymorphism in multiple sclerosis and optic neuritis. J Neuroimmunol 27:85–88, 1990A.

27. Gaiser CA, Johnson MJ, DeLange G, Rassenti L, Cavalli-Sforza LL, and Steinman L: Susceptibility to multiple sclerosis associated with immunoglobulin gamma 3 restriction fragment length polymorphism. Clin Invest 79:309–313, 1987.

28. Garchon HJ, Bedossa P, Eloy L, and Bach JF: Identification and mapping to chromosome 1 of a susceptibility locus for periinsulitis in nonobese diabetic mice. Nature 353:260–262, 1991.

29. Gaudet JPC, Hashimoto L, Sadovnick AD, and Ebers GC: A study of birth disorder and multiple sclerosis in multiple families. Neuroepidemiology 14:188–192, 1995.

30. Ghosh S, Palmer SM, Rodriques NR, et al: Polygenic control of autoimmune diabetes in nonobese diabetic mice. Nat Genet 4:404–409, 1993.

31. Gilbert JJ, and Sadler M: Unsuspected multiple sclerosis. Arch Neurol 40:533–536, 1983.

32. Graham CA, Kirk CW, Nevin NC, et al: Lack of association between myelin basic protein gene microsatellite and multiple sclerosis. Lancet 341:1596, 1993.

33. Gronning M, and Mellgren SI: Multiple sclerosis in the two northernmost counties of Norway. Acta Neurol Scand 72:321–327, 1985.

34. Grufferman S, Barton JW, and Eby NL: Increased sex concordance of sibling pairs with Behcet's disease, Hodgkin's disease, multiple sclerosis and sarcoidosis. Am J Epidemiol 126:365–369, 1987.

35. Hader WJ, Feasby TE, Noseworthy JH, Rice GP, and Ebers GC: Multiple sclerosis in Canadian Native People. Neurology 35:300, 1985.

36. Hashimoto LL: T-cell receptor α chain polymorphism in multiple sclerosis. J Immunol 40:41–48, 1992.

37. Hashimoto LL, Walter MW, Cox DW, and Ebers GC: Immunoglobulin variable region polymorphisms and multiple sclerosis. J Neuroimmunol 44:77-79, 1993.

38. Hauser SL, Doolittle TH, Lincoln R, Brown RH, and Dinarello CA: Cytokine accumulations in CSF of multiple sclerosis patients: frequent detection of interleukin-1 and tumor necrosis factor but not interleukin-6. Neurology 40:1735–1739, 1990.

39. Heltberg A, and Holm NV: Concordance in twins and recurrence in sibships in multiple sclerosis. Lancet 1:1068, 1982.

40. Hofman FM, Hinton DR, Johnson K: Tumor necrosis factor identified in multiple sclerosis brain. J Exp Med 170:607–612, 1989.

41. Jacob CO, and Hwang F: Definition of microsatellite size variants for Tnfa and Hsp70 in autoimmune mouse strains. Immunogenetics 36:182–188, 1989.

42. Jersild C, Svejgaard A, and Fog T: HLA antigens and multiple sclerosis. Lancet 1:1972.

43. Kaufman MD: Conjugal multiple sclerosis. Neurology 42:1644–1645, 1992.

44. Kinnunen E, Juntunen J, Ketonen L, et al: Genetic susceptibility to multiple sclerosis: A co-twin study of a nation-wide series. Arch Neurol 45:1108–1111, 1988.

45. Kuokkanen S, Sundull M, Terwilliger JD et al: A putative vulnerability locus to multiple sclerosis maps to 5p 12-14 in a region syntenic to the murine locus EAE 2. Nature Genetics 13:477–480, 1996.

46. Kurtzke JF, Beebe GW, and Norman JE: Epidemiology of multiple sclerosis in U.S. veterans. I. Race, sex and geographic distribution. Neurology 29:1228–1235, 1979.

47. Leiter EH, Serreze DV, and Prochazka M: The genetics and epidemiology of diabetes in NOD mice. Immunol Today 11:147–149, 1990.

48. Little CC: A possible Mendelian explanation for a type of inheritance apparently non-Mendelian in nature. Science 40:904–906, 1917.

49. Livingstone A, Edwards CT, Shizura JA, and Fathman CG: Genetic analysis of diabetes in the nonobese diabetic mouse. I. MHC and T cell receptor B Gene expression. J Immunol 146:529–534, 1991.

50. Lynch SG, Rose JW, Petajan JH, Stauffer D, Kamerath C, and Leppert M: Discordance of T-cell receptor α chain gene in familial multiple sclerosis. Annals of Neurology 30:402–410, 1991.

51. Lynch SG, Rose JW, Petajan JH, Stauffer D, Kamerath C, and Leppert M: Discordance of T-cell receptor α chain gene in familial multiple sclerosis. Neurology 42:839–844, 1992.

52. Lynch SG, Rose JW, Smoker W, and Petajan JH: MRI in familial multiple sclerosis. Neurology 40:900–903, 1990.

53. Mackay RP, and Myrianthopoulos NC: Multiple sclerosis in twins and their relatives. Final report. Archives of Neurology and Psychiatry 15:449–462, 1966.

54. Malo D, Schurr E, Epstein DJ, Vekemans M, Skameme E, and Gros P: The host resistance locus BcG is tightly linked to a group of cytoskeleton-associated protein genes that include villin and desmin. Genomics 10:356–364, 1991.

55. McCombe PA, Clark P, Frith JA, et al: α-1-antitrypsin phenotypes in demyelinating disease: An association between demyelinating disease and the allele PiM3. Ann Neurol 18:1985.

56. Miyazaki T, Uno M, Uehira M, et al: Direct evidence for the contribution of the unique 1-ANOD to the development of insulitis in nonobese diabetic mice. Nature 345:722–729, 1990.

57. The Multiple Sclerosis Genetics Group: A complete genome screen for multiple sclerosis underscores a role for the major histocompatibility complex. Nature Genetics 13:469–471, 1996.

58. Mumford CJ, Wood NW, Kellar-Wood H, Thorpe J, Miller D, and Compston DAS: The British Isles survey of multiple sclerosis in twins. Neurology 44:11–15, 1994.

59. Nuwer MR, Visscher BR, Packwood JW, and Namerow NS: Evoked potential testing in relatives of multiple sclerosis patients. Ann Neurol 18:30–34, 1985.

60. Oksenberg JR, Sherritt M, Begovich AB, et al: T-cell receptor V α and C α alleles associated with multiple sclerosis and myasthenia gravis. Proc Natl Acad Sci USA 86:988–992, 1989.

61. Olerup O, and Hillert J: HLA Class II-associated genetic susceptability in multiple sclerosis: A critical evaluation. Tissue Antigens 38:1–15, 1991.

62. Olsson T: The immunology of MS. Current Opinion Neurology and Neurosurgery 5:195–202, 1993.

63. Olsson T, Sun J, Hillert J, Hojeberg B, and Ekre HP: Increased numbers of T cells recognizing multiple myelin basic protein epitopes in multiple sclerosis. Eur J Immunol 22:1083–1087, 1992.

64. Popov VS: Clinical picture and epidemiology of disseminated sclerosis. Zhurnal Neuropatologii I Psikhiatrii 83:1330–1334, 1983.

65. Poskanzer DC, Terasaki PI, Prenney LB, Sheridan JL, and Parks MS: Multiple sclerosis in the Orkney and Shetland Islands. III. Histocompatibility determinants. J Epidemiol Community Health 43: 253–257, 1980.

66. Pratt RT, Compston ND, and McAlpine D: The familial incidence of multiple sclerosis and its significance. Brain 74:191–232, 1951.

67. Prochazka M, Leiter EH, Serreze DV, and Coleman DR: Three recessive loci required for insulin-dependent diabetes in nonobese diabetic mice. Science 237:286–289, 1987.

68. Propert DW, Bernard CC, and Simons MJ: Gm allotypes and multiple sclerosis. J Immunogenetics 9:359–361, 1982.

69. Risch N: Linkage strategies for genetically complex traits. I. Multilocus models. Am J Human Genet 46:222–228, 1990.

70. Risch N: Linkage strategies for genetically complex traits. II. The power of affected relative pairs. Am J Human Genet 46:229–241, 1990.

71. Risch N, Ghosh S, and Todd JA: Statistical evaluation of multiple-locus linkage data in experimental species and its relevance to human studies: Application to nonobese diabetic (NOD) mouse and human insulin-dependent diabetes (IDDM). Am J Hum Genet 53:702–714, 1993.

72. Risch and Merikangas K: The future of genetic studies of complex human disease Science 273:1516–1517, 1996.

73. Rose J, Gerken S, Lynch S, et al: Genetic susceptibility in familial multiple sclerosis not linked to the myelin basic protein gene. Lancet 341:1179– 1181, 1993.

74. Sadovnick AD, Armstrong H, Rice GPA, et al: A population based twin study of multiple sclerosis in twins: Update. Ann Neurol 33:281–285, 1993.

75. Sadovnick AD, and Baird PA: The familial nature of multiple sclerosis: Age-corrected empiric recurrence risks of children and siblings of patients. Neurology 38:990–991, 1988.

76. Sadovnick AD, Baird PA, and Ward RH: Multiple Sclerosis: Updated risks for relatives. Am J Med Genet 29:533–541, 1988.

77. Sadovnick AD, Bulman DE, D'Hooghe MB, and Ebers GC: The influence of gender on the susceptibility to multiple sclerosis in sibships. Arch Neurol 48:586–588, 1991.

78. Sadovnick AD, Bulman DE, Ebers GC: Parent-child concordance in multiple sclerosis. Ann Neurol 29: 252–255, 1991.

79. Sadovnick AD, and Ebers GC: Epidemiology of multiple sclerosis: A critical overview. Can J Neurol Sci 20:17–29, 1993.

80. Sadovnick AD, Ebers GC, Dyment D, Risch N and the Canadian Collaborative Study Group. Evidence for the genetic basis of multiple sclerosis. The Lancet 347:1728–1730, 1996.

81. Sawcer S, Jones HB, Feakes R et al: A genome screen in multiple sclerosis reveals susceptibility loci on chromosome 6 pg. 21 and 17g22. Nature Genetics 13: 464–468, 1996.

82. Schapira K, Poskanzer DC, and Millar H: Familial and conjugal multiple sclerosis. Brain 86:315–332, 1963.

83. Seboun E, Robinson MA, Doolittle TH, Ciulla TA, Kindt TJ, and Hauser SL: A susceptibility locus for multiple sclerosis is linked to the T cell receptor β chain complex. Cell 57:1095–1100, 1989.

84. Selmaj K, Raine CS, Cannella B, and Brosnan CF: Identification of lymphotoxin and tumor necrosis factor in multiple sclerosis lesions. J Clin Invest 87:949–954, 1991.

85. Sharief MK, and Hentges R: Association between tumor necrosis factor-α and disease progression in patients with multiple sclerosis. N Engl J Med 326:272–273, 1992.

86. Sharief MK, and Thompson EJ: In vivo relationship of tumor necrosis factor β to blood-brain barrier damage in patients with active multiple sclerosis. J Neuroimmunol 38:27–33, 1992.

87. Skamene E: Genetic control of susceptibility to mycobacterial infections. Rev Infect Dis 11 (suppl 2):393–399, 1989.

88. Skegg DC, Corwin PA, Craven RS, Malloch JA, and Pollock M: Occurrence of multiple sclerosis in the

north and south of New Zealand. J Neurol Neurosurg Psychiatry 50:134–139, 1987.

89. Smith HR, and Steinberg AD: Autoimmunity: A perspective review. Annu Rev Immunol 1:175–210, 1983.

90. Tienari PJ, Wikstrom J, Sajantila A, Palo J, and Peltonen L: Genetic susceptibility to multiple sclerosis is linked to the myelin basic protein gene. Lancet 340:987–991, 1992.

91. Todd JA, Bell JI, and McDevitt HO: A molecular basis for genetic susceptibility to insulin dependent diabetes mellitus. Trends in Genetics 4:129–134, 1988.

92. Vogel F, and Motulsky AG: Human Genetics. Problems and Approaches. Springer-Verlag, Berlin and Heidelberg, 1979, pp 173–186.

93. Walter MW, Gibson WT, Ebers GC, and Cox DW: Susceptibility to multiple sclerosis is associated with the proximal immunoglobulin heavy chain variable region. J Clin Invest 87:1266–1273, 1991.

94. Wei S, Charmley P, Birchfield RJ, and Concannon P: Human T-cell receptor Vβ gene polymorphism and multiple sclerosis. Am J Hum Genet 56:963–969, 1995.

95. Xian-hao X, and McFarlin DE: Oligoclonal bands in CSF: Twins with MS. Neurology 34:769–774, 1984.

96. Wood NW, Holmans P, Clayton D, Robertson N, Compston DAS. No linkage or association between multiple sclerosis and the myelin basic protein gene in affected sibling pairs. J Neurol Neurosurg Psychiat 57:1191–1194, 1994.

CHAPTER 4

DIAGNOSIS OF MULTIPLE SCLEROSIS

Donald W. Paty, MD
John H. Noseworthy, MD
George C. Ebers, MD

Only recently has a high degree of clinical accuracy been achieved in the diagnosis of MS. This development is the result of several factors, including advances in neurological education, imaging, and laboratory testing. Nevertheless, in the absence of an unequivocal diagnostic test, MS remains a clinical diagnosis. In many instances, the combination of fluctuating or persistent sensory or visual symptoms, ataxia, and/or bladder disturbances suggests MS even to the neurologically inexperienced physician. Often, however, the typical clinical profile is not seen, and confirmation of the diagnosis of MS rests on the judgment of an experienced neurologist. The application of strict criteria for diagnosis has important implications for prognosis and treatment as well as for clinical research. Experience shows that once the diagnosis has been made, or even suggested, by a competent neurologist, medical inquisitiveness and imagination may be curtailed. More important, because deterioration of neurological function is often expected and accepted unquestioningly, it is necessary to be as certain as possible in making a clinical diagnosis of MS.

A major factor in arriving at an accurate diagnosis is care in taking the history. To develop an accurate temporal profile of the illness, the clinician must be careful in identifying the dates of onset, the rate of progression or diminution of intensity of symptoms, the waxing and waning of other associated symptoms, and the duration of remission. Questions should be asked about common MS symptoms, and specifically about Lhermitte's symptom[234] and other paroxysmal symptoms, because these symptoms may not be volunteered. Reviewing previous medical records for *reliable* evidence of neurological symptoms or findings that may have been forgotten also may prove beneficial. Such evidence can often help in dating disease onset. Because disease duration may have an impact on prognosis, it is important to be *precise* about the date and character of previous symptoms (see Chapters 5 and 6).

PATIENT CHARACTERISTICS

Multiple sclerosis is largely a disease of young adults with the mean age of onset about 30 years. It is unusual for symptoms to begin before the age of 15 years or after 50 years (see Diagnostic Criteria following). The peak age of onset is from 23 to 24 years (Fig. 4–1). Studies from Great Britain, North America, Australia, northern Europe, southern Europe, and other areas show a remarkable consistency in age of onset. MS tends to affect females more than males at a ratio of almost 2:1.[92,94,124] The age of onset for females is slightly younger than that for males (see Fig. 4–1).

Most patients younger than 40 years old begin with subacute attacks of neurological dysfunction that tend to remit spontaneously. Subsequent relapses then occur with variable frequency, and eventually most of these patients develop permanent neurological impairment (see Chapter 6). In MS that occurs after age 50, relapsing-remitting disease is less common, and chronic progressive spinal cord disease is the more common presentation.[443] Many older patients, because of the monosymptomatic nature of their disease, pose diagnostic problems. Also, because evoked potentials (EPs) and imaging abnormalities become less specific and reliable with age, investigation usually must be more extensive. In our experience, the age at onset of patients who are diagnosed as laboratory-supported definite MS (LSDMS)[338] peaks at age 37 years (Fig. 4–2), reflecting diagnostic problems in older patients. Paraclinical tests such as EPs, computed tomography (CT) and magnetic resonance imaging (MRI) scanning, and cerebrospinal fluid (CSF) analysis for immunoglobulins or oligoclonal banding (OB) are helpful in

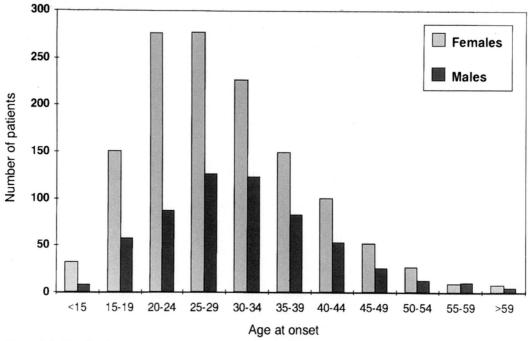

Figure 4–1. The distribution of age at onset against frequency for males and females. Note that the peak age at onset for females is in the early 20s. The peak age of onset for males is in the late 20s. (Data for Figures 4–1 and 4–2 from the MS-COSTAR computerized medical record at the University of British Columbia Multiple Sclerosis Clinic.)

older patients. However, patients who convert from LSDMS to clinically definite MS (CDMS) by developing clinical evidence for dissemination in space are usually in the same age range as typical CDMS patients.[375]

Childhood MS is not very different from adult MS in presentation.[169,421a] Duquette and his colleagues[93] have described the clinical features of childhood MS in a sample of 123 Canadian children. Symptoms tend to be more acute in onset with more rapid recovery after exacerbations. Progressive disease from onset is infrequent. The female-to-male ratio is 3:1. Acute disseminated encephalomyelitis (ADEM) is more common in children; therefore, it is an important part of the differential diagnosis. Olcay and colleagues[310] reported a case of MS at age 6 years. The earliest reported age of onset with autopsy confirmation is 10 months. MRI has been found to be helpful in the diagnosis of MS in childhood and adolescence.[59,149,314]

People of northern European extraction are more susceptible to MS than are other racial groups[100] (see Chapter 2). MS

in blacks living in Africa has been reported.[85,261] Accordingly, the prototype patient is a 24-year-old woman of northern European extraction with symptoms of posterior column involvement (often ascending in hands or feet and trunk) evolving over a few days, followed by a remission in 4 to 6 weeks. Human leukocyte antigens influence risk.[91,251]

Surveys of families with MS have shown some asymptomatic family members to have abnormal MRI scans.[249,413] Multiple cases of MS also occur in some families,[367] sometimes resulting in pseudo-clusters being reported from small communities (H. Millar, personal communication, 1990).

Although a relapsing-remitting course is characteristic of the disease (followed by chronic progressive deterioration), 15 to 30 percent of cases, mostly in the older age group, are chronic progressive from the onset. Minderhoud[281] has proposed that MS could be due to two different mechanisms. The first mechanism, possibly an inflammatory one, could account for relapses, and a second mechanism, such

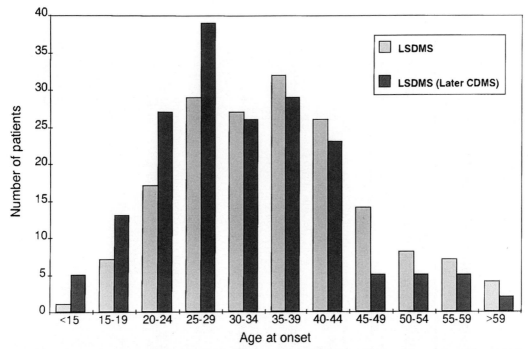

Figure 4–2. The age at onset distribution of all laboratory-supported definite MS (LSDMS) patients and LSDMS patients who converted to clinically definite MS (CDMS). Note that the total cohort of LSDMS patients peaks in onset in the mid-30s. However, if you look only at patients with LSDMS who later convert to CDMS (e.g., by having had a second clinical event), the age distribution becomes exactly the same as in patients who present as CDMS in the first instance. The skew of the curve for all LSDMS toward an older age is due to the inclusion of many patients with chronic progressive myelopathy who satisfy the criteria for LSDMS but may never satisfy the criteria for CDMS.

as axonal loss, could explain chronic disability.

DIAGNOSTIC CRITERIA

Criteria have been drawn up to help ensure some uniformity in diagnosis for clinical research studies. These criteria have lost some of their relevance with the advent of imaging and CSF studies. Incorrect diagnoses continue to be made but can be avoided if the appropriate diagnostic criteria are applied. A review of the approach to the diagnosis of MS has recently appeared.[32]

Table 4–1 summarizes the most frequently used diagnostic classifications and criteria.[210] In North America, the Schumacher criteria[375] have achieved the widest use. These criteria clearly define CDMS. Lesser degrees of certainty can be designated as "probable" or "possible" MS, although the usefulness of these two categories is not immediately apparent today.

When the criteria CDMS cannot be satisfied, perhaps a single category of "suspected" MS should be identified.

All diagnostic criteria require the demonstration of white matter lesions of the central nervous system (CNS), which are disseminated in both time and space. To paraphrase Schumacher's criteria:

I. There should be clinical evidence for lesions that reflect primarily white matter dysfunction disseminated in time and space in a patient in the expected age range (10 to 50 years).

II. There must be objective abnormalities on the neurological examination, preferably but not exclusively demonstrated at the time of making the diagnosis.

III. The dissemination of lesions in time must fit into one of the following patterns:

A. At least two clear-cut episodes of functionally significant symptoms, each lasting over 24 hours and

Table 4–1. CRITERIA FOR VARIOUS CLINICAL DIAGNOSTIC CLASSIFICATIONS SUGGESTED FOR MULTIPLE SCLEROSIS

Allison and Millar[9]	McAlpine, Lumsden, and Acheson[262]	Schumacher et al.[375]	McDonald and Halliday[265]	Rose et al.[360]
CERTAIN: PATHOLOGICAL PROOF			PROVEN: PATHOLOGICAL PROOF	
Probable MS	*Definite MS*	*Clinically Definite MS*	*Clinically Definite MS*	*Clinically Definite MS*
Some physical disability; usually remitting and relapsing; signs of multiple lesions	Remitting and relapsing; ≥2 episodes; signs of multiple lesions	Remitting and relapsing; ≥2 episodes, 1 mo apart or steadily progressive ≥6 mo; signs of lesions at two or more sites; lesions predominantly of white matter; age at onset 10 to 50 years; no better explanation	Some physical disability; remitting and relapsing; ≥2 episodes; signs of lesions at two or more sites; lesions predominantly of white matter; age at onset 10 to 50 years; no better explanation	Remitting and relapsing; ≥2 episodes, 1 mo apart or steadily progressive >6 mo; signs of lesions at 2 or more sites; lesions predominantly in white matter; age at onset 10 to 50 years; no better explanation
Early Probable and Latent MS	*Probable MS*		*Early Probable or Latent MS*	*Probable MS*
Slight or no disability; remitting and relapsing; ≥1 abnormal sign associated with MS; early, single episode suggestive of MS with signs of multiple lesions	Single episode suggestive of MS with signs of multiple lesions at onset; good recovery with subsequent variability in signs		Slight or no disability; remitting and relapsing; ≥1 abnormal signs associated with MS; early, single episode suggestive of MS with signs of multiple lesions	Remitting and relapsing; 1 abnormal sign associated with MS; single episode suggestive of MS with multiple lesions; good recovery; subsequent variability in symptoms and signs; no better explanation

Continued on following page

Table 4–1.—*continued*

Allison and Millar[9]	McAlpine, Lumsden, and Acheson[262]	Schumacher et al.[375]	McDonald and Halliday[265]	Rose et al.[360]
		CERTAIN: PATHOLOGICAL PROOF	PROVEN: PATHOLOGICAL PROOF	
			Progressive Probable MS Progressive history of paraplegia; ≥2 lesions; other causes excluded	
Possible MS Some physical disability; progressive history; insufficient signs of multiple lesions; other causes excluded	*Possible MS* Progressive history; insufficient signs of multiple lesions; other causes excluded			*Possible MS* Relapsing and remitting without signs or with signs insufficient to establish >1 CNS white matter lesion; no better explanation
	Similar to "probable" but with unusual features, paucity of signs, insufficient follow-up		*Progressive Possible MS* Progressive history of paraplegia; evidence of only 1 lesion; other causes excluded.	

Source: Adapted from Kelly RE,[210] pp 49–78. With kind permission of Elsevier Science—NL, Sara Burgerhartstraat 25, 1055 KV Amsterdam, The Netherlands. CNS = central nervous system.

separated by at least 1 month. Remission is not necessary.

B. Slow, progressive development of the same disseminated pattern evolving over at least 6 months.

IV. The diagnosis should be made by a competent clinician (preferably a neurologist), and there must be no better explanation for the diagnosis.

Schumacher's criteria remain the gold standard for MS diagnosis. After the advent of diagnostic tests that are reliably able to reveal asymptomatic lesions, however, Poser and his committee[338] drew up a new set of criteria that recognized paraclinical evidence for dissemination in space. Table 4–2 gives these criteria. Imaging and EP can detect asymptomatic dissemination in space, and CSF analysis can indicate that an abnormal immunologic response is present. A full discussion of the use of paraclinical studies follows later in this chapter. In essence, for research protocols, solid paraclinical evidence can be used for identification of one of the two lesions needed in order to demonstrate dissemination in space. The presence of OB can then increase the likelihood of MS to such a level as to reduce the need for demonstrating dissemination in time, satisfying the criteria for LSDMS. Poser co-edited a book on the diagnosis of MS[337] that explained many of the principles underlying the revised criteria for diagno-sis. The Poser Criteria apply equally well to children and adults[421a]

We would like to propose an additional category (see Table 4–2) for the situation in which a patient has a single clinical episode suggestive of MS and in which the MRI scan or EPs show dissemination in space. CDMS a3 could be then diagnosed if there is unequivocal new development of paraclinical evidence for dissemination in time (for example, a new significant visual evoked potential [VEP] delay or a new MRI lesion greater than 6 mm).

In spite of the caution that there be no better explanation before a diagnosis of MS is accepted, multiple sclerosis is not a "rule-out" diagnosis. In most instances, a clear-cut and positive diagnosis of MS can be made on the basis of a carefully obtained history and physical examination.

Engell[111] and Izquierdo and colleagues[192] published autopsy studies of the accuracy of diagnostic criteria. These are the only studies of which we are aware in which the accuracy of the clinical diagnosis using standard diagnostic criteria has been assessed by autopsy. Izquierdo found that the Poser and colleagues[338] criteria were the most sensitive ones early in the course of the disease. Engell reported that the diagnosis of CDMS was correct in 485 of 518 cases (94 percent), and "probable" MS was accurate in 66 percent.

Table 4–2. DIAGNOSTIC CRITERIA FOR MULTIPLE SCLEROSIS USING BOTH CLINICAL AND PARACLINICAL METHODS

Category	Subcategory	No. of Clinical Attacks	Clinical Evidence (No. of Lesions)	Paraclinical Evidence (No. of Lesions)	CSF OB
Clinically definite MS	CDMS a1	2	2	N/A	N/A
	CDMS a2	2	1	and 1 (or more)	N/A
	CDMS a3*	1	1	2†	N/A
Laboratory-supported definite MS	LSDMS b1	2	1	or 1 (or more)	+
	LSDMS b2	1	2		+
	LSDMS b3	1	1	and 1 (or more)	+

Source: Adapted from Poser CM, Paty DW, Scheinberg L, et al,[338] pp 227–231.
CDMS = clinically definite MS; CSF OB = oligoclonal banding; LSDMS = laboratory-supported definite MS; N/A = not applicable; + = present.
*Category CDMS a3 is a newly proposed category (see text).
†A diagnosis of CDMS a3 requires paraclinical evidence for dissemination in time as well as space.

Goodkin and colleagues[151] refined the diagnostic criteria for familial MS. The refined criteria emphasize the need for greater vigilance to exclude hereditary degenerative disorders.

Diagnostic criteria in the past have excluded patients older than 50 years, but unequivocal MS can certainly begin in the sixth decade or even later. In a recent report,[305] 79 patients with MS were found who presented to the neurologist after the age of 50 years. In 30 (38 percent) of those patients, previous remote neurological symptoms had occurred in the distant past but did not lead to medical assessment. The other 49 (62 percent) could remember no prior neurological episodes, and the onset of neurological symptoms was, therefore, assumed to have been after the age of 50 years. These 79 patients represented 9.4 percent of the total MS clinic population at the University of Western Ontario. Most of the patients with an older age of onset had been previously diagnosed as having something other than MS because of the low index of suspicion for MS when dealing with patients older than 50 years.[325] MS was the initial diagnosis in only 27 (34 percent) of the patients, the majority having carried the diagnosis of spondylotic myelopathy. Hooge and Redekop[181] surveyed the MS clinic population at University of British Columbia (UBC) (N = 2019 CDMS patients) and found 12 (0.6 percent) in whom neurological symptoms began after the age of 60 years. Most of their patients had a slowly progressive motor onset. Younger patients with MS are more likely to have initial sensory symptoms, whereas older patients tend to have a slow motor onset. Patients with late-onset MS also tend to be more rapidly disabled than their younger counterparts.

INITIAL SYMPTOMS CHARACTERISTIC OF MULTIPLE SCLEROSIS

Table 4–3 gives a list of initial symptoms and the frequency with which they were seen in patients attending the MS Clinic at UBC (see also Chapter 5).

Sensory Symptoms

Initially, the most common sensory symptom is the subacute onset of numbness or paresthesias in one or more limbs. Commonly, patients will awaken with abnormal sensation in the distal portion of the limb, which gradually spreads more proximally, increasing in extent and intensity. It may then extend across the lower trunk to involve the opposite leg. It usually reaches its maximum extent in 2 to 4 days and is usually funicular in distribution. Occasionally it can be radicular and, sometimes, dysesthetic. If this symptom begins in both legs, it often gradually ascends to involve the trunk. The trunk involvement may be at a different level on the two sides. Commonly, similar symptoms can begin in both arms simultaneously and may not involve the legs. Symptoms only in the arms suggest bilaterally symmetrical lesions in the lemniscal system or in the posterior columns of the high cervical cord. Occasionally all four limbs develop sensory symptoms, suggesting a sensory polyneuropathy, especially when onset is simultaneous.

Many times when a sensory disturbance begins in the lower extremities, it is not associated with any functional abnormality of the legs or the bladder. Because frequently there are no changes in motor function, such patients may be told that they have "neuritis" or that "stress" is responsible. The fact that such symptoms go away spontaneously reinforces those impressions. A recent report of patients with ON who developed MS[36] found that transient "nonspecific" sensory symptoms before the ON were a significant risk factor for the subsequent development of MS.

A less common sensory onset can be in a radicular distribution, with numbness, paresthesia, dysesthesia, pain, or itching.[304] Such symptoms are probably due to an acute lesion at the sensory root entry zone into the spinal cord or the brain stem. Because such acute onset syndromes involving the spinal roots C5, C6, C7, L5, and S1 can suggest compression of nerve roots, it is not unusual to find patients with MS who have had spinal surgery for attempted relief of root compression. Again, the fact that such syndromes can resolve spontaneously reinforces the im-

Table 4–3. **INITIAL SYMPTOMS IN 1721 PATIENTS WITH CLINICALLY DEFINED MULTIPLE SCLEROSIS FROM THE UNIVERSITY OF BRITISH COLUMBIA MULTIPLE SCLEROSIS CLINIC**

Symptom	Total Number N = 1702	Percentage of Total (% = 100)	Percentage of Females (% = 68.9)	Percentage of Males (% = 31.1)	Mean Age at Onset (Total)
Sensory in limbs	522	30.7	33.2	25.1	28.6
Visual loss*	271	15.9	16.3	15.1	28.2
Motor, slowly developing	152	8.9	8.3	10.4	36.4
Diplopia	115	6.8	6	8.5	26.4
Gait disturbance	81	4.8	3.2	8.3	34.9
Motor, acute onset	74	4.3	4.4	4.2	28.4
Sensory in face	47	2.8	2.9	2.5	30
Balance problem	50	2.9	2.5	4	33.2
Vertigo	29	1.7	1.8	1.5	28.6
Lhermitte's symptom	31	1.8	1.6	2.3	27.4
Bladder symptoms	17	1	0.9	1.1	29.4
Acute transverse myelopathy	12	0.7	0.8	0.6	27.6
Limb ataxia	17	1	0.9	1.3	30.5
Pain	8	0.5	0.3	0.8	39.8
Other	43	2.5	2.6	2.5	30.2
Polysymptomatic onset	233	13.7	14.5	11.9	30.8

Source: These data are derived from the University of British Columbia MS-COSTAR computerized medical records systems, as described in Paty DW, Studney D, Redekop WK, and Lublin FD,[328] pp S134–S135, and Studney and Paty[401] pp145–152.
*Usually unilateral optic neuritis.

pression of nerve root compression that has responded either to conservative management with bedrest or to operative management with decompression. Rarely patients will complain of symptoms suggestive of phantom limb, and phantom limb can be the initial complaint.[260]

Useless Hand Syndrome

Even though useless hand syndrome does not occur frequently in MS, when it does oc-cur it is so characteristic that it is highly suggestive of the diagnosis,[247] although it has been seen in cervical spondylosis.[358b] The "useless hand" is functionally impaired by sensory loss (Table 4–4). The sensory loss is usually confined to discriminatory sensations such as vibration sense, two-point discrimination, graphesthesia, stereognosis, and proprioception. The hand (or hands) becomes useless because of the lack of proprioception and feedback control of movement.

The lesion responsible for the useless hand is usually in the lemniscal system, ei-

Table 4–4. CHARACTERISTICS OF THE SENSORY USELESS HAND

- Vibration and proprioception loss usually profound
- Usually unilateral but can be bilateral
- Acute in onset (80%)
- Strength usually normal (must be examined with visual control of movement)
- Cerebellar function usually normal (must be examined with visual control of movement)
- Recovery is the rule (3–9 mo)

ther in the high cervical posterior columns or in the brain stem. The sensory loss usually occurs unilaterally but is sometimes bilateral. When bilateral, it can be remarkably symmetrical and can spare the legs. Hand function most often recovers spontaneously, although impairment can last for many months. It is unusual to see the useless hand syndrome with subacute onset in other spinal disorders, although we have seen it occasionally in patients with large central cervical disk protrusions. Occasionally patients with spondylitic myelopathy have a preponderance of posterior column deficits and rarely only these.

Lhermitte's Symptom

Another sensory symptom that is seen at the onset in less than 5 percent of patients is the Lhermitte phenomenon. This symptom was first described by Babinski and Dubois in 1891[22] as an electric current–like shock in the back and legs produced by neck flexion in patients with traumatic disease of the cervical spinal cord. Lhermitte and colleagues[234] pointed out that the symptom was most frequently seen in patients with MS. Their patient said: "When I try to lower my head, I feel a violent shock in the nape of my neck, and a pain like an electric current runs throughout my whole body, from my neck to my feet, down my vertebral column." They proposed that this symptom reflected "the inherent excitability of sensory fibers stripped of their insulating myelin sheath." This symptom has been described as a clinical "sign." We think it is better to refer to the symptom only as a symptom, or perhaps as the "Lher-

mitte phenomenon," because it is not a sign of MS. However, in the appropriate clinical context, it is of considerable diagnostic value because of relative specificity and localizability.

In patients with MS, Lhermitte's symptom is not always associated with flexion of the neck. Occasionally it can be brought on by lateral flexion of the neck, flexion or twisting of the dorsal spine, or simply a jolt to the spine while the patient walks over uneven ground. It may also be spontaneous. It usually disappears quickly, even if the neck is kept in flexion, but rarely it will persist. Most often, a brief shocklike sensation will extend from the neck to the base of the spine. Frequently, the sensation will extend down a single limb to the exclusion of the others or will affect both arms and both legs. Lhermitte's symptom commonly fatigues (disappears) after several consecutive neck flexions. This symptom can occasionally become troublesome, even in patients with no other neurological deficit, and if so, these patients often respond to a low dose of carbamazepine (Tegretol).

In neurological practice, most patients who present with Lhermitte's symptom have MS, although Lhermitte's symptom can be seen in subacute combined degeneration (SCD) of the spinal cord, neck trauma, cervical spondylosis, arachnoiditis, cervical disk protrusion, radiation myelitis, syringomyelia, combined systems disease, cisplatin neuropathy,[89] and spinal cord tumor. In cervical spondylosis, a similar symptom is usually elicited by neck extension rather than flexion, a useful differential point because we have not seen extension related to Lhermitte's symptom in MS. It is a reliable indicator of cervical spinal cord disease and therefore worth a specific inquiry.[428]

Optic Neuritis

Optic neuritis is a clinical disorder with a close relationship to MS.[96,98,99,264] It is the initial symptom in 16 percent of patients with MS and is common during the course of the disease. Visual loss in MS has recently been reviewed by McDonald[263] and by Barnes and McDonald.[28] ON usually begins with the acute or subacute onset of monocular visual blurring or loss, the most profound defect being in the central visual field (central scotoma).[301] ON is almost invariably associated with diminished visual acuity. However, Frederiksen and colleagues[128] have called attention to the fact that 18 of 50 patients that they investigated for acute ON had only subtle visual symptoms with normal visual acuity. The maximum loss of vision is usually within the first 4 days, although chronic progressive visual loss can be seen. There may be associated positive visual symptoms such as flashes of light (photopsias), or a "flight of colors"[282] brought on by eye movement (an optic nerve Lhermitte's symptom).

Because ON affects only one eye in most patients, some only become aware of the visual disturbance indirectly, such as when the vision from the other eye has been occluded (for example, in applying eye makeup). Occasionally the scotoma is temporal, peripheral, or hemianopic. Altitudinal defects can be seen. The frequency of involvement of the two eyes is equal. The differential diagnosis of unilateral visual loss can be aided by high-resolution MRI.[134] In a recent report of 75 consecutive patients with optic neuropathy 25 had idiopathic optic neuritis, 10 had ischemic optic neuritis, 5 had central retinal artery occlusion, 4 had Leber's optic neuropathy, 15 had benign intracranial hypertension, and 20 had optic nerve tumors. Uveitis can also cause unilateral visual impairment and is also associated with MS.[23] Therefore, it should be ruled out in atypical cases of visual blurring with ocular pain.

Pain on eye movement occurs frequently and can precede, accompany, or follow the visual loss.[330] The discomfort is usually maximal on eye movement, but there may also be tenderness of the globe. The pain usually resolves before recovery of visual acuity. There is no evidence that the severity or the duration of the pain has any effect on visual outcome. We have seen pain with the characteristics of ON develop and resolve in patients with MS in the absence of any clear visual deficit. The pain of ON may result from distension of the dura by a swollen optic nerve or, alternatively, from inflammation extending outside the confines of the optic nerve to involve pain receptors in the dural sheath. Lepore[233] thought that the

pain was due to traction on the optic nerve sheath by the rectus muscles. Extension beyond the optic nerve may also account for the rare patient with "opticociliary" neuritis, who has transient ciliary ganglion or ciliary nerve dysfunction resulting in pupillary hyporeactivity. MRI and CT studies have visualized the lesions in the optic nerve in optic neuritis.[270] Miller and his colleagues[202,274,279,453] found that the visual loss tends to be proportional to the apparent length of the involved segment of optic nerve as detected by MRI. Figure 4–3 shows a CT scan with enhancement of the optic nerve in a case of bilateral optic neuritis.

A number of studies have shown a loss of the retinal nerve fiber layer (RNFL) in MS and ON.[108,250,387] About one-half of patients with MS have defects in the RNFL. The functional and pathogenic significance of this axonal loss is not known, and the phenomenon requires investigation. The frequency of the finding suggests that loss of the nerve fiber layer could be diagnostically important. The specificity for MS is unknown.

Investigation of patients with acute unilateral ON have shown that up to 70 percent have multiple lesions on MRI scan (Table 4–5). Most of the patients with MRI lesions will have CSF OB as well, allowing a

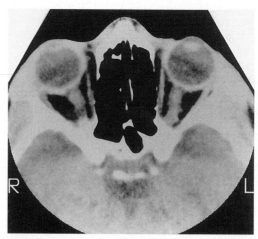

Figure 4–3. This CT is a high volume delayed scan, focusing on the optic nerves, in a young woman with bilateral optic neuritis. Note the intense enhancement and enlargement of both optic nerves. The enlargement suggests edema.

Table 4–5. **INVESTIGATIVE STUDIES OF OPTIC NEURITIS**

Year	Senior Author	No. of Patients with ON	No. (%) of Patients with Investigation Abnormalities to Suggest MS	Abnormal VEP: No. (%)	Abnormal SEP: No. (%)	Abnormal MRI/CT: No. (%)	Abnormal CSF: No. (%)	Comments
1984	Sanders[373]	30	19 (63)	30 (100)	6 (20)	6+ (20)	14 (47)	Only 3/14 patients with OB had an increased IgG Index. Sixty-eight percent of patients who had EP or CT abnormalities were OB-positive.
986	Johns[200]	10	7 (70)	—	—	7 (70)	—	In a 14-month follow-up, two patients had recurrent symptoms.
1986	Ormerod[311]	35	21 (61)	—	8 (30)	21 (61)	—	EP much less sensitive than MRI.
1986	Rudick[364]	8	5 (63)	—	—	4 (50)	5 (63)	Free K-light chains in CSF
1986	Jacobs[194]	16	8 (50)	—	—	8 (50)	—	
1987	Kinnunen[222]	10	4 (40)	10 (100)	1 (10)	4 (40)	1 (10)	Bilateral VEP abnormalities in 3; all had unilateral symptoms.
1987	Yedavally[449]	23	16 (70)	16 (70)	—	15 (65)	—	VEP more sensitive for optic nerve.
1988	Paty[325]	38	25 (60)	33 (87)	13 (34)	25 (66)	23 (61)	Nineteen (50%) were diagnosed as LSDMS.
1988	Miller[274]	37	—	—	—	—	—	MRI of optic nerves revealed abnormalities in 37/44 (84%) of symptomatic nerves and 6/30 (20%) of asymptomatic optic nerves.
1988	Eidelberg[104]	20	4 (20)	—	—	4 (20)	—	All had clinically progressive optic neuropathy, 8/20 (40%) had compression.
1988	Riikonen[354]	14	8 (50)	—	—	8 (57)	—	All children, mean age of 9.3 years.
1989	Staedt[397]	24	19 (79)	24 (100)	—	19 (79)	19/79 (83)	Correlation between CSF and MRI abnormalities was good.
1989	Frederiksen[125]	50	31 (62)	—	—	31 (62)	—	

Continued on following page

Table 4-5.—continued

Year	Senior Author	No. of Patients with ON	No. (%) of Patients with Investigation Abnormalities to Suggest MS	Abnormal VEP: No. (%)	Abnormal SEP: No. (%)	Abnormal MRI/CT: No. (%)	Abnormal CSF: No. (%)	Comments
1991	Frederiksen[127]	50	38/48 (79)	42 (84)	8/46 (17)	30/48 (63)	—	VEP abnormalities increased with time.
1991	Scholl[377]	81	31/43 (72)	74 (91)	—	31/43 (72)	—	Uhthoff's symptom increased the likelihood of developing MS on follow-up.
1991	Jacobs[195]	48	23 (48)	—	—	23 (48)	—	All MRI lesions clinically silent.
1991	Miller[279]	53	34 (64)	—	—	34 (64)	—	Eleven of 18 had transiently enhancing MRI lesions.
1991	Merandi[270]	19	5 (26)	—	—	5 (26)	—	Enhancement in the optic nerve was seen in 7/14.
1992	Hornabrook[184]	28	21 (75)	—	—	21 (75)	—	Lesions were seen in optic radiations.
1993	Beck[34]	418	112 (27)	—	—	112 (27)	—	MRI, 2 or more lesions considered strongly suggestive of MS.
1994	Gass[134]	25/79	25	—	—	—	—	High-resolution MRI diagnosis of optic neuropathies improves the yield.

CSF = cerebrospinal fluid; CT = computed tomography; EP = evoked potentials; LSDMS = laboratory-supported definite MS; MRI = magnetic resonance imaging; OB = oligoclonal banding; ON = optic neuritis; SEP = somatosensory evoked potentials; VEP = visual evoked potentials.

diagnosis of LSDMS.[325] Follow-up of these patients will show the accuracy of the diagnosis of LSDMS. The Optic Neuritis Treatment Trial[358a] found that CSF OB and MRI abnormalities predicted the diagnosis of CDMS. In a short follow-up of 1 year, Miller and his colleagues[276] showed that patients with multiple lesions on MRI were much more likely to develop CDMS (56 percent) than were patients with a normal MRI scan (16 percent). Plant and colleagues[334] found that many patients with ON had retrochiasmal lesions as well.

Youl and colleagues[454] also showed that 11 of 18 patients with acute ON had transient gadolinium enhancement of the optic nerve on MRI scan. The patients with enhancement were likely to have more severe clinical deficits than were those without enhancement. Lee and his colleagues[229] found that the optic nerve could be imaged well by lipid-suppressed chemical shift imaging. Gass and associates[133] have used the fast short T1 inversion recovery (STIR) sequence. Celesia and associates[67] studied 20 patients with acute ON, most of whom (65 percent) improved to normal within 6 months. Of those patients who had initial severe or total visual loss, 60 percent had some residual visual impairment. Scholl and colleagues[377] investigated 81 patients with ON. One-half had increasing loss of vision brought on by exercise or exposure to heat (Uhthoff's phenomenon). The patients with Uhthoff's phenomenon were more likely to have an abnormal MRI scan (87 percent) than did those without this feature (55 percent). They were also more likely (70 percent versus 37 percent) to develop MS in a 3.5-year follow-up.

The results of the Optic Neuritis Treatment Trial (ONTT)[34,35] showed that visual loss continued to improve in both treated and untreated patients over an entire year.

The afferent pupillary defect (APD, Marcus Gunn pupil) can be seen in ON and may be the only hard evidence present (see Chapter 7). One good way to show APD is to examine the patient in dim light using the ophthalmoscope to reveal a magnified red reflex. When the red reflex has been seen, the light can be moved from eye to eye and the pupillary reflex identified by the change in the red reflex. In APD, the pupil from the involved eye will not constrict or will actually dilate in the face of the ophthalmoscope light, showing that the consensual reflex is stronger than the direct reflex. Interesting discussions have occurred concerning the validity of the swinging light sign.[62,74,75] Posterior defects can also occur.[126]

Optic neuritis does not always lead to clinical MS. Older studies indicated that the frequency of the development of MS after ON varied from 13 to 85 percent (Table 4–6). Factors that increase the risk for MS after ON are lower age (younger patients have a high risk), being female, previous nonspecific sensory symptoms, multiple MRI lesions, the presence of DR2 antigen, and the presence of OB in the CSF.[228] Most patients who develop MS after ON will do so within 5 years, but we have seen patients with an interval as long as 35 to 40 years between the initial ON and the second symptom proving dissemination in space.

Our own experience with more than 100 cases of isolated ON indicates that more than half the patients with unilateral visual loss suggesting ON developed MS (especially in females) when cases of non-ON, such as central serous retinopathy and neuroretinitis, are excluded. In addition, the rate of developing MS after an initial symptom of MS in our UBC MS population is plotted in Figure 4–2. The curve is similar for males and females, with the longest intervals in females (data derived from a query run in the MS-COSTAR data base at UBC).[328,401] Non-MS causes of ON that might be confused with MS include lupus erythematosus, sarcoid,[110] Sjögren's syndrome (SS),[408] syphilis, Lyme disease,[196] and human immunodeficiency virus (HIV) infection.[403] One study[320] claims that cases of papillitis which, at follow-up, develop a macular exudate or "star" most likely have a vasculopathy called *neuroretinitis*. Patients with neuroretinitis apparently do not have a significant risk for developing MS.[320]

A study by Ebers and his colleagues[98] of 84 kindreds with familial CDMS found seven patients with isolated ON. The occurrence of isolated ON in the first-degree relatives of patients with MS suggests that MS may exist in a forme fruste as ON alone. Several of these patients with ON have been

Table 4–6. RISK OF MULTIPLE SCLEROSIS IN FOLLOW-UP STUDIES OF PATIENTS WITH ISOLATED OPTIC NEURITIS

Year	Senior Author	No. of Patients with ON	Duration of Follow-up (yr)	No. (%) Going on to MS	Comments
1974	Nikoskelainen[301]	116	10	58 (50)	Another 18 showed evidence of possible MS.
1978	Compston[72]	146	4	58 (40)	Risk of MS increased with HLA-DR2.
1979	Landy[228]	105	9	58 (55)	Those with onset of ON between ages 21 and 40 were at greatest risk for MS.
1979	Cohen[71]	60	7	17 (28)	Risk was higher in females than males.
1983	Kinnunen[221]	296	9	56 (19)	Risk was higher in females than males.
1984	Parkin[319]	31	up to 28	10 (32)	Risk for MS was low after bilateral simultaneous ON in adults.
		11 bilateral simultaneous ON		2/11 (18)	Risk for MS after ON in children was low.
		20 bilateral sequential ON		8/20 (40)	
1986	Hely[174]	82	4.7	26 (32)	Risk for MS increased with HLA-DR2 and -B7 haplotype.
1987	Francis[123]	101	11.6	58 (57)	Risk for MS increased with HLA-DRW3 and DRW2.
1987	Kinnunen[222]	10	11.6	4 (40)	Isolated ON still has multiple lesions.
1987	Lightman[236]	46	3.5	13 (28)	Evidence for ocular inflammation increased the likelihood of developing MS.
	Subgroup 1*	14	3.5	8/14 (57)	
	Subgroup 2†	32	3.5	5/32 (16)	
1988	Rizzo and Lessell[356]	60	14.9	35 (58)	Risk was highest in females.
1988	Miller[276]	34 MRI scans abnormal	1	19 (56)	MRI-positive patients are much more likely to develop MS than MRI-negative ones.
		19 MRI scans normal	1	3 (16)	
1988	Jacobson[197]	14	16 mo	3 (21)	All patients older than 50 years of age; three had recurrent ON.

Continued on following page

Table 4–6.—*continued*

Year	Senior Author	No. of Patients with ON	Duration of Follow-up (yr)	No. (%) Going on to MS	Comments
1988	Riikonen[354]	14	4.6	7 (50)	All children mean age 9.4 years.
1989	Frederiksen[125]	50	11 mo	7 (14)	All that developed MS had an abnormal MRI scan.
1989	Sanders[374a]	48	0.5–3.5	29 (60)	VEP can help predict the risk for MS.
1989	Alvarez[11]	23	9.7	1 (413)	Patients from Chile had a low risk for MS.
1989	Anmarkrud[17]	30	2 to 11	17 (57)	Risk increased with OB (79%). Most developed MS within 3 yrs.
1989	Grønning[159]	36	5.9	4 (42)	One ethnic Lapp had ON.
1990	Sandberg-Wollheim[371]	86	13	33 (38)	Risk increased for MS in younger patients and those with abnormal CSF (9/13).
1991	Jacobs[195]	48	4	9 (18)	Three of 25 MRI-negative patients developed MS.
1991	Scholl[377]	81	3.5	35 (43)	Uhthoff's symptom increased likelihood of developing MS.
1991	Mapelli[254]	40	12	10 (25)	This study suggests a lower than average risk for MS in an Italian population.
1993	Morrissey[290]	44	5	24 (55)	An abnormal MRI scan at outset was present in 23/24. Only 1/16 had a normal MRI scan.
1993	Beck[36]	389	2	47 (12)	Highest risk was in patients with a positive MRI scan. Methylprednisolone treatment delayed the onset of MS at 2 yr (see text).
1994	Rodriguez[358]	156	14.4	64% @ 40 yr follow-up	The conversion rate to MS increases with time to 64%.

CSF = cerebrospinal fluid; MRI = magnetic resonance imaging; ON = optic neuritis.
*Subgroup 1: perivenous sheathing or other evidence for ocular inflammation.
†Subgroup 2: no evidence for ocular inflammation.

followed into the seventh decade and have negative MRI and CSF studies, supporting the concept of monosymptomatic involvement with MS (solitary sclerosis?) (Ebers, 1986).

The question of what to tell the patient with ON about the possibility of MS has not been settled.[394a] There is no unanimity of opinion; the needs of individual patients should dictate whether or not they are told of the suspicion of MS. The current practice in many centers is to fully disclose all risks.

Leber's hereditary optic neuropathy (a mitochondrial DNA disorder)[209] is an important differential in the diagnosis of ON. Harding and colleagues[171] have described an MS-like illness in women who have a Leber's hereditary optic neuropathy mitochondrial DNA mutation. Most such patients present with severe and generally incompletely remitting fellow eye involvement within weeks of the initial attack of visual loss. Patients with Leber's neuropathy can also have spasticity.[60] In addition, some patients with apparent MS have the same mitochondrial DNA mutations as do Leber's patients.[73,209]

Optic neuropathy and myelopathy (neuromyelitis optica) occurring together have been referred to as *Devic's syndrome*. This combination is seen frequently in the Orient as the "oriental form of MS." Some authors, however, believe that the syndrome of neuromyelitis optica has characteristic features that allow it to be diagnosed separately from MS.[57,253] Patients who have the simultaneous onset of ON and acute myelitis probably have either ADEM or the first onset of MS. Only clinical, MRI, and pathological follow-up will decide the question of which is the appropriate diagnosis. Johns and colleagues[201] have described a brother and sister with the Devic's syndrome who had a mitochondrial DNA mutation causing a cytochrome oxidase abnormality.

Jacobson and colleagues[196] examined 20 consecutive patients with ON from a region endemic for Lyme disease for antibodies to *Borrelia burgdorferi*. Four (20 percent) were positive and improved in association with antibiotic treatment. Any relationship between the antibodies and the ON is still uncertain, because ON is a spontaneously resolving disorder.

Bilateral ON differs from unilateral ON in its outcome. As shown in Table 4–6, Parkin and colleagues[319] found that only 2 of 11 adults (18 percent) with simultaneous bilateral ON developed MS, compared with 8 of 20 patients (40 percent) with sequential bilateral ON, in a study with follow-up of up to 37 years. Chiasmal neuritis can sometimes occur and has the same implications for MS as does retrobulbar neuritis.[299]

An interesting exchange of views concerning ON and the risk for MS, including many useful tables, was published in 1985.[96,227] For further discussion of ON, see Chapter 7 and the text by Perkin and Rose.[330]

Motor Deficits of Slow Onset (Chronic Progressive Myelopathy)

Slowly progressive weakness, spasticity, or both of the lower extremities are the essential features of what has come to be known as *chronic progressive myelopathy (CPM)*. The usual patient is older than 40 years with a slowly developing deficit involving isolated motor or combined motor and sensory symptoms in the legs. CPM is often asymmetrical in its onset, although at the time of examination bilateral signs are usually present. The motor deficit is usually slowly progressive. There is usually no clinical evidence for dissemination in space (e.g., optic atrophy or internuclear ophthalmoplegia, INO) in patients with the CPM syndrome. In these patients, it is necessary to obtain reliable paraclinical evidence for dissemination in space to support the diagnosis of MS (see subsequently). Even though a slow onset can occur with any category of MS, the great majority of such chronically progressive patients demonstrate primarily spinal involvement. All such patients should have either complete myelography (including the foramen magnum) or spinal MRI studies to exclude structural and compressive causes of spinal cord dysfunction. Head MRI and VEPs are particularly important if there is no clinical evidence for a lesion above the foramen magnum. If OB is found in the CSF in addition to paraclinical evidence for dissemination in space, LSDMS can be diagnosed. As noted below, a diagnosis of LSDMS has been proved to be as reliable as a diagnosis of CDMS.[231]

Occasionally, spinal cord and dural arteriovenous malformations (AVM), herniated thoracic disks, intramedullary tumors, Arnold-Chiari malformations, or syringomyelia[346] can mimic spinal progressive MS. Tumor or compression in the thoracic region can be missed unless special care is taken at the time of the imaging studies. HTLV-1-associated myelopathy (HAM) or tropical spastic paraplegia (TSP) must also be considered in patients from the Caribbean, Japan, or other endemic areas[141,142,313] or those with known risk factors. Several studies have suggested that HAM or TSP can mimic MS. Rudge and colleagues[362] studied 14 patients from the Caribbean who had MS; none had HTLV-1 antibodies. They did find, however, that some patients with HAM or TSP had cerebral MRI abnormalities that could mimic MS. Of 30 patients with CPM, 27 had HTLV-1 antibodies. Oger and colleagues[309] have recently described HTLV-1 myelopathy in North American Indians. This condition may be more widespread than previously recognized. HTLV-II may also cause a myelopathy.[232a]

Marshall's landmark 1955 paper concerned spastic paraplegia of middle age.[255] In this clinicopathological study of 80 cases, he retrospectively reviewed the history of 52 cases, in about one-half of whom the diagnosis had become apparent over time. The most common diagnosis was MS, although compression from tumor, disk, and cervical spondylosis also occurred. The major differential diagnosis was between MS and spinal tumor. A clear-cut sensory level was highly suggestive of tumor. In retrospect, much of the diagnostic difficulty in Marshall's study was due to the inadequacy of myelography at that time.

Berger and Quencer[39] have reported on a man with pernicious anemia and myelopathy (combined systems disease) who presented with Lhermitte's symptom. A lesion seen on the cervical cord MRI scan resolved after vitamin B_{12} therapy.

In recent years, the application of paraclinical examinations to the evaluation of patients with CPM has shown that a majority of such cases have abnormalities in CSF IgG or OB and abnormal VEPs, CT scan, or MRI scan (Table 4–7).[65,323,325]

In one study,[312] 72 patients with CPM in whom compressive lesions had been ruled out were investigated for evidence of lesions disseminated in time and space and CSF changes that would support a diagnosis of MS. The mean age at onset of CPM was 42 years, with a mean duration of 10 years at the time of examination. The findings suggest that between one-half and three-quarters of patients with CPM have MS. The patients without MS have a variety of infrequently encountered disorders, including primary lateral sclerosis (PLS),[336,342] familial spastic paraparesis, or arachnoiditis. A small number will remain undiagnosed. Clinical follow-up shows that patients with spinal symptoms suggestive of MS who have OB are much more likely to develop CDMS than are those without OB (Table 4–8).[293] Eales disease can also present as a chronic neurological deficit, although occasionally it can present as multifocal disease.[8]

Another study[325] showed that one-half of 42 patients with noncompressive CPM had an abnormal VEP as evidence for dissemination in space. The abnormal VEP in those patients was supported by an abnormal MRI scan. The diagnosis of MS was further supported in the majority of those patients by the presence of OB in the CSF. Unfortunately, a number of false-negative VEPs were seen. Additional information obtained by doing MRI and CSF studies showed that one-half of the patients in whom the VEP was normal had MRI and CSF abnormalities pointing definitely toward a diagnosis of MS. On the other hand, MRI identified all of the patients with CPM who could be diagnosed as LSDMS regardless of the VEP result. VEP did not identify any patients as having LSDMS that were not identified by MRI. This study suggests that in CPM, an MRI examination for dissemination in space is all that is needed, and that the VEP contributes little additional information if an MRI is available.

Weinshenker and colleagues[438] published an autopsy series of four patients who had progressive myelopathy and no clinical evidence of dissemination of lesions. Two had MRI evidence of dissemination. One had a

Table 4–7. **CHRONIC PROGRESSIVE MYELOPATHY: INVESTIGATION WITH IMAGING, EVOKED POTENTIALS, AND CEREBROSPINAL FLUID ANALYSIS**

Year	Senior Author	No. of Patients	Abnormalities Suggesting MS	Abnormal VEP	Abnormal CT	Abnormal MRI	OB Positive CSF	Comments
				NO. (%) OF PATIENTS WITH:				
1977	Bynke[65]	25	21 (84)	19 (76)	—	—	16 (64)	Many CPM patients have MS.
1979	Paty[323]	72	61 (85)	32 (44)	38 (53)*	—	32 (44)	Blink reflex abnormal in 40 (56%): sixty-seven percent diagnosed as LSDMS
1986	Edwards[103]	10	8 (80)	3/10 (30)	—	6 (60)	4/10 (40)	MRI and CSF combined best test.
1987	Miller[273]	89	73 (82)	20 (28)	—	73 (82)	15/40 (37)	MRI alone is helpful.
1987	Miska[285]	20	13 (65)	8/15 (53)	—	13 (65)	12/16 (75)	MRI most sensitive test.
1988	Mauch[259]	18	15 (83)	?	0 (0)	15 (83)	10 (55)	VEP less helpful than MRI, CT unhelpful only CSF done systematically.
1988	Steiner[398]	76	39 (51)	—	—	—	39 (51)	
1988	Paty[325]	52	44 (84)	28 (54)	11 (21)*	31 (60)	32 (62)	Conservative MRI criteria, see text. Twenty-four (46%) LSDMS.
1991	Berger[39]	1	1	—	—	—	—	B$_{12}$ deficiency myelopathy with Lhermitte's phenomenon and an MRI lesion in the cervical cord.

CSF = cerebrospinal fluid; CT = computed tomography; LSDMS = laboratory-supported definite MS; MRI = magnetic ressonance imaging; OB = oligoclonal banding; SEP = somatosensory evoked potential; VEP = visual evoked potential.
*CT abnormalities mostly atrophy.

Table 4–8. **CHRONIC PROGRESSIVE MYELOPATHY: FOLLOW-UP, CLINICAL CHARACTERISTICS, AND DIAGNOSTIC CONSIDERATIONS**

Year	Senior Author	No. of Patients	Age at Onset (yr)	Duration of Follow-up (yr)	No. (%) with MS in Follow-up	Comments
1955	Marshall[255]	52	40	10.4	10 (19)	In 27, the diagnosis remained unknown. Thirteen had structural lesions.*
1955	Marshall[255]	35	43	7	12 (34)	In postmortem series, 31% had tumor.
1971	Gårde[132]	45	45	3.5	7 (15)	Seven patients were diagnosed with CDMS.
					10 (22)	Ten patients showed evidence of possible MS.
1973	Hübbe[186]	24	37	8.9	6 (25)	Six patients were diagnosed with CDMS.
1983	Moulin[293]					
	Subgroup 1	55 OB+	36.3	3	20 (36)	OB+ patients were more likely to develop CDMS on follow-up.
	Subgroup 2	56 OB−	37.5	3	9 (16)	
1989	Martí-Fàbregas[256]	50	38	2.33	29 (58)	In 42%, the diagnosis remained unknown.

CDMS = clinically definite MS; OB− = oligoclonal banding negative; OB+ = oligoclonal banding positive.
*This early study suffered from poor diagnostic techniques, especially myelography, so that when reinvestigated, 13 of 52 (23%) had treatable structural cord lesions.

single demyelinating lesion in the spinal cord and OB. Mixed motor and sensory findings suggest MS, whereas pure motor findings do not.[198a]

Pringle and colleagues[342] proposed specific diagnostic criteria for primary lateral sclerosis. Gieron and colleagues[146] reported a case of transient subacute progressive myelopathy in a 14-year-old girl in whom a spinal MRI lesion resolved as she improved clinically. CSF studies were negative for OB. The ultimate diagnosis is not known. This case could very well turn out to be MS.

The following cases illustrate a number of important principles of MS differential diagnosis:

CASE HISTORY: MS—Solitary Cervical Lesion Causing Chronic Progressive Myelopathy

This 54-year-old man had a 4-year history of the left arm feeling numb, cold, and sore. Seven months after onset of his left arm symptoms, he began to notice progressive weakness of his left leg. Myelography showed a protruding C5–6 disk with slight cord compression. Diskectomy was performed, but his symptoms worsened. Bowel, bladder, and sexual function remained intact. Neck flexion produced nonfatiguing left arm tingling as well as tingling in the left buttock and down the back of the leg. Neck extension allowed improved hand movement

(McArdle's sign). Tone was slightly increased in the right and moderately increased in the left extremities. There was substantial weakness in the left arm, especially distally, and bilateral extensor plantar responses. Minimal vibratory loss was found in the feet and the fifth fingers of both hands. MRI scan showed increased signal at the C2–3 level. The head MRI scan was normal. CSF electrophoresis showed OB. A second head MRI scan 3 years later showed several lesions consistent with MS, including small lesions in the corpus callosum and periventricular region. In this situation, demonstration of dissemination in time and space allowed the diagnosis of CDMS according to the Poser criteria.

Comment: This patient's symptoms appear to have resulted from a single cervical cord (probably demyelinating) lesion in the absence of clinical or laboratory evidence of dissemination in space. At follow-up, however, additional lesions were demonstrated by MRI scan. We also have experience with two autopsy-proven cases of progressive paraplegia in which a single spinal cord plaque was the only evidence for MS in the entire nervous system. Both patients had OB in the CSF.[113,438]

CASE HISTORY: Spinal Arteriovenous Malformation Causing Chronic Progressive Myelopathy Syndrome

A 56-year-old man had a long history of chronic low back pain, interrupted by the sudden onset of severe pain 4 years previously. He subsequently noticed numbness in the outer aspects of both legs, which slowly got worse. He also had bladder urgency without incontinence. Bilateral wasting was seen in the extensor digitorum brevis and the plantar foot muscles. No fasciculations were seen. There was weakness in an L5-S1 distribution, and loss of light touch in an L4-S1 distribution, with sacral sparing. Joint position sense and vibration sense were reduced in both feet. Deep tendon reflexes in the legs were absent except for a brisk left knee jerk. The right plantar response was extensor. A myelogram was normal, but a dural AVM was seen on spinal angiography.

Comment: This man showed no dissemination in space or time, and symptoms were consistent with a single spinal lesion, which was missed on initial prone myelography. Multiple absent reflexes in the lower extremities, very unusual findings in CPM, suggested extensive nerve root involvement.

CASE HISTORY: Spinal Cord Compression due to Osteophyte, Wrongly Diagnosed as Multiple Sclerosis

A 22-year-old man presented with a 2-month history of numb and stiff legs. The only past history was of a motor vehicle accident 2 years previously, in which he had trivial head injuries. When examined, he was found to have spastic legs and vague sensory loss in the legs. CT scan of the head, cervical spine x-rays, and EPs were normal. CSF analysis showed a slightly elevated total protein (TP), normal globulins, and a questionable marked elevation of myelin basic protein (MBP) level. A myelogram was not done. Follow-up examination showed possible temporal pallor in one eye and minimal lateral gaze nystagmus. A diagnosis of MS was made. He subsequently became much worse and, after an apparent relapse, was seen at a second medical center. Re-evaluation, including a supine myelogram, showed a severe compression of the spinal cord at C3 and C4 by a large osteophyte. After decompressive surgery, he improved slowly but remains wheelchair bound and unable to transfer himself. A recent MRI scan has failed to show any head lesions.

Comment: A mistaken diagnosis of MS in this young man resulted in irreversible damage to the cervical spinal cord. An elevated MBP level in the CSF was wrongly interpreted as supporting the diagnosis of MS. In retrospect, this man had a congenitally narrow spinal canal and developed a large osteophyte following a relatively minor head and neck injury 2 years before the onset of neurological symptoms.

Gait and Balance Disturbance

Abnormal gait and balance can result from dysfunction in many different tracts singly or in combination. Unfortunately, many patients are unable to define the nature of their balance disturbance. Subtle neurological findings may be the only clue that such a complaint is actually due to an organic CNS disease such as MS.

Vague lightheadedness, gait disturbance, and instability are seen so frequently with peripheral vestibular disease that vestibulopathy is often the diagnosis made before the clear-cut demonstration of CNS abnormalities on neurological examination.[176] Such symptoms can be due to spasticity or proprioceptive deficits in the legs as well as to subtle vestibulocerebellar brain stem lesions. Careful neurological evaluation, many times done repeatedly, may be necessary to identify the specific lesions causing such vague symptoms.

Vertigo

Vertigo is a common symptom in neurological practice. Most patients who present with vertigo have a peripheral vestibular disturbance. Many of these patients have a paroxysmal onset of symptoms, with a possible residual complaint of positionally induced vertigo. Central vertigo is more chronic than paroxysmal vertigo, but in MS, vertigo can be of either type. Vertigo as a single symptom, without diplopia, certainly occurs in MS, but it is also a frequent symptom in other, more common conditions. Although, in our experience, vertigo has occurred as the initial symptom of MS in only 1.7 percent of patients, vertigo and balance abnormalities are common at some point in the course of the illness. The vertigo seen in acute primary vestibular disorders is often more severe than the vertigo seen in MS. These symptoms are frequently associated with MRI lesions.[157]

Limb Incoordination

Isolated limb incoordination is relatively unusual as an initial symptom. The useless (clumsy) hand due to sensory loss is more common (see earlier). Occasionally, the clinician sees an acute or slowly progressive onset of limb clumsiness and intention tremor without weakness or sensory loss.

Diplopia

Barnes and McDonald[28] have reviewed abnormalities of eye movement in MS. Diplopia is common, and the patient's description may help to determine the likely mechanism underlying this complaint. It is important to determine whether the separation of images is vertical, horizontal, or diagonal and whether the double vision is seen on primary gaze, lateral gaze, or in all directions of gaze. Precision in history taking is important, particularly when the patient was not examined at the time of the symptom in question. Occasionally, sixth nerve palsies and, rarely, third nerve palsies[131,298,421,422] can be the initial presentation of MS. We have seen the latter only on a single occasion. Fourth nerve palsies have been described, but it is not clear that they have actually been due to MS. Vertical diplopia is often related to a skew deviation. The most frequent disturbance presenting as horizontal double vision in MS is an internuclear opthalmoplegia (INO).[24,25] Curiously, diplopia may not be present in some patients with INO. Involvement of the medial longitudinal fasciculus in MS is so frequent that eventually some evidence of INO is seen in close to one-half of all patients.

A fully developed bilateral INO usually presents in a characteristic way. Patients develop double vision that is maximal on lateral gaze in either direction but is minimal on primary gaze. The diplopia is usually horizontal. Patients may volunteer that they experienced oscillopsia, probably due to ataxic nystagmus on lateral gaze. The history of bidirectional gaze evoked horizontal diplopia is so characteristic of INO that it probably can be used on historical grounds alone as a basis for demonstrating lesions disseminated in time and space. Unfortunately, this "typical" history may not be present, and when faced with a remote history of diplopia, the clinician usually must look for evidence that the lesion involved was confirmed on neurological examination by a reliable observer (see Chapter 7). Subtle slowing of adduction of one or both eyes often persists for years after the onset of INO and can be readily detected by having the patient look quickly from side to side. The most subtle residual INO is isolated abduction eye (ataxic) nystagmus. Bilateral INO has also been described in lupus erythematosus, in brain stem tumors including metastases, and in paraneoplastic syndromes.

Acutely Evolving Motor Dysfunction (Including Acute Transverse Myelitis)

Acutely developing motor symptoms are less common than sensory symptoms as the initial presenting feature of MS (Table 4–9). Nevertheless, they may be seen in any extremity, singly or in combinations, and may include hemiparesis and quadriparesis. Even a reversible acute locked-in syndrome has been reported at onset.[385] Certainly, the most dramatic acute motor syndrome is that of acute transverse myelitis (ATM). Fukazawa[129] found 16 patients with CDMS from Japan who had ATM during the course of their illness. Scott and colleagues[380] evaluated 14 patients with ATM retrospectively with MRI and found that spinal cord swelling seen on MRI scan had a poor prognosis. In contrast, a normal head and spinal MRI scan provided a good prognosis with 8 of 10 such patients making a good to complete recovery. None of their patients developed MS after an average follow-up of 3 years. OB was not seen in any of the eight patients so tested. They concluded that spine MRI scan was a better prognostic indicator than the degree of paralysis.

Even though acute spinal cord symptoms are characteristic of MS, the syndrome of complete ATM is unusual as an initial onset of MS. Less than 14 percent of patients with ATM will develop MS.[10] Conversely, only 0.7 percent of our 3500 patients with CDMS or LSDMS had an onset with ATM.

In spite of the fact that acute, complete ATM is infrequent in MS, a number of patients with MS started with an incomplete transverse (predominantly motor) spinal syndrome (see Table 4–3).[168] MRI can be helpful in the diagnosis.[130] Incomplete acute transverse cord syndromes are frequently encountered.[122] Even though sensory levels are often seen during acute MS relapses, it is unusual to find a persistent, sharply defined sensory level. A previous history of subacute or acute onset of sensory loss or weakness, or both, in both legs in a young patient presenting with a second neurological episode involving the optic nerve, brain stem and cerebellum, followed by complete recovery, strongly suggests MS. An incomplete, acute, combined motor-sensory disturbance with a sensory level and good recovery in a young adult is typical of MS. However, the clinician must be careful in using such a history as a reliable indicator of dissemination in time and space, particularly if the patient was not examined at the time of the initial event.

Tippett and colleagues[414] described three patients with relapsing ATM in whom CSF was consistently negative for OB, and cranial MRI scans were normal. They suggested that relapsing ATM is more common than previously thought and that it may have no relationship to MS. It would be interesting to see further follow-up of Tippett's patients. We have never recognized or diagnosed relapsing ATM. Most patients with relapsing spinal syndromes have either MS or some specifically diagnosable condition, such as spinal AVM or thoracic disk.

Tan[406] published a clinical follow-up of 52 patients from Malaysia with acute or subacute transverse myelopathy. Fourteen (27 percent) developed MS at follow-up, a higher proportion than previously suspected. This observation should be followed up with other studies, because it is unclear in Tan's article if some of his patients had partial ATM. If so, then these patients would be at risk for MS. Only patients with acute *complete* ATM have a low risk for developing MS. ATM in children does not carry a risk for MS.[2]

Urinary Bladder Symptoms

Disturbances of bladder function will occur at some time in 80 percent of patients. Bladder symptoms can be seen at the outset in about 10 percent, and they may be the initial, isolated symptoms in 1 percent. Urgency, frequency, and stress incontinence

Table 4–9. **ACUTE TRANSVERSE MYELOPATHY: RISK FOR DEVELOPING MULTIPLE SCLEROSIS**

Year	Senior Author	No. of Patients Studied	Age (yr)	Proportion with Recovery (Partial or Complete)	No. (%) with MS in Follow-Up	Comments
1963	Altrocchi[10]	67	1–65	1/3 good	4 (6)	Most were under age 40 years; 26 under age 15 years.
1973	Lipton[241]	29	15–55	2/3 good	1 (3)	
1978	Ropper[359]	52	4–83 (mean 32)	1/3 good	7 (13)	Mean follow-up was 5 yr. Subacute onset had a better initial prognosis.
1989	Tan[406]	28	33	most	14 (52)	MS more likely in females. Ten had recurrent ATM.
1989	Miller[277]	33	30	—	—	Abnormal MRI increased the risk for MS.
	(MRI abnormal)	18	29	—	13 (72)	
	(MRI normal)	15	32	—	1 (7)	
1991	Tippett[414]	3	15 to 41	3/3	0	Patients had relapsing transverse myelopathy, non-MS.
1994	Scott[380]	14	14 to 72	12/14	0	Patients with normal head and spinal MRI scans recovered. Spinal cord swelling on MRI scan was a poor prognostic sign.

ATM = acute transverse myelopathy; MRI = magnetic resonance imaging.

are frequent in the female non-MS population, even in nulliparous women, so the diagnosis may be elusive.[38] The mere presence of bladder symptoms is insufficient evidence for a neurological lesion. For example, the most common cause of urinary symptoms is infection. Sixty percent of women with frequency and urgency have bacterial infection, but because the combination of neurogenic bladder and urinary tract infection is so common, the analysis of these symptoms can be difficult. It may be hazardous to use bladder symptoms as evidence of dissemination.

Bladder symptoms can be varied, even at the outset of MS, and during the course of the illness, any of the symptoms resulting from neurogenic bladder disturbances can be seen. The most common symptoms are a combination of frequency and urgency, urge incontinence, and hesitancy. Unfortunately, the time-honored concept that frequency and urgency indicate a small, spastic bladder, whereas hesitancy, dribbling, double voiding, and retention suggest bladder neck obstruction, is inexact. Only 45 percent of patients who complain of symptoms suggesting a problem with urinary storage (frequency and urgency) are found to have appropriate pathophysiology.[44] Consequently, investigation must always be undertaken before the diagnosis of isolated neurogenic bladder is made. If patients are unable to produce a clean midstream urine sample for culture voluntarily, bladder catheterization should be done. Residual volume can also be determined at the same time. Clear-cut evidence for a neurogenic bladder can be used as evidence for dissemination in space, but only with caution. It is not always a sign of spinal cord dysfunction. One must remember that a neurogenic bladder can be caused by isolated lesions in the spinal cord, brain stem, or hemispheres, where the involvement causing bladder symptoms would have to be bilateral. Urinary retention can cause bladder stretching and produce a flaccid bladder. A flaccid bladder can occur in MS but also occurs in psychogenic retention. Excessive bladder contractability may be a dysfunctional symptom without an identifiable structural cause.

Sexual Function Evaluation

Sexual function is a relatively new area in the evaluation of patients with MS.[283,404] Patients and physicians vary in their willingness to discuss issues of sexuality, particularly during the initial stages of the doctor-patient relationship. Symptoms of sexual dysfunction are more commonly volunteered by men and are usually manifested by difficulty in erection or ejaculation. In women, typical symptoms include decreased vaginal lubrication, decreased ability to reach orgasm, and vaginal spasm. Because impotence can affect up to 20 percent of otherwise normal males, and 9 percent of otherwise normal females do not reach an orgasm during an entire life span, the clinician must be careful in ascribing sexual dysfunction to MS. Patients being evaluated for a serious disease, such as MS, may also frequently experience sexual dysfunction and decreased libido secondary to depression or anxiety.

Undoubtedly, sexual dysfunction is common in MS and represents a serious problem, which can be a source of considerable stress for both patients and their partners. As many as 80 percent of men with MS have some degree of sexual dysfunction. Thirty to 50 percent of women with MS also may have sexual dysfunction, but women may not spontaneously report sexual dysfunction, and such a history may not be obtained, even after careful inquiry. Careful evaluation of sexual function during the initial evaluation can provide the information necessary to make an accurate diagnosis of sexual dysfunction. Because of the reluctance of most patients to discuss sexual dysfunction, the physician should make a special effort to detect these problems and offer appropriate management.

Heat and Exercise Intolerance

A frequent finding in patients with MS is an exquisite sensitivity to increased body temperature. This sensitivity can be brought out by exercise, sunbathing, hot baths, emotion, fatigue, fever, or other factors associated with an increase in body temperature. Occasionally, the initial symptom occurs only after a hot bath or after exercise.[40] Virtually any MS symptom can present this way. For instance, patients may complain of blurring of vision after a jog. Because such symptoms disappear after rest, they may confuse physicians unfamiliar with this phenomenon. Heat sensitivity is not necessarily specific to MS, but it is more commonly seen in demyelinating disorders (both central and peripheral) than in neurological conditions primarily involving the neuron or axon. For a physiological explanation, see Chapters 5 and 8. Remitting weakness after exercise may be seen in the periodic paralyses. This condition differs from MS in that the weakness may affect the exercised limbs, as in one of our patients whose arm hung limply at his side after throwing a football for a half hour.

Visual symptoms present in this way more frequently than others.[420] Such symptoms as monocular visual loss (Uhthoff's phenomenon), double vision, or simply blurred vision may be seen only after a hot bath or exercise. Some patients learn to deal with this problem by taking cold showers or cooling their body in some other fashion. The authors have seen patients in whom this symptom complex went on for years before the patient sought medical attention. The authors are also aware of two temperature-related deaths in patients with MS. One patient died of scalding because he was unable to get out of a hot shower, whereas another drowned in the bathtub when left unattended. Heat-induced weakness was suspected as the problem, because both were able to walk unaided previously. Heat sensitivity has some diagnostic value, as in the hot bath test.

Scholl and associates[377] have recently looked at Uhthoff's phenomenon in patients with ON. They found that patients with ON who had Uhthoff's phenomenon also had significant MRI abnormalities and an increased risk for MS at follow-up.

UNUSUAL PRESENTATIONS

Pain

Pain has been neglected as a symptom in MS, yet it has been reported as the initial symptom in as many as 11 percent of patients and it also occurs in some form in almost half the patients (Table 4–10).[292] The pain seen at the onset of MS is likely to be radiating or radicular in distribution, such as that seen in root compression syndromes or in tabes dorsalis. The description of pain varies from a tickle to a burning or boring sensation that can be unbearable. If the pain is confined to one nerve root distri-

Table 4–10. **UNUSUAL (BUT NOT RARE) PRESENTATIONS OF MULTIPLE SCLEROSIS**

- Pain
- Paroxysmal symptom
  Visual loss
  Generalized sensory disturbances
  Positive motor disturbances
  Weakness
  Brain stem dysfunction: Dysarthria, diplopia
  Trigeminal neuralgia, etc.
- Dementia and affective disorders
- Fatigue
- Others:
  Movement disorders
  Seizures
  Aphasia
  Hemianopsia
  Autonomic disturbance

bution, the clinician might think of nerve root compression. Vermote and his colleagues[425] did a survey of pain in 83 consecutive patients with MS. Forty-five percent had pain that was not headache or visceral pain. The authors thought that 2 of 45 (4 percent) had psychogenic pain, 17 (38 percent) had tendinoskeletal pain, and 26 (58 percent) had neurogenic pain. Of the 26 patients with neurogenic pain, 12 had persistent extremity pain, 8 had painful tonic spasms, and 6 had paroxysmal pain. The presence of neurogenic pain was not related to the degree of disability, whereas tendinoskeletal pain was seen mostly in disabled patients. Stenager and colleagues[399] also looked at pain syndromes in 117 MS patients and found pain in 65 percent. Thirty-two percent reported that pain was the most severe symptom of MS, and 23 percent had pain at the onset of MS.

In a recent review[292] of a geographically representative sample of 182 patients from Middlesex County, Ontario, Canada, seen at the MS Clinic of the University of Western Ontario, 88 (48 percent) had either acute or chronic pain sometime during their disease, 9 percent had acute paroxysmal pain including trigeminal neuralgia (TN), and 48 percent had chronic pain syndromes. The clinical characteristics of the patients with and without pain were similar. The chronic extremity pain was usually associated with other symptoms of myelopathy. In 5 percent of their patients, pain was the initial symptom of MS.

The following case illustrates TN as the initial symptom of MS: When TN starts before age 50 years, MS should be suspected as the cause.[318,366] However, when TN is the initial symptom after age 50 years, MS is rarely the cause.

CASE HISTORY: Trigeminal Neuralgia at Onset—Exacerbation of Multiple Sclerosis Symptoms with Carbamazepine

A year before examination, this 48-year-old man began to experience sudden jolts of pain in the second division of the right TN associated with the typical triggers of touching, eating, and talking. A diagnosis of idiopathic TN was made. He was given carbamazepine, which stopped the pain but seemed to make him ataxic even in small doses. Six months later, the pain recurred. Neurological examination showed prominent nystagmus, which was thought to be due to the carbamazepine. CSF electrophoresis showed oligonal bands, visual and auditory evoked potentials were abnormal, and CT scan showed mild atrophy. Subsequent neurological examination found bilateral INO (latent) and bilateral corticospinal signs.

Comment: This patient illustrates that in patients younger than 50 years old with tic, MS should be suspected. Many MS patients are very sensitive to the effects of any drug with CNS depressant effects. Often drugs given for one MS-related indication produce neurological side effects in other areas.

Tic-like pains are commonly seen in patients with MS. In patients in whom the diagnosis of MS is established, TN does not produce a diagnostic dilemma. The duration of pain is usually short, but it can be recurrent and disabling. Tic pains will usually respond to carbamazepine, phenytoin (Dilantin), or baclofen (Lioresal). If medication fails, percutaneous trigeminal rhizotomy[56] can be very effective. TN is one of the paroxysmal symptoms described subsequently.

Paroxysmal Symptoms

Paroxysmal symptoms are a fascinating group of motor or sensory symptoms that are by no means rare in MS (see Table 4–10). They may originate in the pathophysiology of demyelination that allows ephaptic transmission.[164] Occasionally when paroxysmal symptoms are present at onset, they are confused with transient ischemia, migraine, or seizures. These paroxysmal episodes are to be distinguished from acute relapses and pseudorelapses.[375] The paroxysmal symptoms of MS are generally abrupt in onset and brief in duration. They can recur up to 100 times a day and are not precipitated by fever. They may be disabling because of intensity and frequency. Because paroxysmal symptoms are not usually identified in the first instance as being due to MS, such patients may be diagnosed as being hysterical.

PAROXYSMAL GENERALIZED SENSORY DISTURBANCES

Paroxysmal generalized sensory disturbances are probably variations on the Lhermitte phenomenon. The symptoms can begin in the feet or at the top of the head. The patient usually describes a sensation that passes through the body in a wave. It can be painful but usually is described as an intense electric tingling sensation. Some patients have even described a flow of sensory abnormality that passes up the body. When the sensation reaches the head, it can occasionally be associated with slurred speech or double vision, the whole episode reportedly lasting less than 30 seconds. These generalized sensory paroxysms suggest an electrical discharge spreading across the brain stem, starting in the lemniscal system. When such transient sensory symptoms are unilateral, they may be difficult to distinguish from sensory seizures or transient ischemia.

PAROXYSMAL POSITIVE MOTOR DISTURBANCES

The most common of the paroxysmal motor symptoms in MS is the painful tonic spasm or seizure (PTS).[390] This symptom is usually characterized by a sudden onset of stiffness and involuntary flexion in the arm or hand with the inability to use the limb. The tension in the muscles can become so great that the limb is painful, associated with very tight clenching of the fist. Sometimes the spasm involves both the arm and leg simultaneously, and rarely, simultaneous bilateral involvement is seen, as in all four limbs or both legs. Each episode can last up to 2 minutes, though most often about 30 seconds, and may recur several times each day. When PTSs occur at the outset of MS, diagnostic error is almost always the rule. The dramatic response to carbamazepine may cement the opinion that this is focal epilepsy. In some patients, it is difficult to distinguish PTS from paroxysmal choreoathetosis. Berger and colleagues[41] reported eight patients with "paroxysmal dystonia" as the initial symptom of MS. This phenomenon is probably identical to what has been described as PTSs.[390] The symptom can be brought on by voluntary movement, tactile stimulation, or startle. In our experience, flexion of the neck or back, hyperventilation, or exercise can precipitate any of these paroxysmal symptoms. Hemifacial spasm can occur as well.[407]

Less than 5 percent of patients present with convulsive seizures. One case of MS has been described in which seizures, preceded by lethargy and headache, mimicked tumor. The MRI scan resembled a butterfly glioma.[206] Paroxysmal hemiballism has also been seen.[355]

CASE HISTORY: Paroxysmal Symptoms (Both Motor And Sensory) At Onset

A 36-year-old housewife was well until 3 months before examination when, while walking up stairs, she experienced pins and needles in both legs. She then had a 1-minute attack in which the fingers of *both* hands tightened into a fistlike posture followed by tonic flexion at the elbows. She also had chest tightness and breathing difficulty. She experienced three attacks within a half an hour. The fourth attack was preceded by a tingling sensation in the right arm. While the fourth attack was similar to the preceding three, it was clearly worse on the right side and began earlier in the right arm than on the left. She also had some curling of her toes. Hyperventilation or panic attacks were considered, but MRI scan showed numerous white matter lesions. CSF electrophoresis was positive for OB. Small doses of carbamazepine immediately and completely abolished her attacks. Follow-up neurological examination showed brisk and asymmetrical knee jerks and a mild decrease in vibration sense in the legs. Hyperventilation could provoke a typical "spell" when carbamazepine was withheld.

Comment: This patient illustrates a rare case of MS with bilateral PTS (PTSs in MS are almost always unilateral), which closely resembled the carpopedal spasms of hyperventilation. PTS can often be precipitated by hyperventilation in MS.

PAROXYSMAL WEAKNESS

In 1961, Zeldowicz[457] reported on several patients who developed recurrent attacks of weakness (usually in the lower extremities) as isolated symptoms, who went on to develop MS. Some of these patients were thought to have psychoneurosis or conversion hysteria when first seen. The weakness was described as an unexplained giving way of the legs, attacks of falling to the ground, or other abrupt symptoms of weaknesses. Paroxysmal weakness should be distinguished from the more common form of focal transient weakness seen in MS, which is brought on by exercise. The paroxysmal weakness of MS comes on abruptly and is usually manifested as a total inability to use the limb. The weakness brought on by exercise is much more gradual in both onset and resolution and is therefore similar to the type of weakness seen in patients with myasthenia gravis (MG). The etiology of these rare attacks is obscure.

PAROXYSMAL BRAIN STEM DYSFUNCTION

Some patients have paroxysmal slurred speech, ataxia, hemifacial spasm,[407] double vision, or some combination of these symptoms (so-called "paroxysmal dysarthria with ataxia") at the onset or later during the clinical course of MS. Episodes of paroxysmal dysarthria with ataxia often are both brief in duration (30 to 60 seconds) and may recur many times a day. When such symptoms occur at the onset, the clinician must consider transient brain stem ischemia in the differential diagnosis. The complex nature of these bouts suggests brain stem ischemia, but in MS, they are carbamazepine responsive (frequently only a very low dose is necessary) and self-limiting and therefore are likely due to physiological mechanisms.

PAROXYSMAL PAINS

Trigeminal neuralgia is the most common paroxysmal pain in MS and when seen in a young adult is suggestive of MS. TN starting after the age of 50 in persons without MS is usually idiopathic. Other radicular pains can also be paroxysmal.[345] (See Pain section previously and in Chapter 5).

DIAGNOSIS AND MANAGEMENT OF PAROXYSMAL PHENOMENA

The evaluation of patients with isolated paroxysmal symptoms is made easier by the advent of paraclinical laboratory studies such as MRI and CSF electrophoresis. Unfortunately, single MRI abnormalities are not any more specific for MS than are single clinical manifestations. Even though helpful, MRI and other paraclinical test abnormalities must be interpreted with caution because of their lack of specificity.

Any of these paroxysmal symptoms can become disabling if persistent, but they can usually be suppressed or stopped by carbamazepine, phenytoin, or benzodiazepines. Because the time course of paroxysmal events is usually one of clusters, prolonged therapy is not usually necessary. The physiology of the paroxysmal disturbances is unknown. Because they are usually not associated with the acute onset of other neurological symptoms, they are commonly thought to be due to a physiological disturbance, perhaps transient changes in the microenvironment of demyelinated axons, causing those axons to discharge and propagate spontaneous electrical discharges across, as well as along, fiber tracts (ephaptic transmission). The fact that they respond to anticonvulsants supports the concept that paroxysmal symptoms in MS are electrical events which are subcortical in origin.

The location of the lesion(s) in patients with these syndromes is not consistent. In three of our patients with PTS, MRI scans showed a single enhancing internal capsule lesion in one, a brain stem lesion in another, and no lesion in a third.

DEMENTIA AND AFFECTIVE DISORDERS

Occasionally MS presents with personality change, loss of memory, inattentiveness, word-finding difficulty, or even dementia.[205,331,332,347,402] For example, Vighetto and colleagues[426] reported on a 37-year-old man with presentation as an amnestic syndrome. Psychological and cognitive features are more likely to be noticed by the family and friends than by the patients themselves. Depression or manic-depressive, or bipolar, disorder (BPD) can be the presenting symptom.[286] Depression is frequently seen in MS and must be distinguished from pseudodepression due to organic involvement of the brain.[47] BPD is an associated disease with familial elements. We have observed quite a few instances in which MS and BPD coexisted. The presentation of BPD after the onset of MS is easily recognized, but BPD followed by MS is more difficult to detect. Aphasia is rare in MS but has been described as the presenting feature.[20a] An encephalopathic onset may be seen in an acute form of MS called Baló's concentric sclerosis.[45a,142a]

CASE HISTORY: Multiple Sclerosis Onset with Dementia in a Young Adult

A 37-year-old nurse was seen for evaluation of memory loss. Over 3½ years she had gradually increasing problems with memory, both recent and long term. Also, at the age of 34 years, she had an episode of right arm weakness that lasted 2 weeks. A diagnosis of "reversible ischemic neurological deficit" secondary to embolus from mitral valve prolapse was made at that time. At age 35 years, after experiencing 1 year of progressive memory failure and personality change, she had an episode of transient left facial numbness and double vision that lasted several days. Eight months later, she developed left leg weakness and gait difficulty, but the neurological examination was normal. Four months later, her memory and spatial deficits were so severe that when she returned to her job at a hospital in which she had worked for 10 years, she had difficulty finding her way around. No neurological abnormality was found on examination save for cognitive impairment. She was admitted to a psychiatric service because of increased anxiety and depression. She was alert and fully oriented, but she had obvious difficulty with her recent memory and could not recall the details of her hospitalization a month previously. Her thinking was very concrete. She had a performance IQ of 80, verbal IQ of 93 and a memory quotient of 86. She had bilateral optic pallor with a mild, right-sided facial droop. Reflexes were brisk in the left arm. The plantar responses were bilaterally flexor. There was some left arm dysmetria. Sensory examination was normal. Gait was slow and deliberate and slightly wide based. She could not do tandem gait. CSF showed OB, and a CT scan showed multiple periventricular hypodensities. A diagnosis of MS was made. The patient became progressively demented and paranoid. By the age of 39 years, she was institutionalized, yet she remained fully ambulatory.

Comment: Cognitive change greatly overshadowed subtle neurological impairment, and hysteria was diagnosed by two experienced neurologists early in this patient's course.

Fatigue and Other Onset Symptoms

Fatigue can be the first symptom in persons who eventually develop MS (see Chapter 5), although focal neurological symptoms and signs are usually present. The fatigue can be either focal muscle fatigability, as in MG, or a generalized sense of lassitude. Most patients with a generalized fatigue syndrome do not have MS; therefore, the clinician does not usually think of MS in the differential diagnosis of fatigue.

Autonomic symptoms and signs are rare as presenting features. Neurogenic pulmonary edema[138] and cardiovascular instability[16] have been seen at onset.

Motor Presentations

AMYOTROPHY

Because the hallmark of MS pathology is demyelination with sparing of the axon, MS is not expected to produce amyotrophy. However, axonal sparing is only relative. Muscle wasting in MS was recognized by Charcot, who noted that the responsible plaques could be located in the anterior horn of the spinal cord. In contrast, Table 4–11 lists reports of CNS involvement in chronic demyelinating neuropathy.

Focal muscle wasting in MS is often due to nerve entrapment. For example, ulnar

Table 4–11. CENTRAL NERVOUS SYSTEM LESIONS IN PATIENTS WITH DEMYELINATING POLYNEUROPATHY OR POLYRADICULOPATHY

Year	Senior Author	Findings
1966	Rosenblum[361]	Two autopsied cases of polyradiculopathy in which there was marked dorsal column demyelination and anterior horn cell loss. Cord changes possibly secondary to the severe dorsal and anterior root axonal damage.
1987	Mendell[269]	Six of 16 patients with chronic inflammatory polyradiculopathy had multiple CNS lesions on MRI scan.
1987	Thomas[409]	Six cases of chronic demyelinating peripheral neuropathy with superimposed relapsing multifocal CNS disorder and abnormal MRI head scans.
1990	Feasby[119]	One of 19 patients with chronic inflammatory demyelinating polyneuropathy had bilateral Babinski signs, whereas 7/19 had two or more lesions on the MRI head scan; 1 had an infarct and 5 were older than 55 years of age. One patient, aged 38, had two small subcortical lesions suggestive of vasculitis or MS.

CNS = central nervous system; MRI = magnetic resonance imaging.

nerve entrapment at the elbow is not unusual in patients with MS, particularly in those who are bedridden or confined to a wheelchair. Nevertheless, several studies have now shown that focal muscle atrophy is frequent in longstanding MS in the absence of entrapment.[83] Pathological studies have shown that atrophy in MS can be due to the involvement of the gray matter of the spinal cord with severe demyelinating lesions that include loss of anterior horn cells or axons. Atrophy can be due to a motor root exit zone lesion. Amyotrophy is not always restricted to severely disabled patients. Occasionally an MS patient can present with regional muscle wasting suggesting amyotrophic lateral sclerosis (ALS).[83] This finding at presentation would suggest that multiple roots or segments are involved in some destructive process. When a single motor nerve root is involved, it will produce a segmental motor syndrome.[304]

In a survey of more than 100 ambulatory patients with MS, one of the authors (Paty, 1978) found a number of patients with evidence for denervation in one or more limbs. None of the patients had nerve or root entrapment by electrophysiological criteria. In addition, there have been several reports of peripheral nerve disease occurring in MS,[107,335,434,435] so one must be aware of the possible coexistence of peripheral nervous system (PNS) and CNS disease (see Tables 4–11 and 4–12).

DROPPED (ABSENT) REFLEXES

Dropped reflexes are uncommon early in the course of MS. An absent biceps jerk is most commonly seen in MS and, only slightly less often, an absent triceps jerk. Inverted upper extremity reflexes are fairly common in patients with disabling spinal MS, and usually this finding implies a root entry zone lesion combined with corticospinal involvement at that segment or at a higher segment (see subsequently). This abnormality may be seen in the form of an inverted triceps reflex, where the triceps jerk is usually absent but the brachioradialis reflex is hyperactive. That sign indicates two separate lesions in the nervous system. The depressed triceps reflex is due to the interruption of the C7 reflex arc, and the

Table 4–12. **SOME CONDITIONS THAT MIGHT BE CONFUSED WITH MULTIPLE SCLEROSIS: DISSEMINATION IN TIME BUT NOT SPACE**

AVM (cerebral, brain stem, or spinal)
Familial cavernous hemangiomata (hemisphere or brain stem)
Tumor (cerebral, brain stem, or spinal)
Thoracic disk protrusion
Cervical spondylosis
Toxic exposure with recurrent neuropathy
Arnold-Chiari malformation
Foramen magnum lesions, arachnoid cysts
Periodic cerebellar ataxias
Leber's optic atrophy
Familial spastic paraplegia
Adult-onset leukodystrophies (metachromatic adrenomyeloneuropathy; Eldridge's, Alexander's disease)

AVM = arteriovenous malformation.

hyperactive reflex is due to a corticospinal lesion above the C6 level. This combination of signs may be an instance where one single tap of a reflex hammer can demonstrate dissemination in space.

With advanced paraparesis or paraplegia, lower extremity reflexes may be lost, and occasional patients appear to be completely areflexic in the absence of signs of peripheral neuropathy. When reflexes are diminished or absent, other causes should be vigorously sought. (We have recognized coexistent disorders such as nitrofurantoin neuropathy, arachnoiditis, or idiopathic demyelinating neuropathy). In many such patients with long-standing, severe MS and paraplegia (quadriplegia) and reduced or absent reflexes, longitudinally extensive MS lesions are clearly visible on spinal MRI scans.

FACIAL MYOKYMIA

When first described, facial myokymia was thought to be an unusual finding in MS,[13] but careful follow-up has shown myokymia to be relatively common. It presents as spontaneous undulating waves of contracting muscle fibers in the facial musculature, either bilateral or unilateral.[162] When severe, it can suggest facial hemispasm. It usually does not persist, although in some patients, it reproducibly reappears with fatigue. Electromyographic investigation suggests continuous spontaneous discharges in the facial nucleus. Although facial myokymia can produce distressing symptoms, it is usually benign in its effects. Facial myokymia responds to therapy with benzodiazepines or anticonvulsants. Facial hemispasm can also occur in MS, but is usually unrelated to myokymia.

THIRD NERVE PALSY

Only a few cases of third nerve palsy have been reported as the initial symptom of MS.[298,421,422] One report was of a patient with a complete third nerve palsy after a flu-like illness of one month's duration. The patient recovered spontaneously and went on to develop unsteady gait, hyperreflexia, ataxia, and extensor plantar responses. The authors have never seen a *complete* third nerve palsy in MS. Pupillary abnormalities other than the afferent pupillary defect are also uncommon in MS (3 percent), and incomplete third nerve palsies may resemble INO. The acute onset of a painful third nerve palsy suggests aneurysmal compression of the third nerve. Because it is so uncommon in MS, patients who develop a third nerve palsy should have the usual investigations to exclude non-MS causes.

CHRONIC PROGRESSIVE OR MONOSYMPTOMATIC RELAPSING SYNDROMES

Accurate diagnosis of chronic progressive and monosymptomatic relapsing syndromes is the most difficult. Most monosymptomatic presentations are spinal cord syndromes, but progressive visual loss or cerebellar or brain stem deficits can also occur. Some patients also have monosymptomatic relapsing-remitting disease, such as recurrent acute myelopathies, without evidence of dissemination in space. The slowly progressive onset is usually seen in older patients, although it can occasionally develop in young adults. In the past, many such patients have been subjected to extensive investigations before the appropriate diagnosis was made. It is in this clinical setting that MRI and other paraclinical tests, including CSF analysis for OB, can be most helpful. Unfortunately, because these monofocal syndromes are seen most frequently in older patients, the problem of nonspecificity of the abnormalities seen in paraclinical tests is a serious problem (see MRI section).

PHYSICAL EXAMINATION OF THE PATIENT WITH SUSPECTED MULTIPLE SCLEROSIS

Multiple sclerosis, being the complex disease that it is, requires meticulous examination to better understand the patient's complaints. Many times no appropriate physical findings accompany the symptoms, or the physical findings indicate lesions other than those suggested by the symptoms. When neurological signs are found that indicate dysfunction in white matter tracts unsuspected from the history, it is diagnostically helpful. For example, when a patient complains of sensory disturbance in one leg, there may be no detectable sensory loss, but an extensor plantar response may be seen in either the symptomatic or the asymptomatic leg or, even more frequently, in both legs. When no appropriate findings accompany the symptoms, EPs or MRI may be helpful in detecting diagnostically important asymptomatic white matter lesions. Certain areas of the neurological examination are particularly difficult and the following points may be helpful:

Nystagmus. Nystagmus at the end point may be physiological or drug induced, but abducting eye nystagmus that is irregular in amplitude and rhythm (ataxic nystagmus) is suggestive of medial longitudinal fasciculus involvement. Subtle abducting eye nystagmus in MS may be made more prominent by position change, especially by lying down. Therefore, examining the patient for nystagmus both sitting and immediately after lying down can be helpful. Also, the lateral gaze or ataxic nystagmus seen in MS may be brought out and sustained if the eyes are first taken to the extreme end point of lateral gaze and then brought back toward the midline by a few degrees.

Eye Movements. The most subtle eye movement disorder is that of loss of smooth pursuit. This finding might be missed if one examines pursuit movements either too fast or too slowly. However, a slow rate of pursuit is probably better than a fast rate because the saccadic pursuit phenomenon can be missed with faster movements. As noted previously, persistent subtle slowness of adduction on lateral gaze strongly suggests INO.

Sensory Testing. Easily detectable and reproducible dissociated pinprick and temperature levels rarely persist beyond the acute relapse. When they do persist, the deficits have a tendency to be patchy and variable and are usually in association with deficits attributed to posterior column involvement. In contrast, vibratory and proprioceptive deficits are very characteristic of MS and frequently persist, although they can be subtle. Therefore, threshold testing is indicated. These deficits also can be selective, such as a vibratory and proprioceptive deficit localized to the ulnar side of the hand but sparing the median fingers.

The clinician must remember that in the useless hand syndrome, the deficit may actually be solely due to loss of proprioception and feedback control of movement. This phenomenon can be shown easily by testing strength both with eyes closed and with eyes open, concentrating on visual control of the movement being tested. A pseudo-motor deficit will improve dramatically under visual control.

Deep Tendon Reflexes (DTRs). When detecting asymmetrical DTRs, the clinician must always confirm the asymmetry, however, especially if the diagnosis depends on the findings. The reflexes should be tested in more than one position, because subtle but physiologically important changes will persist after position changes. Absent or markedly depressed reflexes are important segmental signs. A lost reflex identifies the side and the spinal segment involved and can be useful in identifying dissemination in space. An absent biceps or brachioradialis reflex is best elicited with the patient sitting with the arms in the lap, but an inverted triceps reflex is best elicited by having the examiner support the arm in 90-degree abduction, in order that the medially rotated shoulder can allow the arm to swing dependently. The inverted triceps reflex is due to an absent triceps reflex spreading to a hyperactive biceps and brachioradialis. It is easily seen in the position as described and indicates both a segmental lesion at C7 and a hyperactive response at C5–6. As mentioned, this one test supplies evidence for dissemination in space, with lesions both at the C7 segment and in the pyramidal tract above C7. The inverted brachioradialis reflex is also seen in MS, suggesting both root lesion and cord involvement at C6 with a hyperactive reflex at C7.

Plantar Response. Some patients with very active plantar responses will have triple flexion after stroking the sole of the foot. However, a consistent asymmetry in DTRs is a convincing sign of corticospinal tract damage, even if the plantar responses are normal.

Superficial Reflexes. The abdominal reflexes are commonly lost in early corticospinal disease and an asymmetry helps confirm the meaningfulness of asymmetry of DTRs. It is helpful to know that abdominal reflexes are commonly present despite marked corticospinal involvement in Amyotrophic Lateral Sclerosis (ALS) or Primary Lateral Sclerosis (PLS).

DISEASES THAT MIGHT BE CONFUSED WITH MULTIPLE SCLEROSIS

In this section we describe conditions that might be confused with MS because they can present as lesions disseminated in time, space, or both.[379]

Some Conditions That Might Be Confused with Multiple Sclerosis: Dissemination in Time but Not Space

Conditions that can mimic MS by producing relapsing-remitting disease confined to one focal area of the CNS are listed in Table 4–12. For example, spinal AVM, if diagnosed early, can be treated by surgery or embolization so that serious disability does not develop. To properly identify such treatable diseases, appropriate tests must be done. Dural or spinal AVMs are notoriously difficult to diagnose clinically and even at the time of myelography. The most sensitive myelographic technique is to do the myelogram with the patient in both the supine and prone positions. A direct diagnosis of MS or AVM can be made by using MRI and CSF analysis, avoiding expensive and risky procedures such as spinal angiography, even though MRI can miss spinal AVMs. The following cases indicate how congenital and vascular conditions can mimic MS by producing symptoms and signs that fluctuate over time:

CASE HISTORY: Arnold-Chiari Malformation

This 26-year-old woman had a 7-year history of daily burning headaches. The pain was made worse with noise, excitement, and flexion or rotation of the neck. She considered herself clumsy from the age of 12 years. Her clumsiness worsened when she was tired. She had generalized fatigue and muscle pain, with one 3-day episode of severe muscle pain and weakness several months before examination. Two months before examination, she blacked out at work and had difficulty with speech and facial numbness when she awoke. She then began to experience weekly episodes of dizziness, and over several months, she noticed numbness of her fingers for 3 to 4 hours a day over periods of 3 or 4 days at a time. She also noted double vision on one occasion, which lasted for an evening but cleared by morning, food sticking in her mouth and regurgitating through her nose, dysarthria,

oscillopsia, and episodic hoarseness. She also had urinary urgency and hesitancy. Neurological examination revealed horizontal nystagmus in both eyes on lateral gaze and vertical nystagmus on down gaze. The corneal reflex and nasal tickle were depressed. The gag reflex and uvula movement were poor. Sensory and motor examination were normal. All DTRs were active. The left plantar response was equivocal and the right was downgoing. There was some evidence of truncal ataxia and tandem gait was poor.

Multiple sclerosis was suspected. CSF analysis showed normal IgG, glucose, protein and protein electrophoresis. Blink reflexes were normal. VEPs were delayed in the left eye, with no response in the right. A CT scan showed small areas of slightly increased density in the basal ganglia bilaterally.

One year later, she developed bitemporal headache, sore throat, joint pain, and fatigue. Laboratory investigations again were negative except for the previously seen VEP delay. The CT scan was unchanged. There was no hydrocephalus. Her grossly abnormal eye findings persisted.

The diagnosis of Arnold-Chiari malformation was suggested. A myelogram showed no evidence for syrinx but did show an impression bilaterally at the level of C1 consistent with an Arnold-Chiari malformation type I. A suboccipital craniectomy and upper cervical laminectomy revealed bilateral tonsillar herniation. She was markedly improved postoperatively; headache, tingling in the fingers, and oscillopsia ceased. Gait was gradually improving at the time of discharge.

Comment: Chronic headache is not usual in MS. The symptoms and signs characteristic of lesions at the craniovertebral junction are often interpreted as showing dissemination in space, and when they fluctuate, they may also suggest dissemination in time.

CASE HISTORY: Clivus Chordoma

A 22-year-old male student had progressive ataxia and intermittent diplopia beginning at age 15 years. He subsequently developed urinary urgency, a progressive right hemiplegia, and dysphagia. A CT scan was reported as normal. A diagnosis of MS was made. There was no visual involvement and no acute attacks. He had gross direction-changing horizontal nystagmus, most coarse on left lateral gaze. There was also periodic alternating nystagmus. Visual acuity was

20/20 bilaterally, the fundi were normal, and there were no scotomas. There was left palatal weakness and the patient's tongue deviated to the right. There was mild ataxia in all limbs, with a right spastic hemiparesis and general hyperreflexia. Toes were upgoing. Gait was hemiparetic, spastic, and slightly ataxic. Repeated CT scans, angiography, and subsequent metrizamide myelocisternography showed a vertically oblong, 3.5 × 2.5-cm, partly calcific mass, at the level of the foramen magnum in the left half of the vertebral canal, displacing the cord and the medulla to the right. Pathological features were of a chordoma.

Comment: The asymmetrical findings suggesting both spinal and brain stem involvement plus an initially normal CT scan led to an incorrect diagnosis of MS.

CASE HISTORY: Thoracic Arteriovenous Malformation

A 63-year-old right-handed, retired businessman developed diffuse sore spots in his legs and back 8 months previously. Subsequently, within a period of 30 minutes, he developed saddle numbness, was unable to sit, and lost control of his bowel and bladder. He improved somewhat over 4 months and remained ambulatory. He was found to be moderately weak in the legs. Reflexes were absent, and there was patchy distal loss of pinprick sensation. Over the subsequent 4 months, he became progressively paraplegic and incontinent. He had a flaccid paraplegia with a positive Beevor's sign. Pinprick and light touch sensation were decreased below T10. Position sense was impaired to the hips. Vibration sense was diminished at the anterior superior iliac crest but normal at the sternum. Myelography showed numerous serpiginous vessels extending from the level of T7–12 in the thoracic region, compatible with a thoracic AVM. The spinal cord and nerve roots were normal.

Comment: This myelopathy was relapsing but never disseminated in space. A persistent dense sensory level to pinprick is unusual in MS.

CASE HISTORY: Fourth Ventricular Arteriovenous Malformation

A 26-year-old right-handed woman developed dizziness and double vision. Three weeks previ-

ously, she noted general malaise, positional vertigo, and nausea. She also had double vision on left lateral gaze, dysphagia for liquids, and had several short-lived, mild right frontal headaches. A similar episode without visual complaints occurred 6 months previously with spontaneous remission. She had normal visual fields. Visual acuity was 20/40 on the right and 20/30 on the left. There was an occasional beat of nystagmus at rest, as well as in all directions of gaze. She had a right gaze palsy and a marked right lower motor neuron facial palsy. Tearing was decreased in the right eye. Muscle tone and power were normal. She had slight gait ataxia and decrease in vibration sense on the right side. CSF showed 725 red cells, 5 white cells, and slight xanthochromia. Hematological and biochemistry studies were normal. Auditory EPs and vertebral angiography were normal. CT scan showed a high-density lesion in the fourth ventricle, suggestive of either a hemorrhage or a calcified mass. Four weeks later, she was readmitted with increased dysphagia and ataxia. A second CT scan showed that the lesion had doubled in size. A right pontine fourth ventricle hematoma was successfully removed. The ataxia, facial palsy, and gaze paresis completely resolved.

Comment: The symptoms in this patient were disseminated in time but not in space. MS was suspected in part because she was a 26-year-old woman, the context in which MS often is first seen. Because the brain stem contains a large number of neuronal pathways, dissemination in space is sometimes suggested erroneously.

Some Conditions That Might Be Confused with Multiple Sclerosis: Dissemination in Space but Probably Not in Time

Diseases that can present with a polysymptomatic onset mimicking MS are listed in Table 4–13. Chronically developing degenerative disease such as spinocerebellar degeneration, Strümpell's disease, and Charcot-Marie-Tooth neuropathy can occasionally be associated with subacute optic neuropathy, so that differentiating them from MS could be a problem. Three recently described patients developed multifocal inflammatory leukoencephalopathy

Table 4–13. SOME CONDITIONS THAT MIGHT BE CONFUSED WITH MULTIPLE SCLEROSIS: DISSEMINATION IN SPACE BUT PROBABLY NOT IN TIME

Multiple cerebral emboli

Cerebral vasculitis

Thrombotic thrombocytopenic purpura

Idiopathic thrombocytopenic purpura

Mitochondrial encephalomyopathies

Acute disseminated encephalomyelitis

Glioblastoma

Progressive multifocal leukoencephalopathy

Subacute combined degeneration of the spinal cord

Sarcoidosis

Behçet's disease

Lyme disease

Mycoplasma pneumonia encephalopathy

Adult-onset leukodystrophies

Table 4–14. SOME CONDITIONS THAT MIMIC MULTIPLE SCLEROSIS: DISSEMINATION IN BOTH TIME AND SPACE

Hypertensive cerebrovascular disease

Multiple cerebral emboli: paroxysmal atrial fibrillation, mitral valve prolapse, myocardial infarction, mural thrombus, myxoma of the mitral valve, etc.

Subacute myelo-optic neuritis (SMON)

Familial cavernous hemangiomata

Cerebral lymphoma

Acute intermittent porphyria

Cerebral vasculitis

Lupus erythematosus

Eale's disease

Lyme disease

HIV disease with recurrent encephomyelopathy

Sjögren's syndrome

Mitochondrial disease

Myasthenia gravis

Migratory sensory neuritis

Chronic arachnoiditis

Co-occurrence of two or more neurological diseases, such as diabetic neuropathy with ischemic optic neuropathy

HIV = human immunodeficiency virus.

after treatment of bowel cancer with 5-fluorouracil and levamisole.[182] Adult-onset leukodystrophies and various toxic neuropathies can also present with symptoms disseminated in space but not time.

Some Conditions That Mimic Multiple Sclerosis: Dissemination in Both Time and Space

The conditions most likely to become confused with MS are the cerebrovascular diseases, including hypertensive cerebrovascular disease (CVD) with lacunar infarcts (Table 4–14). Lacunar disease is usually clearly and easily identifiable by the associated significant degree of sustained hypertension and the older age of the patient. The presence of hypertension does not, however, necessarily mean that the symptoms are not due to MS. MS can certainly present after the age of 50 years, so that the differentiation can be difficult. Because the MRI appearance of MS and hypertensive cerebrovascular disease can be very similar, VEP and CSF analysis become important in distinguishing the two.

In addition, the syndromes produced by multiple cerebral emboli from subtle cardiac abnormalities, such as MVP, patent foramen ovale, or subendocardial infarction, can be clinically indistinguishable from MS, particularly when they occur in young adults.[379]

Subacute myelo-optic neuritis (SMON) is a disease of the spinal cord and optic nerve first seen in Japan over 20 years ago.[296] Usually associated with gastrointestinal symptoms, SMON was shown to be neurotoxicity secondary to clioquinol use. The pattern of symptoms could mimic MS, but now that clioquinol use has been limited, this disease is rare. We have seen no examples in the last decade.

Primary lymphomas (T cell or B cell) of the brain can mimic MS by having both symptoms and enhancing multifocal CNS lesions that relapse and remit. CT and MRI scans can look exactly like MS, with the lesions and clinical signs both being steroid responsive. Because of the prolonged clinical course in some of these patients, brain biopsy may be necessary for an accurate diagnosis.

Two HIV-positive patients with a fulminating leukoencephalopathy and pathology compatible with MS have been recently described.[156] The possible relationship between HIV and MS is obscure. Many other diseases listed in Table 4–14 can mimic MS.

In addition to single disease states that mimic MS, a combination of neurological problems evolving over time may easily be misdiagnosed as MS. For example, diabetic neuropathy producing sensory loss associated with diabetic retinopathy or ischemic optic neuropathy causing visual disturbances can suggest MS. Central vascular retinopathy with monocular visual loss and scotoma occurring in someone with cervical spondylosis has also been confused with MS.

Finally, clinicians must not accept previous neurological diagnoses without reservation. They must listen carefully to the history, particularly the symptoms, as a required check for the plausibility of previous diagnostic labels. They must never accept a previous diagnosis of MS until it can be substantiated by either a convincing history, clinical notes, or current investigations—preferably all three.

Hysterical (Psychoneurotic or Functional) Symptoms and the Onset of Multiple Sclerosis

Many patients with MS begin with fleeting sensory symptoms that are not easily described. As mentioned previously, a recent study of patients with ON found that nonspecific sensory symptoms before the onset of ON were a strong risk factor for the subsequent development of MS.[34] The patient is usually experiencing a number of symptoms that, to them, are clearly organic. The early symptoms of MS can be evanescent in nature, and the lack of hard clinical findings may make them poorly understood by both the patient and the physician. Such patients may be labeled as neurotic or hysterical. Under these circumstances, the physician can understand why patients could then become preoccupied with their symptoms. Frustrated and confused patients may develop "overlay" symptoms that suggest conversion reaction or hysteria.[417] In some cases, patients will consciously or unconsciously exaggerate their symptoms and deficits, perhaps because of the fear of not being taken seriously. This new development then makes it even more difficult for the physician, who must interpret which symptoms are due to organic lesions and which are due to psychological mechanisms and introspection. It should be emphasized, however, that "clinical signs of hysteria" (Hoover's sign, etc.) are common in patients with organic CNS disease, especially MS.[20]

CASE HISTORY: Hysterical Paralysis Superimposed on a Relapse of Multiple Sclerosis

A 30-year-old woman, mother of two children, with CDMS had a clinical course characterized by relapses and remissions of sensory loss, ON, and diplopia. Her MS was quite benign until she began to take on more and more responsibility for her husband's and children's leisure activity, in spite of her fatigue. She then had an acute relapse of sensory symptoms in the legs, which was treated with IV-pulsed methylprednisolone. After two doses, she developed an irregular heartbeat and dyspnea. The next day, she developed a paraplegia, even as the sensory loss resolved. She was thought to have had a severe motor relapse of MS and was treated in her local hospital with physical therapy.

When we saw her again, she had been paraplegic for 3 weeks. On examination, she had optic atrophy and some residual vibratory loss in the legs, but the weakness was inconsistent and DTRs were normal. With encouragement, she began to recover, and within 3 days, she could be discharged with almost normal leg function. She was advised to reduce her commitments outside the home.

Comment: This woman developed a hysterical paraplegia precipitated by a reaction to steroids superimposed upon a relapse of MS. The condition was prolonged by her anxiety concerning her ability to continue with her hectic schedule outside the home. Reassurance and a reduction in expectations allowed her to recover to her previously mildly abnormal neurological state.

Unfortunately MS and hysterical overlay are found together so frequently that the skills of even the most experienced clinician are taxed. True physical symptoms are among the most common precipitants of conversion reactions in susceptible individuals. A parallel is found with pseudo-seizures and epilepsy because many patients who have hysterical seizures or pseudoseizures also have epilepsy.[417] At the onset of MS, such hysterical overlay symptoms can be confusing, and it is always best to assume the presence of an underlying organic disorder and to look for it carefully. There is no quicker way to alienate patients and cause emotional turmoil than to tell them that their symptoms, which they know are organic, are due to emotional mechanisms (or, as the patient may interpret it, "in my head"). Finally, one should always consider the cognitive and affective abnormalities common in MS as either causative or contributory to physical or emotional symptoms or both.

Psychophysiological symptoms are a natural phenomenon. It is the emotional reaction to such symptoms that causes so much distress in patients and misunderstanding by the physician. Patients with psychophysiological symptoms, whether superimposed on MS, will respond to sympathetic concern and can worsen significantly if treated with indifference and neglect. Because psychophysiological symptoms and conditions can be severely disabling, early recognition and sympathetic concern and supportive encouragement is important. Referral to a knowledgeable psychiatrist can be helpful, but many neurologists find success in explaining these symptoms in biologic terms that are palatable to patients.

DIFFERENTIAL DIAGNOSIS OF MULTIPLE SCLEROSIS

Acute Disseminated Encephalomyelitis

Acute disseminated encephalomyelitis is characteristically a polysymptomatic syndrome that may begin after an upper respiratory or other viral infection or immuniza-tion.[158,177,203, 226,368] More frequently seen in children than in adults, ADEM is characterized by a multifocal neurological presentation suggesting simultaneous or sequential involvement of the brain stem, spinal cord, optic nerve, or cerebrum and/or cerebellum. Patients with ADEM can be febrile and acutely ill, and the clinical course can be complicated by convulsions, pneumonia, and death. Mortality can be as high as 20 percent, but substantial recovery can be seen in at least half the patients. Large neurological centers in Canada and the northern United States see perhaps two or three well-defined examples of ADEM each year, compared with 150 new cases of MS in a similar period. Table 4–15 gives the salient characteristics that can help the physician to distinguish ADEM from MS.

The best described pathological description of ADEM is the post–rabies vaccination cases from Japan reported by Shiraki and Oani.[391] The pathological process was characterized by inflammatory perivenous demyelination. The changes were indistinguishable from those of acute MS, except that the ADEM lesions tended to be smaller and more widely disseminated throughout the CNS than those of typical MS. Five percent of such patients will develop MS.[158,175] We have seen one case of ADEM in which the MRI scan showed little abnormality in the setting of otherwise unexplained coma, indicating the small size of lesions in some cases. Some of the patients with the syndrome of acute neuromyelitis optica have ADEM and some will demonstrate MS on follow-up.

Acute MS can also present as a fulminating illness that is multifocal in character with subsequent relapses.[341] Cases have been reported associated with herpes virus-6.[66a] Is this disease MS or is it a relapsing form of ADEM? Paraclinical tests are not helpful in making the distinction; lesions detected by MRI in both instances are disseminated throughout the white matter.[216] Unfortunately, the MRI patterns of ADEM and MS cannot be reliably distinguished from each other. OB may be present in both diseases, although in our series of 12 patients with ADEM from London, Ontario, none has had CSF OB during the acute phase of the illness (Ebers, 1990). The early absence of

Table 4–15. **CHARACTERISTICS OF ACUTE DISSEMINATED ENCEPHALOMYELITIS (ADEM) VERSUS MULTIPLE SCLEROSIS**

	ADEM	MS
Age:	Childhood more than adulthood	Usually young adult
Antecedent:	URI or immunization	Can be precipitated by URI and rarely immunization
Onset:	Polysymptomatic	Frequently monosymptomatic
Constitutional symptoms:	Yes	Usually no, except fatigue
Recurrence:	No (rare)	Likely
MRI findings:	Multifocal lesions	Multifocal lesions
CSF findings:	Cells, increased IgG, OB+ (<50%)	Cells, increased IgG, OB+ (95%)
Optic neuritis:	Frequently bilateral	Usually unilateral
Acute transverse myelitis:	Common	Uncommon (partial cord syndromes frequent)
Progressive symptoms:	No	Frequently

URI = upper respiratory infection.
OB+ = oligoclonal banding–positive.

OB in ADEM may be a useful differential point. Occasionally we have seen patients with a relapsing-remitting polysymptomatic CNS disease after vaccination. This disease is probably MS, but some would call it a relapsing form of ADEM.

Acute infectious mononucleosis (IM) has been one of the classic settings for the development of ADEM. A recent study,[237] however, found a relative risk for developing MS of 3.7 in patients who have had IM. Others have recently described a case of encephalopathy due to *Mycoplasma pneumoniae* in which the MRI appearance was similar to ADEM, MS, or both.

Cerebrovascular Disease

Numerous syndromes associated with CVD can mimic MS. The pattern often can satisfy the criterion for dissemination in time and space, and usually only clinical judgment and follow-up can distinguish primary vascular disease from MS in the young adult. Primary cerebral vasculitis, systemic lupus erythematosus, polyarteritis nodosa, and familial cavernous hemangiomata can occasionally mimic MS, as can hypertensive and atheromatous CVD. Eales' disease with neurological involvement (retinal periphlebitis, vitreous hemorrhage, flaccid paraplegia, or myelopathy with a sensory level and sphincteric disturbance) can also produce a similar syndrome.

Inflammatory Central Nervous System Disorders

Inflammatory neurological diseases such as Behçet's,[68] Lyme disease,[120,244] SS,[6,7] neurosarcoidosis,[86,272] and neurobrucellosis[63] can also mimic MS. Because the CSF findings can be similar in all of these conditions, CSF examination is not very helpful in making the differential diagnosis. When Behçet's disease presents with the characteristic mucocutaneous ulcerations, relapsing iridocyclitis, meningoencephalitis, confusion and dementia, thrombophlebitis, arthritis, and erythema nodosum, it is not difficult to distinguish from MS. Diagnostic criteria for Behçet's disease have been clearly established[189] and should aid clinicians in making the distinction from MS. Only about 10 to 25 percent of patients with Behçet's disease have neurological involvement. When Behçet's disease produces oculomotor palsies, spinal cord involvement, and occasionally optic neuropathy, differential diagnosis can be difficult.[3a] Behçet's disease is most frequently seen in the Middle and Far East. It can be associated with intracranial hypertension and papilledema. Such symptoms as headache, signs of meningeal irritation, and prostration are not features of MS and are common in Behçet's disease. The MRI findings include major changes in the basis pontis having some specificity for Behçet's disease.[4,437]

Neurobrucellosis, also known to produce optic neuropathy and cerebellar findings, could possibly be confused with MS. However, relapsing fevers are not part of MS.

Sarcoidosis can produce similar confusion because it can produce multifocal CNS involvement of the optic nerve,[155] brain stem, and spinal cord. Symptomatic hypothalamic involvement is also common in sarcoidosis and rare in MS. The diagnosis of sarcoidosis is a clinical one and ultimately rests on the histological examination of liver, skin, lungs, bone, conjunctiva, or other tissue (noncaseating sarcoid granulomata). Several cases of neurosarcoidosis have been reported to have multiple periventricular lesions similar to MS.[272] The administration of gadolinium shows diffuse leptomeningeal enhancement that is not usually seen in MS.[389]

Lyme disease (infection with *B. burgdorferi*) can produce neurological symptoms that might be confused with MS.[120,135,167,170,244,317] Even though the most frequently seen neurological syndrome in Lyme disease is that of a meningoencephalitis, some patients experience a delayed phase in which mononeuropathies or polyneuropathies, transverse myelopathy, and subacute encephalopathy can occur. MS-like syndromes have occurred in which MRI, EP, and CSF findings were all abnormal. In one study of 14 patients with Lyme disease,[120] 6 (43 percent) had MRI abnormalities, most showing multiple subcortical white matter lesions on the T_2-weighted image. One CNS lesion due to Lyme disease was biopsied[344] and showed reactive astrocytes, spongiform change, and gliosis, in addition to typical spirochetes. Therefore, the clinician should be alert to the possibility of Lyme disease masquerading as MS, especially in areas endemic for Lyme disease. If present, the infection with *B. burgdorferi* should be treated with a 2-week course of penicillin or intravenous ceftriaxone (2 g per day). A survey of patients with MS in an endemic area for Lyme disease, however, revealed only 19 of 283 CDMS patients to be positive for anti-

Table 4–16. **STUDIES OF THE POSSIBLE OVERLAP BETWEEN MULTIPLE SCLEROSIS AND SJÖGREN'S SYNDROME**

Year	Senior Author	Findings
1981	Alexander[7]	Eight patients had SS and CNS involvement. Five patients had aseptic meningitis. One had ATM and one had CPM. Lesions due to vasculitis?
1986	Alexander[6]	Twenty patients had SS and CNS involvement. (Sixteen of 20 were relapsing.) Eight had documented skin vasculitis. Five had oligoclonal banding.
1988	Alexander[5]	Fourteen of 38 SS patients had CNS MRI abnormalities; most patients with MRI abnormalities had CNS symptoms.
1988	Metz[271]	None of 42 patients with MS had SS. All patients with dry eyes and a positive Schirmer's test were on anticholinergic drugs. None of 42 had autoantibodies.
1989	Noseworthy[303]	None of 192 patients with MS had both clinical and serological evidence for SS. Fifty-five of 192 had a positive Schirmer's test, and 3/192 had a positive anti-Ro ELISA test.
1990	Miró[284]	Two of 64 consecutive patients with MS had SS. Seven of 64 had dry eyes. Two of seven with dry eyes had biopsy evidence for SS.
1991	Ellemann[109]	Two of 20 female patients with MS surveyed had SS, not an increased frequency over that expected.

ATM = acute transverse myelitis; CNS = central nervous system; CPM = chronic progressive myelopathy; ELISA = enzyme-linked immunosorbent assay; SS = Sjögren's syndrome.

bodies to *B. burgdorferi*.[76,78] In eight patients, repeated serologic tests were non-confirmatory. Of the others, only five had intrathecal production of antibody, and antibiotic treatment did not prevent subsequent relapses in these patients. The authors did not believe that serologic findings positive for Lyme disease without other features of the disease in MS patients was likely to be of significance.

Sjögren's syndrome is a common disease in which dry eyes and mucous membranes (sicca complex) may be associated with vasculitis of skin, muscle, and peripheral nerve. Twenty percent of SS patients have neurological involvement. Because MRI and CSF abnormalities suggesting MS also may occur,[5] one must be alert to this possibility in the differential diagnosis of MS. However, surveys of 42 and 192 consecutive MS patients[271,303] failed to find a single one that fit accepted diagnostic criteria for SS. A Swedish group[370] found 1 of 30 patients with MS to have primary SS and concluded that SS was not more common among patients with MS than among the general population. Another survey of 64 patients with MS from Spain[284] showed two patients positive for SS. Another survey in Denmark found 2 of 20 female patients with MS to have SS.[109] The possible overlap or association between MS and SS is yet to be clearly established. Table 4–16 cites several papers on the subject. Acute intermittent porphyria has also been described recently as producing reversible, focal white matter lesions that could be confused with MS.[219] Lupus erythematosus, even though the CNS lesions are not inflammatory, can present like MS with recurrent and disseminated neurological symptoms.[37]

MIGRATORY SENSORY NEURITIS

Migratory sensory neuritis (MSN) is a benign condition that Wartenberg[432] described as a syndrome of multifocal sensory symptoms. MSN characteristically migrates from site to site and can be painful, so confusion with MS, particularly early MS, can occur. Fortunately, most of the cases of MSN present with clear-cut cutaneous nerve involvement reminiscent of leprosy. The radial, sural, ulnar, and digital nerves are frequently involved. This pattern of sensory loss is not likely to be confused with MS. MSN causes focal loss of cutaneous sensation in the area of symptoms.

Metastatic and Remote Effects of Cancer (Paraneoplastic Syndromes)

Multiple metastases can occasionally present in such a way as to mimic MS. It is usually the relentless progressive features of metastatic disease, pain, or signs of increased intracranial pressure that allow it to be distinguished clinically from MS. If there is a known primary neoplasm, MS is not a likely diagnosis. MRI can help in distinguishing the focal lesions noted earlier from the typical disseminated lesions seen in MS.

The remote effects of cancer can rarely include bilateral INO, sensory and motor neuropathy, cerebellar ataxia, and ON. These conditions may occur as isolated manifestations but can also occur together, suggesting MS, especially when the lesions are disseminated in time.

Subacute Combined Degeneration of the Spinal Cord (Vitamin B$_{12}$ Deficiency)

Previously a common neurological disorder, SCD of the spinal cord is seen much less frequently now than in the past. This change is probably due to more accurate early diagnosis of anemia. SCD presents more often in older patients than does MS, and the findings are characteristically symmetrical and progressive. Loss of proprioceptive and discriminatory sensation in the legs is accompanied by gradual progression of weakness with pyramidal findings. Peripheral neuropathy with absent ankle jerks is common, and ON can also be seen. Dysesthesias are commonly seen. Even though uncommon, SCD must always be considered in the differential diagnosis of myelopathy, because it is treatable. A blood cell count, vitamin B_{12} levels, and Schilling's test should be done in all suspected cases. One case of pernicious anemia has been reported in which there was a cervical cord MRI lesion that went away after vitamin B_{12} treatment.[39]

Myasthenia Gravis

Myasthenia gravis may be misdiagnosed as MS[300] primarily because relapsing diplopia and weakness are symptoms common to both conditions (Table 4–17). Patients with MG who experience eye muscle weakness may complain of diplopia and have a "pseudo-INO" with abducting eye nystagmus. Another source of confusion is that patients with MG can complain of numbness, without objective sensory findings. MG is usually distinguished from MS by the absence of sensory and pyramidal findings, the tendency to have predominantly proximal rather than distal muscle weakness, the characteristic finding of neck, palatal, and respiratory muscle weakness (unusual in MS), electromyogram changes of jitter and decremental response to repetitive stimuli, and the presence of acetylcholine receptor (AChR) antibody. We have seen five cases of combined MG and MS, all of which were women. In several of our cases, both disorders were mild, suggesting that the combination is due to a benign autoimmune diathesis. One of the cases, a young woman, has had Hashimoto's thyroiditis, MG, and MS[242] and most recently has developed joint complaints and laboratory findings suggestive of rheumatoid arthritis. She is currently doing well except for minor MS symptoms.

HTLV-1-Associated Myelopathy (See Chapter 10)

In recent years a CPM seen in the Caribbean (TSP),[141,142] in Japan (HAM),[313] and in Canada[308a,333a] has been associated with HTLV-1 infection. The pathology of this disease differs from MS, but the clinical manifestations are of a progressive motor sensory myelopathy suggestive of the chronic spinal form of MS. MRI studies can show multiple cerebral lesions, and patients typically have OB in the CSF. Some patients with HAM or TSP have also been described as having ON, intention tremor, and double vision, therefore producing confusion with MS. We have never seen ON in this condition, but our experience is limited. MRI can usually differentiate MS from HAM in Japanese patients.[225a]

The differentiation of HAM or TSP from CPM of MS is a practical clinical problem.

Table 4–17. CHARACTERISTICS OF MYASTHENIA GRAVIS (MG) VERSUS MULTIPLE SCLEROSIS

	MG	MS
Muscle weakness:	Proximal > distal	Distal > proximal
Diplopia:	Yes	Yes
Fatigability:	Proximal greater than distal	Distal greater than proximal
Sensory loss:	No	Frequent
Pyramidal findings:	No	Frequent
Evoked potentials:	Normal	Frequent abnormalities
Single-fiber EMG and repetitive stimulation:	Frequently abnormal	Usually normal
CSF:	Normal	Abnormal
Acetylcholine receptor antibody:	Frequently present	Negative

CSF = cerebrospinal fluid; EMG = electromyogram.

The racial populations that have been found to be susceptible to HAM (blacks from the Caribbean, Japanese from the southern islands of Japan, and natives from the islands of the Indian Ocean) have moved to areas where MS is common and are presenting as cases of possible MS to clinicians who are not used to dealing with this particular problem. In addition, HTLV-1 antibodies are being found in people who have never been to the endemic areas. Some of these are related to transfusion. HTLV-1 myelopathy has been described in several patients in the United States and Europe with no known risk factors,[198] so it is obvious that we must be vigilant for this diagnostic possibility. In addition, a myelopathy associated with HTLV-1 antibodies has been described in native Canadians in British Columbia, Canada.[309] A high frequency of HTLV-1 myelopathy has also been found in an Iranian-born group of Mashhadi Jews[1] with some suggestion of genetic factors. It is necessary to test for antibodies to HTLV-1 in any patient with unexplained chronic myelopathies because transfusion and sexual contact have spread the disorder outside the areas traditionally deemed endemic.

Surveys of MS patients for evidence of HTLV-1 infection have produced conflicting results. Wattel and colleagues[433] could not find evidence for HTLV-1 infection in French patients with MS. Other surveys of HLTV-1 antibodies in patients with MS outside of Japan and other endemic areas[340] have failed to show any significant evidence of HLTV-1 antibody in patients with suspected MS or chronic myelopathy, except for the native indians of British Columbia.[309] In addition, several types of inflammatory neurological disease carry higher than normal levels of antibody to HTLV-1. There have been a few reports of low levels of HTLV-1 antibody in MS patients. The significance to MS of these antibodies has yet to be determined, but their presence must be considered in the context of a convincing body of information showing that patients with MS can have minor elevations of antibodies to a bewildering array of viruses. The antibody levels that have been seen in patients with MS have been low, in contrast to the high antibody levels seen in patients with HAM or TSP.

Acquired Immunodeficiency Syndrome Myelopathy and Other Human Immunodeficiency Virus Syndromes

Recent years have seen the detection of many neurological manifestations of acquired immunodeficiency syndrome (AIDS). The myelopathy of AIDS can present in much the same way as does the myelopathy of MS, and because patients with AIDS can also have multiple white matter lesions on MRI scan, the clinician must be alert to potential confusion with MS. There have been several reports of relapsing-remitting white matter disease in HIV-infected patients[42] in addition to AIDS-related polyradiculopathy.[405]

Herpes Zoster Myelitis

Herpes zoster (HZ) myelitis is another virus-induced myelopathy that occurs primarily in immunosuppressed patients.[88] The recognized cases begin about 12 days after the HZ rash. We have also seen a few MS patients whose onset began with a myelopathy following HZ. The relationship may be coincidental, but the occurrence should be noted.

Arachnoiditis

Arachnoiditis, which is poorly understood, may occur rarely as a familial disorder or, more commonly, as a result of a chronic inflammatory response to hemorrhage, myelography dye, or surgery. It can also be seen as a delayed complication of a previous bacterial or microbacterial cerebral spinal infection. Chronic arachnoiditis is a common cause of myelopathy in parts of Asia where tuberculosis is still endemic.

In North America, it is most commonly seen complicating myelography with the older oil-based contrast agents. Although arachnoiditis usually comes to attention in the clinical context of a progressive painful polyradiculopathy, occasionally the differential diagnosis of MS can be difficult. In one of our patients, myelopathy with thoracic spinal subarachnoid obliteration and block coexisted with progressive bilateral optic neuropathy. Arachnoiditis of the anterior visual pathways (optic nerve and chiasm) is rarely seen, and many of the older examples may have been secondary to syphilis or indeed may have occurred in patients with MS. Optic nerve involvement can occur, though, as part of a more diffuse arachnoiditis, and the presence of OB (commonly seen in this condition)[99,101] can cause even more diagnostic confusion.

In the patient described previously, the optic nerve involvement, myelopathy, and OB made MS seem likely, but MRI scanning of the head was normal; only cord atrophy was seen on spinal MRI. Repeated myelography demonstrated spinal subarachnoid narrowing and block. No evidence was found for extrinsic compression.

Chronic Fatigue Syndrome and Other Conditions

Chronic fatigue syndrome (CFS) is a perplexing condition that has not been clearly defined. A recent report[61] described 159 patients diagnosed with CFS, of whom 78% had MRI high-signal-intensity lesions. In 79 of 113 (70 percent), active replication of human herpesvirus type 6 was detected. These findings, though fascinating, need confirmation and do not yet establish the syndrome as a clinicopathological entity. A recent editorial[439] puts the syndrome into perspective.

Trichlorethelene poisoning has been seen to mimic MS.[306] Some reports have claimed an association between an "MS-like" syndrome and silicone breast implants.[315] We have not recognized such an association and a recent careful study from the Mayo Clinic found no such association.[130a] Adult-onset leukodystrophy can also mimic MS.[378]

CLINICAL AND PARACLINICAL TESTS TO HELP IN DIAGNOSIS

General Principles

The principles involved in the use of paraclinical tests in the diagnosis of MS are no different from those applied to the clinical diagnosis.[217,322,323] The general aim is to satisfy the criterion for dissemination in time and space using critical clinical judgment. Paraclinical studies, including EPs and brain imaging to detect lesions disseminated in space, should be considered extensions of the neurological examination. The evaluation of CSF fluid for OB or laboratory evidence for increased IgG synthesis rates is not relevant to space or time dissemination but is nevertheless highly discriminatory. The clinician should be cognizant of the sensitivity, specificity, and prognostic implications of these tests to maximize their usefulness.

Clinical Tests

Table 4–18 comments on several clinical tests that may be useful in the diagnosis of MS.

HOT BATH TEST AND OTHER PROVOCATIVE TESTS

The hot bath test, rarely done today and described for historical purposes only, was originally proposed by Guthrie[161] and studied by Davis and colleagues.[81,82] It is performed by having a patient recline in a bath tub or a whirlpool bath. Water temperature is gradually increased from 85° to approximately 110°F. Neurological examinations with an emphasis on visual and oculomotor function are performed at regular intervals. Body temperature usually begins to rise after 10 to 15 minutes. Small changes in body temperature (less than 2°F) can be associated with the appearance of previ-

Table 4–18. **CLINICAL TESTS FOR THE DIAGNOSIS OF MULTIPLE SCLEROSIS (Most of the ones listed are nonspecific but can be helpful.)**

Test	Comment
Hot bath test	A positive result strongly suggests demyelination but is nonspecific for MS (of historical value only).
Neuropsychological testing	This kind of testing can be very useful in managing MS, but the use in diagnosis is not well substantiated. Sixty percent of patients with MS have abnormalities in neuropsychological tests, but the defects may be subtle. The defects seen in MS are subcortical and nonspecific. They may be missed by many standard screening tests, such as the Mini–Mental State Examination.
Visual psychophysical tests	These tests are sensitive but are nonspecific for MS. Of MS patients with normal visual acuity, 40% may have a decreased contrast threshold.
Urologic evaluation	This evaluation is very nonspecific, especially in females. Patients must be free of infection, if possible, at the time of investigation.
Sexual function	Even though sexual dysfunction is common in MS, this area of evaluation is the most nonspecific of all. However, it is important to evaluate sexual function for proper MS management.

ously unapparent signs. In using the hot bath test, just as in the performance of a tensilon test for MG, the clinician must have a definite endpoint, and the findings, if they are to be used diagnostically, must be unequivocal. The endpoint can be the emergence of a clear-cut sign or signs not seen in the basal state. It is helpful if the signs correspond to symptoms that have previously been known to increase or appear during hot weather or exercise. The test should be terminated at the earliest possible moment, and patients should never be left unattended.[40,436]

The "hot bath test" is also considered positive when it produces evidence of a previously unsuspected lesion that satisfies the criterion for dissemination in space. An example of such evidence would be the appearance of an INO in a patient who previously had only signs and symptoms suggesting a spinal cord lesion. This additional finding would then give clinical evidence for two lesions, one in the spinal cord and a second in the dorsal brain stem.

The test uses the exquisite temperature sensitivity seen in some patients with MS. Exercise, fever, and increased ambient temperature can all be associated with an increase in neurological deficit or the development of previously unapparent neuro-

logical signs and symptoms. However, temperature sensitivity is not specific to MS. About 60 percent of patients with MS will show increased symptoms when subjected to a hot bath,[252] probably because of reversible conduction block in temperature-sensitive demyelinated fibers.[348] The safety factor for conduction in a normal nerve is about five times in excess of what is needed to maintain conduction. In demyelinated nerves, the safety factor is reduced considerably, so that a small additional impediment to conduction, such as increased temperature, can block the propagation of the impulse. Lidocaine, a sodium channel blocker, has been used to induce clinical symptoms in 30 MS patients.[369] Twenty-five of the 30 developed new clinical signs or showed an increase in pre-existing clinical signs after the injection of lidocaine. This study, if confirmed, might turn out to be less cumbersome and time consuming than the hot bath test in unmasking clinical signs to demonstrate dissemination in space.

NEUROPSYCHOLOGICAL TESTING

Neuropsychological testing is neither a specific nor sensitive test in the diagnosis of MS, however, it may be helpful in the diagnosis[33a]. It can, however, be helpful in the management of MS, especially in understanding behavioral problems. Neuropsychological testing, which is discussed in detail in Chapter 5, may also become an accepted outcome measure in clinical trials, although the tests are so time consuming that their use may not be realistic.

VISUAL PSYCHOPHYSICAL TESTS

Recent years have seen a great increase in research and understanding of the psychophysical aspects of vision. Such studies as visual contrast sensitivity, perceptual delays, and flicker fusion frequency can now be applied to the evaluation of patients with suspected MS and may show abnormalities in the presence of normal visual acuity. Patients with MS who have optic nerve involvement often complain of poor vision yet have normal visual acuity on the Snellen test. Many of these patients describe their vision as "washed out" in character.

Regan and his associates[350] have found that contrast sensitivity in MS can be grossly impaired in 40 percent of patients while standard visual acuity is normal. The test for contrast sensitivity measures the threshold for determination of contrast by using graded intensity black or gray bars against a white background. More complex tests such as perceptual delay, flicker fusion, and double flash tests are more difficult to administer and are not widely available. However, they do give clinical information beyond that available from ordinary acuity testing.

BLADDER EVALUATION (URODYNAMICS)

Although only 5 percent of patients with MS will manifest urinary symptoms[190] at onset, at least 80 percent will have bladder dysfunction later during the course of the disease. However, because bladder disturbances are prevalent in the non-MS population, especially among females, the clinician should be cautious in using urinary symptoms to establish evidence for dissemination in space. Urodynamic and electrophysiological studies may be helpful in determining whether a neurogenic bladder is present, but even detailed testing can be ambiguous (see Chapter 12).

Nonimaging Tests (Cerebrospinal Fluid Analysis, Evoked Potentials)

Approximately 50 percent of patients suspected of having MS at presentation will require laboratory studies to confirm the diagnosis or to rule out other diagnoses. Table 4–19 lists some CSF studies that may be helpful.

CEREBROSPINAL FLUID ANALYSIS FOR OLIGOCLONAL BANDING

Cerebrospinal fluid (CSF) analysis in MS has recently been reviewed several times.[95,238,268, 416,441] A consensus report from Europe[14] has concluded that OB is the most specific CSF test for MS. Some patients with MS have a CSF pleocytosis. It is unusual to find more than 20 cells per cubic millimeter. They are mostly lymphocytes with a few macrophages. TP can be elevated, but values above 1000 mg per liter should suggest an additional coexistent problem or an alternative diagnosis. CSF electrophoresis can resolve the components of TP that are most important for diagnosis. Alterations in albumin and beta globulins are nonspecific to MS, but the gamma globulins are most important to understand.

One of the hallmarks of MS is an increased production of immunoglobulin within the CNS. This increase is caused by excessive IgG synthesis on the brain side of the blood-brain barrier (BBB). Forty years ago, it was shown that 70 percent of patients with MS had high levels of the gamma globulin fraction of TP of CSF.[204] Increased IgG levels can be measured in several ways. Evidence for quantitative abnormalities in IgG production is based on ratios between albumin and IgG in the CSF and the serum.[45] The presence of OB in the CSF together with its absence in the serum is pathognomonic of an immune response localized to the CNS. OB is the presence of two or more distinct IgG bands in the gamma region of the electrophoresis.[95,101,240,372,458]

Table 4–19. **CSF STUDIES THAT MAY BE HELPFUL IN THE DIAGNOSIS OF MULTIPLE SCLEROSIS**

CSF Evaluation	Comment on Findings
Cells	Can be elevated (10–50/mm³)
Protein	
Total protein	May be mildly elevated
Gamma globulin	Elevated in 70% of CDMS
IgG	Elevated in 70% of CDMS

Oligoclonal banding	Most specific abnormality
	    Positive in 85%–95% of CDMS
	    Positive in 40%–50% of suspected MS
	    Pattern usually remains the same over time

IgG synthesis rates	Sensitive but less specific than oligoclonal banding
Kappa light chains	May be very sensitive, but specificity is yet to be determined
MBP and antibodies to MBP	Diagnostically nonspecific; changes may reflect disease activity
Glucose	Normal
Culture	Normal
Enzymes	May be elevated, nonspecific

CDMS = clinically definite MS; CSF = cerebrospinal fluid; MBP = myelin basic protein.

Lowenthal[246] was the first to show that specific bands in the gamma globulin region were found in MS. Some of the bands can be IgM.[394] The more recent application of agarose electrophoresis and isoelectric focusing (IEF) have shown that abnormal bands, probably representing multiple monoclonal globulins (mostly IgG), can be seen in the CSF of more than 90 percent of patients with CDMS. OB is not specific to MS and can occur in any condition that has an immune response component, such as viral meningitis or encephalitis, bacterial meningitis, syphilis, idiopathic polyneuropathy, MS, ADEM, or HAM (Table 4–20). It has even been reported recently in as unlikely a situation as Huntington's disease.[393]

Not only is the sensitivity for MS high (greater than 90 percent), but the specificity for MS also seems to be high.[267] The appearance of OB specific to the CSF can be taken as proof that there is an abnormality in IgG production in the CNS. Interestingly, the application of CSF electrophoresis to the diagnosis of MS took many years to become uniformly available. The reason for this delay is not immediately apparent, but one factor may be that the detection of OB rests almost entirely on visual inspection of the electrophoresis strip. Densitometer readings are usually insensitive for

the detection of OB. Figure 4–4 shows the characteristic pattern of OB in the CSF in MS.

A prospective follow-up study of 183 patients with monosymptomatic suspected MS[293] showed that the presence of OB was associated with a 24 percent conversion rate to CDMS within 34 months. In contrast, only 9 percent of patients with monosymptomatic disease that were OB-negative developed CDMS during the same follow-up period. This study provides evidence that the presence of OB in monosymptomatic disease is a good but not exclusive predictor for the development of CDMS. In that particular study, a large number of the patients had CPM. As noted previously, CPM is a particularly difficult group of patients for diagnostic evaluation. Ebers[97] has provided some context for the use of CSF electrophoresis in the diagnosis of MS. He points out that false-negatives and false-positives in OB are of concern but that the specificity for MS is quite good. When we compare the use of OB in MS to other diagnostic tests it is helpful to be reminded that the sensitivity of the electrocardiogram for myocardial infarction is about 60 to 70 percent and that approximately 20 percent of patients with angiographically proven triple-vessel coronary artery disease have

Table 4–20. **DIAGNOSES IN NON–MULTIPLE SCLEROSIS PATIENTS POSITIVE FOR OLIGOCLONAL BANDING (N = 36 of 1000 done = 3.6%)***

Diagnosis	No. of Patients
DISORDERS ASSOCIATED WITH A LOCAL IMMUNE RESPONSE OR SERUM BANDS	
Viral meningitis	3
Viral encephalitis	3
Arachnoiditis	2
Neuropathy (chronic)	1
Guillain-Barré syndrome	1
Neurosyphilis	1
Chronic hepatitis (serum bands present)	1
Polycythemia (serum bands present)	1
Sarcoidosis	1
Fungal meningitis	1
Lymphomatoid granulomatosis	1
Chronic encephalitis	1
Post epidural paraplegia	1
Chronic focal encephalitis	1
Total	19
DISORDERS NOT ASSOCIATED WITH LOCAL IMMUNE RESPONSE OR SERUM BANDS	
Headache	3
Stroke	2
Lumbar disk disease	2
Diabetic neuropathy	1
Cervical spondylosis	1
Vertigo, ? etiology	1
Arnold-Chiari malformation	1
Supranuclear palsy	1
CNS leukemia	1
Psychosis	1
Syncope	1
Acoustic neuroma	1
Amyotrophy, ? cause	1
Total	17

Source: Ebers GC, and Paty DW,[101] pp 275–280, with permission.

CNS = central nervous system.

*Nineteen with expected local immune response; 12 not expected to have local immune response.

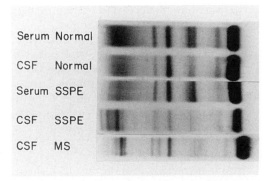

Figure 4–4. Agarose electrophoresis of serum and cerebrospinal fluid (CSF) showing oligoclonal bands in subacute sclerosing panencephalitis (SSPE) serum and CSF and in MS CSF. The bands are on the left side of the strip. Albumin is on the right.

normal stress electrocardiograms, yet few physicians are deterred by this low sensitivity. Also, one-third of patients with early or late syphilis have a negative VDRL, 30 percent of rheumatoid arthritis patients have no rheumatoid factor, 10 percent of patients with MG are negative for AChR, and temporal lobe spikes are seen during the first electroencephalogram (EEG) tracing in only one-half of the patients with temporal lobe epilepsy.

McLean and colleagues[267] and Ratnaike and colleagues[349] have looked at the impact of CSF biochemistry upon the diagnosis of MS. Both groups found that OB was more sensitive than IgG levels. They also found that abnormal CSF findings frequently influenced the certainty with which the diagnosis of MS was made.

In Ebers and Paty's series,[101] 8 percent of neurological patients without MS had OB. These patients were equally divided into those with and without an expected local CNS immune response (see Table 4–20). The diagnoses in those patients expected to have OB were viral infections of the CNS and other inflammatory conditions, including idiopathic polyneuropathy and neurosyphilis. In most of these instances, the clinical presentation would not be confused with that of MS. The appearance of OB had no obvious explanation in 4 percent of patients without MS, at least one of whom developed MS on follow-up. It is possible that the presence of unanticipated OB in most such patients is associated with previously occurring but unrecorded inflammatory CNS disease such as viral meningitis.

In spite of a 4 percent false-positive rate, systematic study has shown that patients with monosymptomatic disease that eventually turns into MS can have totally normal spinal fluid on repeated occasions. Eventually some of these patients will develop OB, so that repeated CSF evaluation may be necessary to detect OB (see Chapter 11 for more details).

An autopsy study looking at OB-positive versus OB-negative patients[113] has shown a clear correlation between OB and the presence of plasma cells in brain lesions. The study also showed clearly that OB can be absent in autopsy-proven MS. Those patients without OB had few plasma cells in the brain lesions. OB, once it is present, usually persists throughout the course of the disease, and the qualitative banding pattern changes little if at all over time. This stability suggests that the process that dictates the pattern of banding is present early in the course of the disease and then persists as a continuing stimulus for abnormal intrathecal IgG synthesis. One study[372] has shown some change in the OB pattern over time, but if true, such changes must be unusual. Coyle[77] has claimed to find OB in the tears of MS patients, but it is not consistently present and others[386] have failed to find it.

Isoelectric focusing (IEF) has become more generally available. IEF is a much more sensitive technique than agarose electrophoresis for separating IgG bands. Unfortunately, IEF is so sensitive that it can actually separate a myeloma protein produced by a single clone of plasma cells into several bands. When used in routine diagnosis, the false-positive rate with IEF is considerably higher than that with agarose electrophoresis. Therefore, many laboratories reserve IEF for doubtful cases and for reanalysis of specimens in which routine agarose electrophoresis is negative. The high false-positive rate with IEF must be kept in mind when interpreting these results.[95]

One report[456] found that the frequency of OB in Hong Kong Chinese with CDMS was low (33%). This study confirms the impressions that the authors have obtained from many different Asian centers and our own experience in Vancouver with many nonwhite patients with MS.

A more recent investigation[364] of CSF abnormalities in MS has suggested that free kappa light chains could be even more specific for MS than is OB. Rudick and his colleagues claim that free kappa chains are frequent in MS, and that they are not seen with any regularity in other neurological diseases. However, others have not been able to confirm that this test is any more sensitive or specific for MS than is OB. Sindic and Laterre[393] looked at free kappa and lambda light chains in the CSF of a number of patients. They were not found in normal control subjects (N = 26). Oligoclonal free kappa bands restricted to the CSF were seen in 92 percent of patients with MS (44 of 48). This finding was similar to that for IgG OB, which was seen in 40 of 48, and for free lambda IgG OB, which was seen in 33 of 48. OB was seen in three of five unrelated patients with Huntington's disease.

In addition, recent studies have also shown that MBP can be detected in the CSF of patients with MS.[440] Unfortunately, the presence of MBP is not diagnostically specific; it does seem to be more likely to appear in the CSF during periods of disease activity.[442] In addition, antibody to MBP,[239,431] especially free antibody, has now been shown to be markedly elevated in patients with MS, particularly in those with clinical evidence for disease activity.

IgG INDEX AND SYNTHESIS RATE

Both Link[238] and Tourtelotte and colleagues[415] have made important contributions to the study of immunoglobulins in MS CSF. Link has developed an IgG index that rivals OB in sensitivity and specificity, as does the IgG synthesis rate derived by Tourtelotte and colleagues.

Comparison of OB, the IgG index, and the IgG synthesis rate shows relatively little difference in sensitivity.[245] Most hospital laboratories do electrophoresis for OB in CSF, although optimally for MS specificity, OB should also be shown to be absent in serum. When done properly, CSF electrophoresis for OB is probably more specific for MS than the other two tests.[14] Several critical reviews of this area have been published.[179,232,268,441] McLean and colleagues[267] compared electrophoresis and quantitative IgG measurements in the diagnosis of MS. They found that both the sensitivity and specificity of electrophoresis was much higher than the quantitative IgG measurements and suggested that the quantitative measures be abandoned for routine purposes. IgM has also been studied.[147]

EVOKED POTENTIALS (EP)

The application of neurophysiological techniques to the evaluation of MS accelerated in the 1980s but is decelerating in North America with the wide availability of MRI. Electroencephalogram (EEG) findings can be abnormal in MS, but no specific EEG abnormality has been described. Perhaps abnormal EEG findings could suggest that there are cerebral hemisphere abnormalities in a patient who otherwise exhibits brain stem, optic nerve, or spinal cord symptoms, but because nonspecific EEG abnormalities are common in the normal population, the clinician must approach the use of the EEG in this setting with caution. The most useful physiological studies in the diagnosis of MS have been the EPs.[374] Table 4–21 gives some principles to be followed in the use of EP in the diagnosis of MS. The use of EP in neurological diagnosis has also been the subject of several reviews.[12,69,105,434] Abnormal EPs may have a role in predicting both the diagnosis of MS and clinical deterioration.[187] Figure 4–5 illustrates the principles of the use of EP in diagnosis.

Visual Evoked Potentials. Visual evoked potentials were the first EPs to be studied, by Richey and his colleagues.[353] These authors looked at 50 patients with MS and found a considerable delay in the VEP. They suggested that VEP studies could be useful in detecting otherwise occult cerebral lesions. This suggestion was made because they did not find much difference between patients who did or did not have other objective signs of optic nerve involvement.

Table 4–21. **PRINCIPLES FOR THE USE OF EVOKED POTENTIALS IN THE DIAGNOSIS OF MULTIPLE SCLEROSIS**

Use evoked potentials to:
1. Confirm suspicious but not definite symptoms such as numbness in arms and legs, or "blurred vision" when there are no physical findings
2. Look for asymptomatic lesions disseminated in space, such as:
    Do a VEP study in a patient with clinical spinal abnormalities
    Do SEP studies in a patient with optic symptoms, diplopia, or ataxia

Remember that:
1. Latency prolongation suggests demyelination.
2. Morphological dispersion or decreased amplitude are clearly abnormal but do not specifically suggest demyelination.
3. Abnormalities, as with neurological findings, are nonspecific (see text).
4. If clear-cut clinical findings are present in a system (e.g., the visual system), that system need not be studied with evoked potentials.
5. The *pattern* of abnormalities, both clinical and paraclinical, makes the diagnosis of MS, not any one finding.

The first study to show that an abnormal VEP could be taken as evidence for a subclinical lesion in the optic nerve was by Halliday and his colleagues.[165,166] In one of their studies, 17 of 19 patients with acute unilateral ON were found to have delayed latencies. The VEP was produced by a novel stimulus, a checkerboard pattern of light and dark squares that were reversed twice per second. They went on to study 73 patients with suspected MS and found a delayed VEP in 52 (70 percent). Abnormal VEPs and CDMS were almost 100 percent correlated. They also found that 23 (45 percent) of 51 patients with MS who had normal optic disks had abnormal VEPs. Thus, they rightly proposed that the pattern-reversal VEP could be used as a test for subclinical lesions in the anterior visual pathways.

The technique of recording VEPs depends on the ability to average numerous cortical responses to visual stimuli.[145] This average is necessary to be precise about the

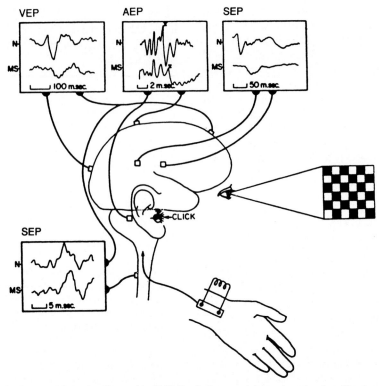

Figure 4–5. Evoked potentials in the diagnosis of MS. Evoked potentials can be stimulated in the visual (VEP), auditory (AEP), or the somatosensory (SEP) systems, as illustrated by computer averaging techniques (see text), and the subsequent latency to the brain then measured. (Adapted from an illustration provided by Dr. T. Feasby, personal communication, June 1980).

time of appearance of the EP following a standard stimulus. Flashes of light have been used for VEPs, but flashes produce a complex waveform with high intersubject variability and high trial-to-trial variability. This variability makes the flash VEP less useful than the pattern-reversal VEP. The pattern-reversal technique holds background luminance constant and alternates black and white in a checkerboard configuration. This alteration was initially done by using slide projectors and mirrors, but more recently it has been performed using a television screen. The pattern-reversal occurs at 1 to 2 Hz, while the subject views the screen by fixing vision at a specific target at the center of the screen.

The potentials that are measurable at the occipital cortex are subjected to computer averaging and the delay between the stimulus and the peak of the major positive deflection is measured. This peak is usually referred to as the *P100* because it occurs at about 100 ms following the stimulus. The range of normality varies from laboratory to laboratory, so it is important that local standards for normality are derived before one pronounces the findings of a specific study to be abnormal.

A number of variables can occur normally.[15,71] For instance, latency tends to be prolonged after the age of 50 years. Before age 50 years, the normal latency range is quite stable. Latency in women may be shorter than in men. Hyperthermia can prolong the latency in MS.[333] The major problem in variability derives from the patient's state of attention. The patient must be wide awake and free of ocular disease. Vision must be corrected to 20/20 with lenses if possible. Drowsiness, lack of cooperation, and general inattention can prolong the latency. Factitious delay can be produced by defocusing or by using transcendental meditation. Interocular symmetry is usually very precise. A latency difference of greater than 10 ms between eyes is usually considered to be abnormal, even though both latencies may be within the normal range.

Visual evoked potential abnormalities are not specific for ON or MS. Ocular disease, including congenital amblyopia, is the most common cause of non–optic nerve abnormalities. Compressive lesions of the anterior visual pathways can cause a delay. Other diseases known to have abnormalities in the VEP include Charcot-Marie-Tooth, hereditary ataxias, and spinocerebellar degenerations. Patients with Parkinson's disease can show decreased amplitude but normal latency. Metabolic disturbances such as chronic renal failure and chronic alcoholism have also been reported as occasionally showing abnormal VEP studies.

Somatosensory Evoked Potentials and Other Limb Neurophysiological Tests. Somatosensory evoked potentials (SEPs) are also used to detect subclinical evidence for dissemination in space.[105] The subject has recently been reviewed.[106,434] Unlike the VEP, whose pathways are confined to optic nerve and posterior cerebral hemisphere structures, SEP transverses spinal cord, brain stem, and cerebral hemisphere. Even though original studies used sensory nerve stimulation of the arm, experience has shown that leg stimulation samples the entire spinal cord and is more productive for detecting asymptomatic lesions.

SEP is obtained by stimulating a mixed motor-sensory nerve while the patient relaxes in a dimly lit room. EPs are recorded using cephalic bipolar electrodes. Patients are stimulated at about 5 Hz, and EPs are averaged over 500 to 1000 stimuli. Cutaneous recordings over the cervical spine and dorsal spine can also be obtained, allowing calculation of conduction times between these sites. Interpretation of SEP assumes that the PNS is intact. Therefore, in questionable circumstances, it is important that peripheral nerve conduction velocities, sensory action potentials, and other peripheral nerve studies be performed before doing SEPs.

A delay in the latency of SEPs at the cerebral cortex is suggestive of demyelination as a pathological process. One usually thinks of SEP prolonged latencies as suggesting spinal cord lesions, but delays can result from lesions in the brain stem and the cerebral hemispheres. Interpretation of the morphology and dispersion of SEP is a more difficult problem. This process involves an analysis of the configuration of the potential. Unlike prolonged latencies, abnormalities of configuration or amplitude are not specifically suggestive of demyelination as a pathological process, although in competent hands, such abnormalities are probably valid indicators of organic disease.

It is advisable to under-interpret evoked potential abnormalities because of the danger of supporting a false-positive diagnosis of MS. Prolonged latency (greater than 3 SD above the normal mean) or a side-to-side difference of greater than 2 ms is highly suggestive of demyelination. Total absence of SEP on one side with normal components on the other side is also very suspicious. Absence of a single component of SEP or increased dispersion are much softer findings and should not be taken as indicating demyelination.

Yokota and colleagues[451] have compared SEP to clinical findings and found that SEP abnormalities were better correlated to selective loss of position sense than to vibration sense. They also measured the sympathetic skin responses (SSRs) in 28 patients with MS[452] and found that 75 percent had abnormalities. They suggested that the SSR could be used as a sensitive detector of myelopathy because it was abnormal in 14 percent of patients who had a normal SEP.

Brain Stem Auditory Evoked Potentials and Blink Reflex. The auditory evoked potential was first shown in 1970 by Jewett and colleagues.[199] Brain stem auditory evoked potentials (BAEPs) are small cortical potentials stimulated by a repetitive click in the ear. Reliable recording is technically difficult and requires considerable expertise and care. A standardized monaural click is used to stimulate the cochlea.[69] The rate of stimulation is usually 10 Hz, and abnormalities suggest a block or delay in conduction through the auditory sensory pathways. Because of the complexity of the waveform, recognition of specific waves can be a problem, so that assigning specific latencies to specific peaks can be difficult. As in other EPs, each laboratory must work out its own normal ranges for latencies and amplitudes.

Anatomical correlations suggest that the first wave represents the eighth nerve activation potential. Wave II originates from either the proximal eighth nerve or cochlear nucleus. Waves III, IV, and V are generated within or near the superior olivary complex, the lateral lemniscus, and the inferior colliculus, respectively. It is not known if these waves are derived from white matter tracts or nuclear complexes. The other waves are variable in their expression in normal subjects. Therefore, waves I through IV are considered useful for clinical purposes.

Brain stem auditory evoked potentials may be used to detect asymptomatic, ipsilateral MS lesions.[33] The BAEP is abnormal in 67 percent of patients with CDMS. It is abnormal in fewer patients in other diagnostic categories. Enthusiasts have suggested that from one-fifth to one-half of patients with MS without brain stem symptoms have abnormal BAEP studies. The experience of our laboratories[343] has suggested that the BAEP is less sensitive than VEP and SEP in the diagnosis of MS and is probably not cost-effective. For that reason, we have stopped doing BAEP studies in MS diagnostic evaluations.[325]

Blink reflexes have also been used to detect physiological abnormalities in the brain stem in patients suspected of having MS.[218] The blink reflex is rarely abnormal when the BAEP is normal and therefore does not add much to the use of the BAEP. A recent study,[183] however, has described the blink reflex as being helpful in localizing lesions to either the midbrain or the rostral pons.

General Approach to Evoked Potentials

As outlined on Table 4–21, each of these physiological tests must be used selectively, and applied in a systematic fashion in order to identify subclinical lesions. EPs must not be used if either clinical findings or information available from other tests makes them unnecessary.

Diagnostic Imaging

Computed tomography and particularly MRI have developed a secure place in the diagnostic evaluation of MS. MRI is the most sensitive method for revealing asymptomatic dissemination in space.[295,308,325] Recent evidence has shown that repeated MRI scans can be highly sensitive and specific for showing dissemination in time as well (see previous section, Diagnostic Criteria).[207] The following review covers diagnostic imaging, dealing with historical and less sensitive techniques first.

RADIONUCLIDE BRAIN SCANNING

This technique is insensitive to the lesions of MS. The appearance of abnormalities on the brain scan depends on leakage of a radioactively labeled material through the BBB into brain substance. The first report of an MS-positive brain scan was in 1954.[382] In a review of patients with neoplastic disease and positive brain scans, one case of MS was found and was later pathologically documented. The next report was of a single case in 1965.[316] This study was also a survey, this time looking at patients with non-neoplastic disease. A 1970 study[148] reported that 5 of 28 patients with MS had positive brain scans. All of these 28 patients had "active" MS. Of 14 patients with MS in acute relapse surveyed in 1972, none had positive brain scans.[291] In 1973, serial scans in several patients showed that the scan lesions in MS could come and go.[280] Nuclear brain scans' lack of sensitivity for MS was revealed in 1974 when a review of 160 scans on patients with MS found only 3 that were abnormal.[19] Interesting serial observations were recorded in 1978[294] on a young woman who was eventually found to have MS in which two lesions in the left hemisphere and two lesions in the right hemisphere came and went over a 10-month period. She presented with headaches, anxiety, and depression and subsequently developed unsteadiness of gait, memory loss, and some paresthesia in her extremities. Her physical examination findings were normal at the time that her first brain scan was abnormal. Therefore, the radioactive brain scan is able to detect quite large acute cerebral lesions in MS, but the sensitivity of the technique is not great enough to be useful for diagnostic purposes.

POSITRON EMISSION TOMOGRAPHY

Research applications of positron emission tomography (PET) have shown that oxygen utilization and blood flow in both white matter and gray matter can be abnormal in MS. Moreover, the reduction in oxygen utilization and cerebral blood flow seem to be coupled.

A diffusible lipophilic alcohol, 11-C-diphenylmethanol, has also been used to assess the distribution of myelin.[178] This material, labeled with a positron emitter, can be seen in large lesions. These studies show that brain abnormalities in MS can be detected by PET, but the sensitivity is insufficient to be useful for diagnostic purposes.[388] The changes seen in cerebral blood flow and glucose metabolism in the cerebral hemispheres probably reflect decreased neuronal activity secondary to interruption of conduction in the underlying white matter pathways. Perhaps when a sensitive quantitative measure of BBB disruption is available, PET studies will be able to add significantly to our understanding of the evolution of acute MS lesions.

COMPUTED TOMOGRAPHY

In 1974, low-density CT lesions were reported in patients with MS.[80] In 1976, a strikingly positive CT scan with several large low-density lesions was found in a patient with biopsy-proven demyelination.[430] This patient developed very aggressive MS, and subsequent autopsy confirmation of the diagnosis was obtained. In the same year, 6 of 19 CT scans (32 percent) in MS were reported to be abnormal.[66] Large low-density CT lesions that were pathologically confirmed to be acutely inflammatory MS lesions were also reported.[430] All of those studies detected low-density lesions. Similarly, 36 percent of 110 patients with MS had low-density lesions in the periventricular white matter.[163] The distribution of this periventricular low density was similar to the distribution of demyelination seen in

the pathology of MS, suggesting that lesions detected by CT were indeed demyelinating.

Enhancing CT lesions in patients with MS were found in 1976.[448] Other investigators showed multiple enhancing lesions in MS and suggested that enhancing lesions were a sign of active disease.[3,383,384] The appearance of multiple areas of enhancement in the white matter without mass formation is thought to be highly suggestive of MS, but the finding is, of course, nonspecific. Subsequent studies have shown that the enhancing lesions can resolve quickly; two cases were reported with enhancing lesions in which resolution of the enhancement and improvement of the clinical symptoms occurred in parallel.[243] Subsequently, enhancing lesions in MS were reported to be steroid sensitive, particularly when steroids were administered intravenously.[418]

A number of studies have confirmed that enhancing CT lesions can be seen in acute relapses of MS, and that a high-volume delayed CT(HVDCT) is probably the most sensitive of all CT studies for showing enhancing lesions. HVDCT is produced when a double dose of contrast is given 1 hour before the scan is done. The use of the high-volume delayed enhancement technique has generally been well tolerated by patients. The majority of patients under investigation for MS are young and have normal renal function. Theoretically, the osmotic changes associated with leakage through the BBB could have negative clinical effects. After 6 years of using this technique, the authors have yet to see a single case of clinical deterioration that could be ascribed to the use of HVDCT. Figures 4–6, 4–7, and 4–8 show typical low-density and enhanced CT lesions in MS. Vinuela and associates[427] concluded that in 72 percent of cases, more information could be derived from the HVDCT than from the ordinary single-dose immediate contrast CT scan. Ebers and colleagues[102] showed that 53% of enhanced CT scans could be abnormal in acute relapsing MS, with lesser degrees of abnormality in clinically stable patients. In their paper, the authors suggested that enhanced CT could be used as an outcome measure for MS clinical trials. Our own experience is that 72 percent of patients in

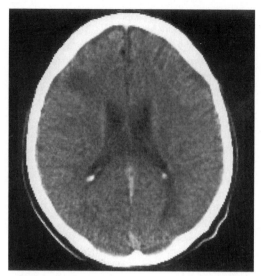

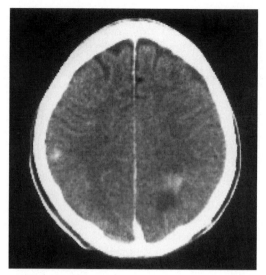

Figure 4–6. Unenhanced CT showing a single low density lesion in the frontal area of the right hemisphere in a patient with MS. (Figs. 4–6 through 4–8 courtesy of Dr. David Li, Department of Radiology, Vancouver Hospital and Health Sciences Center, University of British Columbia site).

Figure 4–8. HVD CT at a higher level on the same patient, showing multiple enhancing lesions, one adjacent to a low density lesion.

acute relapse show multiple enhancing lesions. The frequency of enhancing lesions is lower in clinically stable patients. Ebers and colleagues[102] in 1984 reported a case with autopsy confirmation of demyelination in several previously seen CT-enhancing lesions.

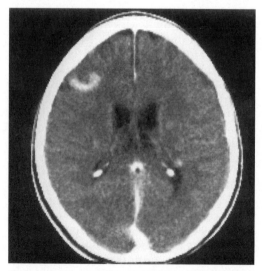

Figure 4–7. Post-infusion CT (HVD) on the same patient as in Figure 4–6, showing a crescent of enhancement in the previously identified low density lesion.

One caution should be noted: The administration of contrast material may convert a previously hypodense lesion seen on the unenhanced CT scan to isodense. Under these circumstances, an enhanced scan might actually become "normalized."

Unfortunately, the use of CT scanning in the diagnosis of MS is not always helpful. Many of the patients who come for diagnosis, particularly at the time of tertiary referral, have already passed through periods of clinical activity and can be symptom-free at the time of examination. Therefore, the yield for enhancing lesions is considerably less than in patients who are studied during an acute attack. The enhancement seen on CT is obviously related to a disturbance in the BBB. This disturbance can be transitory and seems to be responsive to steroid therapy.[383] Wolinsky and colleagues[447] have shown that triple-gadoteridol increased the yield of enhancing lesions by as much as 50 percent.

The enhancement seen on CT tells us something about the acute evolving lesion. We know that acute MS lesions can be markedly enhancing and that the intensity of enhancement is reduced over time. There is local, intense disruption of the BBB in MS, but this disruption is not associated with significant elevations in CSF albumin and may be a selective disturbance. Multifocal enhancing lesions are not, of course, specific for MS. Multiple metastases, infarcts, abscesses, multicentric glioblastomas, cerebral lymphoma, sarcoidosis, cerebral Whipple's disease, and lymphoid granulomatosis can all produce a similar appearance.

MAGNETIC RESONANCE IMAGING

The use of MRI in MS diagnosis has been reviewed extensively.[266,312,325] MRI has proved to have a sensitivity perhaps 10 times that of CT in detecting MS lesions (Table 4–22). In 1981, one group investigated eight patients with CDMS and found 100 percent of them to have low-intensity lesions on inversion

recovery (IR) scans.[455] The same laboratory[64] then looked at three additional patients with suspected MS and found MRI lesions in all three.

Subsequent studies[235,248,302,365] reported a total of 70 patients with CDMS, all of whom showed lesions, particularly using the spin echo (SE) technique. Since then, a number of other studies have shown that MRI can reveal multiple asymptomatic lesions in the white matter in patients suspected of having MS.[58] The standard approach to doing MRI examinations for the diagnosis of MS has been to do axial T_2-weighted scans. Fast spin echo technique may be as good as the conventional SE technique.[411]

The current MRI technique that is being used for diagnostic studies is based on the

Table 4–22. **SELECTED STUDIES OF THE FREQUENCY OF MAGNETIC RESONANCE IMAGING ABNORMALITIES IN PATIENTS WITH CLINICALLY DEFINITE MULTIPLE SCLEROSIS**

Year	Senior Author	No. of MS Patients Studied	No. MRI Positive	Percent MRI Positive	Comments
1981	Young[455]	8	8	100	All inversion recovery
1983	Lukes[248]	10	10	100	Spin echo technique better than inversion recovery
1983	Brant-Zawadzki[52]	13	12	93	
1984	Runge[365]	42	42	100	
1985	Kirshner[223]	27	27	100	
1985	Gebarski[137]	30	26	87	
1985	Jackson[193]	25	19	76	
1986	Farlow[112]	18	15	83	
1986	Scotti[381]	30	30	100	
1987	Robertson[357]	36	36	100	Conservative UBC criteria*
1987	Stewart[400]	56	43	77	
1987	Ormerod[312]	114	102	89	Periventricular lesions alone not considered positive
1988	Grenman[157]	21	16	76	Ultra-low field-strength MRI
1988	Honig[180]	41	31	76	
1988	Boné[46]	40	34	85	
1990	Osborn[314]	12	12	100	Adolescents
1990	Noakes[302]	42	38	90	
1991	Yetkin[450]	92	83	90	MRI specificity for the diagnosis of MS was 95%–99%
1992	Haughton[173]	39	39	100	

*See text for University of British Columbia (UBC) criteria for strongly suggestive of multiple sclerosis.

magnetic resonance of hydrogen nuclei. Because water is by far the most common source of hydrogen nuclei in living tissue, it is likely that the water content of tissue is producing most of the signal seen on the scans. The relaxation time of hydrogen in lipid is short when compared with that in non-lipid tissue. The MS plaque is lipid deficient compared with white matter and is known to contain increased amounts of water. Thus, the magnetic resonance image in MS probably reflects, to a great degree, the distribution of water.

Studies have emphasized the importance of the corpus callosum in making the diagnosis.[392] Investigators[136,446] have shown that sagittal T_2-weighted scans can pick up more lesions than axial ones and that the findings are probably more specific for MS than are axial views only. Figures 4–9 through 4–18 show typical MRI lesions in several patients with MS. The reader should note the characteristics of the lesions in different planes. In the axial slice, the lesions have a "lumpy-bumpy," usually symmetrical appearance along the superior lateral ventricle. Parasagittal views show that the lesions mostly originate in the corpus callosum and tend to "point" away from the corpus callosum. This appearance is characteristic of MS. The atlas of MRI in MS by Kesselring and his colleagues[217] shows many excellent examples of both typical and atypical lesions.[58] Quantitative magnetic resonance may be helpful as well.[173]

Magnetic resonance imaging cannot distinguish between intracellular and extracellular water, however, nor can it distinguish between acute and chronic MS lesions. Because the enhanced CT or MRI scan is probably identifying the most active lesions, because of a disrupted BBB, there is reason to believe that MRI (with and without enhancement) combined with evoked potentials can provide more useful information than one modality alone. Experimental magnetic resonance imaging studies are producing information on the characteristics of edema,[30] demyelination,[31] inflammation,[208] gliosis,[29] and axonal loss.[208]

Recent studies using MRI contrast agents have provided insight into the factors un-

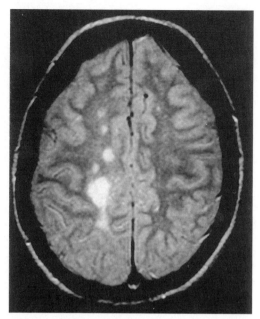

Figure 4–9. MRI axial SE-40 view taken above the level of the lateral ventricle from a young woman with MS. Note the large, white lesions with a lumpy appearance adjacent to the right lateral ventricle (see text). (Figs. 4–9 and 4–10 courtesy of Dr. R. Nugent, Department of Diagnostic Radiology, Vancouver Hospital and Health Sciences Center, Vancouver General Hospital site).

derlying the changes seen in MS. Gadolinium-DTPA (Gd-DTPA) is a chelate between a DTPA molecule and the paramagnetic metal ion gadolinium. Gd-DTPA is distributed within the intravascular compartment. It does not cross the intact BBB in man but will penetrate into neural tissue in areas where the BBB has been disturbed.[150,160,213] Gadolinium-enhanced images may also have advantages over ordinary T_2 images, especially with a triple dose of gadoteridol.[120b]

One study of serial head MRI scanning (intervals 3 to 5 weeks) showed that 12 of 12 new MRI-detected lesions enhanced with Gd-DTPA.[278] The majority of the new lesions were asymptomatic. Contrast-enhanced MRI was able to detect cortical lesions previously unrecognized by standard MRI. The increased sensitivity of enhanced MRI in detecting gray matter lesions is probably explained by a higher concentration of Gd-DTPA in the cortex, where blood flow is

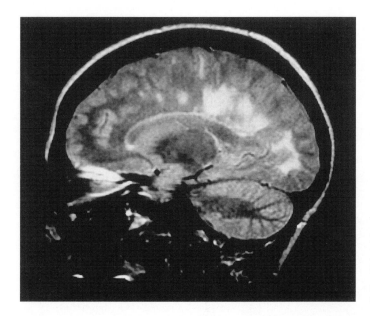

Figure 4–10. A parasagittal SE-40 view from the patient in Figure 4–9. Note that most of the lesions tend to be "ovoid" in appearance (see text) and appear to be "pointing" away from the corpus callosum.

known to be fourfold greater than in white matter.

Using quantitative dynamic Gd-DTPA–enhanced MRI, investigators found that the degree and pattern of gadolinium en-

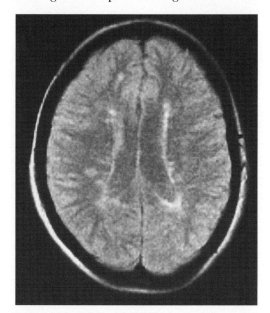

Figure 4–11. MRI axial SE-40 view showing subtle periventricular distribution of lesions. Note the tendency for the periventricular lesions to be symmetrical. (Figs. 4–11 through 4–13 courtesy of Dr. David Li, Department of Radiology, Vancouver Hospital and Health Sciences Center, University of British Columbia site).

hancement varies with the age of the lesion.[214,415] Gadolinium enhancement was seen to precede T_2-detected changes in 3 of 11 cases studied, again suggesting that this technique detects early BBB disruption. The time to peak enhancement was shortest in acute lesions and became more prolonged on follow-up studies performed several weeks later. With time (usually 6 to 12 weeks), the degree of enhancement gradually lessened and then disappeared. Chronic lesions tended to enhance only on their periphery, suggesting that the active inflammation is on the periphery of the lesion and that there is restoration of the BBB in its center. It appears likely, therefore, that gadolinium-enhanced MRI scanning of brain, and possibly of the spinal cord, may be useful in serial MRI studies to detect dynamic changes in BBB permeability. In addition, Moreira and colleagues[288] have suggested that an "open-ring" appearance on enhanced MRI may be characteristic of MS.

Some patients with MS manifest a tumor-like mass lesion on MRI.[144,206] Meningeal enhancement has also been seen.[27]

Kappos and his colleagues[207] have suggested that the simultaneous finding of both unenhanced and enhanced MRI lesions increases the likelihood that the pattern is due to MS and might be taken as

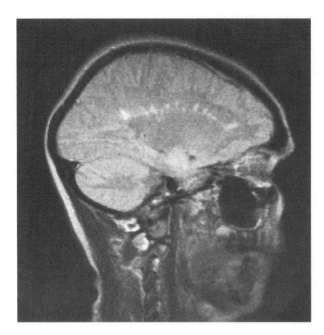

Figure 4–12. A parasagittal SE-40 view of the patient in Figure 4–11, showing the same tendency for the lesions to point away from the corpus callosum. This appearance is very characteristic of MS.

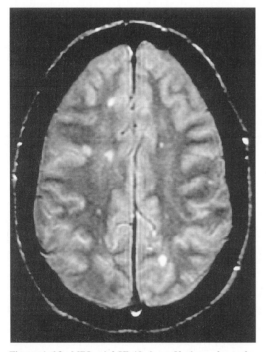

Figure 4–13. MRI axial SE-40 view of lesions above the ventricular level in a young man with MS. Note the small, white lesions scattered throughout the white matter.

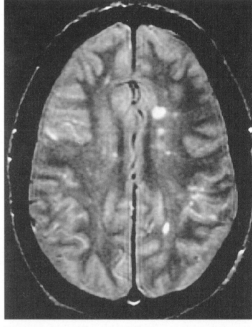

Figure 4–14. MRI axial SE-40 view of multiple lesions in a slice at the level of the superior edge of the lateral ventricle in the patient in Figure 4–13. (Figs. 4–14 through 4–18 courtesy of Dr. R. Nugent, Department of Diagnostic Radiology, Vancouver Hospital and Health Sciences Center, Vancouver General Hospital site).

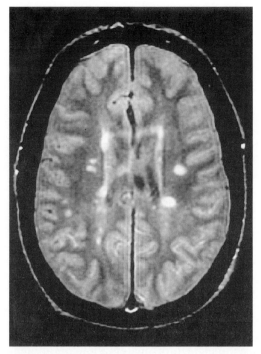

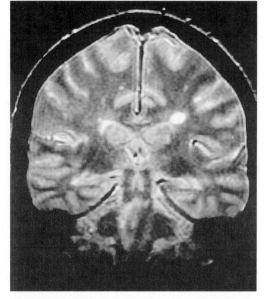

Figure 4–17. MRI posterior coronal view of the patient in Figures 4–13 through 4–16, showing more periventricular and brain stem lesions. Note the large ovoid lesion in the left cerebral hemisphere, the same one noted in Figure 4–15.

Figure 4–15. MRI axial SE-40 slice at the mid-lateral ventricle level in the patient in Figures 4–13 and 4–14, showing scattered periventricular lesions. Note the large, round lesion at the posterior end of the left lateral ventricle. This lesion is seen in Figure 4–17 in a coronal slice taken in the same patient.

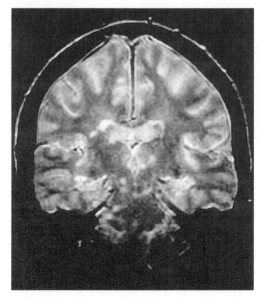

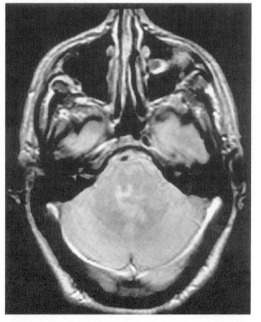

Figure 4–16. MRI anterior coronal view of the patient in Figures 4–13 through 4–16. Note the periventricular distribution of several lesions, as well as the presence of several brain stem and cerebellar lesions.

Figure 4–18. MRI axial SE-40 slice at the level of the fourth ventricle in the patient in Figures 4–13 through 4–17. Note the bright lesion in the floor of the fourth ventricle.

evidence for the lesions being of different ages. This concept might satisfy the criterion of dissemination in time as well as space. Even though it is an intriguing concept, one must be careful in relying solely on MRI in the diagnosis, because of the danger of overdiagnosing rather than underdiagnosing MS.

Systematic natural history studies of MRI activity and the quantitation of the extent of MRI scan abnormalities in area or volume of lesions may yield an objective measure of the activity and extent of the disease process.[120a,321,410] (See Chapter 12 for a discussion of MRI as an outcome measure in clinical trials.) As more becomes known about the tissue characteristics that produce the MRI signal, one may be able to accurately follow and define intrinsic changes in lesions as well as their size and intensity. The concept of area quantitation is already being applied to the adjudication of therapeutic trials in MS.[326] In the future, MRI not only will add to our knowledge of the evolution of the MS process but also will give us an accurate and objective way of measuring the extent and severity of the process.

Table 4–23 shows the 5-year follow-up of a number of patients with isolated clinical syndromes who had MRI evaluations at onset. The reader will note that an abnormal head MRI greatly increases the risk for MS at 5 years and 10 years.[310a] Spinal MRI may also be useful when the head MRI is normal.[412a]

Many have believed that the use of MRI would change the epidemiology of MS by increasing confidence in the diagnosis. In a systematic study of the impact of MRI on the epidemiology of MS, Poser and her colleagues[339] found that only 3 of 69 patients diagnosed between 1986 and 1990 in South Lower Saxony would have been missed without MRI. They did find, however, that MRI tended to change the diagnostic classification to a more positive one. Another study[249] found that MRI studies can also be abnormal in asymptomatic family members of patients with MS.

Even though some still think MRI has not demonstrated overall clinical usefulness,[211] cost-impact studies on the use of MRI in medical decision making have begun.[287] Giang and colleagues[143] found that MRI and EPs both had impact on clinical decision making in MS but that MRI had the greatest impact. Unfortunately after comprehensive testing, half of the patients still had a tentative diagnosis. As O'Connor and colleagues[307] found, patient health perceptions were altered by diagnostic testing in MS; consequently, these authors recommended that patients be informed that a negative test result does not completely rule out MS.[307a] They also found that the clinical severity of the patients introduced a bias in the application of the MRI data to

Table 4–23. FIVE-YEAR FOLLOW-UP OF PATIENTS WITH ISOLATED CLINICAL SYNDROMES: MAGNETIC RESONANCE IMAGING PREDICTION FOR THE DIAGNOSIS OF MULTIPLE SCLEROSIS

Clinical Syndrome	MRI Result	Number/ Total	(Percentage)	Number with MS at 5 Yr	(Percentage)
ON	Abnormal	28/44	(64)	23	(82)
	Normal	16/44	(36)	1	(6)
Brain stem	Abnormal	12/17	(71)	8	(67)
	Normal	5/17	(29)	0	(0)
Spinal cord	Abnormal	17/28	(61)	11	(65)
	Normal	11/28	(39)	1	(9)
Overall	Abnormal	57/89	(64)	41	(72)
	Normal	32/89	(36)	2	(6)

Source: Morrissey SP, Miller DH, Kendall BE, et al,[290] pp 135–146, with permission.
MRI = magnetic resonance imaging; ON = optic neuritis.

the diagnosis.[307a] Such studies will be very important for determining the overall need for access to MRI technology in the future. Despite some drawbacks, there is no doubt that MRI is the most useful test in the diagnosis of MS.[363]

One study[230] looked at the relative sensitivity of spinal and head MRI in 22 patients with MS who had spinal cord symptoms. Twenty (91 percent) had a positive head MRI scan, whereas only 12 (55 percent) had a positive spinal MRI scan. This study confirms that head MRI is the preferred study to do in suspected cases, even those with strictly spinal symptoms. New advances in spinal imaging should help in future studies.[412]

Using both STIR and SE pulse sequences of the head, one study[429] found that the lesions were somewhat better seen by STIR, but that the final diagnostic impression was not changed over that determined by SE technique alone. Ultrafast sequences such as Turbo-flair,[87] Fast Flair,[172a] and Flair-Haste (3.7 seconds) may turn out to be as good as ordinary T_2 sequences.[43] (See Chapter 9 for a full discussion of new MRI techniques.)

The majority of the lesions seen on MRI are asymptomatic.[191] Serial studies* have shown that these asymptomatic lesions can appear over 2 weeks to a month and then begin to fade. Some of these new lesions appear to resolve completely when followed sequentially with a low-field (0.15 T) MRI machine. They are not so likely to resolve completely with higher strength magnet machines. Some pulse sequences may be better than others for identifying and measuring MS lesions.[329] Fast SE technique may be as good as conventional SE technique.[411] Typically, new, large lesions will shrink to a much smaller size on followup. Some MS lesions present as a cerebral mass lesion.[212] Overall, MRI provides the most reliable paraclinical data for the diagnosis of MS.[295] However, Schiffer and his colleagues[376] call attention to the many pitfalls in relying too much on the MRI for diagnosis. Goodkin and associates[152] reviewed all aspects of the use of MRI in MS. They suggested that MRI should not be used as a screen for MS in populations at risk be-cause of the nonspecificity. They also called for development of precise MRI criteria for the diagnosis of MS. Precise criteria may be too suggestive that MS can be diagnosed by MRI. MRI evidence must remain only a supportive factor in what is ultimately a clinical diagnosis.

Pathological Correlation. Pathological correlation studies with MRI[31,400] have shown that demyelinated lesions as small as 3 mm in diameter can be detected, but the correlation seems to be quite variable.[297] Pathological correlation has also shown that in the chronic lesion, gliosis is associated with a stronger magnetic resonance signal, particularly on the T_1-weighted image. If systematic variability in the signal is consistent in pathological correlation studies, there is hope for the concept that magnetic resonance techniques, especially magnetic resonance spectroscopy (MRS), will eventually be able to detect specific tissue characteristics reliably. This information not only will improve diagnostic specificity in MS but also will help the clinician to observe the pathological process by identifying both the degree of severity of lesions and the extent of disease (see Chapter 9). Richards[352] has reviewed MRS in the diagnosis and evaluation of MS.

Principles of MRI Interpretation. The recent wave of enthusiasm for the use of magnetic resonance in the diagnosis of MS has led some clinicians to believe that a specific diagnosis of MS can be made using MRI alone, but this is not possible. Yetkin and colleagues[450] found that even though as many as 20 percent of control subjects have periventricular foci of high-signal intensity on MRI, the diagnostic specificity of MRI was 95 to 99 percent, and the sensitivity was 80 percent. They looked at 92 patients with CDMS and compared them with 60 patients with hypertension and with 100 healthy control subjects. They also found that up to 4 percent of healthy control subjects of all ages can have periventricular changes that cannot be distinguished from MS. However, if the MRI head scan shows disseminated lesions at the time of clinical presentation, the probability of MS being the correct diagnosis is high,[231] and the clinical prognosis may also be poorer than if the MRI head scan were normal.[46,290]

---

*References 160, 172, 191, 224, 278, 445.

With increasing age, nonspecific MRI abnormalities, especially on the SE scan of the periventricular area, become increasingly common (Table 4–24). Therefore, the clinician must be cautious in interpreting periventricular lesions in patients after age 50 years.[188] In pathological correlation studies on brains from elderly patients, some investigators[49,154] found little in the way of specific pathological changes in the MRI-detected lesions in the deep cerebral white matter. Other investigators[115,116] have also done pathological correlations on incidental white matter abnormalities and found them to represent mostly vascular lesions. One study[423] looked at 42 elderly patients with hypertension and found 10 with confluent white matter lesions on MRI scan. Only 1 of the 42 age-matched controls had similar changes. The patients with the MRI changes also had decreased cognitive abilities. Another study[55] of older patients correlated cerebrovascular risk factors and cognitive changes with white matter lesions on MRI scans.

Table 4–25 lists a number of studies of non-MS conditions that can be confused with MS on an MRI scan. Table 4–26 gives the characteristics of lesions on MRI scan that favor MS. Table 4–27 lists a number of studies that have looked at the usefulness of MRI in the diagnosis of conditions that are likely to be onset symptoms of MS, such as ON, CPM, and isolated brain stem syndromes. In one study,[269] 6 of 16 patients (38 percent) with chronic inflammatory polyneuropathy had CNS white matter lesions indistinguishable from those seen in MS. Reversible white matter lesions have also been reported in porphyria.[219]

Magnetic Resonance Imaging Criteria For Diagnosis. The authors strongly suggest that a conservative approach be taken to the evaluation of the MRI. Finding one or two MS-like lesions is not enough. Following the UBC criteria,[325] we suggest that the following findings are *strongly suggestive of MS*:

1. Four white matter lesions (Barkof and colleagues[26] have suggested eight.)
2. Three white matter lesions, one periventricular

3. Diameter of all lesions greater than 3 mm and predominantly in the white matter

In addition to these criteria, other characteristics that give a greater *specificity for MS* include:

1. Diameter greater than 6 mm[118,308]
2. An ovoid shape of the long axis of the lesions usually 90 degrees to the plane of the lateral ventricle, especially arising near the lateral ventricle and pointing toward the cortex (see Figs. 4–10 and 4–17)[185]
3. White matter lesions in the brain stem (see Figs. 4–16 and 4–18)[116,280]
4. Lesions along the corpus callosum best seen on sagittal T_2-weighted scans (see Figs. 4–10, 4–12, 4–16, and 4–17).[392]
5. An open ring appearance on enhanced MRI.[257a]

Table 4–28 provides some guidelines for the use of CT and MRI in diagnosis.

The concept of four or more white matter lesions being strongly suggestive of MS has received support recently.[290,308] Four or more lesions at onset was associated with a higher rate of progression to MS, more frequent development of moderate to severe disabilities, and a greater number of new MRI lesions at 5-year follow-up.

Multimodality Paraclinical Testing

Evoked potentials, CT scanning, and MR scanning have been found, in varying degrees, to be sensitive methods for detecting asymptomatic lesions. This sensitivity has been reflected in a wave of enthusiasm for the use of paraclinical evidence in the diagnosis of MS.[327] It is important to point out that none of these tests can reliably distinguish between various tissue pathologies. Some studies can be highly suggestive of demyelination as a pathological event, but they are all nonspecific. For example, a prolonged latency in the EP can be used as evidence for neurological abnormality, probably demyelinating and probably restricted to the white matter, but the diagnostic implications of that finding must then be assessed using critical clinical judgment.[273]

Table 4–24. **STUDIES OF AGE-RELATED MRI ABNORMALITIES**

Year	Senior Author	No. of Patients	Mean Age (yr)	No. (%) of Abnormal MRI	Diagnosis	Comments
1983	Brant-Zawadzki[52]	5	71	5 (100)	Dementia	Non-Alzheimer's
		5	62	2 (40)	Controls	Mild abnormality
		9	77	6 (67)	Controls	More severe abnormality
1984	Bradley[48]	20	Over 60	6 (30)	Controls	Patients with UBOs* were older (82 years) than those without (68 years).
1985	Kinkel[220]	23	72	12 (52)	Seven stroke Eight dementia Eight vague symptoms	Hypertension and diabetes were risk factors.
1985	Brant-Zawadzki[53]	19	71	9 (47)	Dementia and elderly normals	Nonspecific MRI findings increase with age and CVD risk factors.
1986	Gerard[140]	151	Over 50	?(31)	CVD risk factors or symptoms	
			Over 50	?(7.8)	No CVD risk factors or symptoms	
1986	George[139]	35	<45	0	Controls	
		9	65	8 (89)	Controls	
		8	74	7 (88)	Alzheimer's	
1987	Fazekas[114]	9	68	6 (67)	Controls	
		12	69	10 (83)	Alzheimer's	
		4	70	4 (100)	Multi-infarct dementia	

Continued on following page

Table 4-24.—*continued*

Year	Senior Author	No. of Patients	Mean Age (yr)	No. (%) of Abnormal MRI	Diagnosis	Comments
1988	Kertesz[215]	58	60	45 (77)	Controls	Most changes were periventricular rims and caps.
1988	Braffman[49]	23	Over 60	7 (30)	Controls	1. Lesions were demonstrated on postmortem fixed brain studies. 2. Most lesions were vascular. 3. One of the seven control patients with abnormal MRI scans had asymptomatic MS.
1989	Hunt[188]	46	78	34 (74)	Controls	Frequency increased with older patients.
1989	Masdeu[258]	40	83	20 (50)	Falling elderly	CT lesions were correlated with gait disturbance.
1990	Breitner[54]	8	Over 63	8 (100)	Late-onset paranoid psychosis	All psychotic patients had white matter abnormalities on MRI scan.
1991	van Swieten[422]	10 12 13 3	60–69 70–79 80–89 >90	1 (10) 6 (50) 4 (31) 2 (67)	Some patients with dementia; all brains examined post mortem	Pathological correlation existed between MRI lesions and vascular lesions with secondary demyelination.
1991	Fazekas[115]	101	31–84 yr 30–39 40–49 50–59 60–69 70–79	48 (47) (11) (29) (54) (65) (71)	Controls	Patients with CVD risk factors had an increased frequency of UBOs.
1993	Fazekas[116]	11	52–82	11 (100)		Postmortem correlations with MRI: ischemia.
1993	Fisher[121]	60	76	37 (60)		All ambulatory controls.

CT = computed tomography; CVD = cardiovascular disease; MRI = magnetic resonance imaging; UBOs = unidentified bright objects.

Table 4–25. **DIFFERENTIAL DIAGNOSIS OF MULTIPLE SCLEROSIS ON MAGNETIC RESONANCE IMAGING AND COMPUTED TOMOGRAPHY: NON-AGE-RELATED MAGNETIC RESONANCE IMAGING ABNORMALITIES**

Year	Author	No. of Patients	Diagnosis	MRI/CT Features
1983	Vermess[424]	9	Systemic lupus erythematosus	Eight had abnormal MRI, both focal and periventricular lesions.
1985	Ansink[18]	1	Diffuse sclerosis	Multiple areas of low density with marked enhancement MCT were present in this patient.
1986	Zimmerman[459]	365	Consecutive cases, mixed diagnosis	Periventricular hyperintensity was seen in 94% of cases (nonspecific)
1986	Atlas[21]	3	ADEM (ages 5, 24, 55)	Patchy periventricular and deep white matter lesions were present.
1986	Dunn[90]	5	ADEM (children)	Multifocal reversible white matter lesions were apparent in all.
1987	Mendell[269]	16	Idiopathic polyneuropathy	Six patients, all over 50 yrs of age, had multiple lesions on MRI scan.
1987	Thomas[409]	5	Idiopathic polyneuropathy	All patients had relapsing CNS disease and MRI changes.
1987	Miller[275]	24	10 SLE 9 Behçet's 5 Other Vasculitis	Periventricular, deep white matter and cortical lesions.
1988	Alexander[5]	38	Sjögren's	Fourteen had abnormal MRI with subcortical and periventricular lesions; most had neuropsychiatric symptoms.
1988	Miller[272]	21	Sarcoid	Seventeen had MRI abnormalities: mixed focal and periventricular. Two of 18 had diffuse meningeal enhancement on CT.
1988	Soges[396]	24	Migraine	Eleven (46%) had small, periventricular white matter lesions on T_2 weighted scans; 3 had large cortical infarcts.
1989	Smith[395]	5	Sarcoid	Five had periventricular and 2 had focal subcortical lesions.
1990	Kesselring[216]	12	ADEM	Ten of 12 had multifocal white matter lesions.

Continued on following page

Table 4–25.—*continued*

Year	Author	No. of Patients	Diagnosis	MRI/CT Features
1989	Halperin[167]	33	Lyme disease	Five of six patients with an MS-like illness had MRI lesions. Seven of 17 patients with encephalopathy had MRI lesions. None of the others had MRI lesions.
1990	Williams[444]	2	Sarcoid	Meningeal enhancement distinguished sarcoid disease from MS.
1990	DeAngelis[84]	2	Primary CNS lymphoma	Looks like MS.
1990	Moriwaka[289]	1	Lupus erythematosus (SLE)	Lesions disseminated in space.
1990	Sherman[389]	17	Sarcoid	Meningeal enhancement present.
1990	Feasby[119]	19	CIDP	Seven of 19 (37%) had two or more lesions on MRI scans, mostly in older patients. Lesions were not "typical of MS."
1990	Kesselring[216]	12	ADEM	
1991	Bell[37]	19	SLE	Some steroid responsive.
1991	King[219]	1	Acute intermittent porphyria	Reversible lesions were present in a patient with cerebral symptoms.
1992	Hook[182]	3	Colon cancer with 5-fluorouracil and levamisole	Multifocal "inflammatory" white matter lesions were present. The lesions went away after withdrawal of the chemotherapy.
1992	Fazekas[117]	38	Migraine	Focal white matter lesions seen in fifteen (39%)

ADEM = acute disseminated encephalomyelitis; CIDP = chronic idiopathic demyelinating polyneuropathy; CNS = central nervous system; CT = computed tomography; MRI = magnetic resonance imaging; SLE = systemic lupus erythematosus.

Prospective studies* have shown that in patients suspected by neurologists of having MS, typical asymptomatic abnormalities in appropriate EPs are generally supported as significant by abnormalities in both MRI and CSF studies.[79,180] Unfortunately, normal EP studies are not helpful in this same way. Patients suspected of having MS can have completely normal EPs in one, two, or three regions and still have grossly abnormal MRI studies, plus OB. These same reports have also shown that in selected monosymptomatic clinical presentations, such as ON and CPM, MRI identified 100 percent of patients that could be diagnosed as LSDMS. Appropriate EP studies did not add diagnostically useful information. At one year follow-up, MRI accurately predicted the conversion to CDMS in 18 of the 19 patients in who did so.[325] A subsequent follow-up study[231] showed that 38 of 85 patients (45 percent) originally diagnosed as LSDMS developed CDMS. In contrast, only 17 percent of the 100 patients who re-

*References 34, 35, 275, 276, 279, 311, 325.

Table 4–26. **SPECIFICITY OF MAGNETIC RESONANCE IMAGING CRITERIA FOR MULTIPLE SCLEROSIS**

Year	Senior Author	Criteria	Specificity
1986	Simon[392]	Corpus callosum involvement common	Suggestive of MS
		Corpus callosum atrophy common	Nonspecific finding
1987	Brainin[50,51]	Brain stem lesions: most tend to involve the inner or outer brain surfaces	Brain stem lesions are characteristic of MS; they are not likely to be seen in normal elderly patients.
1988	Fazekas[118]	Size ≥6 mm	These features are characteristic of MS; they are not likely to be seen in normal elderly patients.
		Location	
		Abutting ventricles	
		Infratentorial	
1988	Paty[325]	Four or more white matter lesions, at least one in periventricular region	Four or more white matter lesions are characteristic of MS (conservative criteria).
1988	Reider-Groswasser[351]	White matter lesions are correlated with ventricular dilatation in MS	Ventricular dilatation is characteristic of MS.
1989	Horowitz[185]	Oval-shaped high-signal lesions perpendicular to the A-P axis of the brain (probably perivascular)	Fifty-one of 59 (86%) MS patients had "ovoid" lesions. When these lesions are near the corpus callosum, they are characteristic of MS.
1989	Uhlenbrock[419]	Lesions around the fourth ventricle	Characteristic of MS
		Deep white matter lesions in watershed territory	Characteristic of vascular lesions
1991	Youl[453]	MS or ADEM lesions can look like tumor	Inspection cannot distinguish lesions from tumor; but the time course can.
1991	Paty and Li (unpublished observations)	Corpus callosum	MS lesions in the supraventricular region seem to originate in the corpus callosum. They are clearly seen on a parasagittal T_2-weighted sequence.
1991	Gean-Marton[136]	Corpus callosum	Confluent and focal lesions involving the corpus callosum were found in 93% of 42 MS patients and only 2.4% of patients with other diseases.
1991	Wilms[446]	Sagittal scans	Sagittal scans pick up more lesions than do axial ones and are better for seeing lesions of the corpus callosum.
1993	Offenbacher[308]	Fazekas criteria	Follow-up shows that these criteria have a 90% sensitivity and a 81% specificity.
1994	Barkhof[26]	MRI number of lesions	Eight lesions are more specific for MS than four.
1996	Masdeu[257a]	Open ring	An open ring on enhanced MRI is very suggestive of MS.

ADEM = acute disseminated encephalomyelitis; AP = anteroposterior; CT = computed tomography; MRI = magnetic resonance imaging.

Table 4–27. STUDIES OF THE USE OF MAGNETIC RESONANCE IMAGING IN ISOLATED NEUROLOGICAL SYNDROMES ASSOCIATED WITH MULTIPLE SCLEROSIS ONSET

Year	Senior Author	No. of Patients	No. (%) Positive MRI Scans	Comments
			OPTIC NEURITIS (ON)	
1986	Jacobs[194]	16	8 (50)	
1991	Johns[201]	10	7 (70)	Patients with neuroretinitis were excluded.
1986	Ormerod[311]	35	21 (60)	Six of the positive patients developed CDMS on follow-up.
1987	Yedavally[449]	23	15 (65)	Conservative criteria were used in this study: Six white matter lesions were required for a positive MRI scan.
1987	Kinnunen[222]	10	4 (40)	
1988	Paty[325]	38	25 (66)	Conservative (UBC) criteria were used in this study.*
1988	Eidelberg[104]	7	4 (57)	Nontumor or compressive ON. Two patients had sarcoidosis.
1988	Riikonen[354]	14	8 (57)	All patients were children (4–14 years).
1989	Frederiksen[125]	50	31 (62)	
1991	Martinelli[257]	43	21 (49)	
1991	Scholl[377]	43	31 (72)	Uhthoff's Symptom increased the likelihood of a positive MRI scan.
1992	Christiansen[70]	19	14 (74)	50% of lesions were old ones.
1993	Beck[34]	389	47 (12)	Conservative (UBC) criteria were used in this study.
	Total	697	236 (34)	
			CHRONIC PROGRESSIVE MYELOPATHY (CPM)	
1986	Edwards[103]	10	6 (60)	MRI superior to EP.
1987	Miller[273]	89	73 (82)	LSDMS was diagnosed in 28/89 (31%).
1987	Miska[285]	20	13 (75)	
1987	Ormerod[312]	24	20 (83)	All 20 had cord MRI abnormalities.
1988	Paty[325]	52	31 (60)	Conservative (UBC) MRI criteria were used in this study.*
1988	Mauch[259]	18	15 (83)	
	Total	213	158 (74)	
			ACUTE MYELOPATHY	
1989	Miller[277]	38	18 (56)	MRI lesions predicted CDMS on follow-up.
			BRAIN STEM SYNDROMES	
1987	Ormerod[312]	44	30 (68)	Four patients had tumor.
1988	Paty[325]	54	26 (48)	Conservative (UBC) MRI criteria were used in this study.*
1989	Miller[277]	23	17 (74)	Of 17 patients with acute lesions, 5 developed CDMS in 15 months: all had an abnormal MRI scan when first studied.
	Total Brain Stem	121	73 (60)	

CDMS = clinically definite MS; LSDMS = laboratory-supported definite MS; MRI = magnetic resonance imaging; ON = optic neuritis; UBC = University of British Columbia; EP = evoked potentials.
*See text and Table 4–28.

Table 4–28. USE OF COMPUTED TOMOGRAPHY AND MAGNETIC RESONANCE IMAGING IN THE DIAGNOSIS OF MULTIPLE SCLEROSIS

CT: The enhanced CT scan can show a defective BBB, but enhanced CT is not as sensitive as MRI, and plain CT is even less sensitive. Enhanced CT is also not likely to be positive in clinically inactive patients.

MRI: MRI is the most sensitive paraclinical examination for showing asymptomatic dissemination in space. Results should be interpreted with caution, however, because of the frequency of false-positives, especially in older normal individuals, and because of the nonspecificity for demyelination. Conservative (UBC) criteria propose that four white matter lesions are strongly suggestive of MS (see text).

Comments:

Features that are considered to increase the specificity for MS are:

1. White matter lesions >6 mm in diameter
2. Presence of at least one periventricular lesion adjacent to the body of the lateral ventricle
3. Presence of at least one lesion in the brain stem or cerebellum
4. Ovoid lesions (these lesions are near the lateral ventricles and oval in shape, with the long axis of the lesion 90° to the plane of the lateral ventricle)*
5. Lesions that originate in the corpus callosum and radiate outwards and upwards
6. Eight white matter lesions

BBB = blood-brain barrier; CT = computed tomography; MRI = magnetic resonance imaging; UBC = University of British Columbia.

*See text for explanation.

mained as clinically suspected MS but who did not initially satisfy the criteria for LSDMS went on to develop CDMS. Of the 55 patients who developed CDMS on follow-up, 46 (84 percent) had had an MRI scan that was strongly suggestive of MS when first studied. Ninety-five percent (52 of 55) had had at least one abnormal white matter area on MRI scan when first studied. Three patients were falsely diagnosed as strongly suggestive of MS on MRI scan who went on to have other diagnoses made. All of these patients were older than 65 years, and none had CSF OB. Long-term clinical follow-up studies are the only way that we will know just how accurately the patterns of abnormality seen in paraclinical tests predict a diagnosis of CDMS.

Because of the nonspecificity of MRI in the diagnosis of MS, in 1987, a committee made up of a number of MS investigators published a policy statement for the use of MRI in the diagnosis of MS.[322] In addition, the proper use of paraclinical tests has been reviewed.[327] The cautions expressed in relation to the use of MRI in the 1987 statement should be applied to the interpretation of all paraclinical tests.[36a]

We wish to emphasize that MS is still a clinical diagnosis and that tests are carried out to support the clinical impression or to exclude unlikely alternatives. The reader should *not* leave with the impression that all suspected MS patients need all or any of the aforementioned diagnostic examinations.

In a tertiary care setting with active clinical research programs, one must emphasize the certainty of diagnosis as well as the identification of non-MS disorders. We take the position that we must be certain of the diagnosis in every patient referred to us. We would always prefer to make the diagnosis of something other than MS, because a premature diagnosis of MS, especially by an MS clinical center, stops critical thinking and may allow treatable conditions to be overlooked. Table 4–29 lists some of the non-MS diagnoses made on patients referred to our MS clinics.

In summary, the principles of MS diagnosis rest on showing the dissemination of white matter lesions in time and space. Unfortunately, when taken in isolation, no finding on history, physical examination, or laboratory studies is entirely specific to MS. When the pattern of dissemination in time

Table 4–29. SOME NON–MULTIPLE SCLEROSIS FINAL DIAGNOSES IN PATIENTS REFERRED TO THE UNIVERSITY OF BRITISH COLUMBIA AND UNIVERSITY OF WESTERN ONTARIO MULTIPLE SCLEROSIS CLINICS

Adrenoleukodystrophy
AIDS myelopathy
Amyotrophic lateral sclerosis
Vitamin B_{12} deficiency
Bell's palsy
Benign fasciculations
Cerebellar degeneration
Chronic spinal arachnoiditis
Eales' disease
Functional illness
Hereditary spastic paraplegia
HTLV-1 associated myelopathy (HAM)
Hydrocephalus
Migraine
Myasthenia gravis
Non-MS chronic myelopathies (including primary lateral sclerosis)
Relapsing idiopathic demyelinating neuropathy
Spinal AVM
Spinal tumor (cervical, thoracic)
Thoracic disk disease

AIDS = acquired immunodeficiency syndrome; AVM = arteriovenous malformation.

and space is identified in the proper setting, however, especially when seen in the presence of supportive laboratory studies such as CSF electrophoresis and MRI, the diagnosis is about 95 percent secure. Prognosis is difficult to determine at onset.[324]

TELLING THE DIAGNOSIS

Gorman and her colleagues[153] surveyed 100 patients with MS concerning the telling of the diagnosis. More than 90 percent definitely wanted to know the diagnosis at the earliest time that it was certain. More than one-half wanted to know even suspicions of the diagnosis.

When the diagnosis is conveyed to the patient, we suggest the following guidelines:

• The spouse or a significant other should be present.

• The diagnosis should be given with encouragement and hope for either a benign prognosis or for good news from future research.

• A follow-up session should be scheduled to give information about the disease.

Many patients do not remember very much of their first encounter after being told of the diagnosis of MS, but they do respond positively to the physician's taking the time to explain the disease. The diagnosis is best received if given by the physician, and if the specific name "multiple sclerosis" is used, rather than some vague term such as "demyelinating disease" or "inflammation of the spinal cord." We also believe, as do others, that if the physician identifies specific, short-term goals for the patient, the response will be positive. The physician must avoid showing disinterest in either the disease or the patient or expressing a sense of hopelessness. We also suggest that medical jargon be avoided.

In our experience, it is best to explain that the clinical course of MS is somewhat unpredictable. Although, at the moment, it is incurable, the natural tendency to remission shows that the body is able to cure itself in the majority of attacks. When patients are getting worse over the short term, there is at least a 70 percent chance that they will improve spontaneously. In addition, in as many as 40 percent of patients observed after 15 years of disease, the disease is still relatively benign and may remain so (Redekop and Paty, 1995). Also, there is no clear indication that the severity of attacks influences the eventual outcome, so long as there is full recovery between attacks. This kind of information should be stressed at the beginning of the encounter, so that the patient can understand that there is considerable hope, if only in relation to the body's ability to control the process spontaneously.

Factors that might support a delay in telling the diagnosis are youth (patient younger than 20 years old), decreased intelligence or emotional instability, and perceived lack of support, particularly emotional support from friends and relatives. When patients do not ask about their diagnosis, they are usually expressing a considerable amount of fear and apprehension. However, just giving the diagnosis of MS to a patient can result in significant impairment of their quality of life (Canadian Burden of Illness Study, Montreal, Quebec, 1996).

SUMMARY

The diagnosis of MS can be made purely on clinical grounds in the majority of patients. The clinical demonstration of white matter lesions disseminated in time and space in a young adult strongly suggests MS. Showing asymptomatic MRI and EP abnormalities in young adult patients who are monosymptomatic also suggest MS. Many treatable diseases can mimic MS in both clinical and laboratory features. For this reason, the diagnosis of MS should be made only by an experienced clinician who is well aware of the nonspecificity of both clinical and paraclinical findings. In our

MS clinics, we consider MS to be a most serious diagnosis; therefore, we first try to prove that each patient sent to us does *not* have MS. Over the years, we have diagnosed many patients referred to us by both general physicians and neurologists with a diagnosis of MS as having other diseases. Nonetheless, we believe that the diagnosis of MS is being made with greater frequency and greater accuracy in recent years.

REFERENCES

1. Achiron A, Pinhas-Hamiel O, Doll L, et al: Spastic paraparesis associated with human T-lymphotropic virus type I: A clinical, serological, and genomic study in Iranian-born Mashhadi Jews. Ann Neurol 34:670–675, 1993.
2. Adams C, and Armstrong D: Acute transverse myelopathy in children. Can J Neurol Sci 17:40–45, 1990.
3. Aita JF, Bennett DR, Anderson RE, and Ziter F: Cranial CT appearance of acute multiple sclerosis. Neurology 28:251–255, 1978.
3a. Akman-Demir G, Baykan-Kurt B, Serdaroglu, P, et al: Seven-year follow-up of neurologic involvement in Behçet Syndrome. Arch Neurol 53:691–694, 1996.
4. Al Kawi MZ, Bohlega S, and Banna M: MRI findings in neuro-Behçet's disease. Neurology 41:405–408, 1991.
5. Alexander EL, Beall SS, Gordon B, et al: Magnetic resonance imaging of cerebral lesions in patients with the Sjogren Syndrome. Ann Intern Med 108:815–823, 1988.
6. Alexander EL, Malinow K, Lejewski JE, Jerdan MS, Provost TT, and Alexander GE: Primary Sjogren's syndrome with central nervous system disease mimicking multiple sclerosis. Ann Intern Med 104:323–330, 1986.
7. Alexander GE, Provost TT, Stevens MB, and Alexander EL: Sjögren syndrome: Central nervous system manifestations. Neurology 31:1391–1396, 1981.
8. Alfieri G, Barontini F, Brogelli S, and Maurri S: Unusual association of Eales disease with multifocal neurological deficit. Ital J Neurol Sci 5:461–462, 1984.
9. Allison RS, and Millar JHD: Prevalence and familial incidence of disseminated sclerosis (a report to the Northern Ireland Hospitals Authority on the results of a three-year survey): Prevalence of disseminated sclerosis in Northern Ireland. Ulster Med J 23(suppl 2):5–27, 1954.
10. Altrocchi PH: Acute transverse myelopathy. Arch Neurol 9:21–29, 1963.
11. Alvarez G, and Cardenas M: Multiple sclerosis following optic neuritis in Chile. J Neurol Neurosurg Psychiatry 52:115–117, 1989.

12. Aminoff MJ: Evoked potential studies in neurological diagnosis and management. Ann Neurol 28:706–710, 1990.

13. Andermann F, Cosgrove JB, Lloyd-Smith DL, Gloor P, and McNaughton FL: Facial myokymia in multiple sclerosis. Brain 84:31, 1961.

14. Andersson M, Alvarez-Cermeño J, Bernardi G, et al: Cerebrospinal fluid in the diagnosis of multiple sclerosis: A consensus report. J Neurol Neurosurg Psychiatry 57:897–902, 1994.

15. Andersson T, Siden A, and Persson A: A comparison of clinical and evoked potential (VEP and median nerve SEP) evolution in patients with MS and potentially related conditions. Acta Neurol Scand 84:139–145, 1991.

16. Anema JR, Heijenbrok MW, Faes TJ, Heimans JJ, Lanting P, and Polman CH: Cardiovascular autonomic function in multiple sclerosis. J Neurol Sci 104:129–134, 1991.

17. Anmarkrud N, and Slettnes ON: Uncomplicated retrobulbar neuritis and the development of multiple sclerosis. Acta Ophthalmol Scand 67:306–309, 1989.

18. Ansink BJJ, Davies AG, Bellot SM, and Stam FC: Diffuse sclerosis. Clinical Neuroradiological and Neuropathological Findings. Neuroradiology 27:360–361, 1985.

19. Antunes JL, Schlesinger EB, and Michelsen WJ: The abnormal brain scan in demyelinating diseases. Arch Neurol 30:269–271, 1974.

20. Aring CD: Observations on multiple sclerosis and conversion hysteria. Brain 88:663–667, 1965.

20a. Arnett PA, Rao SM, Hussain M, Swanson SJ, and Hammeke TA: Conduction aphasia in multiple sclerosis: A case report with MRI findings. Neurology 47:576–578, 1996.

21. Atlas SW, Grossman RI, Goldberg HI, Hackney DB, Bilaniuk LT, and Zimmerman RA: MR diagnosis of acute disseminated encephalomyelitis. J Comput Assist Tomogr 10:798–801, 1986.

22. Babinski J, and Dubois R: Douleurs a forme de decharge electrique, consecutive aux tramatismes de la nuque. Presse Med 26:64, 1891.

23. Bachman DM, Rosenthal AR, and Beckingsale AB: Granulomatous uveitis in neurological disease. Br J Ophthalmol 69:192–196, 1985.

24. Baloh RW, Yee RD, and Honrubia V: Internuclear ophthaloplegia. II. Pursuit, optokinetic nystagmus, and vestibulo-ocular reflex. Arch Neurol 35:490–493, 1978(b).

25. Baloh RW, Yee RD, and Honrubia V: Internuclear ophthalmoplegia. I. Saccades and dissociated nystagmus. Arch Neurol 35:484–489, 1978(a).

26. Barkhof F, Filippi M, Tas MW, et al: Towards specific MR imaging criteria for early MS. 10th Congress of the European Committee for Treatment and Research in Multiple Sclerosis, Athens, Greece. Book of Abstracts, 1994, p 9.

27. Barkhof F, Valk J, Hommes OR, and Scheltens P: Meningeal Gd-DTPA enhancement in multiple sclerosis [see comments]. Am J Neuroradiol 13:397–400, 1992.

28. Barnes D, and McDonald WI: The ocular manifestations of multiple sclerosis. II. Abnormalities of eye movements: Review. J Neurol Neurosurg Psychiatry 55:863–868, 1992.

29. Barnes D, McDonald WI, Landon DN, and Johnson G: The characterisation of experimental gliosis by quantitive nuclear magnetic resonance imaging. Brain III(pt 1):83–94, 1988.

30. Barnes D, McDonald WI, Tofts PS, Johnson G, and Landon DN: Magnetic resonance imaging of experimental cerebral oedema. J Neurol Neurosurg Psychiat 49:1341–1347, 1986.

31. Barnes D, Munro PMG, Youl BD, Prineas JW, and McDonald WI: The longstanding MS lesion. Brain 114:1271–1280, 1991.

32. Bates D (chairman): Proceedings of the MS Forum Modern Management Workshop: The Diagnosis of Multiple Sclerosis. (Editorial) Int. MSJ, Vol. 1(1):4–5, 1994, Worthing, U.K.

33. Baum K, Scheuler W, Hegerl U, Girke W, and Schorner W: Detection of brainstem lesions in multiple sclerosis: Comparison of brainstem auditory evoked potentials with nuclear magnetic resonance imaging. Acta Neurol Scand 77:283–288, 1988.

33a. Beatty WW, Paul RH, Wilbanks SL, Hames KA, Blanco CR, and Goodkin DE: Identifying multiple sclerosis patients with mild or global cognitive impairment using the Screening Examination for Cognitive Impairment (SEFCI). Neurology 45:718–723, 1995.

34. Beck RW, Arrington J, Murtagh FR, Cleary PA, Kaufman DI, and the Optic Neuritis Study Group: Brain MRI in acute optic neuritis experience of the Optic Neuritis Study Group. Arch Neurol 50:841–846, 1993.

35. Beck RW, Cleary PA, Anderson MM, and Keltner JL: A randomized, controlled trial of corticosteroids in the treatment of acute optic neuritis. N Engl J Med 326:581–588, 1992.

36. Beck RW, Cleary PA, Trobe JD, et al: The effect of corticosteroids for acute optic neuritis on the subsequent development of multiple sclerosis: The Optic Neuritis Study Group [see comments]. N Engl J Med 329:1764–1769, 1993.

36a. Beer S, Rösler KM, and Hess CW: Diagnostic value of paraclinical tests in multiple sclerosis: Relative sensitivities and specificities for reclassification according to the Poser committee criteria. Journal of Neurology, Neurosurgery, and Psychiatry 59:152–159, 1995.

37. Bell CL, Partington C, Robbins M, Graziano F, Turski P, and Kornguth S: Magnetic resonance imaging of central nervous system lesions in patients with lupus erythematosus: Correlation with clinical remission and antineurofilament and anticardiolipin antibody titers. Arthritis Rheum 34:432–441, 1991.

38. Bemelmans BL, Hommes OR, Van Kerrebroeck PE, Lemmens WA, Doesburg WH, and Debruyne FM: Evidence for early lower urinary tract dysfunction in clinically silent multiple sclerosis. J Urol 145:1219–1224, 1991.

39. Berger JR, and Quencer R: Reversible myelopathy with pernicious anemia: Clinical/MR correlation. Neurology 41:947–948, 1991.

40. Berger JR, and Sheremata WA: Persistent neurological deficit precipitated by hot bath test in multiple sclerosis. JAMA 249:1751–1753, 1983.

41. Berger JR, Sheremata WA, and Melamed E: Paroxysmal dystonia as the initial manifestation of multiple sclerosis. Arch Neurol 41:747–750, 1984.

42. Berger JR, Tornatore C, Major EO, et al: Relapsing and remitting human immunodeficiency virus-associated leukoencephalomyelopathy. Ann Neurol 31:34–38, 1992.

43. Berry I, Clanet M, Franconi JM, and Manelfe C: Ultra-fast MRI sequence for MS lesions visualization: Flair-haste. 10th Congress of the European Committee for Treatment and Research in MS, Athens, Greece. Book of Abstracts, 1994, p 52.

44. Blaivas JG, Bhimani G, and Labib K: Vesicourethral dysfunction in multiple sclerosis. J Urol 122:342, 1979.

45. Blennow K, Fredman P, Wallin A, et al: Formulas for the quantitation of intrathecal IgG production. Their validity in the presence of blood-brain barrier damage and their utility in multiple sclerosis. J Neurol Sci 121:90–96, 1994.

45a. Bolay H, Karabudak R, Tacal T, Önol B, Selekler K, and Saribas O: Balo's Concentric Sclerosis: Report of two patients with magnetic resonance imaging follow-up. J Neuroimag 6:98–103, 1996.

46. Boné G, Ladurner G, Artmann W, and Bsteh C: Correlations between clinical and magnetic resonance imaging findings in multiple sclerosis. Eur Neurol 28:212–216, 1988.

47. Boyle EA, Clark CM, Klonoff H, Paty DW, and Oger JJF: Empirical support for psychological profiles observed in multiple sclerosis. Arch Neurol 48:1150–1154, 1991.

48. Bradley WG, Waluch V, Brant-Zawadzki M, Yadley RA, and Wycoff RR: Patchy, periventricular white matter lesions in the elderly: Common observation during NMR imaging. Noninvasive Medical Imaging 1:35–41, 1984.

49. Braffman BH, Zimmerman RA, Trojanowski JQ, Gonatas NK, Hickey WF, and Schlaepfer WW: Brain MR: Pathologic correlation with gross and histopathology. II. Hyperintense white-matter foci in the elderly. AJNR 9:629–636, 1988.

50. Brainin M, Reisner T, Neuhold A, Omasits M, and Wicke L: Topological characteristics of brainstem lesions in clinically definite and clinically probable cases of multiple sclerosis: An MRI study. Neuroradiology 29:530–534, 1987.

51. Brainin M, Reisner T, Neuhold A, Omasits M, and Wicke L: Topological characteristics of brainstem lesions in clinically definite and clinically probable cases of multiple sclerosis: an MRI study. J Neurol Neurosurg Psychiatry 52 (12):1355–1359, 1989.

52. Brant-Zawadski M, Davis PL, Crooks LE, et al: NMR demonstration of cerebral abnormalities: Comparison with CT. AJR 140:847–854, 1983.

53. Brant-Zawadski M, Fein G, and Van Dyke C: MR imaging of the aging brain: Patchy white matter lesions and dementia. AJNR 6:675–682, 1985.

54. Breitner JC, Husain MM, Figiel GS, Krishnan KR, and Boyko OB: Cerebral white matter disease in late-onset paranoid psychosis. Biol Psychiatry 28:266–274, 1990.

55. Breteler MMB, van Swieten JC, Bots ML, et al: Cerebral white matter lesions, vascular risk factors, and cognitive function in a population-based study: The Rotterdam study. Neurology 44:1246–1251, 1994.

56. Brett DC, Ferguson GG, Ebers GC, and Paty DW: Percutaneous trigeminal rhizotomy: Treatment of trigeminal neuralgia secondary to multiple sclerosis. Arch Neurol 39:219–221, 1982.

57. Breukelman AJ, Polman CH, de Slegte RGM, and Koetsier JC: Neuromyelitis optica (Devic's syndrome): Not always multiple sclerosis. Clin Neurol Neurosurg 90(4):357–360, 1988.

58. Brownell B, and Hughes JT: The distribution of plaques in the cerebrum in multiple sclerosis. J Neurol Neurosurg Psychiatry 25:315–320, 1962.

59. Bruhn H, Frahm J, Merboldt KD, et al: Multiple sclerosis in children: Cerebral metabolic alterations monitored by localized proton magnetic resonance spectroscopy in vivo. Ann Neurol 32:140–150, 1992.

60. Bruyn GW, Bots GTAM, Went LN, and Klinkhamer PJJM: Hereditary spastic dystonia with Leber's hereditary optic neuropathy: Neuropathological findings. J Neurol Sci 113:55–61, 1992.

61. Buchwald D, Cheney PR, Peterson DL, et al: A chronic illness characterized by fatigue, neurologic and immunologic disorders, and active human herpesvirus Type 6 infection. Ann Int Med 116:103–113, 1992.

62. Burde RM, and Landau WM: Shooting backward with Marcus Gunn: A circular exercise in paralogic. Neurology 43:2444–2447, 1993.

63. Bussone G, La Mantia L, Grazzi L, Lamperti E, Salmaggi A, and Strada L: Neurobrucellosis mimicking multiple sclerosis: A case report. Eur Neurol 29:238–240, 1989.

64. Bydder GM, Steiner RE, Young IR, et al: Clinical NMR imaging of the brain: 140 cases. AJR 139: 215–236, 1982.

65. Bynke H, Olsson J, and Rosen I: Diagnostic value of visual evoked response, clinical eye examination and CSF analysis in chronic myelopathy. Acta Neurol Scand 56:55–69, 1977.

66. Cala LA, and Mastaglia FL: Computerised axial tomography in multiple sclerosis. Lancet 1:689, 1976.

66a. Carrigan DR, Harrington D, and Knox KK: Subacute leukoencephalitis caused by CNS infection with human herpesvirus-6 manifesting as acute multiple sclerosis. Neurology 47:145–148, 1996.

67. Celesia GG, Kaufman DI, Brigell M, et al: Optic neuritis: A prospective study. Neurology 40: 919–923, 1990.

68. Chajek T, and Fainaru M: Behçet's disease: Report of 41 cases and a review of the literature. Medicine 54:179–196, 1975.

69. Chiappa KH: Brainstem auditory evoked potentials in multiple sclerosis. In Poser CM (ed): The Diagnosis of Multiple Sclerosis. Stratton-Verlag, New York, 1983, pp 120–130.

70. Christiansen P, Frederiksen JL, Henriksen O, and Larsson HB: Gd-DTPA-enhanced lesions in the brain of patients with acute optic neuritis. Acta Neurol Scand 85:141–146, 1992.

71. Cohen MM, Lessell S, and Wolf PA: A prospective study of the risk of developing multiple sclerosis in uncomplicated optic neuritis. Neurology 29: 208–213, 1979.

72. Compston DAS, Batchelor JR, Earl CJ, and McDonald WI: Factors influencing the risk of multiple sclerosis developing in patients with optic neuritis. Brain 101:495–511, 1978.

73. Cortelli P, Montagna P, Avoni P, et al: Leber's hereditary optic neuropathy: Genetic, biochemical and phosphorus magnetic resonance spectroscopy study in an Italian family. Neurology 41:1211–1215, 1991.

74. Cox TA: Relative afferent pupillary defects in multiple sclerosis. Can J Ophthalmol 24:207–210, 1989.

75. Cox TA: Pupillary escape. Neurology 42:1271–1273, 1992.

76. Coyle PK: Borrelia burgdorferi antibodies in multiple sclerosis patients. Neurology 39:760–761, 1989.

77. Coyle PK: Oligoclonal bands in tears versus CSF of early multiple sclerosis patients. Neurology 41:148, 1991.

78. Coyle PK, Krupp LB, and Doscher C: Significance of reactive Lyme serology in multiple sclerosis. Ann Neurol 34:745–747, 1993.

79. Cutler JR, Aminoff MJ, and Brant-Zawadzki M: Evaluation of patients with multiple sclerosis by evoked potentials and magnetic resonance imaging: A comparative study. Ann Neurol 20:645– 648, 1986.

80. Davis DO, and Pressman BD: Computerized tomography of the brain. Radiol Clin North Am 12:297–313, 1974.

81. Davis FA: Hot bath test in the diagnosis of multiple sclerosis. Journal of Mount Sinai Hospital 33:280–282, 1966.

82. Davis FA, Michael JA, and Neer D: Serial hyperthermia testing in multiple sclerosis: A method of monitoring subclinical fluctuations. Acta Neurol Scand 49:63–74, 1973.

83. Davison C, Goodhart SP, and Lander J: Multiple sclerosis and amyotrophies. Arch Neurol 31: 270–289, 1934.

84. DeAngelis LM: Primary central nervous system lymphoma imitates multiple sclerosis. J Neurooncol 9:177–181, 1990.

85. Dean G, Bhigjee AIG, Bill PLA, et al: Multiple sclerosis in black South Africans and Zimbabweans. J Neurol Neurosurg Psychiatry 57:1064–1069, 1994.

86. Delaney P: Neurologic manifestations of saroidosis. Ann Intern Med 87:79–85, 1977.

87. Den Boer JA, Salverda P, Peters TR, and Prevo RL: Multislice Turbo-FLAIR in brain studies of multiple sclerosis. Proceedings of the Society for Magnetic Resonance in Medicine. Vol. 1, 12th Annual Meeting Aug. 14-20, New York. (USA) p328, 1993.

88. Devinsky O, Cho E, Petito CK, and Price RW: Herpes zoster myelitis. Brain 114(PT3) 1181–1196, 1991 Jan.

89. Dewar J, Lunt H, Abernathy DA, Dady P, and Haas LF: Cisplatin neuropathy with L'hermitte's sign. J Neurol Neurosurg Psychiatry 49:96–99, 1986.

90. Dunn V, Bale JF, Zimmerman RA, Perdue Z, and Bell WE: MRI in children with postinfectious disseminated encephalomyelitis. Magn Reson Imaging 4:25–32, 1986.

91. Duquette P, Decary F, and Pleines J: Clinical subgroups of multiple sclerosis in relation to HLA: DR alleles as possible markers of disease progression. Can J Neurol Sci 12:106–110, 1985.

92. Duquette P, and Girard M: Hormonal factors in susceptibility to multiple sclerosis. Current Opinion in Neurology and Neurosurgery 6: 195–201, 1993.

93. Duquette P, Murray TJ, Pleines J, et al: Multiple sclerosis in childhood: Clinical profile in 125 patients. J Pediatr 111:359–363, 1987.

94. Duquette P, Pleines J, Girard M, Charest L, Senecal-Quevillon M, and Masse C: The increased susceptibilty of women to multiple sclerosis. Can J Neurol Sci 19:466–471, 1992.

95. Ebers GC: Cerebrospinal fluid electrophoresis in multiple sclerosis. In Poser CM (ed): The Diagnosis of Multiple Sclerosis. Stratton-Verlag, New York, 1983, pp 179–184.

96. Ebers GC: Controversies in Neurology: Optic neuritis and multiple sclerosis. Arch Neurol 42:702–704, 1985.

97. Ebers GC: Multiple sclerosis. In Ashbury AK, McKhann GM, McDonald WI (eds): Diseases of the Nervous System. WB Saunders, Philadelphia, 1986, pp 1268–1281.

98. Ebers GC, Cousin HK, Feasby TE, and Paty DW: Optic neuritis in familial MS. Neurology 31: 1138–1142, 1981.

99. Ebers GC, and Feasby TE: Optic neuritis and multiple sclerosis. Can J Neurol Sci 10:79–80, 1983.

100. Ebers GC, and Paty DW: The major histocompatibility complex, the immune system and multiple sclerosis. Clin Neurol Neurosurg 81:69, 1979.

101. Ebers GC, and Paty DW: CSF electrophoresis in one thousand patients. Can J Neurol Sci 7:275–280, 1980.

102. Ebers GC, Vinuela FV, Feasby TE, and Bass B: Multifocal CT enhancement in MS. Neurol 34:341–346, 1984.

103. Edwards MK, Farlow MR, and Stevens JC: Cranial MR in Spinal Cord MS: Diagnosing patients with isolated spinal cord symptoms. Neuroradiology 1003–1005, 1986.

104. Eidelberg D, Newton MR, Johnson G, et al: Chronic unilateral optic neuropathy: A magnetic resonance study. Ann Neurol 24(1):3–11, 1988.

105. Eisen AA: The somatosensory evoked potential. Can J Neurol Sci 9:65–77, 1982.

106. Eisen AA: Use of the somatosensory evoked potential in multiple sclerosis. In Poser CM (ed): The Diagnosis of Multiple Sclerosis. Stratton-Verlag, New York, 1983, pp 131.

107. Eisen AA, and Odusote K: Central and peripheral conduction times in multiple sclerosis. Electroencephalogr Clin Neurophysiol 48:253–265, 1980.

108. Elbol P, and Work K: Retinal nerve fiber layer in multiple sclerosis. Acta Ophthalmologica 68: 481–486, 1990.

109. Ellemann K, Krogh E, and Arlien-Soeborg P: Sjögren's syndrome in patients with multiple sclerosis. Acta Neurol Scand 84:68–69, 1991.

110. Engelken JD, Huh WT, Carter DK, and Nerad JA: Optic nerve sarcoidosis: MR findings. American Journal of Neuroradiology 13:228–230, 1992.

111. Engell T: A clinico-pathoanatomical study of multiple sclerosis diagnosis. Acta Neurol Scand 78:39–44, 1988.

112. Farlow MR, Markand ON, Edwards MK, Stevens JC, and Kolar OJ: Multiple sclerosis: Magnetic resonance imaging, evoked responses and spinal fluid electrophoresis. Neurology 36:828–831, 1986.

113. Farrell MA, Kaufmann JCE, Gilbert JJ, Noseworthy JH, Armstrong HA, and Ebers GC: Oligoclonal bands in multiple sclerosis: Clinical-pathologic correlation. Neurology 35:212–218, 1985.

114. Fazekas F, Chawluk JB, Alavi A, Hurtig HI, and Zimmerman RA: MR signal abnormalities at 1.5 T in Alzheimer's dementia and normal aging. AJNR 8:421–426, 1987.

115. Fazekas F, Kleinert R, Offenbacher H, et al: The morphologic correlate of incidental punctate white matter hyperintensities on MR images. AJNR 12:915–921, 1991.

116. Fazekas F, Kleinert R, Offenbacher H, et al: Pathologic correlates of incidental MRI white matter signal hyperintensities. Neurology 43:1683–1689, 1993.

117. Fazekas F, Koch M, R. Schmidt R, et al: The prevalence of cerebral damage varies with migraine type: A MRI study. Headache 32:287–291, 1992.

118. Fazekas F, Offenbacher H, Fuchs S, et al: Criteria for an increased specificity of MRI interpretation in elderly subjects with suspected multiple sclerosis. Neurology 38:1822–1825, 1988.

118a. Fazekas F, Schmidt R, Offenbacher H, et al: Prevalence of white matter and periventricular magnetic resonance hyperintensities in asymptomatic volunteers. J Neuroimag 1:27–30, 1991.

119. Feasby TE, Hahn AF, Koopman WJ, and Lee DH: Central lesions in chronic inflammatory demyelinating polyneuropathy: An MRI study. Neurology 40(3 pt 1):476–478, 1990.

120. Fernandez RE, Rothberg M, Ferencz G, and Wujack D: Lyme disease of the CNS: MR imaging findings in 14 cases. AJNR 11:479–481, 1990.

120a. Filippi M, Yousry T, Baratti C, et al: Quantitative assessment of MRI lesion load in multiple sclerosis—a comparison of conventional spin-echo with fast fluid-attenuated inversion recovery. Brain 119:1349–1355, 1996.

120b. Filippi M, Yousry T, Campi A, Kandziora C, Colombo B, and Voltz R: Comparison of triple dose versus standard dose gadolinium-DTPA for detection of MRI enhancing lesions in patients with MS. Neurology 46:379–384, 1996.

121. Fisher M, Brant-Zawadzki M, Ameriso S, et al: Subcortical magnetic resonance imaging changes in a healthy elderly population: Stroke risk factors, ultrasound, and hemostasis findings. J Neuroimag 3:28–32, 1993.

122. Ford B, Tampieri D, and Francis G: Long-term follow-up of acute partial transverse myelopathy. Neurology 42:250–252, 1992.

123. Francis DA, Compston DAS, Batchelor JR, and McDonald WI: A reassessment of the risk of multiple sclerosis developing in patients with optic neuritis after extended follow-up. J Neurol Neurosurg Psychiatry 50:758–765, 1987.

124. Francis DA, Thompson AJ, Brookes P, et al: Multiple sclerosis and HLA: Is the susceptibility gene really HLA-DR or -DQ. Hum Immunol 32:119–124, 1991.

125. Frederiksen JL, Larsson HB, Henriksen O, and Olesen J: Magnetic resonance imaging of the brain in patients with acute monosymptomatic optic neuritis. Acta Neurol Scand 80:512–517, 1989.

126. Frederiksen JL, Larsson HB, Nordenbo AM, and Seedorff HH: Plaques causing hemianopsia or quadrantanopsia in multiple sclerosis identified by MRI and VEP. Acta Ophthalmol Suppl 69:169–177, 1991.

127. Frederiksen JL, Larsson HB, Olesen J, and Stigsby B: MRI, VEP, SEP and biothesiometry suggest monosymptomatic acute optic neuritis to be a first manifestation of multiple sclerosis. Acta Neurol Scand 83:343–350, 1991.

128. Frederiksen JL, Larsson HB, Ottovay E, Stigsby B, and Elesen J: Acute optic neuritis with normal visual acuity. Acta Ophthalmol Suppl 69:357–366, 1991.

129. Fukazawa T: Acute transverse myelopathy in multiple sclerosis: Clinical and laboratory analyses. Hokkaido Igaku Zasshi 68:79–95, 1993.

130. Fukazawa T, Miyasaka K, Tashiro K, Hamada T, Moriwaka F, Yanagihara T, et al: MRI findings of multiple sclerosis with acute transverse myelopathy. J Neurol Sci 110:27–31, 1992.

130a. Gabriel SE, O'Fallon WM, Kurland LT, Beard CM, Woods JE, and Melton LJ: Risk of connective-tissue diseases and other disorders after breast implantation (see comments). N Engl J Med 330(24):1697–1702, 1994.

131. Galer BS, Lipton RB, Weinstein S, Bello L, and Solomon S: Apoplectic headache and oculomotor nerve palsy: An unusual presentation of multiple sclerosis. Neurology 40:1465–1466, 1990.

132. Gårde A, and Kjellin KG: Diagnostic significance of cerebrospinal-fluid examinations in myelopathy. Acta Neurol Scand 47:555–568, 1971.

133. Gass A, Barker GJ, Moseley IF, MacManus D, Miller DH, and McDonald WI: Clinical evaluation of fast STIR imaging in optic neuritis (abstract). Society for Magnetic Resonance in Medicine 3:1263, 1993.

134. Gass A, Barker GJ, Moseley IF, Miller DH, Sanders MD, and McDonald WI: High-resolution MRI of optic neuropathies. Neurology 44(suppl 2):A267, 1994.

135. Gay D, and Dick G: Spirochaetes, Lyme disease, and multiple sclerosis. Lancet 2:685, 1986.

136. Gean-Marton AD, Vezina LG, Marton KI, et al: Abnormal corpus callosum: A sensitive and specific indicator of multiple sclerosis. Radiology 180:215–221, 1991.

137. Gebarski SS, Gabrielsen TO, Gilman S, Knake JE, Latack JT, and Aisen AM: The initial diagnosis of multiple sclerosis: Clinical impact of magnetic resonance imaging. Ann Neurol 17(5): 469–474, 1985.

138. Gentiloni N, Schiavino D, Della Corte F, Ricci E, and Colosimo C: Neurogenic pulmonary edema: A presenting symptom in multiple sclerosis. Ital J Neurol Sci 13:435–438, 1992.

139. George AE, de Leon MJ, Kalnin A, Rosner L, Goodgold A, and Chase N: Leukoencephalopathy in normal and pathologic aging: MRI of brain lucencies. AJNR 7:567–570, 1986.

140. Gerard G, and Weisberg LA: MRI periventricular lesions in adults. Neurology 36:998–1001, 1986.

141. Gessain A, Barin F, and Vernant JC: Antibodies to human T-lymphotropic virus type 1 in patients with tropical spastic paraparesis. Lancet 2: 407–410, 1985.

142. Gessain A, and Gout O: Chronic myelopathy associated with human T-lymphotropic virus type I (HTLV-I). Ann Int Med 117:933–946, 1992.

142a. Gharagozloo AM, Poe LB, and Collins GH: Antemortem diagnosis of Baló Concentric Sclerosis: Correlative MR imaging and pathologic features. Radiology 191:817–819, 1994.

143. Giang DW, Grow VM, Mooney C, et al: Clinical diagnosis of multiple sclerosis. The impact of magnetic resonance imaging and ancillary testing: Rochester-Toronto Magnetic Resonance Study Group. Arch Neurol 51:61–66, 1994.

144. Giang DW, Poduri KR, Eskin TA, et al: Multiple sclerosis masquerading as a mass lesion. Neuroradiology 34:150–154, 1992.

145. Gibson WF, and Broughton RJ: Techniques in computerized evoked potential recording. Electroencephalogr Clin Neurophysiol 26:633, 1969.

146. Gieron MA, DiPasquale KJ, Martinez CR, and Korthals JK: Transverse myelitis mimicking intramedullary spinal cord tumor. J Neuroimaging 2:39–41, 1992.

147. Giles PD, and Wroe SJ: Cerebrospinal fluid oligoclonal IgM in multiple sclerosis: Analytical problems and clinical limitations. Ann Clin Biochem 27:199–207, 1990.

148. Gize RW, and Mishkin FS: Brain scans in multiple sclerosis. Radiology 97:297–299, 1970.

149. Golden GS, and Woody RC: The role of nuclear magnetic resonance imaging in the diagnosis of MS in childhood. Neurology 37:389–393, 1987.

150. Gonzalez-Scarano F, Grossman RI, Galetta S, Atlas SC, and Silberberg DH: Multiple sclerosis disease activity correlates with gadolinium-enhanced magnetic resonance imaging. Ann Neurol 21:300–306, 1987.

151. Goodkin DE, Doolittle TH, Hauser SS, Ransohoff RM, Roses AD, and Rudick RA: Diagnostic criteria for multiple sclerosis research involving multiply affected families. Arch Neurol 48: 805–807, 1991.

152. Goodkin DE, Rudick RA, and Ross JS: The use of brain magnetic resonance imaging in multiple sclerosis. Arch Neurol 51:505–516, 1994.

153. Gorman E, Rudd A, and Ebers GC: Giving the diagnosis of multiple sclerosis. In Poser CM (ed): The Diagnosis of Multiple Sclerosis. Thieme-Stratton, New York, 1984, pp 216–222.

154. Grafton ST, Sumi SM, Stimac GK, Alvord EC, Shaw C, and Nochlin D: Comparison of postmortem magnetic resonance imaging and neuropathologic findings in the cerebral white matter. Arch Neurol 48:293–298, 1991.

155. Graham EM, Ellis CJ, Sanders MD, and McDonald WI: Optic neuropathy in sarcoidosis. J Neurol Neurosurg Psychiatry 49:756–763, 1986.

156. Gray F, Chimelli L, Mohr M, Clavelou P, Scaravilli F, and Poirier J: Fulminating multiple sclerosis-like leukoencephalopathy revealing human immunodeficiency virus infection. Neurology 41: 105–109, 1991.

157. Grenman R, Aantaa E, Katevuo KV, Kormano M, and Panelius M: Otoneurological and ultra low field MRI findings in multiple sclerosis patients. Acta Otolaryngol (Stockh) 449:77–83, 1988.

158. Griffin DE, Ward BJ, and Jaurequi E: Immune activation in measles. N Eng J Med 320:1667–1672, 1989.

159. Grønning M, Mellgren SI, and Schive K: Optic Neuritis in the two northernmost counties of Norway. A study of incidence and the prospect of later development of multiple sclerosis. Arct Med Res 48:117–121, 1989.

160. Grossman RI, Braffman BH, Brorson JR, Goldberg HI, Silberberg DH, and Gonzalez-Scarano F: Multiple sclerosis: Serial study of Gadolinium-enhanced MR imaging. Radiology 169:117–122, 1988.

161. Guthrie TC: Visual and motor changes in patients with multiple sclerosis: A result of induced changes in environmental temperature. Archives of Neurology and Psychiatry 65: 437–451, 1951.

162. Gutmann L, Thompson HG Jr, and Martin JD: Transient facial myokymia: An uncommon manifestation of multiple sclerosis. JAMA 209:389–391, 1969.

163. Gyldensted C: Computer tomography of the cerebrum in multiple sclerosis. Neuroadiology 12:33–42, 1976.

164. Halliday AM, and McDonald WI: Pathophysiology of demyelinating disease (review). Br Med Bull 33(1):21–27, 1977 Jan.

165. Halliday AM, McDonald WI, and Mushin J: Delayed visual evoked response in optic neuritis. Lancet 3:982–985, 1972.

166. Halliday AM, McDonald WI, and Mushin J: Visual evoked response in diagnosis of multiple sclerosis. Br Med J 4:661–664, 1973.

167. Halperin JJ, Luft BJ, Anand AK, et al: Lyme neuroborreliosis: Central nervous system manifestations. Neurology 39:753–759, 1989.

168. Hamada T, Tashiro K, Moriwaka F, and Yanagihara T: Acute transverse myelopathy in multiple sclerosis. J Neurol Sci 100:217–222, 1990.

169. Hanefeld F: Multiple sclerosis in childhood. Current Opinion in Neurology and Neurosurgery 5:359–363, 1992.

170. Hansen K, and Lebech AM: The clinical and epidemiological profile of lyme neuroborreliosis in Denmark 1985–90. A prospective study of 187 patients with Borrelia burdorferi specific in-

trathecal antibody production. Brain 115 (pt 2): 399–423, 1992.

171. Harding AE, Sweeney MG, Miller DH, et al: Occurrence of a multiple sclerosis-like illness in women who have Leber's hereditary optic neuropathology mitochondrial DNA mutation. Brain 115:979–989, 1992.

172. Harris JO, Frank JA, Patronas N, McFarlin DE, and McFarland HF: Serial gadolinium-enhanced magnetic resonance imaging scans in patients with early, relapsing-remitting multiple sclerosis: Implications for clinical trials and natural history. Ann Neurol 29: 548–555, 1991.

172a. Hashemi RH, Bradley WG, Chen DY, et al: Suspected multiple sclerosis: MR imaging with a thin-section fast FLAIR pulse sequence. Radiology 196:505–510, 1995.

173. Haughton VM, Yetkin FZ, Rao SM, et al: Quantitative MR in the diagnosis of multiple sclerosis. Magn Reson Med 26:71–78, 1992.

174. Hely MA, McManis PG, Doran TJ, Walsh JC, and McLeod JG: Acute optic neuritis: A prospective study of risk factors for multiple sclerosis. J Neurol Neurosurg Psychiatry 49:1125–1130, 1986.

175. Hemachudha T, Phanuphak P, Johnson RT, Griffin DE, Ratanavongsiri J, and Siriprasomsup W: Neurologic complications of semple-type rabies vaccine: Clinical and immmunologic studies. Neurology 37:550–556, 1987.

176. Herrera WG: Vestibular and other balance disorders in multiple sclerosis. Diagnostic Neurotology 8:407, 1990.

177. Herroelen L, de Keyser J, and Ebinger G: Central-nervous-system demyelination after immunization with recombinant hepatitis B vaccine. Lancet 338:1174–1175, 1991.

178. Herscovitch P, Trotter JL, Lemann W, and Raichle ME: Positron emission tomography (PET) in active MS: Demonstration of demyelination and diaschisis. Neurology 34:78, 1984.

179. Hershey LA, and Trotter JL: The use and abuse of the cerebrospinal fluid IgG profile in the adult: A practical evaluation. Ann Neurol 8: 426–434, 1980.

180. Honig LS, Siddharthan R, Sheremata WA, Sheldon JJ, and Sazant A: Multiple sclerosis: Correlation of magnetic resonance imaging with cerebrospinal fluid findings. J Neurol Neurosurg Psychiatry 51:277–280, 1988.

181. Hooge JP, and Redekop WK: Multiple sclerosis with very late onset. Neurology 42:1907–1910, 1992.

182. Hook CC, Kimmel DW, Kvols LK, et al: Multifocal inflammatory leukoencephalopathy with 5 fluorouracil and levamisole. Ann Neurol 31: 262–267, 1992.

183. Hopf HC, Thomke F, and Gutmann L: Midbrain vs. pontine medial longitudinal fasciculus lesions: The utilization of masseter and blink reflexes. Muscle Nerve 14:326–330, 1991.

184. Hornabrook RSL, Miller DH, Newton MR, et al: Frequent involvement of the optic radiation in patients with acute isolated optic neuritis. Neurology 42:77–79, 1992.

185. Horowitz AL, Kaplan RD, Grewe G, White RT, and Salberg LM: The ovoid lesion: A new MR observation in patients with multiple sclerosis. AJNR 10:303–305, 1989.

186. Hübbe P, and Mouritzen-Dam A: Spastic paraplegia of unknown origin: A follow-up of 32 patients. Acta Neurol Scand 49:536–542, 1973.

187. Hume AL, and Waxman SG: Evoked potentials in suspected multiple sclerosis: Diagnostic value and prediction of clinical course. J Neurol Sci 83:191–210, 1988.

188. Hunt AL, Orrison WW, Yeo RA, et al: Clinical significance of MRI white matter lesions in the elderly. Neurology 39:1470–1474, 1989.

189. International Study Group for Behçet's Disease: Criteria for diagnosis of Behçet's disease. Lancet 335:1078–1080, 1990.

190. Ioannidis E, Dimitriadis G, Hatzichristou D, Milonas I, and Kalinderis A: Micturition and sexual disturbances as cardinal symptomatology in multiple sclerosis. 10th Congress of the European Committee for Treatment and Research in MS, Athens, Greece. Book of Abstracts, 1994, p19.

191. Isaac C, Li DKB, Genton M, et al: Multiple sclerosis: A serial study using MRI in relapsing patients. Neurology 38:1511–1515, 1988.

192. Izquierdo G, Hauw JJ, Lyon-Caen O, et al: Value of multiple sclerosis diagnostic criteria: 70 autopsy-confirmed cases. Arch Neurol 42:848–850, 1985.

193. Jackson JA, Leake DR, Schneiders NJ, et al: Magnetic resonance imaging in multiple sclerosis: Results in 32 cases. AJNR 6:171–176, 1985.

194. Jacobs L, Kinkel PR, and Kinkel WR: Silent brain lesions in patients with isolated idiopathic optic neuritis: A clinical and nuclear magnetic resonance imaging study. Arch Neurol 43:452–455, 1986.

195. Jacobs L, Munschauer FE, and Kaba SE: Clinical and magnetic resonance imaging in optic neuritis. Neurology 41:15–19, 1991.

196. Jacobson DM, Marx JJ, and Dlesk A: Frequency and clinical significance of Lyme seropositivity in patients with isolated optic neuritis. Neurology 41:706–711, 1991.

197. Jacobson DM, Thompson HS, and Corbett JJ: Optic neuritis in the elderly: Prognosis for visual recovery and long-term follow-up. Neurology 38:1834–1837, 1988.

198. Janssen RS, Kaplan JE, Khabbaz RF, et al: HTLV-I associated myelopathy/tropical spastic paraparesis in the United States. Neurology 41: 1355–1357, 1991.

198a. Jeffery DR: Chronic progressive myelopathy: diagnostic analysis of cases with and without sensory involvement. (Short Report) J Neurological Sciences 142:153–156, 1996.

199. Jewett DL, Romano MN, and Williston JS: Human auditory evoked potentials: Possible brain stem components detected on the scalp. Science 167:1517–1518, 1970.

200. Johns K, Lavin P, Elliot JH, and Partain CL: Magnetic resonance imaging of the brain in isolated optic neuritis. Arch Ophthalmol 104:1486–1488, 1986.

201. Johns DR, Hurko O, Attlardi J, and, Giffin JN: Molecular basis of a new mitochondrial disease:

Acute optic neuropathy and myelopathy. Ann Neurol 30:234, 1991.

202. Johnson G, Miller DH, MacManus D, et al: STIR sequences in NMR imaging of the optic nerve. Neuroradiology 29:238–245, 1987.

203. Johnson RT, Griffin DE, and Gendelman HE: Post infectious encephalomyelitis. Semin Neurol 5:180–190, 1985.

204. Kabat EA, Gusman M, and Knaub V: Quanitative estimation of the albumin and gamma globulin in normal and pathologic cerebrospinal fluid by immunochemical methods. Am J Med 4:653, 1948.

205. Kahana E, Leibowitz U, and Alter M: Cerebral multiple sclerosis. Neurology 21: 1179–1185, 1971.

206. Kalyan-Raman UP, Garwacki DJ, and Elwood PW: Demyelinating disease of corpus callosum presenting as glioma on magnetic resonance scan: A case documented with pathological findings. Neurosurg 21:247–250, 1987.

207. Kappos L, Gold R, Heun R, and Keil W: MS: Definite diagnosis at first presentation? The role of Gd-enhanced MRI. Neurology 41:168, 1991.

208. Karlik SJ, Strejan G, Gilbert JJ, and Noseworthy JH: NMR studies in experimental allergic encephalomyelitis (EAE): Normalization of T1 and T2 with parenchymal cellular infiltration. Neurology 36:1112–1114, 1986.

209. Kellar-Wood H, Robertson N, Govan GG, Compston DAS, and Harding AE: Leber's hereditary optic neuropathy mitochondrial DNA mutations in multiple sclerosis. Ann Neurol 36:109–112, 1994.

210. Kelly RE: Clinical aspects of multiple sclerosis. In Vinken P, Bruyn G, Klawans H, et al (eds): Handbook of Clinical Neurology. Elsevier, Amsterdam, 1985, pp 49–78.

211. Kent DL, Haynor DR, Longstreth WT Jr, and Larson EB: The clinical efficacy of magnetic resonance imaging in neuroimaging. Ann Intern Med 120:856–871, 1974.

212. Kepes JJ: Large focal tumor-like demyelinating lesions of the brain: intermediate entity between multiple sclerosis and acute disseminated encephalomyelitis? A study of 31 patients. Ann Neurol 33:18–27, 1993.

213. Kermode AG, Thompson AJ, Tofts P, et al: Breakdown of the blood-brain barrier precedes symptoms and other MRI signs of new lesions in multiple sclerosis. Brain 113:1477–1489, 1990.

214. Kermode AG, Tofts PS, Thompson AJ, et al: Heterogeneity of blood-brain barrier changes in multiple sclerosis: an MRI study with gadolinium-DTPA enhancement. Neurology 40:229–235, 1990.

215. Kertesz A, Black SE, Tokar G, Benke T, Carr T, and Nicholson L: Periventricular and subcortical hyperintensities on magnetic resonance imaging: "Rims, caps and unidentified bright objects." Arch Neurol 45:404–408, 1988.

216. Kesselring J, Miller DH, Robb SA, et al: Acute disseminated encephalomyelitis. MRI findings and the distinction from multiple sclerosis. Brain 113:291–302, 1990.

217. Kesselring J, Ormerod IEC, Miller DH, du Boulay EPGH, and McDonald WI: Magnetic resonance imaging in multiple sclerosis: An atlas of diagnosis and differential diagnosis. Verlas, Stuttgart, 1989.

218. Kimura J: Electrically elicited blink reflex in diagnosis of multiple sclerosis. Brain 98:413–426, 1975.

219. King PH, and Bragdon AC: MRI reveals multiple reversible cerebral lesions in an attack of acute intermittment porphyria. Neurology 41:1300–1302, 1991.

220. Kinkel WR, Jacobs L, Polachini I, Bates V, and Heffner RR Jr: Subcortical arteriosclerotic encephalopathy (Binswanger's disease): Computed tomographic, nuclear magnetic resonance and clinical correlations. Arch Neurol 42:951–959, 1985.

221. Kinnunen E: The incidence of optic neuritis and its prognosis for multiple sclerosis. Acta Neurol Scand 68:371–377, 1983.

222. Kinnunen E, Larsen A, Ketonen L, Koskimies S, and Sandstrom A: Evaluation of central nervous system involvement in uncomplicated optic neuritis after prolonged follow-up. Acta Neurol Scand 76:147–151, 1987.

223. Kirshner HS, Tsai SI, Runge VM, and Price AC: Magnetic resonance imaging and other techniques in the diagnosis of multiple sclerosis. Arch Neurol 42:859–863, 1985.

224. Koopmans RA, Li DKB, Oger JJF, et al: Chronic progressive multiple sclerosis: Serial magnetic resonance brain imaging over six months. Ann Neurol 26:248–256, 1989.

225. Koudrivtseva T, Pozzilli C, De Biasi C, et al: Comparative study of gadolinium-DTPA and gadoteridol in MRI of patients with acute MS. 10th Congress of the European Committee for Treatment and Research in Multiple Sclerosis, Athens, Greece. Book of Abstracts, 1994, p11.

225a. Kuroda Y, Matsui M, Yukitake M, et al: Assessment of MRI criteria for MS in Japanese MS and HAM/TSP. Neurology 45:30–33, 1995.

226. Kuroiwa H: Neuromyelitis optica (Devic's disease, Devic's syndrome). Handbook of Clinical Neurology: Demyelinating Diseases, Vol 3. Elsevier, Amsterdam, 1985, p397.

227. Kurtzke JF: Optic neuritis or multiple sclerosis. Arch Neurol 42:704–710, 1985.

228. Landy PJ, Innis M, and Boyle R: Factors likely to affect the development of multiple sclerosis in patients presenting with optic neuritis in a tropical and suptropical area. Clinical and Experimental Neurology, Proceedings of the Association of Neurologists 16:175–182, 1979.

229. Lee DH, Simon JH, Szumowski J, et al: Optic neuritis and orbital lesions: Lipid-suppressed chemical shift MR imaging. Radiology 179: 543–546, 1991.

230. Lee HJ, Bansil S, Cook SD, et al: MRI of the spine in multiple sclerosis. J Neuroimaging 2:61, 1992.

231. Lee KH, Hashimoto SA, Hooge JP, et al: Magnetic resonance imaging of the head in the diagnosis of multiple sclerosis: A prospective 2-

year follow-up with comparison of clinical evaluation, evoked potentials, oligoclonal banding, and CT. Neurology 41:657–660, 1991.

232. Leffert AK, and Link H: IgG production within the central nervous system: A critical review of proposed formulae. Ann Neurol 17:13–20, 1985.

232a. Lehky TJ, Flerage N, Katz D, et al: Human T-cell lymphotropic virus type II–associated myelopathy: Clinical and immunologic profiles. Ann Neurol 40:714–723, 1996.

233. Lepore FE: The origin of pain in optic neuritis: Determinants of pain in 101 eyes with optic neuritis. Arch Neurol 48:748–749, 1991.

234. Lhermitte J, Bollak G, and Nicholas M: Les douleurs a type de decharge electrique consecutives a la flexion cephalique dans la sclerose en plaques. Rev Neurol 42:56–62, 1924.

235. Li DKB, Mayo J, Fache S, Robertson WD, Paty DW, and Genton M: Early experience in nuclear magnetic resonance imaging of multiple sclerosis. Ann NY Acad Sci 436:483–486, 1984.

236. Lightman S, McDonald WI, Bird AC, et al: Retinal venous sheathing in optic neuritis: Its significance for the pathogenesis of multiple sclerosis. Brain 110:405–414, 1987.

237. Lindberg C, Andersen O, Vahlne A, Dalton M, and Runmarker B: Epidemiological investigation of the association between infectious mononucleosis and multiple sclerosis. Neuroepidemiology 10:62–65, 1991.

238. Link H: Immunoglobulin G, and low molecular weight proteins in human cerebrospinal fluid. Acta Neurol Scand 43(Suppl. 28):1–136, 1967.

239. Link H, Baig S, Olsson O, Jiang YP, Höjeberg B, and Olsson T: Persistent anti-myelin basic protein IgG antibody response in multiple sclerosis cerebrospinal fluid. J Neuroimmunol 28:237–248, 1990.

240. Link H, and Laurenzi MA: Immunoglobulin class and light chain type of oligoclonal bands in CSF in multiple sclerosis determined by agarose gel electrophoresis and immunofixation. Ann Neurol 6:107–110, 1979.

241. Lipton HL, and Teasdall RD: Acute transverse myelopathy in adults: A follow-up study. Arch Neurol 28:252–257, 1973.

242. Lo R, and Feasby TE: Multiple sclerosis and autoimmune diseases. Neurology 33:97–98, 1983.

243. Lodder J, de Weerd AW, Koetsier JC, and van der Lugt PJ: Computed tomography in acute cerebral multiple sclerosis. Arch Neurol 40:320–322, 1983.

244. Logigian EL, Kaplan RF, and Steere AC: Chronic neurologic manifestations of lyme disease. N Engl J Med 323:1438–1444, 1990.

245. Losy J, Mehta PD, and Wisniewski HM: Identification of IgG subclasses oligoclonal bands in multiple sclerosis CSF. Acta Neurol Scand 82:4–8, 1990.

246. Lowenthal A: Agar Gel Electrophoresis in Neurology. Elsevier North-Holland, Amsterdam, 1964.

247. Lu CS, Tsai CH, Chiu HC, and Yip PK: Pseudoathetosis as a presenting symptom of spinal multiple sclerosis. Journal of the Formosan Medical Association, 91(1):106–109, 1992.

248. Lukes SA, Crooks LE, Aminoff MJ, et al: Nuclear magnetic resonance imaging in multiple sclerosis. Ann Neurol 13:592–601, 1983.

249. Lynch SG, Rose JW, Smoker W, and Petajan JH: MRI in familial multiple sclerosis. Neurology 40:900–903, 1990.

250. MacFadyen DJ, Drance SM, Douglas GR, Airaksinen PJ, Mawson DK, and Paty DW: The retinal nerve fiber layer, neuroretinal rim area, and visual evoked potentials in MS. Neurology 38:1353–1358, 1988.

251. Madigand M, Oger JJF, Fauchet R, Sabouraud O, and Genetet B: HLA profiles in multiple sclerosis suggest two forms of disease and the existence of protective haplotypes. J Neurol Sci 53:519–529, 1982.

252. Malhotra AS, and Goren H: The hot bath test in the diagnosis of multiple sclerosis. JAMA 246:1113, 1981.

253. Mandler RN, Davis LE, Jeffery DR, and Kornfeld M: Devic's neuromyelitis optica: A clinicopathological study of 8 patients. Ann Neurol 34:162–168, 1993.

254. Mapelli G, Pavoni M, De Palma P, Modestino R, and Pavoni V: Progression of optic neuritis to multiple sclerosis: A prospective study in an Italian population. Neuroepidemiology 10:117–121, 1991.

255. Marshall J, and Manc MD: Spastic paraplegia of middle age: A clinicopathological study. Lancet 7:643–646, 1955.

256. Marti-Fabregas J, Martinez JM, Illa I, and Escartin A: Myelopathy of unknown etiology: A clinical follow-up and MRI study of 57 cases. Acta Neurol Scand 80:455–460, 1989.

257. Martinelli V, Comi G, Filippi M, et al: Paraclinical tests in acute-onset optic neuritis: Basal data and results of a short follow-up. Acta Neurol Scand 84:231–236, 1991.

257a. Masdeu JC, Moreira J, Trasi S, Visintainer P, Cavaliere R, and Grundman M: The Open Ring: A new imaging sign in demyelinating disease. J Neuroimag 6:104–107, 1996.

258. Masdeu JC, Wolfson L, Lantos G, et al: Brain white-matter changes in the elderly prone to falling [see comments]. Arch Neurol 46:1292–1296, 1989.

259. Mauch E, Schroth G, Kornhuber HH, and Voigt K: Importance of cranial magnetic resonance imaging in diagnosis of multiple sclerosis without supraspinal signs. The Lancet 822–823, 1988.

260. Mayeux R, and Benson DF: Phantom limb and multiple sclerosis. Neurology 29:724–726, 1979.

261. Mbonda E, Larnaout A, Maertens A, et al: Multiple sclerosis in a black Cameroonian woman. Acta Neurol Belg 90:218–222, 1990.

262. McAlpine D, Lumsden CE, and Acheson ED: Multiple Sclerosis: A reappraisal. Churchill Livingstone, Edinburgh, 1972.

263. McDonald WI: Demyelinating diseases of the optic nerve. Neurology and Neurosurgery 2:179–182, 1989.

264. McDonald WI, and Barnes D: The ocular manifestations of multiple sclerosis. I. Abnormalities

of the afferent visual system. J Neurol Neurosurg Psychiatry 55:747–752, 1992.

265. McDonald WI, and Halliday AM: Diagnosis and classification of multiple sclerosis (review). Br Med Bull 33:4–9, 1977.

266. McDonald WI, Miller DH, and Barnes D: The pathological evolution of multiple sclerosis. Neuropathol Appl Neurobiol 18:319–334, 1992.

267. McLean BN, Luxton RW, and Thompson EJ: A study of immunoglobulin G in the cerebrospinal fluid of 1007 patients with suspected neurological disease using isoelectric focusing and the Log IgG-Index: A comparison and diagnostic applications. Brain 113 (pt 5):1269–1289, 1990.

268. Mehta PD: Diagnostic usefulness of cerebrospinal fluid in multiple sclerosis. Crit Rev Clin Lab Sci 28:233–251, 1991.

269. Mendell JR, Kolkin S, Kissel JT, Weiss KL, Chakeres DW, and Rammohan KW: Evidence for central nervous system demyelination in chronic inflammatory demyelinating polyradiculoneuropathy. Neurology 37:1291–1294, 1987.

270. Merandi SF, Kudryk BT, Murtagh FR, and Arrington JA: Contrast-enhanced MR imaging of optic nerve lesions in patients with acute optic neuritis. AJNR 12:923–926, 1991.

271. Metz LM, Fritzler MJ, and Seland TP: Sjögren's syndrome infrequently mimics multiple sclerosis. Can J Neurol Sci 15:198, 1988.

272. Miller DH, Kendall BE, Barter S, et al: Magnetic resonance imaging in central nervous system sarcoidosis. Neurology 38:378–383, 1988.

273. Miller DH, McDonald WI, Blumhardt LD, et al: Magnetic resonance imaging in isolated noncompressive spinal cord syndromes. Ann Neurol 22:714–723, 1987.

274. Miller DH, Newton MR, van der Poel JC, et al: Magnetic resonance imaging of the optic nerve in optic neuritis. Neurology 38:175–179, 1988.

275. Miller DH, Ormerod IEC, Gibson A, du Boulay EPGH, Rudge P, and McDonald WI: MR brain scanning in patients with vasculitis: Differentiation from multiple sclerosis. Neuroradiology 29:226–231, 1987.

276. Miller DH, Ormerod IEC, McDonald WI, et al: The early risk of multiple sclerosis after optic neuritis. J Neurol Neurosurg Psychiatry 51:1569–1571, 1988.

277. Miller DH, Ormerod IEC, Rudge P, Kendall BE, Moseley IF, and McDonald WI: The early risk of multiple sclerosis following isolated acute syndromes of the brainstem and spinal cord. Ann Neurol 26:635–639, 1989.

278. Miller DH, Rudge P, Johnson G, et al: Serial gadolinium enhanced magnetic resonance imaging in multiple sclerosis. Brain 111:927–939, 1988.

279. Miller DH, Youl BD, Turano G, Kendall BE, Halliday AM, and McDonald WI: Acute optic neuritis: Relationship between clinical, electrophysiological, and MRI abnormalities. Neurology 41 (Suppl):168, 1991.

280. Miller SW, and Potsaid MS: Focal brain scan abnormalities in multiple sclerosis. J Nucl Med 15:131–133, 1973.

281. Minderhoud JM: On the pathogenesis of multiple sclerosis: A revised model of the cause(s) of multiple sclerosis, especially based on epidemiological data. Clin Neurol Neurosurg 96:135–142, 1994.

282. Minderhoud JM, Boonstra S, Kuks J, and ter Stege G: The flight of colours test in multiple sclerosis, retrobulbar neuritis and healthy controls. Clin Neurol Neurosurg 86:89–94, 1984.

283. Minderhoud JM, Leemhuis JG, Kremer J, Laban E, and Smits PM: Sexual disturbances arising from multiple sclerosis. Acta Neurol Scand 70:299–306, 1984.

284. Miró J, Peña-Sagredo JL, Berciano J, Insúa S, Leno C, and Velarde R: Prevalence of primary Sjögren's syndrome in patients with multiple sclerosis. Ann Neurol 27:582–584, 1990.

285. Miska RM, Pojunas KW, and McQuillen MP: Cranial magnetic resonance imaging in the evaluation of myelopathy of undetermined etiology. Neurology 37:840–843, 1987.

286. Moller A, Wiedemann G, Rohde U, Backmund H, and Sonntag A: Correlates of cognitive impairment and depressive mood disorder in multiple sclerosis. Acta Psychiatr Scand 89:117–121, 1994.

287. Mooney C, Mushlin AI, and Phelps CE: Targeting assessments of magnetic resonance imaging in suspected multiple sclerosis. Med Decis Making 10:77–94, 1990.

288. Moreira J, Masdeu JC, Trasi S, and Grundman M: The open ring: A new imaging sign in demyelinating disease. Paper presented at the 119th Annual Meeting of the American Neurological Association, San Francisco, 1994. Ann Neurol 36:302, 1994.

289. Moriwaka F, Tashiro K, Fukazawa T, et al: A case of systemic lupus erythematosus: Its clinical and MRI resemblance to multiple sclerosis. Japanese Journal of Psychiatry and Neurology 44:601–605, 1990.

290. Morrissey SP, Miller DH, Kendall BE, et al: The significance of brain magnetic resonance imaging abnormalities at presentation with clinically isolated syndromes suggestive of multiple sclerosis. Brain 116:135–146, 1993.

291. Moses DC, Davis LE, and Wagner HN Jr: Brain scanning with 99mmTcO4- in multiple sclerosis. J Nucl Med 13:847–887, 1972.

292. Moulin DE: Pain in multiple sclerosis. Neurol Clin 7:321–331, 1989.

293. Moulin D, Paty DW, and Ebers GC: The predictive value of cerebrospinal fluid electrophoresis in 'possible' multiple sclerosis. Brain 106:809–816, 1983.

294. Murray S, and Veidlinger OF: Serial radionuclide scans in multiple sclerosis. Can J Neurol Sci 5:321–323, 1978.

295. Mushlin AI, Mooney C, Grow V, and Phelps CE: The value of diagnostic information to patients with suspected multiple sclerosis: Rochester-Toronto MRI Study Group. Arch Neurol 51:67–72, 1994.

296. Nakae K, Yamamoto S, Shigematsu I, and Kono R: Relation between subacute myelo-optic neu-

ropathy (S. M. O. N.) and clioquinol: Nationwide survey. Lancet 1:171–173, 1973.

297. Newcombe J, Hawkins CP, Henderson CL, et al: Histopathology of multiple sclerosis lesions detected by magnetic resonance imaging in unfixed postmortem central nervous system tissue. Brain 114:1013–1023, 1991.

298. Newman NJ, and Lessell S: Isolated pupil-sparing third-nerve palsy as the presenting sign of multiple sclerosis. Arch Neurol 47:817–818,1990.

299. Newman NJ, Lessell S, and Winterkorn JM: Optic chiasmal neuritis. Neurology 41:1203–1210, 1991.

300. Newson-Davis J: Myasthenia gravis and myasthenic syndrome. In Appel SH (ed): Current Neurology. Year Book Medical Publishers, Chicago, 1986, pp 47–72.

301. Nikoskelainen E, and Riekkinen P: Opitic Neuritis: A sign of multiple sclerosis or other diseases of the central nervous system. Acta Neurol Scand 50:690–718, 1974.

302. Noakes JB, Herkes GK, Frith JA, McLeod JG, and Jones MP: Magnetic resonance imaging in clinically-definite multiple sclerosis. Med J Aust 152:136–140, 1990.

303. Noseworthy JH, Bass BH, Vandervoort MK, et al: The prevalence of primary Sjögren's syndrome in multiple sclerosis population. Ann Neurol 25:95–98, 1989.

304. Noseworthy JH, and Heffernan LPM: Motor radiculopathy: An unusual presentation of multiple sclerosis. Can J Neurol Sci 1:207–209, 1980.

305. Noseworthy JH, Paty DW, Wonnacott T, Feasby TE, and Ebers GC: MS after age 50. Neurology 33:1537–1544, 1983.

306. Noseworthy JH, and Rice GPA: Trichlorethylene poisoning mimicking multiple sclerosis. Can J Neurol Sci 15:87–88, 1988.

307. O'Connor P, Detsky AS, Tansey C, and Kucharczyk W: Effect of diagnostic testing for multiple sclerosis on patient health perceptions: Rochester-Toronto MRI Study Group. Arch Neurol 51:46–51, 1994.

307a. O'Connor PW, Tansey CM, Detsky AS, Mushlin AI, and Kucharczyk W: The effect of spectrum bias on the utility of magnetic resonance imaging and evoked potentials in the diagnosis of suspected multiple sclerosis. Neurology 47:140–144, 1996.

308. Offenbacher H, Fazekas F, Schmidt R, et al: Assessment of MRI criteria for a diagnosis of MS. Neurology 43:905–909, 1993.

308a. Oger J, and Dekaban G: HTLV-I associated myelopathy: A case of viral-induced auto-immunity. Autoimmunity Vol. 21, pp. 151–159, 1995.

309. Oger JJF, Werker DH, Foti DJ, and Dekaban GA: HTLV-I associated myelopathy: An endemic disease of Canadian aboriginals of the Northwest Pacific Coast? Can J Neurol Sci 20:302–306, 1993.

310. Olcay L, Renda Y, Bakkaloglu A, Topcu M, Diren B, and Besim A: Multiple sclerosis in a six-year-old boy (case report). Turk J Pediatr 36:81–85,1994.

310a. O'Riordan JI, McDonald WI, and Miller DH: The predictive value of MRI in clinically isolated syndromes suggestive of demyelination. Multiple Sclerosis 2:29–30, 1996.

311. Ormerod IE, McDonald WI, du Boulay EPGH, et al: Disseminated lesions at presentation in patients with optic neuritis. J Neurol Neurosurg Psychiatry 49:124–127, 1986.

312. Ormerod IE, Miller DH, McDonald WI, et al: The role of NMR imaging in the assessment of multiple sclerosis and isolated neurological lesions. Brain 110:1579–1616, 1987.

313. Osame M, Usuku K, and Izumo S: HTLV-1 associated myelopathy: A new clinical entity. Lancet 1:1031–1032, 1986.

314. Osborn AG, Harnsberger HR, Smoker WRK, and Boyer RS: Multiple Sclerosis in Adolescents: CT and MR findings. AJNR 155:385–391, 1990.

315. Ostermeyer Shoaib B, and Patten BM: A multiple sclerosis-like syndrome in women with breast implants or silicone fluid injections into breasts. Neurology 44 (suppl 2):A158, 1994.

316. Overton MC III, Haynie TP, and Snodgrass SR: Brain scans in nonneoplastic intracranial lesions: Scanning with chlormerodrin Hg 203 and chlormerodrin Hg 197. JAMA 191:431–436, 1965.

317. Pachner AR, Duray P, and Steere AC: Central nervous system manifestations of Lyme Disease. Arch Neurol 46:790–795, 1989.

318. Parker HL: Trigeminal neuralgic pain associated with multiple sclerosis. Brain 51:46–62, 1928.

319. Parkin PJ, Hierons R, and McDonald WI: Bilateral Optic Neuritis: A long-term follow-up. Brain 107:951–964, 1984.

320. Parmley CP, Schiffman MA, Maitland CG, Miller NR, Dreyer RF, and Hoyt WF: Does neuroretinitis rule out multiple sclerosis? Arch Neurol 44:1045–1048, 1987.

321. Paty DW: Multiple sclerosis: Assessment of disease progression and effects of treatment. Can J Neurol Sci 14:518–520, 1987.

322. Paty DW, Asbury AK, Herndon RM, et al: Use of magnetic resonance imaging in the diagnosis of multiple sclerosis: Policy statement. Neurology 36:1575, 1986.

323. Paty DW, Blume WT, Brown WF, Jaatoul N, Kertesz A, and McInnis W: Chronic progressive myelopathy: Investigation with CSF electrophoresis, evoked potentials and CT scan. Ann Neurol 6(5):419–424, 1979.

324. Paty DW, Ebers GC, and Wonnacott TH: Prognostic Markers in Multiple Sclerosis, Vol 548. Excerpta Medica,World Congress of Neurology, Hamberg, Germany, 1981, p. 56.

325. Paty DW, Oger JJF, Kastrukoff LF, et al: Magnetic resonance imaging in the diagnosis of multiple sclerosis (MS): A prospective study with comparison of clinical evaluation, evoked potentials, oligoclonal banding and CT. Neurology 38:180–185, 1988.

326. Paty DW, and Li DKB: Interferon beta-1b is effective in relapsing-remitting multiple sclerosis. II. MRI analysis results of a multicenter, randomized, double-blind, placebo-controlled trial: UBC MS/MRI Study Group and the IFNB

Multiple Sclerosis Study Group [see comments]. Neurology 43:662–667, 1993.

327. Paty DW, McFarlin DE, and McDonald WI: Magnetic resonance imaging and laboratory aids in the diagnosis of multiple sclerosis. Ann Neurol 29:3–5, 1991.

328. Paty DW, Studney D, Redekop WK, and Lublin FD: MS COSTAR: A computerized patient record adapted for clinical research purposes. Ann Neurol 36 (suppl):134–135, 1994.

329. Pennock JM, Bydder GM, Hajnal JV, and Thomas DJ: A five sequence comparison of the number, size and conspicuity of lesions in the brain in patients with clinically definite multiple sclerosis (abstract). Society for Magnetic Resonance in Medicine, 12th Annual Scientific Meeting, N.Y., N.Y., 1993.

330. Perkin GD, and Rose FC: Optic Neuritis and Its Differential Diagnosis. Oxford University Press, New York, 1979.

331. Peyser JM, and Becker B: Neuropsychologic evaluation in patients with multiple sclerosis. In Poser CM (ed): The Diagnosis of Multiple Sclerosis. Stratton-Verlag, New York, 1983, pp 143–158.

332. Peyser JM, Edwards KR, Poser CM, and Filskov SB: Cognitive function in patients with multiple sclerosis. Arch Neurol 37:577, 1980.

333. Phillips KR, Potvin AR, Syndulko K, Cohen SN, Tourtellotte WW, and Potvin JH: Multimodality evoked potentials and neurophysiological tests in multiple sclerosis: Effects of hyperthermia on test results. Arch Neurol 40:159–164, 1983.

333a. Picard FJ, Coulthart MB, Oger J, et al: Human T-lymphotropic virus type 1 in coastal natives of British Columbia: Phylogenetic Affinities and Possible Origins. Virology 69(11):7248–7256, 1995.

334. Plant GT, Kermode AG, Turano G, et al: Symptomatic retrochiasmal lesions in multiple sclerosis: Clinical features, visual evoked potentials, and magnetic resonance imaging. Neurology 42: 68–76, 1992.

335. Pollock M, Calder C, and Allpress S: Peripheral nerve abnormality in multiple sclerosis. Ann Neurol 2:41–48, 1977.

336. Polo JM, Calleja J, Combarros O, and Berciano J: Hereditary "pure" spastic paraplegia: A study of nine families. J Neurol Neurosurg Psychiatry 56:175–181, 1993.

337. Poser CM: The Diagnosis of Multiple Sclerosis. Stratton-Verlag, New York, 1983.

338. Poser CM, Paty DW, Scheinberg L, et al: New diagnostic criteria for multiple sclerosis: Guidelines for research protocols. Ann Neurol 13: 227–231, 1983.

339. Poser S, Scheidt P, Kitz B, Luer W, Schafer U, Nordmann B, Stichnoth FA: Impact of magnetic resonance imaging (MRI) on the epidemiology of MS. Acta Neurol Scand 83:172–175, 1991.

340. Prayoonwiwat N, Pease LR, and Rodriguez M: Human T-cell lymphotropic virus type I sequences detected by ensted polymerase chain reactions are not associated with multiple sclerosis [see comments] (Review). Mayo Clin Proc 66:665–680, 1991.

341. Prineas JW, Kwon EE, Sharer LR, and Cho ES: Massive early remyelination in acute multiple sclerosis. Neurology 37:109, 1987.

342. Pringle CE, Hudson AJ, Munoz DG, Kiernan A, Brown WF, and Ebers GC: Primary lateral sclerosis: Clinical features, neuropathology, and diagnostic criteria. Brain 115:495–520, 1992.

343. Purves SJ, Low MD, Galloway J, and Reeves B: A comparison of visual, brainstem auditory, and somatosensory evoked potentials in multiple sclerosis. Can J Neurol Sci 8:15, 1981.

344. Rafto SE, Milton W, Galetta SL, and Grossman RI: Biopsy-confirmed CNS Lyme disease: MR appearance at 1.5 T. AJNR 11:482–484, 1990.

345. Ramirez-Lassepas M, Tulloch JW, Quinones MR, and Snyder BD: Acute radicular pain as a presenting symptom in multiple sclerosis. Arch Neurol 49:255–258, 1992.

346. Ransohoff RM, Whitman GJ, and Weinstein MA: Noncommunicating syringomyelia in multiple sclerosis: Detection by magnetic resonance imaging. Neurology 40:718–721, 1990.

347. Rao SM: Neuropsychology of multiple sclerosis: A critical review. J Clin Exp Neuropsychol 8: 503–542, 1986.

348. Rasminsky M: The effects of temperature on conduction in demyelinated single nerve fibers. Arch Neurol 28:287–292, 1973.

349. Ratnaike S, Kilpatrick T, Tress B, et al: Cerebrospinal fluid biochemistry in the diagnosis of multiple sclerosis. Ann Clin Biochem 27:195–198, 1990.

350. Regan D, Raymond J, Ginsburg A, and Murray TJ: Contrast sensitivity, visual acuity and the discrimination of Snellen letters in multiple sclerosis. Brain 104:333–350, 1981.

351. Reider-Groswasser I, Kott E, Benmair J, Huberman M, Machtey Y, and Gelernter I: MRI parameters in multiple sclerosis patients. Neuroradiology 30:219–223, 1988.

352. Richards TL: Proton MR spectroscopy in multiple sclerosis: Value in establishing diagnosis, monitoring progression, and evaluating therapy. AJR 157:1073–1078, 1991.

353. Richey ET, Kooi KA, and Tourtellotte WW: Visual evoked responses in multiple sclerosis. J Neurol Neurosurg Psychiatry 34:278–280, 1971.

354. Riikonen R, Ketonen L, and Sipponen J: Magnetic resonance imaging, evoked responses and cerebrospinal fluid findings in a follow-up study of children with optic neuritis. Acta Neurol Scand 77:44–49, 1988.

355. Riley D, and Lang AE: Hemiballism in multiple sclerosis. Mov Disord 3:1:88–94, 1988.

356. Rizzo JF, and Lessell S: Risk of developing multiple sclerosis after uncomplicated optic neuritis: A long-term prospective study. Neurology 38: 185–190, 1988.

357. Robertson WD, Li DKB, Mayo JR, Fache JS, and Paty DW: Assessment of multiple sclerosis lesions by magnetic resonance imaging. Can Assoc Radiol J 38:177–182, 1987.

358. Rodriguez M, Siva A, Cross S, O'Brien P, and Kurland L: Optic Neuritis: A population-based study in Olmsted County, Minnesota. Neurology 44(suppl 2):A374, 1994.

358a. Rolak LA, Beck RW, Paty DW, Tourtellotte WW, Whitaker JN, and Rudick RA: Cerebrospinal fluid in acute optic neuritis: Experience of the optic neuritis treatment trial. Neurology 46: 368–372, 1996.

358b. Romano JG, Bradley WG, and Green B: High cervical myelopathy presenting with the numb clumsy hand syndrome (short report). Journal Neurol Sciences 140:137–140, 1996.

359. Ropper AH, and Poskanzer DC: The prognosis of acute and subacute transverse myelopathy based on early signs and symptoms. Ann Neurol 4:51–59, 1978.

360. Rose AS, Ellison GW, Myers LW, and Tourtellotte WW: Criteria for the clinical diagnosis of multiple sclerosis. Neurology 26(6 pt 2):20–22, 1976.

361. Rosenblum WI, Budzilovich G, and Feigin I: Lesions of the spinal cord in polyradiculoneuropathy of unknown aetiology and a possible relationship with the Guillain-Barré syndrome. J Neurol Neurosurg Psychiatry 29:69–76, 1966.

362. Rudge P, Ali A, and Cruickshank JK: Multiple sclerosis, tropical scastic paraparesis and HTLV-1 infection in Afro-Caribbean patients in the United Kingdom. J Neurol Neurosurg Psychiatry 54:689–694, 1991.

363. Rudick RA: The value of brain magnetic resonance imaging in multiple sclerosis (editorial and comment). Arch Neurol 49:685–686, 1992.

364. Rudick RA, Jacobs L, Kinkel PR, and Kinkel WR: Isolated idiopathic optic neuritis. Analysis of free kappa-light chains in cerebrospinal fluid and correlation with nuclear magnetic resonance findings. Arch Neurol 43:456–458, 1986.

365. Runge VM, Price AC, Kirshner HS, Allen JH, Partain CL, and James AE Jr: Magnetic resonance imaging of multiple sclerosis: A study of pulse-technique efficacy. AJR 143: 1015–1026, 1984.

366. Rushton JG, and Olafson RA: Trigeminal neuralgia associated with multiple sclerosis. Arch Neurol 13:383–384, 1965.

367. Sadovnick AD, and Macleod PM: The familial incidence of multiple sclerosis: Empiric recurrence risks for first, second and third degree relatives of patients. Neurology 31: 1039–1041, 1981.

368. Saito H, Endo M, Takase S, and Itahara K: Acute disseminated encephalomyelitis after influenza vaccination. Arch Neurol 37:564–566, 1980.

369. Sakurai M, Mannen T, and Tanabe H: Lidocaine test: A new method to detect subclinical demyelinative lesions in multiple sclerosis. Ann Neurol 30:268, 1991.

370. Sandberg-Wollheim M, Axell T, Hansen BU, et al: Primary Sjögren's syndrome in patients with multiple sclerosis. Neurology 42:845–847, 1992.

371. Sandberg-Wollheim M, Bynke H, Cronqvist S, Holtoas S, Platz P, and Ryder LP: A long-term prospective study of optic neuritis: Evaluation of risk factors. Ann Neurol 27:386–393, 1990.

372. Sandberg-Wollheim M, Vandvik B, Nadj C, and Norrby E: The intrathecal immune response in the early stage of multiple sclerosis. J Neurol Sci 81:45–54, 1987.

373. Sanders EA, Reulen JPH, and Hogenhuis LAH: Central nervous system involvement in optic neuritis. J Neurol Neurosurg Psychiatry 47:241–249, 1984.

374. Sanders EA, Reulen JPH, Hogenhuis LAH, and van der Veld EA: Electrophysiological disorders in multiple sclerosis and optic neuritis. Can J Neurol Sci 12:308–313, 1985.

374a. Sanders EACM, and Van Lith GHM: Optic neuritis, confirmed by visual evoked response, and the risk for multiple sclerosis: a prospective survey. J Neurol, Neurosurg and Psychiatry 52: 799–810, 1989.

375. Schumacher GA, Beebe G, Kibler RF, et al: Problems of experimental trials of therapy in multiple sclerosis: Report by the panel on the evaluation of experimental trials of therapy in multiple sclerosis. Ann NY Acad Sci 122:552–568, 1965.

376. Schiffer RB, Giang DW, Mushlin A, et al: Perils and pitfalls of magnetic resonance imaging in the diagnosis of multiple sclerosis. J Neuroimaging 3:81–88, 1993.

377. Scholl GB, Song HS, and Wray SH: Uhthoff's symptom in optic neuritis: Relationship to magnetic resonance imaging and development of multiple sclerosis. Ann Neurol 30:180–184, 1991.

378. Schwankhaus JD, Katz DA, Eldridge R, Schlesinger S, and McFarland H: Clinical and pathological features of an autosomal dominant, adult-onset leukodystrophy simulating chronic progressive multiple sclerosis. Arch Neurol 51:757–766, 1994.

379. Scott TF: Diseases that mimic multiple sclerosis. Postgrad Med 89:187–191, 1991.

380. Scott TF, Weikers N, Hospodar M, and Wapenski J: Acute transverse myelitis: A retrospective study using magnetic resonance imaging. Can J Neurol Sci 21:133–136, 1994.

381. Scotti G, Scialfa G, Biondi A, Landoni L, Caputo D, and Cazzullo CL: Magnetic resonance in multiple sclerosis. Neuroradiology 28:319–323, 1986.

382. Seaman WB, Ter-Pogossian MM, and Schwartz HG: Localization of intracranial neoplasms with radioactive isotopes. Radiology 62:30–36, 1954.

383. Sears ES: Nuclear magnetic resonance versus computerized tomographic enhancement imaging in multiple sclerosis: An apples and oranges comparison (letter)? Ann Neurol 15: 309–310, 1984.

384. Sears ES, Tindall RS, and Zarnow H: Active multiple sclerosis. Arch Neurol 35:426–434, 1978.

385. Seeldrayers PA, Borenstein S, Gerard JM, and Flament-Durand J: Reversible capsulo-tegmental locked-in state as first manifestation of multiple sclerosis. J Neurol Sci 80:153–161, 1987.

386. Servalli C, Grimaldi LM, Martino GV, et al: Absence of IgG, IgA or IgM oligoclonal bands in tears from multiple sclerosis patients. Neurology 41:147, 1991.

387. Sharpe JA, and Sanders MD: Atrophy of myelinated nerve fibers in the retina in optic neuritis. Br J Ophthalmol 59:229–232, 1975.

388. Sheremata WA, Sevush S, Knight D, and Ziajka P: Altered cerebral metabolism in MS. Neurology 34:118, 1984.

389. Sherman JL, and Stern BJ: Sarcoidosis of the CNS: Comparison of unenhanced and enhanced MR images. AJNR 11:915–923, 1990.

390. Shibasaki H, and Kuroiwa Y: Painful tonic seizure in multiple sclerosis. Arch Neurol 30:47–51, 1974.

391. Shiraki H, and Otani S: Clinical and pathological features of rabies postvaccinal encephalomyelitis in man. In Kies MW, and Alvord EC Jr. (eds): 'Allergic' Encephalomyelitis. Charles C Thomas, Springfield, Ill, pp 58–129, 1959.

392. Simon JH, Holtas SL, Schiffer RB, et al: Corpus callosum and subcallosal-periventricular lesions in multiple sclerosis: Detection with MR. Radiology 160:363–367, 1986.

393. Sindic CJM, and Laterre EC: Oligoclonal free kappa and lambda bands in the cerebrospinal fluid of patients with multiple sclerosis and other neurological diseases. An immunoaffinity-mediated capillary blot study. J Neuroimmunol 33:63–72, 1991.

394. Sindic CJM, Monteyne P, and Laterre EC: Occurrence of oligoclonal IgM bands in the cerebrospinal fluid of neurological patients: An immunoaffinity-mediated capillary blot study. J Neurol Sci 124:215–219, 1994.

394a. Slamovits TL, Macklin R, Beck RW, Frankel M, Lim JI, and Hillman DS: What to tell the patient with optic neuritis about multiple sclerosis. Survey of Ophthalmology 36(1):47–50, 1991.

395. Smith AS, Meisler DM, Weinstein MA, et al: High-signal periventricular lesions in patients with sarcoidosis: Neurosardoidosis or multiple sclerosis? AJR 153:147–152, 1989.

396. Soges LJ, Cacayorin ED, Petro GR, and Ramachandran TS: Migraine: Evaluation by MR. AJNR 9:425–429, 1988.

397. Staedt D, Kappos L, Rohrbach E, and Heun R: Contributions of magnetic resonance imaging to the diagnosis of MS in isolated optic neuritis. Psychiatry Res 29:295–296, 1989.

398. Steiner I, Feir G, Soffer D, Pleet AB, and Abramsky O: Chronic progressive myelopathy: Its relation to the spinal progressive form of multiple sclerosis. Acta Neurol Scand 77:152–157, 1988.

399. Stenager E, Knudsen L, and Jensen K: Acute and chronic pain syndromes in multiple sclerosis. Acta Neurol Scand 84:197–200, 1991.

400. Stewart JM, Houser OW, Baker HL, O'Brien PC, and Rodriguez M: Magnetic resonance imaging and clinical relationships in multiple sclerosis. Mayo Clin Proc 62:174–184, 1987.

401. Studney O, Lublin F, Marcucci L, et al: MS COSTAR: a computerized record for use in clinical research in multiple sclerosis. J Neurol Rehab 7(3–4):145–152, 1993.

402. Surridge D: An investigation into some psychiatric aspects of multiple sclerosis. Br J Psychiatry 115:749–764, 1969.

403. Sweeney BJ, Manji H, Gilson RJC, and Harrison MJG: Optic neuritis and HIV-1 infection. J Neurol Neurosurg Psychiatry 56:705–707, 1993.

404. Szasz G, Paty DW, and Maurice WL: Sexual dysfunctions in multiple sclerosis. Ann NY Acad Sci 436:443–452, 1984.

405. Talpos D, Tien RD, and Hesselink JR: Magnetic resonance imaging of AIDS-related polyradiculopathy. Neurology 41:1996–1997, 1991.

406. Tan CT: Prognosis of patients who present with an episode of myelopathy of unknown origin in Malaysia: A retrospective study of 52 patients. Aust NZ J Med 19:297–302, 1989.

407. Telischi FF, Grobman LR, Sheremata WA, Apple M, and Ayyar R: Hemifacial spasm: Occurrence in multiple sclerosis. Arch Otolaryngol Head Neck Surg 117:554–556, 1991.

408. Tesar JT, McMillan V, Molina R, and Armstrong J: Optic neuropathy and central nervous system disease associated with primary Sjögren's syndrome. Am J Med 92:686–692, 1992.

409. Thomas PK, Walker RWH, Rudge P, et al: Chronic demyelinating peripheral neuropathy associated with multifocal central nervous system demyelination. Brain 110:53–76, 1987.

410. Thompson AJ, Kermode AG, Wicks D, et al: Major differences in the dynamics of primary and secondary progressive multiple sclerosis. Ann Neurol 29:53–62, 1991.

411. Thorpe JW, Halpin SF, Barker GJ, et al: A comparison of fast spin echo and conventional spin echo in multiple sclerosis. Paper presented at the Annual Meeting of the Society for Magnetic Resonance in Medicine, 12th Annual Scientific Meeting, N.Y., N.Y., 1993.

412. Thorpe JW, Kidd D, Kendall BE, et al: Spinal cord MRI using multi-array coils and fast spin echo. I. Technical aspects and findings in healthy adults. Neurology 43:2625–2631, 1993.

412a. Thorpe JW, Kidd D, Moseley IF, et al: Spinal MRI in patients with suspected multiple sclerosis and negative brain MRI. Brain 119:709–714, 1996.

413. Tienari PJ, Salonen O, Wikström J, Valanne L, and Palo J: Familial multiple sclerosis: MRI findings in clinically affected and unaffected siblings. J Neurol Neurosurg Psychiatry 55:883–886, 1992.

414. Tippett DS, Fishman PS, and Panitch HS: Relapsing transverse myelitis. Neurology 41:703–706, 1991.

415. Tofts PS, and Kermode AG: Measurement of the blood-brain barrier permeability and leakage space using dynamic MR imaging. I. Fundamental concepts. Magn Reson Med 17:357–367, 1991.

416. Tourtellotte WW, Staugaitis SM, Walsh MJ, et al: The basis of intra-blood-brain-barrier IgG synthesis. Ann Neurol 17:21–27, 1985.

417. Trimble MR: Pseudoseizures. Neurol Clin 4:531–548, 1986.

418. Trojano R, Hafstein M, Ruderman M, Dowling PC, and Cook SD: Effect of high-dose intravenous steroid administration on contrast-enhancing computed tomographic scan lesions in multiple sclerosis. Ann Neurol 15:257–263, 1984.

419. Uhlenbrock D, and Sehlen S: The value of T1-weighted images in the differentiation between MS, white matter lesions, and subcortical arte-

riosclerotic encephalopathy (SAE). Neuroradiology 31:203–212, 1989.

420. Uhthoff W: Untersuchungen uber bei multiplen Herdsklerose vorkommenden Augenstorungen. Archiv Fur Psychiatrie und Nervenkrankheiten 21:55–116, 303–410, 1890.

421. Uitti RJ, and Rajput AH: Multiple sclerosis presenting as isolated oculomotor nerve palsy. Can J Neurol Sci 13:270–272, 1986.

421a. van Lieshout HBM, van Engelen BGM, Sanders EACM, and Renier WO: Diagnosing multiple sclerosis in childhood. Acta Neurol Scand 88:339–343, 1993.

422. van Swieten JC, van den Hout JHW, van Ketel BA, Hijdra A, Wokke JHJ, and van Gijn J: Periventricular lesions in the white matter on magnetic resonance imaging in the elderly—a morphometric correlation with arteriosclerosis and dilated perivascular spaces. Brain 114:761–774, 1991.

423. van Swieten JC, Geyskes GG, Derix MMA, et al: Hypertension in the elderly is associated with white matter lesions and cognitive decline. Ann Neurol 30:825–830, 1991.

424. Vermess M, Bernstein RM, Bydder GM, Steiner RE, Young IR, and Hughes GRV: Nuclear magnetic resonance (NMR) imaging of the brain in systemic lupus erythematosus. J Comput Assist Tomogr 7:461–467, 1983.

425. Vermote R, Ketelaer P, and Carton H: Pain in multiple sclerosis patients: A prospective study using the McGill pain questionnaire. Clin Neurol Neurosurg 88:87–93, 1986.

426. Vighetto A, Charles N, Salzmann M, Confavreaux C, and Aimard G: Korsakoff's syndrome as the initial presentation of multiple sclerosis. J Neurol 238:351–354, 1991.

427. Vinuela FV, Fox AJ, Debrun GM, Feasby TE, and Ebers GC: New perspectives in computed tomography of multiple sclerosis. AJR 139:123–127, 1982.

428. Vollmer TL, Brass LM, and Waxman SG: Lhermitte's sign in a patient with herpes zoster. J Neurol Sci 106:153–157, 1991.

429. Walicke PA, Stuart WH, and Gilbert RW Jr: STIR imaging in multiple sclerosis. J Neuroimaging 2:61, 1992.

430. Warren KG, Ball MJ, Paty DW, and Banna M: Computer tomography in disseminated sclerosis. Can J Neurol Sci 3:211–216, 1976.

431. Warren KG, and Catz I: Synthetic peptide specificity of anti-myelin basic protein from multiple sclerosis cerebrospinal fluid. J Neuroimmunol 39:81–89, 1992.

432. Wartenberg R: Neuritis, Sensory Neuritis, and Neuralgia. New York. Neuritis and Multiple Sclerosis, Oxford University Press, New York, 1958, pp 296–305.

433. Wattel E, Mariotti M, Bignon JD, et al: No evidence of HTLV-I infection in French patients with multiple sclerosis using the polymerase chain reaction. J Clin Pathol 44:871–872, 1991.

434. Waxman SG: Clinical course and electrophysiology of multiple sclerosis. In Waxman SG (ed): Advances in Neurology: Functional Recovery in Neurological Disease. Raven Press, New York, 1988, pp 157–184.

435. Waxman SG: Peripheral nerve abnormalities in multiple sclerosis (editorial). Muscle Nerve 16:1–5, 1993.

436. Waxman SG, and Geschwind N: Major morbidity related to hyperthermia in multiple sclerosis. Ann Neurol 13:348, 1983.

437. Wechsler B, Dell'Isola B, Vidaihet M, et al: MRI in 31 patients with Behçet's disease and neurological involvement: Prospective study with clinical correlation. J Neurol Neurosurg Psychiatry 56:793–798, 1993.

438. Weinshenker BG, Gilbert JJ, and Ebers GC: Some clinical and pathologic observations on chronic myelopathy: A variant of multiple sclerosis. J Neurol Neurosurg Psychiatry 53:146–149, 1990.

439. Wesseley S: Chronic fatigue syndrome (editorial). J Neurol Neurosurg Psychiatry 54: 669–671, 1991.

440. Whitaker JN: Myelin encephalitogenic protein fragments in cerebrospinal fluid of persons with multiple sclerosis. Neurology 27:911–920, 1977.

441. Whitaker JN, Benveniste EN, and Zhou S: Cerebrospinal fluid. In Cook SD (ed): Handbook of Multiple Sclerosis New York, N.Y. Marcel Dekker, 1990, pp 251–270.

442. Whitaker JN, Layton BA, Herman PK, Kachelhofer RD, Burgard S, and Bartolucci AA: Correlation of myelin basic protein-like material in cerebrospinal fluid of multiple sclerosis patients with their response to glucocorticoid treatment. Ann Neurol 33:10–17, 1993.

443. White AD, Swingler RJ, and Compston DAS: Features of multiple sclerosis in older patients in South Wales. Gerontology 36:159–164, 1990.

444. Williams DW III, Elster AD, and Kramer SI: Neurosarcoidosis: Gadolinium-enhanced MR imaging. J Comput Assist Tomogr 14:704–707, 1990.

445. Willoughby EW, Grochowski E, Li DKB, Oger JJF, Kastrukoff LF, and Paty DW: Serial magnetic resonance scanning in multiple sclerosis: A second prospective study in relapsing patients. Ann Neurol 25:43, 1989.

446. Wilms G, Marchal G, Kersschot E, et al: Axial vs sagittal T2-weighted brain MR images in the evaluation of multiple sclerosis. J Comput Assist Tomogr 15:359–364, 1991.

447. Wolinsky L, Bardini J, Cook SD, Zimmer A, Sheffet A, and Lee HJ: Triple-dose versus single-dose gadoteridol in multiple sclerosis patients. J Neuroimaging 4:141–145, 1994.

448. Wuthrich R, Gigli H, Wiggli U, Muller HR, Elke M, and Hunig R: CT scanning in demyelinating diseases. In Lanksch W, and Kafner E (eds): Cranial Computerized Tomography. Springer-Verlag, New York, 1976, pp 239–243.

449. Yedavally S, Pernicone J, and Kaufman D: MRI demonstrates that a higher percentage of patients with acute optic neuritis have multiple sclerosis than has previously been documented. Journal of the Society for Magnetic Resonance Medicine p.297(Abstract Book), 1987.

450. Yetkin FZ, Haughton VM, Papke RA, Fischer ME, and Rao SM: Multiple sclerosis: Specificity of MR for diagnosis. Radiology 178:447–451, 1991.

451. Yokota T, Hirose K, Tsukagoshi H, and Tanabe H: Somatosensory evoked potentials in patients with selective impairment of position sense versus vibration sense. Acta Neurol Scand 84: 201–206, 1991(a).

452. Yokota T, Matsunaga T, Okiyama R, et al: Sympathetic skin response in patients with multiple sclerosis compared with patients with spinal cord transection and normal controls. Brain 114(pt 3):1381–1394, 1991(b).

453. Youl BD, Kermode AG, Thompson AJ, et al: Destructive lesions in demyelinating disease. J Neurol Neurosurg Psychiatry 54:288–292, 1991.

454. Youl BD, Turano G, Miller DH, et al: The pathophysiology of acute optic neuritis: An association of gadolinium leakage with clinical and electrophysiological deficits. Brain 114:2437–2450, 1991.

455. Young IR, Hall AS, Pallis CA, Bydder GM, Legg NJ, and Steiner RE: Nuclear magnetic resonance imaging of the brain in multiple sclerosis. Lancet 2:1063–1066, 1981.

456. Yu YL, Woo E, Hawkins BR, Ho HC, and Huang CY: Multiple sclerosis amongst Chinese in Hong Kong. Brain 112:1445–1467, 1989.

457. Zeldowicz L: Paroxysmal motor episodes as early manifestations of multiple sclerosis. Can Med Assoc J 84:937–941, 1961.

458. Zeman AZJ, Keir G, Luxton R, Thompson EJ, Miller DH, and McDonald WI: Oligoclonal bands in multiple sclerosis. Paper presented at the 119th Annual Meeting of the American Neurological Association, San Francisco, 1994. Ann Neurol 36:325, 1994.

459. Zimmerman RD, Fleming CA, Lee BCP, Saint-Louis LA, and Deck MDF: Periventricular hyperintensity as seen by magnetic resonance: Prevalence and significance. AJNR 7:13–20, 1986.

CHAPTER 5

CLINICAL FEATURES

Donald W. Paty, MD
George C. Ebers, MD

135

The clinical features of MS are of bewildering variability.[148,199] Although there are some reasonably predictable features, the pattern in which visual, motor, sensory, and autonomic abnormalities combine results in remarkable clinical variation. The severity of clinical signs and symptoms is more often related to the location of the areas of damage than to the severity and extent of the MS pathological process. Some patients with severe disability due to MS carry a relatively low total volume of damaged areas, but the damage is strategically located in "eloquent" areas of the nervous system, such as the brain stem, spinal cord, and optic nerve. Even small lesions in these regions are more likely to produce disabling symptoms than are lesions in the cerebral hemispheres. For example, involvement of the periventricular region near the lateral ventricles is often asymptomatic. On the other hand, frontal periventricular involvement may contribute significantly to spasticity in the legs and to bladder disturbances, because this is the region of pyramidal fibers.

The severity of the pathological process in MS depends on many variables. Present methodologies do not permit determination of the relative contributions of edema, inflammation, blood-brain barrier (BBB) disruption, demyelination, and gliosis to clinical expression. Demyelination impairs but does not necessarily block axonal conduction. However, axonal loss and gliosis are likely to be irreversible changes. The plasticity and redundancy of the central nervous system (CNS) may partly protect against permanent deficit. We do not know all of the factors that determine whether a given lesion will become symptomatic, even if placed in an anatomically eloquent location.

Specific demyelination has always been defined as the hallmark of MS. Although that statement is probably true, can we say that demyelination is responsible for the continued symptoms? Instances of a total loss of function (for example, in optic neuritis, ON), after which patients can recover to a functionally normal or near normal state, are common. This recovery may occur in spite of the presence of striking residual optic atrophy and grossly impaired visual evoked potential (VEP) latencies in the affected eye. Nondemyelinating elements in the pathological process, such as edema, inflammation, gliosis, and axonal loss, all play a part in determining the clinical expression of a particular lesion.

PATHOPHYSIOLOGY OF DEMYELINATION

The pathophysiology of experimental demyelination is well understood (see reviews[149,287,288,289,290]). This knowledge helps to explain some of the clinical phenomenology of MS (see Chapter 8).

Conduction in a normally myelinated nerve is made possible by the presence of sodium channels mostly located at the nodes of Ranvier. Saxitoxin (STX) binds specifically to sodium channels.[216] STX binding has been used to show low sodium channel density in the internodal region (that region of the membrane under the myelin sheath) and high density at the nodes of Ranvier. These sodium channels are responsible for the sodium ion shifts that occur with depolarization. Depolarization that occurs at the node produces an electrical charge which can then be conducted through the myelinated segment by the cable properties of the nerve. At the next node, depolarization occurs again, facilitated by the presence of sodium channels, to propagate the impulses farther.

In demyelinated segments of nerve, sodium channels proliferate along the demyelinated surface of the membrane, allowing propagation of the depolarization wave along that membrane. Since the days of Charcot, symptom production in MS has been thought to be due to blockade or some other disturbance of conduction in demyelinated fibers. More recently, it has also been proposed that circulating factors may interfere significantly with conduction. In addition, it is known that conduction can persist in demyelinated fibers. Bostock and Sears[27] have shown in a series of elegant studies that depolarization potentials can be propagated along the demyelinated axon membrane. Conduction under these conditions is slow, and it is this slow conduction along the demyelinated portions of the nerve that is probably responsible for the general slowness of conduction in all forms of demyelination, whether peripheral or central.

Propagation of conduction, made possible by the proliferation of sodium channels along the demyelinated axon membrane, is sensitive to small changes in temperature and electrolytes, which can quickly produce conduction block. In normally myelinated nerve, small increases in temperature will speed up conduction. However, Rasminsky[212] and later Rasminsky and Sears[213] showed that increased temperature could produce conduction block in demyelinated fibers. They also showed that trains of impulses could result in conduction block in these same fibers. The trains of impulses apparently produce conduction block by the mechanism of prolongation of the refractory period of the axon. These investigators were also able to show that decreased calcium concentration could inhibit the tendency of increased temperature to cause conduction block. In addition, lowering the temperature or pharmacologically shortening the refractory period (such as by the use of ouabain) could have a similar effect.[110]

Some aspects of the focal muscle fatigue seen in MS may be explained by these characteristics of demyelinated fibers. Demyelinated fibers fail to conduct rapid trains of stimuli as well as do normal fibers. A "myasthenic phenomenon" is commonly seen in patients with MS, characterized by increasing weakness usually in distal muscles after repeated contractions of that specific muscle. The tendency for demyelinated fibers to go into conduction block when they have been subjected to repeated trains of stimuli might underlie this clinical phenomenon.

This physiological change, related to temperature and electrolyte disturbance, probably explains Uhthoff's phenomenon,[291] originally described as a reduction of visual acuity associated with hyperthermia. It also occurs with exercise, probably because of increased core body temperature. It is not specific to MS, but its presence certainly suggests demyelination. Many other neurological symptoms in patients with MS can be susceptible to minor body temperature changes as well. The influence of temperature on MS has recently been reviewed.[87a]

The phenomenon of slow conduction in demyelinated fibers accounts for the prolonged latency in evoked potential (EP) studies. McDonald[151] calculated that a 1-cm plaque in the optic nerve could produce a 25-ms delay in VEP latency. The EP abnormalities could also be explained by conduction loss in the faster conducting fibers, which, in turn, would prolong the peak latency.

Schauf and Davis[235] suggested that pharmacological modification of sodium and potassium channels might help to produce increased current density in demyelinated fibers, which in turn would help to minimize the tendency to conduction block. They also showed that lowering serum ionized calcium, which increases axonal excitability, facilitated conduction in demyelinated fibers and could also lead to transient improvement in the clinical status of patients.

A potassium channel blocker, 4-aminopyridine (4-AP), can temporarily improve neurological symptoms such as gait ataxia, limb ataxia, and weakness (see Chapter 12).[51]

ACUTE EXACERBATION

An acute attack or exacerbation, as defined by Schumacher and colleagues,[238] is a focal disturbance of function, affecting a white matter tract, lasting for more than 24 hours. Typically, an acute exacerbation tends to progress over a period of a few days, reaching a maximum in less than 1 week and then slowly resolving. Complete recovery from an attack is common early in the disease. The centrifugal spread of a pathological disturbance from a focus is implied by the pattern of development of symptoms. Curiously, symmetrical lesions in both posterior and lateral columns are often implicated by the march of symptoms beginning in the legs and moving to the arms in many spinal exacerbations. Attacks may be unifocal or multifocal. Recent evidence from imaging studies, however, suggests that most MS disease activity is asymptomatic.[300]

RECOVERY OF FUNCTION

The recovery mechanism after relapse is poorly understood and is probably multifactorial. It has generally been thought that recovery of the BBB, resolution of edema, the reduction of inflammation, and changes in production of accompanying mediators (cytokines) all underlie the recovery process. In addition, until about 10 years ago it was thought that remyelination did not occur in the CNS. We now know from the studies of Ludwin[137] and Prineas[205] that remyelination can occur quite readily in the CNS. Remyelination is probably responsible for the restoration of function in some instances, although the shortened internode length characteristic of remyelination shows that the process is imperfect. The pathological phenomenon of "shadow plaques" was previously believed to represent partial demyelination. Neuropathologists now believe shadow plaques represent remyelination rather than partial demyelination (see Chapter 8). However, many patients show improvement after relapse that is too rapid to be explained by remyelination. In these instances, improvement has been attributed to physiological recovery in fibers that have not been morphologically altered (perhaps not even demyelinated).

The paroxysmal symptoms so frequently seen in MS also suggest abnormal physiological rather than structural mechanisms (see later). Ekbom and his colleagues[63] described focal motor seizures of "spinal origin." They proposed the mechanism of ephaptic transmission as the cause. Ephaptic transmission is the lateral spread of electrical activity between axons in a demyelinated zone. Pathological studies have shown that demyelinated axons in the MS plaque are in close proximity to one another with little intervening neuropil. Drugs such as benzodiazapines and anticonvulsants, which reduce sodium and potassium conductances, block paroxysmal attacks (see Chapter 12), apparently by blocking the ephaptic spread of axonal discharges.

POSITIVE SENSATIONS

The production of myokymia, paresthesia, Lhermitte's symptom, photopsias, and other positive symptoms in MS[5] may well reflect movement-induced or other physiologically stimulated discharges in demyelinated fibers. These symptoms are probably caused by mechanical or chemical changes along the demyelinated membrane that evoke either focal or spreading discharges. Smith and colleagues[254] showed that partial demyelination with lysolecithin produced demyelinated fibers that were abnormally sensitive to mechanical deformation.

Andermann and his colleagues[4] have pointed out the relative frequency of the occurrence of myokymia in MS. Electromyographic studies have shown that there are brief runs of spontaneous firing of individual motor units. This phenomenon can occur in many muscle groups, but it is seen most commonly in the facial muscles.

CLINICAL CATEGORIES OF MULTIPLE SCLEROSIS

Table 5–1 lists and defines the most commonly used clinical categories in MS. Although not clearly established, most clinicians believe that relapsing-remitting MS (RRMS) and secondary progressive MS (SPMS) are just two sequential phases of the same disease. However, a minority of patients (15 percent) have primary chronic progressive MS (CPMS), with worsening of disability unassociated with relapse. It is possible that this form of MS entails different pathogenic mechanisms (see discussion

Table 5–1. **CLINICAL CATEGORIES OF MULTIPLE SCLEROSIS**

Name of Clinical Category	Definition
DIAGNOSTIC CATEGORIES (SEE CHAPTER 4)	
Clinically definite MS (CDMS)	Patients who satisfy the Schumacher criteria of dissemination of white matter lesions in time and space.
Laboratory-supported definite MS (LSDMS)	Patients who do not satisfy the CDMS criteria but who have paraclinical evidence for dissemination in space plus oligoclonal banding in the CSF.
Probable MS	Patients who have dissemination in time or space alone without other supporting evidence.
CLINICAL COURSE CATEGORIES	
Relapsing-remitting MS (RRMS)	Patients who have attacks of the disease with subsequent recovery and who have little or no residual neurological deficit between attacks. Some patients have a stepwise increase in neurolgical deficit.
Secondary Progressive MS (SPMS) (Relapsing progressive)	Patients who start with attacks but develop significant neurological deficits that increase during follow-up. Most patients slowly get worse.
Primary chronic progressive (I°CPMS)	Patients who have a slow and steady progression of a chronic neurological deficit from onset without any attacks.
Acute (malignant) MS	Patients who have polysymptomatic disease that progresses to severe disability and/or death in a few months.
Benign MS (a subcategory of RRMS)	Relapsing patients who do not develop a significant residual neurological deficit (usually defined as <EDSS 3) after 10–15 yr of disease.

CSF = cerebrospinal fluid; EDSS = Extended Disability Status Scale.

following). A consensus article on the various clinical courses has been published recently.[136a]

Relapsing-Remitting Multiple Sclerosis

Seventy percent of patients with MS begin with a relapsing-remitting clinical course (see Table 5–1). Relapse symptoms develop in an acute or subacute manner, and the tendency is toward recovery. Schumacher and colleagues'[238] criteria state that true relapses must last more than 24 hours and must be associated with significant changes in functional ability. Also, relapses cannot occur more frequently than one per month. This stipulation is somewhat arbitrary; certainly focal sensory symptoms can be seen that have the temporal characteristics of exacerbations elsewhere but do not produce a change in functional ability. The cooperative trial of therapy with adrenocorticotropic hormone (ACTH) in MS[220] showed that 75 percent of untreated patients recover within 6 weeks after an acute relapse. Patients frequently report clear-cut relapses and remissions that have occurred over many years. From patient interviews, the impression is that relapses can be defined and quantitated in a relatively precise fashion. In practice, however, attempts at prospectively describing relapses and remissions have turned out to be difficult. For example, it is not uncommon for patients to experience episodes of an overwhelming fatigue without having any significant change in neurological findings. Paty and

Ebers have seen such patients who did not have any changes in neurological symptoms or findings who did have large new lesions seen on serial magnetic resonance imaging (MRI) studies which eventually resolved at follow-up.

Clinical relapse frequency has been studied by many authors (see Table 6–4). The mean annual frequency has been shown to vary between 0.4 and 1.1 relapses per patient per year. The rate reported depends on the age and type of patient population, duration of disease, and frequency of follow-up, among other factors. The more frequently patients are seen, the greater the frequency of identified attacks. We have found that the relapse frequency decreases by the second year of disease. The range of relapse rates is from 0 to a theoretical limit of 12 relapses per patient per year. The relapse rate may decline with duration of disease, but at least one prospective study has suggested that relapse rates do not decline.[189] The relapse rate also may be independent of the clinical outcome. However, in severely disabled patients, new relapses may be less easy to define because of the overwhelming neurological deficit that is chronically present.

In a population-based study from London, Ontario,[293] the average attack rate in the first year was found to be 1.5 to 2.3 relapses per patient per year. The attack rate fell with age and duration of disease. Some uncontrolled clinical trials have reported a dramatic decline in relapse rate as a significant therapeutic effect, but one carefully controlled randomized and blinded clinical trial showed a dramatic reduction in relapse rate in both treatment and placebo groups, with no significant difference between the two groups.[38] Goodkin and colleagues[83] did not find a decline in attack rates in a short follow-up (2.6 years) of 254 patients from North Dakota. They did find, however, that patients frequently changed from stable to progressive and back again. They also found that relapses occurred most frequently in the spring and summer months. Previous studies from Switzerland had shown relapses to be most frequent in the winter months,[302] and a prospective study from northern England found no seasonal trend.[233] Some reports had stressed the spring as the most frequent time for relapses.[249] Bamford and associates[13] followed up 178 patients with MS prospectively for 5 years to determine the monthly exacerbation rate. They found that relapses were more common in the warmer months.

The interval between bouts can be from a minimum of 1 month (by definition from the Schumacher criteria) to more than 35 years. The prognosis for good recovery is best (90 percent) when the acute-onset relapse begins to abate within 2 to 4 weeks. With increasing duration of the bout, the potential for recovery diminishes. The recovery potential decreases to less than 10 percent when the duration of the attack has been over 1 year. The identification of a relapse is not always straightforward. As noted previously and in Chapter 9, not only is MRI activity in the cerebral hemispheres usually asymptomatic in neurological terms, but occasionally the patient can have fatigue as the only clinical manifestation of a new MS lesion.[120a,300] Therefore, the arbitrary clinical decisions made concerning relapses are probably not precise.

Pseudorelapses are seen when a change in neurological function occurs that appears to be due to MS activity but is actually due to a physiological change. Such physiological changes are usually due to intercurrent episodes such as urinary tract infection with fever, changes in body temperature from other sources, electrolyte abnormalities, and drugs. In general, pseudorelapses (Table 5–2) are usually characterized by the following features:

1. A recurrence of old symptoms
2. Short duration
3. A definable accompanying metabolic or toxic change
4. Disappearance of symptoms and signs when the aggravating metabolic change has been corrected

For example, a patient with a previous history of spasticity and leg weakness can be precipitated into paraplegia or even quadriplegia by the fever accompanying a urinary tract infection. The mechanism for this exacerbation of the neurological deficit involves elevated temperature (1° or 2°C) and other microenvironmental changes adjacent to the demyelinated ax-

Table 5–2. **TRUE RELAPSES VERSUS PSEUDORELAPSES**

	True Relapses	Pseudorelapses
Onset:	Acute or subacute	Acute more likely
Duration:	Weeks likely	Days rather than weeks
Previous deficit:	Not necessary	Likely
Fever associated:	Not likely	Usually

ons producing reversible conduction block. The conduction block, in turn, produces a temporary recurrence of old symptoms or, if asymptomatic lesions have developed in the interim, the acute development of new ones. If truly due to physiological events, pseudorelapses should resolve when the offending abnormal metabolic factor has been reversed. The most helpful rule for distinguishing a true relapse from a pseudorelapse is that if there is an abrupt change in symptoms or signs in an area of the nervous system known to be previously damaged, perhaps the relapse is due to a physiological event and not a true pathological change. In such a case, the physician must look carefully for the primary cause of the pseudorelapse.

TRIGGERING EVENTS FOR RELAPSES

Multiple sclerosis is a reasonably common disorder that is not protective against most of the other ills of human beings. Accordingly, considerable literature has attempted to relate virtually any naturally occurring event to the precipitation of relapses (see Chapter 2). Many of these event data are retrospective and speculative. We review here the best-studied factors that have been suspected to influence onset and relapse. (See Chapter 11 for a discussion of the mechanism of relapses.)

Pregnancy and Delivery (See Chapter 2). The subject of pregnancy in MS has been recently reviewed.[23,24,75,170] Pregnancy has been shown, largely in prospective studies, to be associated with a reduction in relapse rates, and the same studies have shown an increased risk of exacerbation in the 3 months after delivery. Another common clinical impression is that relapses tend to occur in women after delivery. Nelson and her colleagues[170] interviewed 435 women regarding their pregnancies and relapses. They found that the exacerbation rate during the 9 months postpartum was 34 percent compared with 10 percent during the 9 months of pregnancy. The highest exacerbation rate was in the 3 months postpartum. Breast-feeding did not seem to influence the postpartum exacerbation rate. Because those same women seem to do well during pregnancy, it could be said that the pregnancy holds back the relapse, which then expresses itself after delivery.[121] In addition, a woman with MS (as is any other mother) is subject to a great deal of stress when caring for a new baby. Perhaps the stress, the anticlimax, and the hormonal changes that occur postpartum come together to create a particularly vulnerable time for the mother with MS. Table 5–3 cites several retrospective studies[75,80] of the relationship between pregnancy and attacks of MS.

In 1959, Millar and his colleagues[153] were the first to draw attention to the effect of pregnancy on MS, reporting a significant increase in the number of relapses seen during pregnancy years as opposed to nonpregnancy years. Schapira and his colleagues[234] studied 321 women, 255 of whom had had pregnancies. Even though they found that the relapse rate in women who had been pregnant was not significantly different from those who had not been pregnant, they confirmed that the relapse rate in pregnancy years was greater than in nonpregnancy years. Further study of this phenomenon showed that the risk of relapses was particularly high during the 3 months after delivery. Of relapses that occurred during a pregnancy year, 85 percent occurred in the 3 months after delivery. Their study also found that if the onset of MS was after delivery, the risk of relapse was high

Table 5–3. POSSIBLE PRECIPITATING FACTORS FOR RELAPSES IN MULTIPLE SCLEROSIS: PREGNANCY AND DELIVERY

Year	Senior Author	Type of Study	No. of Patients	Findings
1959	Millar[153]	R	262	Relapse in pregnancy year was two times that of nonpregnancy year. Most relapses occurred in puerperia.
1966	Schapira[234]	R	321	The relapse rate in pregnancy years was higher than that in nonpregnancy years. Most relapses occurred in the puerperium. Disability was greatest in women who had their first relapse after a delivery.
1981	Sibley[249]	R	141	Exacerbation rate or worsening of MS was high after delivery compared with low exacerbation rate during pregnancy.
1981	Ghezzi[80]	R	119	A higher relapse rate occurred in the puerperium. Long term outcome was not influenced by pregnancy.
1983	Poser[200]	R	512	Risk of onset, relapse, and other worsening were higher (×3) during 6 mo after delivery. Pregnancy did not influence outcome.
1984	Korn-Lubetzki[121]	R	338	Relapse rate decreased in third trimester and increased in the puerperium.
1986	Thompson[270]	R	178	Pregnancy had no influence on outcome. Those with initial symptoms during pregnancy had less disability on follow-up.
1988	Frith[75]	R	52	No increase in relapse was associated with pregnancy. There was a decrease in relapse rate in the first two trimesters.
1988	Nelson[170]	R	435	Exacerbation rate in puerperium was three times the rate during pregnancy. Breast-feeding had no effect.
1989	Weinshenker[295]	R	185	No association occurred between outcome disability and pregnancy.
1990	Birk[23]	P	8	Six of eight patients had relapses after delivery.
1994	Sadovnick[228]	P	53	Relapse rate was low in third low trimester. No increase in relapse rate occurred after delivery.
1994	Worthington[301]	P	15	Relapse rate increased in first 6 mo postpartum but below expected in the period 6–24 mo postpartum. Overall (over 1–3 yr), there was no difference from controls.

P = prospective; R = retrospective.

with subsequent deliveries. In other words, women who have had an exacerbation after delivery of a child are likely to have further relapses associated with subsequent deliveries. Some clinicians have used this observation as a basis to advise against further pregnancies or to terminate subsequent pregnancies in such women. Poser and Poser[200] found that exacerbation or progression of disease was three times higher during the 6 months after childbirth than at other times during the course of MS in those same patients. However, they did not find evidence that the long-term outcome was influenced by pregnancy and childbirth. Weinshenker and colleagues[295] did a retrospective study of 185 women and found no association between disability and total number of term pregnancies, timing of pregnancy relative to the onset of MS, and either onset or worsening of MS in relationship to a pregnancy.

Could pregnancy have a protective effect in MS? Perhaps the same immunological factors that protect the fetus against rejection suppress the autoimmune attack against the nervous system during pregnancy. This speculation led Abramsky[1] to study the effects of alpha-fetoprotein (AFP) in experimental allergic encephalitis (EAE). He found that AFP could protect animals against EAE if administered before the provocative immunization.

The data just cited come largely from retrospective studies. A prospective study recently was carried out by Sadovnick and colleagues (see Table 5–3).[228] She studied 46 women with MS through 55 pregnancies resulting in liveborn infants. She used as control subjects both female patients with MS (matched to the mothers by MS clinical category, clinical course, and initial symptoms) who did not become pregnant during the study period, and the prospective mothers' clinical course, documented in the clinic, before the pregnancy. The following findings were reported (Table 5–4):

1. The mean exacerbation rate in the study patients before the pregnancies in question was 0.71 relapses per patient per year.
2. The prospectively followed mothers had a reduced relapse rate during the third trimester but no increase in the relapse rate after delivery.

3. The matched control subjects had a relapse rate of 0.81 per patient per year. They also had, on the average, more children than did the study patients.
4. None of the changes were statistically significant.

Pregnancy had no long-term adverse effect on the outcome of MS (except for the variable relapse rate in the third trimester), and the MS had no adverse effects on the pregnancy (e.g., no increase in miscarriages). Two retrospective studies found that the number of pregnancies had no influence on long-term outcome of the MS.[270,295]

One prospective study[301] reported an increase over expected numbers of relapses in the first 6 months postpartum, but below expected rates at 6 to 24 months postpartum. Over the entire period of up to 3 years postpartum, there were no significant differences between delivery patients and control subjects in relapse rates, disability scores, and functional scores.

The practical requirements of patient counseling dictate that the possible association between delivery and exacerbation be brought to the attention of young couples when the question of having a child is discussed. (See section on reproductive counseling in Chapter 12.)

Immunizations and Infections. Because immunizations and infections stimulate the immune system, it might be anticipated that such events would be risk factors for triggering relapses in MS (Table 5–5).[248] Miller and his colleagues[156] described nine

Table 5–4. RELAPSE RATES DURING AND AFTER PREGNANCY IN A PROSPECTIVE STUDY

Time Period	Number of Relapses[†]	Comparison with Expected Rate
First trimester	11	1.2 times expected*
Second trimester	6	0.76 times expected*
Third trimester	3	0.33 times expected*
Up to 3 mo postdelivery	14	1.09 times expected*
Four to 6 mo postdelivery	8	1.09 times expected*

Source: Sadovnick AD, Eisen KA, Farquhar, et al, Pregnancy and multiple sclerosis: A prospective study. Arch Neurol 51(11):1120–1124, 1994,[228] and are based upon a prospective study of 55 pregnancies in 46 women with MS; (see text).
  *Expected rates from data on matched controls.
  [†]None of the changes were statistically significant.

Table 5–5. **POSSIBLE PRECIPITATING FACTORS FOR RELAPSES IN MULTIPLE SCLEROSIS: IMMUNIZATION AND INFECTIONS**

Year	Senior Author	Type of Study	Results
1965	Sibley[248]	P	Forty-eight percent of relapses were associated with infection, and 40% of infections were associated with relapse. No risk with immunization.
1967	Miller[156]	R	Five cases demonstrated onset of MS shortly after vaccination, and four cases, relapse shortly after vaccination.
1977	Myers[167]	P	A controlled study showed no increase in relapse rates after influenza vaccination
1978	Bamford[12]	P	A controlled study showed no relationship existed between swine flu immunization and relapse.
1981	Andersen[6]	R	Immunization was not a risk factor for relapse in 92 patients (N) with MS compared with matched control subjects (N ×3).
1989	Berr[22]	R	Immunization was not a risk factor in 63 patients with MS compared with matched control subjects.
1985	Sibley[246]	P	Twenty-seven percent of relapses were related to infection, mostly upper respiratory viral ones. MS patients had fewer infections than did matched controls.

P = prospective; R = retrospective.

cases of onset or exacerbation of MS after immunization. Their opinion was that the association was a significant one. Paty and Ebers have also seen the onset of MS after immunization, but it has been a relatively uncommon observation.

Andersen and associates[6] surveyed 92 patients with MS and an equal number of matched control subjects from the Copenhagen register of school health records. They were unable to find any significant relationship between routine vaccinations, bacterial infections of childhood, or surgical operations and the onset of MS. They did find a significant association between a negative tuberculin skin test at age 7 years and the later development of MS. They interpreted this finding as revealing a low incidence of early exposure to tuberculosis (TB), rather than showing an intrinsic poor skin reactivity to tuberculin or a deficient immune response in patients with MS.

After the 1976 swine influenza epidemic in the United States, there were a number of secondary cases of Guillain-Barré syndrome[125] due to the immunization. If immunization were to precipitate MS, 1976 would be the year that one would expect a sudden surge in new cases.[12] No such change in incidence occurred. A retrospective analysis of the swine flu epidemic has failed to show any clear-cut association with the onset or exacerbation of MS. Myers and associates[167] did a double blind placebo-controlled study to evaluate the safety and efficacy of *inactivated* influenza virus vaccine in 66 patients with MS. The clinical relapse rate was the same for the vaccine-immunized and placebo-immunized groups. The unimmunized control group had a slightly higher relapse rate than did either of the immunized groups. Nevertheless, it is not unusual for neurologists to observe the onset of MS or relapses after immunization. We have seen exacerbations in two patients with MS after hepatitis B vaccination. Herroelen and colleagues[92] reported on two patients who had CNS episodes after hepatitis B vaccination. One patient had pre-existing MS; the other had no previous history of neurological disease. Both patients had HLA-DR2 and B7. It is therefore wise to approach the topic of immunization in MS with caution and to recommend against nonessential immunizations (see Chapter 12).

Another long-standing clinical impression has been that MS relapses can be precipitated by intercurrent infections. Similar to the known onset of postinfectious acute disseminated encephalomyelitis (ADEM) after specific virus infections, it is reasonable to think that the immune stimulation that occurs as a reaction to infection could result in the reactivation of the MS process. Chronic sinus infection is probably common.[142] In a prospective study, Sibley and his colleagues[244,246] reported a clear-cut temporal relationship between infections and relapses. They followed 170 patients with MS prospectively over 6 years, reviewing them at monthly intervals. The relapse rate after infection was significantly higher than at any other periods of time in both the same patient (historical self-control subjects) or in noninfected patients (control subjects). To determine whether or not postinfectious relapses occur only in selected susceptible cases or as a general phenomenon will require additional study. They also found that viral infections were significantly less common in the more disabled patients with MS than in non-MS control subjects and less disabled patients with MS. This phenomenon could be due to less exposure to infectious contacts in the more disabled group. It also could be because MS patients have a "superior" immune system.[248] Bray and colleagues[33,34] described four of five patients with neurologically complicated Epstein-Barr virus (EBV) infection who went on to develop MS on follow-up. They did not suggest a causal relationship between EBV and MS. A review of their cases suggests that the symptoms could have been due to MS and that the EBV infection could have been the trigger for the attack. Previous studies by the same group had shown that 99 percent of 313 patients with MS had EBV antibodies at an elevated level compared with an 89 percent antibody-positive rate in control subjects.

Surgery, Stress, and Trauma. The relationship between traumatic events and activity of MS is a controversial area of study and speculation, particularly in the United States, where attribution of blame and damages are commonly pursued with vigor. Another common clinical impression has been that patients with MS can have relapses or deterioration in function after anesthesia, surgery, or both (Table 5–6). McAlpine and Compston[146] found a relapse rate of one per patient per year during the 3 months after surgery in 36 surgical cases compared with a rate of 0.39 relapses per patient per year in the entire clinic population. This finding led them to conclude that there was an increased risk of relapse after surgery. Other studies have suggested that previous surgery and traumatic events are more frequent in patients with MS than in control subjects. Siemkowicz[250] reported 16 anesthetics in 11 patients with MS over a period of 3 years. Five of those patients (45 percent) developed marked deterioration after anesthesia and surgery. However, prospective studies have failed to confirm this clinical impression. Bamford and colleagues[14] followed up 130 patients with MS prospectively for 3½ years and documented both relapses and traumatic events including surgery. They found the exacerbation rate during the 6 months after surgery (N = 38) to be the same as in non-postsurgery months. In addition, these authors found no correlation between trauma and relapses. More recently, the same authors have extended these studies and, again, found no association between surgery and relapses.[247]

The relationship between traumatic events and the general level of life stress and clinical deterioration seen in MS has

Table 5–6. **POSSIBLE PRECIPITATING FACTORS FOR RELAPSES IN MULTIPLE SCLEROSIS: SURGERY**

Year	Senior Author	Type of Study	Findings
1976	Siemkowicz[250]	R	Five exacerbations in 11 patients after 16 anesthetics
1981	Bamford[14]	P	No increase in relapse rate after surgery

P = prospective; R = retrospective.

been difficult to examine, especially retrospectively (Tables 5–7 and 5–8)[168]. In 1875, Moxon[165] recorded eight cases of MS. Two of the patients claimed that their first symptoms had followed an emotional shock.

In addition, Charcot suggested in his writings that grief and anger could precipitate MS symptoms. Warren and her colleagues[284] interviewed and compared 100 patients with MS with hospital control patients. However, the reader must realize that appropriate controls for such a study are almost impossible to identify. The reseachers recorded events thought to be stressful before the onset of MS. More patients with MS than control patients reported that they were under unusual stress during the 2 years before the onset of their disease or during a similar period for the control patients. The patients with MS also reported a total greater number of stressful life situations than did the control patients. The authors drew attention to the diary of Augustus d'Este, one of the earliest descriptions of MS.[69] D'Este recorded the onset of his visual symptoms at the funeral of a father figure.

Warren and her colleagues[285] also looked at stress levels in 95 patients with clinically definite MS (CDMS) with a recent exacerbation and compared them with 95 patients with CDMS in remission. She found that the patients in exacerbation scored higher than the control patients in emotional disturbance and intensity of stressful events.

The patients who experienced an exacerbation also tended to use emotion-focused coping techniques as opposed to problem-solving or social support techniques. She recommended counseling patients on stress reduction techniques.

Interestingly, stress is known to cause immunosuppression in some situations.[45,116] There is reason to believe that autoimmunity can be influenced by stress and vice versa.[260] In addition, even though stress is commonly reported by patients as being a significant factor in precipitating worsening of symptoms, having MS is stressful in its own right. Remarkably, the reduction in quality of life just in knowing the diagnosis appears to approximate that attributed to a change of some 3 points in the Kurtzke Disability Status Scale (I. Brownscombe, 1989) as assessed by the time trade-off technique. The effects of this stress are seen in both family disruption and in the frequent episodes of depression that occur. If patients with MS see their lives as generally stressful, a retrospective survey would find that patients with MS interpret prior events as being stressful as well. However, a non-MS control subject might judge a similar event as not stressful. A blinded prospective study using subjective and semiobjective scales of stressors should be done, looking at the question of exacerbations associated with stress. The researchers experience shows that even though some patients will equate relapses with stressful events in their lives, most patients do not have true

Table 5–7. **POSSIBLE PRECIPITATING FACTORS FOR RELAPSES IN MULTIPLE SCLEROSIS: STRESS**

Year	Senior Author	Type of Study	Findings
1982	Warren[284]	R	Patients with MS recalled an increased frequency of unusual stress before onset of the disease when compared to hospital control patients.
1983	Dalos[50]	P	Sixty-four patients with MS experienced an increased emotional state during relapse. Emotional state was not associated with the degree of disability.
1989	Grant[85]	R	A high proportion of patients with MS reported marked life adversities in the year before onset of MS symptoms, most markedly in the 6 mo prior.

R = retrospective; P = prospective.

Table 5–8. **POSSIBLE PRECIPITATING FACTORS FOR RELAPSES IN MULTIPLE SCLEROSIS: TRAUMA**

Year	Senior Author	Type of Study	Findings
1952	McAlpine[146]	R	Fourteen percent of his patients had a traumatic event within 3 mo before the onset of MS. In many of these (22/36), there was a correlation between the site of the trauma and the site of the lesion. Twenty-nine of 80 traumatic incidents were followed by relapses.
1964	Miller[157]	R	Seven cases were reported in which MS symptoms started after trauma.
1969	Namerow[168]	R	Four cases were reported in which MS symptoms or relapses followed trauma.
1981	Bamford[14]	P	No association was found between trauma and relapses, worsening or onset of MS in 120 patients followed up for 3.5 yr. Electrical shock was weakly associated with an increased relapse rate.
1991	Sibley[247]	P	No correlation was found between traumatic events and relapses or disability in 170 patients with MS followed up for 8 yr.
1993	Siva[252]	R	Disability status of patients with and without trauma was the same. Also, previous trauma was not associated with the onset of MS. No head injury patients (N = 819) developed MS within 6 mo of the trauma.

P = prospective; R = retrospective.

exacerbations that are temporally related to stressful events.

In recent years, a number of claims and studies have suggested that disease activity in multiple sclerosis can be triggered or caused by a number of external factors, all probably independent of the actual cause of the disease. Relapses were clearly defined by the Schumacher committee in 1965.[238] Relapses in MS are probably mediated by autoimmune assault on oligodendrocytes or myelin of the CNS.

Several studies have suggested that life events of various kinds can trigger attacks of MS or make MS worse.[50,86,284] The natural history of relapses is that many patients with MS stop having them, and most develop a disease course that is chronically progressive, either with or without superimposed relapses. The onset of the chronic progressive phase is thought to be a poor prognostic sign.[48,292]

Most neurologists have seen patients with MS who have developed a relapse or have deteriorated in some way after an environmental event such as a virus infection or a particularly stressful physical or emotional trauma. Popular contemporary theories of disease of unknown cause commonly accommodate a role for these factors without much supporting evidence. It is plausible that external events can act as triggers to cause a temporary upset in homeostatic mechanisms that would allow a relapse of the MS to proceed. Perhaps the immune system in patients with MS could be upset by external factors. However attractive such notions might be, we must rely on, or at least consider, the data derived from prospective and systematic studies. The most clear-cut demonstration that an environmental event can trigger activity in MS was from a study clearly implicating viral infections as a trigger for relapses.[246]

A particularly controversial proposal has been that physical trauma can precipitate relapses of MS or produce significant worsening of disease that may otherwise remain benign throughout life.[146,157,197] At present, there are few data to substantiate this allegation, and the weight of evidence is against it.

McAlpine and Compston[146] suggested a number of years ago that trauma could exacerbate MS. They believed that the frequency of relapses seen during a 3-month period after physical injury was significantly increased over other 3-month periods in the lives of patients with MS. They reported five cases in which MS relapses followed within 24 hours of injury. They drew attention to what they thought was a tendency for the location of the trauma to determine the anatomical localization of the initial neurological symptoms in their patients. They also suggested that injury to a certain area of the nervous system might precipitate a relapse confined to that area. Miller and Durh[157] subsequently reported on seven patients who developed significant neurological deterioration after injury. They acknowledged that these associations could be by chance and that the vast majority of injuries to patients with MS were not followed by relapses. However, it was still their belief that there was a significant association between trauma and episodes of activity in MS. Namerow[168] also suggested that trauma could exacerbate MS. McAlpine's text[148] also suggested that trauma could exacerbate MS activity. Poser[197] claimed that trauma can precipitate temporary and perhaps even permanent deterioration. He speculated that head trauma could cause focal disruption in the BBB, which, in turn, could result in a localized active lesion of MS. Kelly[112] reported that 14 patients subjected to thalamotomy all deteriorated afterwards. In addition, one pathological report showed new lesions of MS scattered along the needle tract after biopsy of MS lesions.[197]

The only prospective controlled studies of the possibility of a link between trauma and activity of MS have been done by Bamford and colleagues[14] and by Sibley and colleagues.[247] These authors have examined the effect of traumatic events on patients with MS and compared them with age- and sex-matched nonfamilial control subjects. They first did a retrospective analysis of previous events in which they found only two cases in which MS symptoms had started shortly after traumatic events. They then studied 137 patients in a prospective fashion, recording both traumatic events, relapses, and overall neurological status. They found no clear evidence that the onset of MS, relapses of MS, or chronic clinical deterioration

could be linked to physically or emotionally traumatic events.

Sibley and his colleagues[247] have published another paper describing their extended prospective experience with traumatic events in MS. They followed up 170 patients with MS and 130 normal control subjects for 8 years. There were 1407 instances of trauma. They found no significant correlation between all trauma and disease activity. Interestingly, a significantly low level of disease activity was seen in the 3-month period after surgical procedures and fractures. In addition, they found a significant association between electrical injury and relapse. No linkage was found between the frequency of trauma, the incidence of trauma, and the onset of progressive disability. They did, however, find that their patients had more than two times the control rate of trauma.

A different approach to this question was given by Siva and colleagues,[252] who showed no increased risk of MS in a large population of brain-injured individuals. Sibley's editorial that accompanied the Siva article[245] and Jellinek's editorial in *Lancet*[104] review the issues, pointing out that anecdotal evidence cannot suffice. Otherwise, the doctrine of *post hoc, ergo propter hoc* could be used to prove that virtually any environmental factor could exacerbate MS. An interesting set of letters to the editor[123b, 127a, 198a, 280] appears in the July 1994 issue of *Neurology*. It is clear from the discussion that some practitioners will grasp at any statistical possibility to justify linking trauma to worsening of MS. The authors worry that most of such linkage is to seek compensation and not to seek the truth.

In a recent review, Poser[198] proposed that disruption of the BBB was an obligatory prelude to any relapse of MS. He also proposed that the BBB changes that trigger relapses could be nonspecific in etiology. He argued that completely asymptomatic MS could be converted to symptomatic disease by an incident of trauma that disrupted the BBB.

Recent studies involving MRI study of MS have shown that disruption of the BBB is an early and perhaps even an obligatory change that occurs before the development of new lesions. The majority of these new lesions seen on serial MRI studies were located in the white matter of the cerebral hemispheres. Also, most investigators would interpret the BBB (gadolinium enhancement) findings as indicating that opening the BBB in early MS lesions is a vital and integral part of the specific MS process, not a nonspecific event produced by factors independent of the MS process.

Poser[198] cited experimental studies by Povlishock and colleagues[201] to support his claim that alterations in the BBB can occur after mild concussive trauma and that the BBB alterations can occur quite far displaced from the anatomical site of injury. The experiments by Povlishock and colleagues involved a protocol for studying the effects of rapidly increasing intracranial pressure (ICP) in experimental animals. Microscopic evidence for breakdown in the BBB was seen after modest abrupt changes in ICP, but the effects were limited to several localized areas of grey matter in the brain stem. In order for the experiments to be relevant to the MS issue, the BBB changes should be predominantly seen in the white matter, where the majority of MS lesions are seen. In addition, the BBB changes must also involve the cerebral hemispheres, where the majority of acute MS lesions are known to be preceded by BBB disruption. There is no mention of white matter being involved in the BBB changes seen by Povlishock and colleagues. The cerebral hemispheres were also not involved. Therefore, though interesting, Poser's reference to these studies seems to have no relevance to the problem of BBB disruption in MS.

There is no experimental or empirical reason to believe that the disruption of the BBB seen in MS is not a specific and intrinsic part of the MS process. The contention that minor trauma precipitates MS is very reminiscent of the claims that trauma caused cancer, a debate that transiently resulted in large plaintiff awards some decades ago. (This subject is entertainingly reviewed in Peter Huber's excellent monograph, *Galileo's Revenge: Junk Science in the Courtroom.*[99])

Also, no evidence has been found that lumbar puncture (LP) or myelography has any long-term effect on the clinical course of MS. However, some patients have complained that their symptoms were temporarily worse after either LP or myelography.

In summary, there is no evidence that the long-term clinical outcome of MS is influenced by any of the putative precipitating factors of stress and trauma. The entire issue has become clouded by the litigation factor that accompanies personal injury, especially in relation to motor vehicle accidents. Based on our experience, trauma or other stressful events do not influence the long-term outcome in MS unless there has been direct traumatic injury to the brain or spinal cord, and even then it is unclear whether the outcome of the MS process is accelerated. Large prospectively controlled studies (perhaps with MRI monitoring) are needed to examine the question of trauma as a precipitating factor for the onset of MS or for relapses.

In spite of the lack of proof of an association between relapses and stress, many neurologists counsel patients to organize their lives in such a way that stress is minimized, because it probably does influence symptoms if not outcome. A drawback to suggesting that stress provokes relapses is that some patients will become convinced that they are somehow to blame for their disease and any subsequent deterioration. This assumption of guilt can have a negative effect on their quality of life. In addition, if patients refrain from physical or mental activity because of fear of making their MS worse, they would be unnecessarily reducing the scope and variety of their activities.

Menstruation. Some patients report that their symptoms are worse during the premenstrual period. However, no consistent effect of menstruation on the long-term clinical course of MS has been demonstrated.

Chronic Progressive Forms of Multiple Sclerosis

About 15 percent of patients with MS begin with chronic progressive neurological dysfunction, and most patients with RRMS will eventually become chronic progressive (see Table 5–1). The time of development of chronic progression is highly correlated with age.[178] Once a chronic progressive course has begun, stabilization can certainly occur, but the typical patient then develops a slow, relentless progression of neurological impairment. The rate of progression can vary from time to time, and exacerbations can punctuate the clinical course in some patients. The clinical categories appropriate to chronic progressive deterioration follow.

SECONDARY PROGRESSIVE MULTIPLE SCLEROSIS (RELAPSING PROGRESSIVE MULTIPLE SCLEROSIS)

Secondary progressive multiple sclerosis (SPMS) or relapsing progressive multiple sclerosis (RPMS), is most commonly seen after 3 or more years of relapsing disease (Fig. 5–1). The figure shows the curves for age at onset in patients with RRMS and age at onset of the progressive phase for the University of British Columbia (UBC) clinic

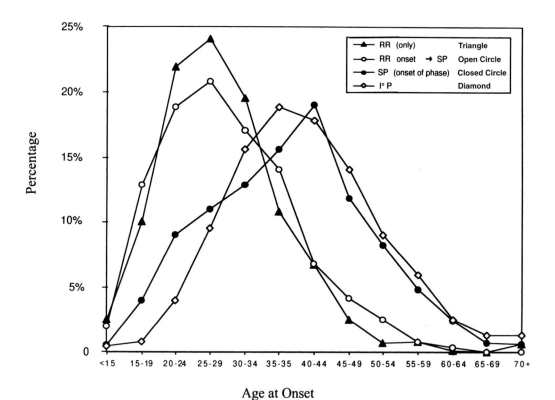

Age at Onset

Figure 5–1. These four curves display the onset time of the following phases of MS based on a cohort of patients from the MS Clinic at the University of British Columbia.

1. **Triangle (RR):** this is the age of onset curve for patients who were relapsing at onset and who remained **relapsing and remitting** (RR) after 10 years follow-up.
2. **Open Circle (SP):** this is the age of onset curve for patients who started as RR and converted in follow-up to **secondary progressive** (SP) (previously known as **Relapsing Progressive** [RP]).
3. **Closed Circle (SP Conversion):** this is the curve of the age of conversion from RR to a **progressive phase** of the patients (from #2 above) who started out as RR but after 10 year follow-up eventually became **progressive** (SP).
4. **Diamond (I°P):** this is the age of onset curve for patients who began as **primary progressive** (I°P). These patients have never had a relapse and were previously labelled **chronic progressive** (CP).

Note that the age for onset of the **progressive phase** of patients who eventually were categorized as secondary progressive is the same as for the primary progressive patients, suggesting that the age for starting the progressive aspect of the disease is the same regardless of whether there was a relapsing onset. Note also that the peak age of the SP conversion (closed circle) is about 8 years after the onset of the RR phase of SP (open circle), showing that the average duration of the relapsing phase is 8 years.

patients with CDMS. Patients begin with relapses and remissions and subsequently convert to a chronic progressive phase (with or without superimposed relapses). Some of these patients will stabilize or even temporarily improve, but the general tendency is towards deterioration. Conversion from a relapsing-remitting course to a chronic progressive course is an indicator of a poor prognosis (see Chapter 6).

PRIMARY PROGRESSIVE MULTIPLE SCLEROSIS (CHRONIC PROGRESSIVE MULTIPLE SCLEROSIS)

Primary progressive multiple sclerosis or chronic progressive multiple sclerosis (CPMS), is not as common as is the relapsing-remitting pattern. Many of these patients never have a relapse. They usually get worse at a somewhat steady rate. These patients experience little variability in clinical course, but they may reach a plateau. In addition, the patients that are steadily progressive from outset tend to be older and male. The prognosis for the accumulation of neurological deficit per year of disease in these older patients is not as good as for younger patients with RRMS.

Two recent reports suggest that primary CPMS is an entity distinct from RPMS. Olerup and his colleagues[180] found different major histocompatibility complex (MHC) associations in the two categories. Primary CPMS was associated with the DQB1 restriction fragment pattern seen in DR4, DQw8, DR7, DQw9, DRw8, and DQw4 haplotypes. Relapsing disease was associated with the DQB1 allelic pattern seen in the DRw17 and DQw2 haplotypes. In addition, Thompson and his colleagues[268] have reported major differences in the MRI pattern between CPMS and SPMS. The patients studied with primary CPMS had low levels of MRI activity with almost no gadolinium enhancement seen. In contrast, patients with RRMS and SPMS had many new and enhancing lesions that were larger than those seen in CPMS. Recently, Sharief and Hentges[240] reported that tumor necrosis factor-α (TNF-α) is elevated in the CSF of 53 percent of patients with CPMS.

TNF may turn out to be a marker for a primary chronic progressive clinical course, but confirmation is necessary. Claim has also been made toward serum antiganglioside antibodies being a marker for progressive disease.[163] An autopsy study has been reported[215a] which showed more similarities than differences between primary and secondary progressive disease. SPMS cases had more inflammation in the lesions than did primary progessive cases.

Many patients with CPMS from outset fall into monosymptomatic categories, such as chronic progressive myelopathy (CPM) or chronic cerebellar ataxia. Follow-up over time will frequently show that dissemination in space can eventually be detected. In the early stages of such monosymptomatic syndromes, however, such patients present difficult diagnostic problems. In these patients, paraclinical diagnostic tests are of most value (see Chapter 4).

The degree of severity seen in the chronic spinal and cerebellar types of MS probably reflects the "eloquence" of the spinal cord and cerebellum in producing clinical signs and symptoms. A few strategically placed active plaques can apparently produce severe disability without wide dissemination occurring in other areas of the nervous system.[294]

Sometimes patients with chronic spinal MS have a purely motor syndrome, especially in the early stages. Although asymmetry of findings is common, the overwhelming majority of chronic MS patients will eventually have a combination of both motor and sensory deficits. When an exclusive motor chronic progressive pyramidal disorder is seen, the physician must consider familial spastic paraparesis and primary lateral sclerosis, both of which tend to follow a relatively slow course.

Benign Multiple Sclerosis (a subcategory of RRMS)

Many patients with MS have a relatively benign clinical course (see Chapter 6). However, the total number of patients with benign disease is difficult to determine. Autopsy studies[81] have shown that undiagnosed MS can be present in the non-neurological autopsy population at a rate of approximately 1 per 500. An extrapolation from these findings to the general population suggests that undiagnosed MS exists at least at the same prevalence as does diagnosed disease (1 per 1000 in Canada). In a clinical and laboratory study of benign MS, Thompson and colleagues[267] found that younger-onset patients did best. They also found that sensory-onset patients tended to have a more benign course.

Unfortunately the clinician cannot reliably predict the development of benign disease based on initial signs and symptoms. In general, patients with benign MS tend to be women with a younger age of onset. They have relapsing-remitting disease and usually begin with sensory symptoms, including ON. McAlpine[145] drew attention to benign MS in 1961, but Bramwell in 1917[31] had identified several patients with benign disease, a state that he called "permanent arrest." McAlpine described his benign patients as "unrestricted." They made up 32 percent of his total series. His unrestricted patients usually started with ON or sensory or brain stem symptoms in a relapsing pattern with a low relapse rate.

D. Paty and K. Redekop (unpublished data; these data come from a Ph.D. thesis by K. Redekop at UBC 1995) studied patients with a duration of over 10 years, seen in the MS clinic at UBC. In their experience, 130 (24 percent) of the 536 patients who had MS for more than 10 years had an Extended Disability Status Scale score of 3 or less, which they consider relatively benign. The authors think that this clinic population is representative of the British Columbia MS population as a whole, although conclusions drawn from the observation of these patients will be flawed because of the loss of follow-up of patients with the most aggressive disease, who either died before 10 years elapsed or were confined to chronic care institutions and lost to the survey.

Koopmans and colleagues[120] did an MRI comparison of a group of 32 patients with benign disese and 32 disabled patients with SPMS matched for age, sex, and duration of disease. The burden of disease in the patients with SPMS was greater than in the patients with benign disease in 81 percent of the matched pairs. Considerable overlap in the extent of involvement was found between the two groups, but it is impressive that in 19 percent of the matched pairs, the extent of the MS as determined by the MRI scan was greater in the benign patients of the pairs. The most consistent MRI difference between the two groups was the high degree of periventricular confluence of lesions found in the patients with SPMS as compared with the patients with benign disease. In a serial MRI study of 10 patients with benign disease, Thompson and colleagues[267,269] found that the benign patients had less MRI activity and less gadolinium enhancement than a comparative early relapsing group.

Acute Malignant Multiple Sclerosis

A particularly tragic form of MS is that unusual case in which a young patient, often with a polysymptomatic onset, progresses rapidly to severe disability, death, or both within months (very rare) or a few years (uncommon).[108] Even this most malignant clinical course cannot be reliably predicted at outset. These rapidly progressive young patients are the ones that should be selected for the most aggressive trials of therapy. Fortunately, this very aggressive form of MS is not common. Therefore, controlled study of treatment in this population will require pooling of patients from many centers. (See Chapter 8 for a detailed discussion of acute malignant MS.)

The distinction between acute malignant MS and acute disseminated encephalomyelitis (ADEM) can be difficult. Progression, with the development of new lesions (clinical or MRI), beyond a period of 2 months is much more likely to be due to MS than to ADEM. In addition, in the adult, ADEM is much less common than MS, so that most patients with the acute malignant progression described will turn out to have MS.

Childhood Multiple Sclerosis

Childhood MS is rare (less than 4 percent of cases). In 1958 Gall[78] reported 40 cases found in the Mayo Clinic records with an onset before age 15 years. There were eight patients (six females and two males) with onset before 10 years of age. The symptoms and clinical course, however, resembled those seen in adults. Others have reported vertigo as a frequent initial symptom in childhood.[91] The youngest age of onset reported was 10 months.[242] Other very young cases reported began at age 24 months[20] and 4 years.[58]

Duquette and his colleagues[60] collected data on 125 patients whose MS started before the age of 16 from the combined experience of several Canadian MS clinics (total MS population 4623). This experience showed that childhood MS occurred in 2.7 percent of the total Canadian MS population. Childhood MS was more frequent in females (3:1 ratio), with a remitting sensory onset in most. They found a tendency towards slower clinical deterioration than that seen in adult-onset patients. As in adult patients, the family history was positive in 21 percent. Eighty-two percent had oligoclonal banding (OB) in the CSF. Perniola and associates[191] studied 14 cases of childhood MS. They also found that the youngest children had the best prognosis for impairment over time.

LESS COMMON CLINICAL PRESENTATIONS OF MULTIPLE SCLEROSIS

Despite the fact that most patients with MS will eventually become polysymptomatic and have multiple areas of the nervous system involved, a single anatomical localization or a single neurological system seems to be predominantly affected in several clinical subcategories. Subsequent pathological examination in such patients always shows that the lesions are much more widespread than would be suspected on the basis of clinical symptoms alone.[138,168] As noted previously, the mechanisms that determine which lesions will become or remain symptomatic is not known (see section on pathophysiology of demyelination, at the beginning of this chapter).

Progressive Spinal Multiple Sclerosis

A form of myelogram-negative or noncompressive CPM is a common clinical problem, particularly in older patients. Many of those patients have a chronic spinal form of MS in which it is impossible to satisfy the usual clinical criteria for dissemination in time and space. CPM is one of the clinical syndromes in which the use of paraclinical laboratory examinations such as EPs, MRI scanning, and CSF analysis is most helpful. Most of the chronic spinal MS cases have an older age of onset and tend to be male. Most CPM patients will have a combined motor and sensory deficit, but pure motor deficits can be seen. Familial cases also can occasionally be seen, producing confusion with familial spastic paraparesis. A study of 52 patients with CPM[188] has shown that MRI and spinal fluid analysis can identify laboratory supported definite MS (LSDMS) in about half of them. Of 52 patients, 41 (78 percent) had evidence for disseminated lesions on VEP or MRI examination, and 32 (62 percent) had OB. However, only 24 (48 percent) had both OB and evidence for lesions disseminated in space that would satisfy the criteria for LSDMS.

Cerebral Multiple Sclerosis

Even though neurologists expect cerebral involvement in patients who have severe and disabling disease, such manifestations are predominant in cerebral MS (see section following on cognitive and psychiatric changes). For example, the onset of dementia in a young patient must suggest MS as a diagnosis, particularly if metabolic causes and mass lesions have been excluded. Rarely personality change and impaired judgment can appear without other neurological symptoms and in the presence of otherwise preserved cognition. Also rarely, patients manifest an isolated but striking inability to form new memories (amnestic state). MRI will obviously play a major role in the evaluation of such patients.

Careful assessment of cognitive function in patients with neurologically nondisabling MS has shown that such deficits can occur frequently (approximately 50 percent).[192] Neurologists have tended to downplay this particular type of involvement in MS. Therefore, the neurological literature does not recognize early cognitive deficits in MS as readily as does the psychological or psychiatric literature.[193] It is also apparent that cognitive deficits, even very subtle ones, can have a major impact on employment.[126] Therefore, when symptomatic cognitive dysfunction develops in MS, the physician must recognize it and deal with it in a straightforward fashion. If the physician does not acknowledge that cognitive impairment is present when the patient and family know that it is a problem, strains on the doctor–patient relationship can develop. The patient and the family know that something serious is going wrong. To be told that the patient is neurotic or "acting out" only increases the frustration level of both the patient and the family. In this light, it is not surprising to see that many such patients lose confidence in their doctor and seek better understanding elsewhere.

Kahana and his colleagues[109] called attention to the perplexing problem of patients who exhibit primarily cerebral signs such as hemiparesis, hemianopsia, psychosis, dementia, and convulsions. They found that 101 of 295 patients (34 percent) had cerebral signs at some time during the disease. Six of their patients (2 percent) had dementia.

Chronic Cerebellar Multiple Sclerosis

The early onset of cerebellar dysfunction is usually a poor prognostic sign. Very small lesions in cerebellar pathways can cause major deficits. When progressive, cerebellar manifestations are one of the most disabling features of MS. Truncal ataxia is particularly disabling and unlikely to remit once it develops. The intention tremor described by Charcot in MS is usually secondary to involvement of the cerebellar outflow pathways (dentato-rubro-thalamic tract). The tremor can be so severe that it results in self-injury. Occasionally, the entire body will shake violently while the patient is awake. Cerebellar dysarthria can make speech unintelligible.

Chronic Visual Impairment in Multiple Sclerosis

The clinical presentation of MS as visual impairment is thoroughly explored in Chapter 7.

CLINICAL FINDINGS IN MULTIPLE SCLEROSIS

Table 5–9 lists clinical findings with their frequencies of occurrence as seen in the MS clinics at the Universities of British Columbia and the Western Ontario.

Depressed Level of Consciousness

Depressed level of consciousness is a rare finding in MS. The few instances in which the authors have seen it occur have been either in patients with an acute major brain stem relapse or in patients with acute widespread cerebral demyelination. All of the patients had serious accompanying neurological deficits with some combination of paraplegia, quadriplegia, or brain stem abnormalities. The mechanism for the depressed level of consciousness is probably the involvement of the reticular activating system or its connection with the cortex. Depressed level of consciousness in MS is so rare that when it occurs in a patient with MS it warrants a thorough search for other etiologies before MS is considered the cause.

Sleep Disturbances

Recent studies have shown that patients with MS are more likely than control subjects to have sleep disturbances.[46] The sleep problems may be due to nocturnal spasms

Table 5–9. CLINICAL FINDINGS IN MULTIPLE SCLEROSIS

Symptom or Finding	Percentage at Onset*	Percentage Anytime*	Comments
Hemispheric Functions			
Depression of level of consciousness	Rare	Rare	Depressed level of consciousness is usually associated with severe brain stem relapses.
Sleep disturbances	Rare	Common	
Cognitive changes	<5	70	Cognitive changes are much more common than previously thought; most are subtle, some severe.
Euphoria	<5	10–60	Euphoria is associated with dementia.
Focal cortical deficits	Rare	Unusual	Occasionally stroke-like syndromes can be seen.
Psychiatric disease			
Psychosis	Unusual	Unusual	Psychosis is usually related to drugs.
Depression	<5	25–54	Many can be effectively treated.
Bipolar disease	<5	13–40	There is a possible genetic link.
Seizures	<5	5	Half are probably due to MS.
Headache	<10	30	There is no clear-cut link with MS.
Fatigue	20	80	Fatigue can be very disabling
Brain Stem and Visual Functions			
Horner's syndrome	Rare	<2	Autonomic fibers are not myelinated.
Pupillary defects	16	common	See text.
Visual loss			
Optic neuritis	16	65	Most recover spontaneously; symptoms can be subtle.
Optic atrophy	Uncommon	77	Optic atrophy can be present with normal visual function.
Legal blindness	Rare	<10	
Retinal perivenous sheathing	Unknown	20	Why should inflammation be present in the retina where there is no myelin?
Retinal nerve fiber loss	Unknown	80	The retina is the only place in which the axons can be seen and loss directly visualized. The time course of this phenomenon is unknown.

Continued on following page

155

Table 5–9.—*continued*

Symptom or Finding	Percentage at Onset*	Percentage Anytime*	Comments
Diplopia—3rd Nerve	Rare	Rare	
—4th Nerve	Rare	Rare	
—6th Nerve	3	10	
—Internuclear ophthalmoplegia	17	30	This condition is usually bilateral; some patients have mixed brain stem syndromes.
Parinaud's syndrome	Rare	Rare	We have seen two cases due to MS.
Primary position nystagmus	Rare	5	This form of nystagmus can be vertical, horizontal, or circular.
Nystagmus	20	85	Ataxic nystagmus is the most specific to MS.
Facial palsy	<2	4–16	Facial palsy is usually transient.
Trigeminal sensory decrease	3	10	
Trigeminal neuralgia	5	10–30	Patients usually do not have decreased sensation.
Deafness	<2	5–17	Deafness is usually transient; poor discrimination is common.
Vertigo	4–14	5–50	Vertigo can mimic peripheral vertigo.
Dysphagia	2	10	Dysphagia is usually associated with dysarthria and poor control of lips, tongue, pharynx, and/or larynx.
Dysarthria	2	50	Dysarthria can be cerebellar and/or spastic.
Paroxysmal dysarthria	<2	<5	
Cerebellar or Basal Ganglia Function			
Tremor			
Action	<2	10	
Intention	<5	50	Intention tremor is a major disabling feature.
Titubation	<2	20	
Ataxia of gait and trunk	18	50–80	
Movement disorder	Unusual	<5	
Spinal Cord Function			
Sensory loss	30–50	90	Sensory loss is rarely persistent; it can be seen in acute relapse, even suspended and disassociated type.
Sensory level	<10	<10	
Lower limbs—post col	30	85	
Upper limbs—post col	10	30	
Lower limbs—pain and temp	<5	30	Sensory loss at this level is usually patchy.
Upper limbs—pain and temp	<5	10	Sensory loss at this level is usually patchy.

Continued on following page

Table 5–9.—*continued*

Symptom or Finding	Percentage at Onset*	Percentage Anytime*	Comments
Useless hand syndrome	2	5	
Lhermitte's phenomenon	3	30	Lhermitte's phenomenon can fluctuate in intensity and resolve for long periods.
Paroxysmal sensory	Unusual	20	When hemicorporeal in distribution, mimics transient ischemia.
Paroxysmal motor	Unusual	15	
Pain (neurogenic)	<5	40	Neurogenic pain can be the major disabling feature. See Tables 5–10 and 5–11.
Radicular	2	10	See Tables 5–10 and 5–11.
Diffuse	2	20	See Tables 5–10 and 5–11.
Increased deep tendon reflexes	20	90	
Lost deep tendon reflexes	<2	5–10	Single lost reflexes are not unusual, but inverted reflex patterns are more common.
Weakness			
Legs	10	90	Legs rarely can be flaccid.
Arms	5	22	Arm weakness can be asymmetrical.
Hemiplegia	2	9	
Spasticity	10	90	Spasticity can be a major problem in nursing care.
Spasms, extensor or flexor	<5	50	Paraplegia in flexion a particularly difficult problem.
Cramps	<5	50	Vague symptom, probably related to spasticity.
Amyotrophy	<2	50	Amyotrophy can be due to compression or entrapment at root or peripheral nerve or secondary to central axon loss.
Peripheral neuropathy	Rare	Probably more common than currently acknowledged.	Recent MRI studies have shown CNS lesions in several inflammatory PNS diseases.
Autonomic Functions			
Bladder disturbance	3–10	80	Patients may require specialist's evaluation.
Urgency		80	Urgency usually means small bladder.
Frequency		80	Frequency can mean small or large bladder.
Hesitancy		20	Hesitancy is due to dyssynergia.

Continued on following page

Table 5–9.—*continued*

Symptom or Finding	Percentage at Onset*	Percentage Anytime*	Comments
Incontinence		50	Incontinence can be due to spastic overflow.
Nocturia		80	
Mixed		60	Mixed bladder disturbance is due to dyssynergia.
Bowel disturbance			
Constipation	20	70	Constipation can vary over time; it is more common in females.
Incontinence	Rare	20–50	Exclude impaction.
Mixed		10	
Sexual disturbance	<2	Female: 50	Female patients rarely complain spontaneously.
		Male: 75	
Decreased sensation		25	Decreased sensation is usually seen in spinal form.
Decreased libido		40	
Male—poor erection		63	
—poor ejaculation		37	
Female—decreased lubrication (occasionally painful)		21	
Others:			
Cardiac	Rare	?	
Sweating	Rare	?	
Blood pressure	Rare	?	
Hypothermia	Rare	Rare	
Neurogenic pulmonary edema	Rare	Very rare	
Miscellaneous Functions			
Other syndromes	Rare	Rare	See text.
Charcot's triad (nystagmus, ataxia, and scanning speech)	Rare	<10	Charcot's triad is no longer considered typical of MS.

Sources: These data are a composite from the University of British Columbia and University of Western Ontario MS clinics' experience and are adapted from Poser S,[199] and Studney D, et al,[261] pp 145–152.

*Percentages are approximate.

CNS = central nervous system; MRI = magnetic resonance imaging; PNS = peripheral nervous system; post col = posterior column; temp = temperature.

and may also be a major factor for some patients in the fatigue that is so common in MS. Ferini-Strambi and colleagues[67] used 8-hour polysomnography to study 25 patients with CDMS who had no mood disorder and were drug-free. They found the patients with MS to have poor sleep efficiency, awakening frequently during sleep. Periodic leg movements were probably a factor, being seen in nine (36 percent) of the patients (8 percent in control subjects). Poirier and colleagues[194] studied 70 patients with MS and found that narcoleptic symptoms were common.

Cognitive and Psychiatric Changes

Recent studies in both Europe and North America have shown that minor defects in cognition are quite common (up to 70 percent), even in early MS (up to 50 percent).[119,208] It has long been recognized that dementia can be an accompaniment of severe disabling MS of long-term duration. However, the more recent recognition that cognitive defects can be seen in the early stages of MS has stimulated more activity in the investigation of this phenomenon. This research area has been thoroughly reviewed in a number of papers[85,86,105,192,209,211] and addressed briefly in a recent editorial.[219] MRI has helped considerably in the assessment of these patients. Recent studies have shown that lesions seen in the corpus callosum on MRI scan are not only helpful in diagnosis but are also well correlated with cognitive defects.[203] Pozzilli and colleagues[202] have compared single-photon emission computed tomography (SPECT), MRI, and cognitive functions in 17 patients with CDMS. Periventricular lesions and the width of the third ventricle were the most frequent MRI correlates with cognitive deficits. The SPECT changes were most likely to be seen in the frontal lobes (left greater than right).

Euphoria is always a manifestation of subtle or obvious cognitive change.[192] In spite of the fact that cognitive abnormalities appear to be common in MS, focal "cortical" deficits such as aphasia, apraxia, and agnosia are uncommon, although oc-

casionally such defects have been reported.[2,9a,53,84] Subtle language disorders may predict cognitive impairments.[123a] At least one study[264] has found some correlations between regional cerebral involvement and specific neuropsychological deficits. The most frequent cognitive abnormalities in MS are subtle defects in abstraction, and memory,* attention and word finding,[161] are usually associated with emotional lability and decreased speed of information processing. Not all investigators agree.[218,219] Ron and her colleagues found that patients with single lesion clinical syndromes suspected to be MS had significant cognitive abnormalities, but not as frequently as did the patients with CDMS. Boné and colleagues[26] have also reported good correlation between cognitive changes and the severity of abnormalities on the MRI scan. Feinstein and colleagues[66] reported on a serial psychometric study monitored by MRI in which they found correlation between clinical and MRI changes over time. Pozzilli and associates[202,204] reported that defects in the anterior portion of the corpus callosum seen on MRI were well correlated with verbal fluency abnormalities. Arnett and colleagues[9] showed that frontal lesions on MRI were associated with conceptional reasoning deficits. Amato and colleagues[3] found that verbal memory and abstract reasoning remained stable over 4 years, but new deficits appeared. Kujala and colleagues[123] looked at information processing in detail. Huber[100] found MRI lesion load to correlate with neuropsychological abnormalities.

Traditional tests for dementia designed for use in neuronal degenerative diseases such as Alzheimer's disease are not sensitive to the changes seen in MS.[140] For example, most patients with MS have normal scores on the Mini-Mental State Examination, but appropriate neuropsychological tests can show that significant cognitive deficits do indeed exist.[236] The most sensitive bedside measures for cognitive defects in MS have been tests such as repetition of seven numbers forward and backward, serial sevens or serial threes, and visual recog-

---

*References 19, 29, 30, 39, 134, 135, 185, 210.

nition tests.[134,135] Peyser and colleagues[193] proposed guidelines for neuropsychological testing in MS, hoping to bring some uniformity into the methods of assessment. The concept of uniformity becomes important because neuropsychological testing may become an important aspect of monitoring clinical trials. In addition, Newton and colleagues[173] looked at the cognitive event–related EPs in MS and found very frequent abnormalities that correlated with the cerebral lesion load by MRI, degree of disability, and duration of disease. Ruchkin and colleagues[223] studied event-related brain potential in 10 patients with MS and found that verbal working memory is especially susceptible to impairment in MS. They proposed that this deficit could be due to impairment in the phonological loop important for the retention of verbal information in working memory. Rao and his colleagues[210] and others[29,192] have pointed out that the cognitive aspects of MS are the most likely to determine work status and other quality of life features.

Recent surveys have also shown that mood disorders are frequent in patients with MS. An association may exist between MS and manic-depressive disease (bipolar disorder).[107,215,232,236] A recent survey in the UBC MS Clinic shows that 38 percent of patients with MS have been depressed or could suffer from bipolar disorder.[215] Other forms of psychosis are rare but can be seen. Reactive depression is common, and hypomania sometimes occurs. The fact that some patients respond to steroid therapy with hypomanic behavior could be an indication of an underlying predisposition toward manic-depressive disease (bipolar disorder). Mitchell and colleagues[161] looked at mood state and MRI findings in 40 CDMS patients. They found some lobar correlates with mood disorders, particularly frontal lobe ones. Swirsky-Saccheti and associates[264] also found similar lobar correlates. Moller and colleagues[162] found some correlations between depressive mood disorders and cognitive impairment. A mixed mood (depression and euphoria) may also carry a poor prognosis. Boyle and her colleagues[29] found that the coping strategies of patients with MS could be categorized according to one of four labels: "depression,"

"denial," "exaggerated somatic," and "severity related."

Fatigue

Fatigue (see Chapter 12), a frequent and disabling feature of MS,[72,231] can be divided into two types as follows:

1. Fatigability: A single muscle or group of muscles becomes weaker after repetitive use and recovers after rest. This type of muscle fatigue resembles that of myasthenia gravis (MG). It is akin to Uhthoff's phenomenon, which occurs with increased body temperature.

2. Lassitude: In this form of fatigue, the patients have a persistent sense of tiredness. Sleep may make a difference in some patients, but many find that even extensive sleep does not restore well-being. This type of fatigue is commonly seen during neurological exacerbations. We have also seen it occur in patients without any change in neurological symptoms, but with new large MRI lesions.

Each form of fatigue may be an indicator of disease activity in MS. Fatigue can be a manifestation of depression, but studies have shown that fatigue in MS is unrelated to the degree of neurological impairment[72,122] and that it has a negative impact on mental health and general health status. However, there are many patients with MS and severe fatigue who are not depressed.[231] Coyle and her colleagues[49] have measured immune activation markers in MS patients with severe fatigue and found elevated levels of several markers suggesting that fatigue could be a clinical marker for immune activation in MS. Fatigue has also been found to be associated with poor nocturnal sleep. De Castro[55] found that all patients with MS and fatigue had alterations of immune status, mood, or neurological function. The measurement of fatigue remains difficult.[278a]

Seizures

Convulsive seizures occur in about 5 percent of patients. Half of the seizures are probably due to the MS lesion itself, and the other half due to chance association. When convulsive seizures occur in MS, they are usually easily controlled with anticonvulsants. However, anticonvulsant therapy is usually required indefinitely. Several instances of recurrent convulsions after withdrawal of anticonvulsant medication have been seen.[93] The other paroxysmal symptoms associated with MS are described later on. Spinal seizures are also seen.[63] Truyen and colleagues[271] found that patients with seizures had a tendency to have more subcortical or temporal lobe lesions or both than did control MS patients without seizures.

Headache

Patients with MS frequently complain of headaches.[217] Occasionally acute headache can occur in the pseudotumor acute-onset type of relapse. Some of these patients have CT or MRI evidence of a mass lesion that suggests tumor. One type of headache, seen occasionally in MS, is that of hemicranial headache, sometimes in association with an acute pontine lesion (D. Paty and G. C. Ebers, personal observations 1980). It can be associated with any or all of the following findings: (1) ipsilateral INO, (2) acute sixth or seventh nerve palsy, or (3) an acute ataxic syndrome. Whether or not this headache results from the interruption of pathways to and from brain stem neurons that have dihydroergotamine receptors is unknown. However, in our experience, most patients with MS and headache do not have evidence of cerebral edema.

The headache of ON has a typical pattern characterized by increased intensity of pain due to movement of the eye[150] (See Chapter 7). Most patients with MS who suffer from headache probably have tension headaches due to muscle spasm in the neck and the scalp muscles or migraine, or are depressed.

VISUAL FINDINGS (See Chapter 7)

Pupillary Defects

Pupillary abnormalities are frequent in MS. Most are related to the afferent pupillary defect (APD) (Marcus Gunn pupil). One very sensitive way of showing APD is to examine the patient in dim light with an ophthalmoscope; the pupillary reaction is revealed by the rate of reflex observed through the ophthalmoscope lens. In this way, the red reflex observed with magnification, reveals a precise margin to the pupil. In this instance, especially in patients with a dark iris, the fact that the consensual response is greater than the direct light response can be easily shown. In contrast, fixed dilated pupils associated with or independent from other elements of a third nerve palsy are extremely rare. (We have not observed fixed dilated pupils, although we have seen several patients with coexistent Adie's pupil.) Central Horner's syndrome is occasionally seen.[15] The rarity of efferent pupillary deficits probably reflects the fact that autonomic fibers in the CNS are thinly myelinated or not myelinated at all.

Loss of Vision

Acute loss of vision due to ON is a common feature of MS. Many patients recover functionally normal vision after ON, even in the face of severe residual optic atrophy.[182,241,253] Visual field deficits in MS tend to be central, but occasionally the clinician can encounter paracentral or peripheral scotomata or quadrantopic and hemianopic defects. Homonymous hemianopsias can occur in MS but are unusual; when seen, they should raise the possibility of coexistent tumor or vascular disease. Fortunately legal blindness in MS is unusual[79] (less than 5 percent). When it does occur, numerous low vision aids are available. In addition to loss of vision, many patients with MS have loss of fibers in the retinal nerve fiber layer,[64,139] suggesting death of retinal ganglion cells. Why such proximal axonal loss should occur is not apparent, except to suggest that there are retrograde detrimental effects on the nerve bodies, secondary to demyelination of the axon, or that retinal changes associated with perivenous sheathing[68] are functionally important.

Many patients experience a dimming or obscuring of vision associated with exercise and heat. This symptom was first described by Uhthoff.[274]

Gross nonscotoma visual field deficits are uncommonly seen, but subtle ones can occur. Recent MRI studies[74] have shown that there are lesions in the occipital lobes and other appropriate locations in patients who have vague visual symptoms. Chiasmatic lesions can also occur, suggesting pituitary or suprachiasmatic masses compressing the crossing fibers in the chiasm. Pain is usually seen as an accompaniment to acute ON[129] and may be due to traction of the origins of the superior and medial recti on the optic nerve sheath.

Eye Movement Disorders (Quality of Movement)

The most frequently encountered eye movement disorder in MS is that of impaired smooth pursuit (saccadic pursuit). Often saccadic pursuit is prominent in the absence of any paresis of gaze or nystagmus, and its presence probably reflects involvement of the medial longitudinal fasciculus (MLF), the cerebellum, or cerebellar outflow pathways. However, in spite of its frequency in MS, the finding of saccadic pursuit must be used with caution as a sign of focal disease, because it is readily produced by a variety of drugs, including benzodiazepines, anticonvulsants, and other hypnotics.

Third and Fourth Nerve Palsy

Third and fourth nerve palsies are extremely rare.[77,172,275,276] Lack of adduction is common in MS as part of an internuclear ophthalmoplegia (INO), but third nerve palsy involving paresis of elevation, and depression along with ptosis and pupillary dilitation is distinctly unusual. Fourth nerve palsies are similarly rare. Even though reported in the literature, we have not seen either as an isolated finding.

Sixth Nerve Palsy

Sixth nerve palsies are relatively unusual when compared with the frequency of INO, but are not rare. They are usually unilateral except when seen in association with horizontal gaze palsies, INO, or both, but we have seen bilateral cases. One and one-half syndromes are not uncommon (e.g., a unilateral INO and ipsilateral sixth nerve palsy resulting in ipsilateral loss of adduction and abduction with preserved elevation and depression along with contralateral ataxic nystagmus). It is relatively rare for paresis of abduction or a gaze palsy to be total and persistent, but we have seen a few examples.

Internuclear Ophthalmoplegia and Nystagmus

Internuclear ophthalmoplegia is common in MS. It occurs in as many as 17 percent of patients at outset and at least double that number during the course of the disease. If findings such as saccadic pursuit, slow adduction, and abduction eye nystagmus can be taken as subtle manifestations of INO, it occurs in more than 60 percent of patients.

The lesion that produces INO is in the medial longitudinal fasciculus (MLF). When an INO occurs in MS it tends to be bilateral. This fact probably reflects the anatomical proximity of the two MLF tracts and the fact that MS lesions do not respect the midline. The fully developed INO is manifested by ipsilateral paralysis of adduction, and contralateral irregular nystagmus of inconstant amplitude and rhythm in the abducting eye. This particular form of nystagmus has been referred to as *ataxic* because of the ataxic features, which include irregularity in rate, rhythm, and amplitude of the movements suggesting cerebellar involvement. Another descriptive name for the nystagmus is "jellylike," again reflecting the same irregular features.

Other forms of nystagmus are frequently seen. Patients with a combination of severe visual loss and cerebellar deficits frequently develop a pendular type of nystagmus in the primary position that may be unique to MS. When attempting fixation or resting, these patients have pendular nystagmus in which the central axis of the eye describes a circular or elliptical path with the long axis either vertical or horizontal. The movements closely resemble the postural tremor seen in the extremities with severe involvement of cerebellar outflow pathways. They may occasionally be unilateral. The degree of visual impairment due to optic nerve disease is difficult to determine when this kind of nystagmus is present because of the constant movement. In the authors' opinion, the nystagmus is secondary to impaired fixation due to optic nerve disease combined with cerebellar deficits that interfere with the control of movement. However, we have on at least one occasion seen this kind of acquired pendular nystagmus in the presence of normal visual acuity.

Nystagmus can be convergence-induced. Also, a syndrome of periodic alternating nystagmus (PAN) can be seen. We have recognized PAN in only three or four cases. We have also seen two cases of Parinaud's ophthalmoplegia syndrome due to MS.

Retinal Perivenous Sheathing and Loss of Nerve Fiber Layer of the Retina

Retinal perivenous sheathing occurs in as few as 5 percent of patients with MS and in as many as 30 percent.[68, 131,224] Casual direct ophthalmoscopic examination is not likely to detect it. Inspection through a widely dilated pupil with the indirect ophthalmoscope is usually necessary to see the subtle manifestations in the retina. The pathological process is characterized by infiltration with lymphocytes and plasma cells. Exactly what stimulates the cellular infiltration is unclear. It is worth noting that myelin and myelin antigens are not present in the retina (see Chapter 7 for a more complete description), raising nontrivial questions about specificity of the immune response in MS.

Sharpe and Sanders[241] described loss of the nerve fiber layer of the retina in patients with MS. New techniques allow precise measurement of this phenomenon.[139] The retina is the only place where CNS axons can be observed, and the study of this phenomenon will be important for the future understanding of axonal loss in MS.

OTHER CRANIAL NERVE AND BRAIN STEM FINDINGS

Anosmia

Anosmia is not a common complaint in patients with MS. Nonetheless, careful evaluation will reveal some degree of loss of smell in a number of patients.[8]

Loss of Taste

Unilateral or bilateral loss of taste is infrequent. Paty and Ebers have observed several examples, and in one patient, it was the sole presenting complaint. The symptom has always remitted. Surveys of taste and smell in MS have been reported.[8,44] Although smell is usually normal, taste is slightly reduced, especially in older patients. Kurtzke found that only 1.3 percent of 525 men with MS had decreased taste.[124]

Facial Palsy

The acute development of a peripheral facial nerve palsy (Bell's palsy) is an uncommon but recognized feature of MS. It occurs in less than 4 percent of patients and almost always recovers spontaneously and completely. Recovery from an MS-associated facial palsy is usually not associated with autonomic abnormalities such as crocodile tears; however, aberrant renervation, myokymia, and the phenomenon of intrafacial synkinesis are all commonly seen. Sometimes the acute facial palsies are accompanied by other brain stem findings, such as a sixth nerve palsy, lateral gaze palsy, or deafness. Facial myokymia was first reported by Andermann and colleagues.[4] Paty and Ebers have seen one case with remitting bilateral facial myokymia that was disabling because the patient could not open his eyes. The symptom responded to carbamazepine therapy.

Trigeminal Motor and Sensory Symptoms

Sensory loss in the face can occur in as many as 10 percent of patients, but its persistence is unusual. When trigeminal neuralgia (TN) occurs in MS (see description of paroxysmal symptoms), it usually occurs in the absence of objective evidence of trigeminal nerve sensory loss. Trismus has also been reported.[54]

Deafness

The otolaryngologic features of MS have been reviewed.[28] Central lesions resulting in impaired hearing commonly occur,[175] but persistent complete deafness is unusual in the absence of another etiology. The clinicopathological correlation is unclear. When deafness does occur, it is usually unilateral and is seen in patients who also have instability of gait, double vision, or vertigo in the setting of an acute brain stem relapse.[70,76] Patients often complain of poor auditory discrimination.[206] This problem may be due to defects in central processing of frequency changes.[175] At least one MRI study has shown eighth nerve root entry zone lesions in a patient with bilateral sequential temporary deafness,[17] and we have seen "cortical deafness" in one patient with bilateral acute temporal lobe lesions.

Vertigo

Vertigo is a relatively common symptom. As many as 50 percent of patients have intermittent episodes of vertigo. Vertigo may occur as the initial symptom, although it is also a common enough symptom in the non-MS population that the coincidental occurrence of an episode of non-MS vertigo might be seen in some patients. Herrera[91] has reviewed the subject of vestibular and other balance disorders in MS.

In a review of initial symptoms in MS done by Paty and Ebers, it was found that onset with vertigo was a symptom that favored a long-term, more benign outcome. Vertigo at onset has also been suggested as an indicator of a more benign prognosis in children.[60] A possible interpretation of this finding is that some patients had a coincidental remote episode of vertigo that was incorrectly thought to be the initial symptom of MS.

Dysphagia

Mild dysphagia is common. It usually coexists with dysarthria, often in the setting of pseudobulbar palsy. In this instance, the dysphagia is a manifestation of bilateral involvement of upper motor neuron pathways leading to a desynchronization of the swallowing mechanism.

Dysphagia may also be associated with pharyngeal sensory loss. Such patients have reduced sensation to touch and pinprick in the posterior pharynx and may have lost their gag reflex. Pseudobulbar palsy, along with loss of pharyngeal sensation and gag reflex, and cerebellar disease can singularly or in combination lead to recurrent dysphagia and aspiration.

Dysarthria

Dysarthria of the cerebellar type with scanning speech is part of the Charcot triad. Scanning speech is characterized by monotonous speech interspersed with explosive consonants resulting in irregular volume and indistinct articulation.

Many patients with cerebellar involvement not only develop elements of scanning speech but also develop an intention tremor of the voice. The voice tremor can be demonstrated by having the patient sustain a vowel sound for 10 to 15 seconds. Under such circumstances, the variation in intensity and sometimes pitch of the sound is easily heard. This variation oscillates at a frequency of about 5 to 7 Hz, similar to the oscillation frequency seen in the cerebellar intention tremor.

Patients may show elements of combined cerebellar and pseudobulbar (spastic) dysarthria. Some patients have only spastic speech. Pseudobulbar dysarthria is caused by spastic vocal cords, which result in a high-pitched, low-volume speech in which consonants are slurred. These patients do not have the oscillating tremor or the explosive variability associated with cerebellar speech.

Paroxysmal dysarthria can be either spastic or scanning in nature. It is characterized by short duration and stereotyped recurrence (see following). Paroxysmal dysarthria is to be distinguished from the dysarthria that occurs with fatigue. Some patients with MS develop dysarthria after several minutes of sustained speech. This effort-induced symptom tends to recover after a few minutes of rest. When present, it can suggest myasthenia gravis (MG). In one patient, marked dysarthria was reliably precipitated by physical exercise.

Breathing Disturbance

Some patients find themselves with a peculiar kind of air hunger. Even though lung function seems to be normal, they develop oxygen debt easily after exercise. Some patients get tachycardia as well, suggesting an autonomic abnormality (see section on autonomic disturbances following). Serious respiratory problems, other than pneumonia and bronchitis, are uncommon. Howard and his colleagues[98] reported on 19 patients who developed respiratory complications an average of 5.9 years after onset. Twelve required mechanical ventilatory support, five of whom recovered. Six died after an average of 17.7 months.

SPINAL CORD AND MOTOR FINDINGS

Sensory Loss

Sensory loss is the most frequent of all neurological findings in MS. It is present in 90 percent of patients at some time during the clinical course. The distribution of sensory loss between upper and lower extremities can vary. In addition, isolated transient facial numbness is frequently seen. Unremitting unilateral facial numbness is more likely due to isolated trigeminal neuropathy, as seen in collagen vascular diseases, or schwannoma of the trigeminal nerve. It is also unusual for a sensory segmental level of pain or temperature loss to persist, even in advanced cases. However, during acute exacerbations, a sensory level can be seen in 10 to 15 percent of patients. Persistent changes in touch sensation are also unusual early in the disease. When per-

sistent abnormalities in touch, pain, and temperature sensation do occur, the pattern of loss is likely to be a patchy one. Therefore, it is usually not efficient to spend much time in a detailed examination of crude sensations (pain, temperature, and touch) in patients with MS.

In contrast, posterior column or discriminatory sensation testing can be very useful. Eighty-five to 95 percent of patients with MS will have an abnormality in posterior column sensation at some time during their clinical course. The predominant sensory loss in this sphere is detected by vibratory testing, joint position sense testing, two-point discrimination, or directional touch localization. Occasionally any of these functions can be impaired in isolation. The sensation loss is often prominent in the lower extremities, but bilateral predominant upper extremity impairment is common. Predominant involvement in the arms with relative sparing of the legs probably represents bilateral and symmetrical lesions in the lateral portions of the cuneate fasciculi in the high cervical cord.

The useless hand syndrome is a particularly interesting sensory manifestation, usually seen in patients with predominant upper extremity proprioceptive loss[181] (see Chapter 4). Even though the useless hand syndrome can occur in other disorders, it is highly characteristic of MS. It is common to see young adults with MS develop lack of discriminatory sensation in one upper extremity to the extent that the extremity becomes functionally useless in spite of normal crude sensation, motor, and cerebellar function. The useless hand syndrome in MS usually resolves spontaneously, although it can be extremely disabling while present. It usually begins with either tingling or lack of fine sensory discrimination in the fingers. The patient usually notices an inability to recognize objects in the pocket or purse. The patient can then develop impairment of hand function because of the inability to distinguish various subtleties in tactile sensation, and lack of feedback control of movement.

The useless hand syndrome is typically accompanied by pseudoathetosis, a situation in which the hand cannot be maintained in a steady position with the eyes closed. The lack of proprioceptive sense, even to a subtle degree, will result in or exacerbate spontaneous movement of the hands when visual feedback is removed. At its most severe, pseudoathetosis can mimic a movement disorder reminiscent of drug-induced dyskinesia.

Lhermitte's Symptom

Lhermitte's symptom is the occurrence of tingling and "electric current–like" sensation in the arms, down the back, into the legs, or in all three areas, associated with forward flexion of the neck.[10,130] This symptom occurs in 3 percent of patients at the onset of the disease and probably occurs in 30 to 40 percent of patients overall at sometime during the clinical course. It is most frequently associated with MS, although it is not specific to this disease. Symptoms are usually precipitated by forward flexion of the neck but can also be brought on by forward flexion of the spine, or even other minor movements. The symptoms can, in some instances, occur spontaneously. In unusual circumstances, Lhermitte's symptom, usually because of its frequency, duration, or intensity, can be disabling in the absence of other significant neurological deficits. Such disabling symptoms will usually respond somewhat to carbamazepine or benzodiazepine therapy.

Paroxysmal Symptoms

Careful interviews with patients with MS will frequently identify brief symptoms of a paroxysmal nature. If these paroxysmal symptoms are the only ones present, the situation can be confusing and transient cerebral ischemia, neuralgia, or hysteria might be considered as the cause. Transient symptoms such as hemiparesis, positive or negative sensory phenomena, or dysarthria are not well recognized by non-neurologists as features of MS.

In 1955, McAlpine[147] first drew attention to paroxysmal symptoms as being characteristic of MS. Subsequently, in his textbook,[146] he enlarged on the concept and subdivided short-lived attacks into two groups. The first group consisted of truly paroxysmal symptoms, unassociated with other factors. The second group of transient symptoms were those brought on by other illnesses and exogenous factors such as increased temperature (pseudorelapses). Andermann and his colleagues[5] reported several cases of paroxysmal dysarthria in 1959. Subsequently, a number of other paroxysmal symptoms have been clearly identified, such as ataxia, vertigo, painful and disturbing paresthesia, dysesthesias, monocular blindness, pain and weakness. Paroxysmal motor phenomena include not only weakness, but also spasticity and spasms, tonic seizures, akinesia, diplopia, dysarthria, and chorea in addition to focal and generalized seizures.[93,96]

Paroxysmal symptoms in MS characteristically have an abrupt onset, short duration, and a tendency to stop spontaneously. They can recur up to 50 times per day or more. The true prevalence of paroxysmal symptoms in MS is unknown, but they are seen frequently. Our experience has been that the more frequently one specifically inquires about such symptoms, the more frequently they are found. Because paroxysmal symptoms in MS are usually benign and self-limiting, many times they are not reported spontaneously. In contrast, in some patients, paroxysmal symptoms can be very frightening, disabling, or both. Disabling paroxysmal symptoms usually involve an overwhelming sensation of tingling, numbness, or weakness coursing through the body. The episode can climax in a brief period of akinesia. If the symptom happens frequently, it is understandable that it could be disabling, in the same way that transient ischemic attacks or focal seizures can be disabling. Fortunately paroxysmal symptoms in MS respond well to benzodiazepines or anticonvulsants. In addition, because they tend to be self-limited, prolonged therapy is usually unnecessary. The underlying pathophysiological mechanism is unknown. There is reason to believe that ephaptic transmission[149] across fiber tracts could be responsible. Ephaptic transmission is known to occur in areas of extensive demyelination. Perhaps there are changes in the microenvironment of these demyelinated nerve fibers that produce spontaneous electrical discharges that in turn result in such dramatic paroxysmal motor or sensory episodes.

The best known of these paroxysmal disturbances is the painful tonic spasm (PTS). PTS is usually manifested by tonic flexion or extension of a limb with a writhing movement reminiscent of paroxysmal athetosis.[243] The tension in the muscles of the limb is so great that it becomes quite painful. Luckily the episodes are usually transient, and as in other paroxysmal episodes, they usually respond to therapy. A particularly difficult situation can be due to the paroxysmal loss of neurological function, as in paroxysmal monoparesis or hemiparesis or paroxysmal blindness. At the outset of MS, these symptoms are usually most perplexing (see Chapter 4). When paroxysmal symptoms occur in a patient with well-established disease, even though they can be frustrating, they usually do not produce major problems with added disability or emotional tension. Certainly the onset of paroxysmal symptoms implies a physiological change, perhaps brought on by more extensive pathology. In spite of that likelihood, in the authors' experience, the onset of paroxysmal symptoms has not usually been associated with other objective evidence of exacerbation.[96]

There have been two reports[130a,141] of tonic spasms occurring during acute relapses with MRI correlation in the internal capsule and cerebral peduncle. These findings suggest that the spasms occurred because of new inflammatory lesions that then resolved. Paroxysmal itching has also been described.[183]

Pain

Moulin[164] has reviewed pain in MS (Table 5–10 on page 168 and Table 5–11). There are two major categories of pain: paroxysmal (such as TN) and chronic. The frequency of MS-associated pain has been underestimated in the neurological literature. Such symptoms as TN were well described in the older literature, but the conventional wisdom has been that other pain syndromes are unusual in MS. We now know that TN occurs in approximately 4 to 7 percent of patients, and PTSs occur in about

10 percent (see previous discussion of PTSs). In addition to those relatively uncommon pains, recent surveys have shown that half or more of patients have pain at some time or another. Pain can be the presenting feature.[196]

Vermote and associates[279] found that 54 percent of patients experienced pain at some time during their disease. Slightly less than half of those patients had musculoskeletal pain of various types. The musculoskeletal pain seen in MS is directly related to the degree of disability. It makes sense that patients with weak muscles and poor support of the spine would get such pains, (e.g., low backache, neckache, joint pains). Pain can be seen at the onset of MS.[196]

Thirty-one percent of surveyed patients had pain that could be classified as neurogenic. Clifford and Trotter[47] found 29 percent of patients to have neurogenic pain. Stenager and associates[257] interviewed 117 patients with CDMS and found only 35 percent to be pain-free. Pain complaints were more frequently seen in patients with MS of longer duration and with spasticity. However, there was no correlation between pain and depression.

Warnell[282] found that 64 percent of 364 patients surveyed had pain at some time during their disease. Females were most likely to experience pain, and many reported pain before the onset of other neurological symptoms.

The most common form of this neurogenic pain is usually described as "persistent extremity pain." The descriptors that patients use for this kind of pain include "pricking," "constrictive," "tingling," "dull," "burning," "nagging," and "troublesome." The pain is usually greatest in the lower extremities, although occasionally a painful radicular syndrome in the upper extremities can be present.

The underlying pathophysiology of this kind of pain is unknown, but as in paroxysmal symptoms, ephaptic transmission has been considered as a possible cause. Transmission of abnormal electrical discharges laterally across a demyelinated plaque might produce painful symptoms that could be either paroxysmal or chronic.

The development of radicular pains can also produce confusion between nerve root

Table 5–10. **SOME STUDIES OF NONHEADACHE PAIN IN MULTIPLE SCLEROSIS**

Year	Senior Author	No. of Patients with MS	NUMBER (%) WITH PAIN				Comments
			TN	PTS	RP	PEP	
1928	Parker[184]	1	1	—	—	—	Autopsy showed trigeminal root entry zone lesion.
1965	Rushton[225]	3880	—	—	—	—	Of 1735 cases of TN, 2% had MS.
1982	Jensen[105]	22	39(1)	—	—	—	Of 900 cases of TN, 2.4% had MS. One autopsy case had 5th nerve root entry lesions.
1974	Shibasaki[243]	64	16(100)	—	—	—	Carbamazepine suppressed the spasms.
1984	Bocock[25]	21	—	11(20)	—	—	Survey was conducted by UK MS Society.
1984	Clifford[47]	317	5(2)	6(12)	7(2)	33(10)	Overall, 29% had significant nonheadache pain.
1986	Vermote[279]	83	3(4)	8(10)	3(4)	12(14)	Emphasis was on neurogenic pains.
1989	Moulin[164]	159	7(4)	24(15)	—	46(29)	Pain was unrelated to disability or depression but increased with age.

PEP = persistent extremity pain; PTS = painful tonic spasm (seizure); RP = radicular pain; TN = trigeminal neuralgia.

Table 5–11. **TYPES OF PAIN IN MULTIPLE SCLEROSIS**

		Frequency in MS	Ref
Paroxysmal or phasic	1. Trigeminal neuralgia	4%	Parker, 1928;[184] Jensen et al., 1982; [106] Moulin et al., 1989[164]
	2. Radicular	2%–4%	Vermote et al., 1986[279] Clifford and Trotter, 1984[47]
	3. Pelvic	Rare	Miró et al., 1988[160]
	4. Itchiness	Rare	Osterman, 1979[183]
	5. Painful tonic spasms	2%–20%	Shibasaki, 1974;[243] Vermote et al., 1986[279]
	6. Pain on eye movement	Common	McDonald, 1980[150]
Chronic neurogenic	1. Dysesthetic in legs	10%–20%	Vermote et al., 1986;[279] Clifford and Trotter, 1984[47]
	2. Radicular	Unusual	Portenoy et al., 1988[196]
	3. Phantom limb	Unusual	Mayeux and Benson, 1979[144]

compression pains and those due to MS. Patients with MS are not protected from herniated intervertebral disk and nerve root compression. Therefore, such patients should be given the benefit of the doubt. Since radicular syndromes can also be seen, MS patients should not be subjected to surgery unless the condition is clearly due to nerve root compression. Finally, arachnoiditis must be considered in patients who have had oil myelography or have been subjected to intrathecal steroid injections. Radicular pains can be particularly confusing if they are the initial symptoms of MS. Pelvic pain[160] and phantom limb pain[144] have also been described.

Trigeminal neuralgia is probably the most well-described pain seen in MS. The characteristics of TN in MS are exactly the same as those seen in idiopathic TN.[225] TN is usually manifested as a paroxysm of pain in the distribution of the trigeminal nerve. Usually no objective evidence can be uncovered for motor or sensory deficit of the involved nerve.[106] Trigger zones are common. Touching the involved area, even washing the face, can set off a paroxysm. Chewing, talking, or swallowing can also set it off. The pain itself is usually described as sharp and intense, typically lasting only a few seconds to a few minutes. Intervals between paroxysms are usually pain-free. There is

also a natural tendency for spontaneous remissions to occur with interim years of pain-free existence between episodes.

Ninety percent of patients with idiopathic TN are older than 40 years of age. When TN occurs in patients younger than 40 years, MS must be suspected as the cause. TN in MS is bilateral more frequently (32 percent) than is idiopathic TN (4 percent). Brisman[35] found 6 of 18 patients with bilateral TN to have MS. When TN occurs, it can be extremely severe, and if unresponsive to therapy can produce suicidal tendencies.

The physiology of TN in MS is unknown, but Oppenheim[181] and others have described plaques at the root of the appropriate fifth nerve just as it enters the pons (root entry zone lesion). Such root entry zone lesions may be responsible for many of the radicular types of pain and other paroxysmal symptoms seen in MS.

Pain is also seen on movement of the eye associated with acute ON.[129] Eighty percent of patients with ON have pain at some stage. The pain can precede the onset of visual symptoms but more frequently begins at approximately the same time. Occasionally one sees patients with well-established MS who complain of similar remitting pain on motion of the globe but who do not develop any visual symptoms.[150] The appearance of such characteristic pain on eye movement without visual loss suggests that subclinical ON not only can occur but may be manifested by pain alone. Uveitis or pars planitis (PP), which occasionally is associated with MS, must be excluded as a cause of eye pain. We have seen one patient with acute angle-closure glaucoma where ON had been assumed.

The pain in ON is usually self-limited and is characteristically present only with eye movements.[129] Therefore, to minimize the pain, patients will usually turn their head to look to the side rather than turn their eyes. Treatment for the pain is usually unnecessary. Mild analgesics can be helpful if required. If steroids are used to treat the ON, the pain usually disappears within hours.

Weakness and Spasticity

Weakness in MS is usually pyramidal in distribution but occasionally can be remarkably focal. For example, marked interosseous weakness can occur with preservation of thenar muscle strength. The weakness is usually more distal than proximal. In the arms, weakness tends to be most prominent in the extensors, and in the legs, most prominent in the flexors. Footdrop may be seen in the presence of normal proximal strength. The reverse pattern is also occasionally found. Also in the legs, relatively isolated knee flexion paralysis can be seen, probably due to a focal lesion within the cord.

Spasticity is one of the more frequent symptoms encountered in MS. As many as 90 percent of patients will develop some features of spasticity during the clinical course. The degree of spasticity can vary considerably from patient to patient, and it can also fluctuate over time in patients who otherwise have reasonably stable disease (see section on management of spasticity). The pathophysiology of spasticity has been reviewed.[37]

In some patients with severely weak legs, spasticity is actually beneficial for walking or standing. Weak legs may be able to support considerable weight because of involuntary contraction of the antigravity muscles. Therefore, attempts to treat the spasticity may be counterproductive in those

patients. Relief of the spasticity may actually result in deterioration in functional capacity. However, when spasticity is manifested as paroxysms of flexion or extension, antispastic drugs are almost always helpful. When flexion or extension spasms or both occur primarily at night, benzodiazepines can be useful because of their ability not only to reduce spasticity but also to act as a hypnotic.

Occasional patients have a syndrome of severe increase in muscle tone with a paradoxical reduction in deep tendon reflexes. The exact physiology of this severe rigidity associated with MS is unknown, but perhaps it is due to a combination of extrapyramidal and pyramidal lesions. Severe rigidity is usually seen in patients who are extremely weak or paraplegic, so it is not necessarily a problem for ambulation. However, severe spasticity or rigidity can be a significant problem in nursing care and for the maintenance of stability in wheelchair patients. Spasticity in MS is usually maximal in extension, although as it becomes more severe, spasticity in flexion can predominate. With advancing disease, the spasticity may remit, presumably due to additional spinal cord lesions interrupting segmental reflex pathways.

Severe "paraplegia in flexion" may, at times, be temporary. Many patients recover spontaneously. Some are left with profound weakness, probably because of increasing degrees of neurological damage in the spinal cord. In any event, severe persistent flexor spasticity is a difficult problem. It often is painful as well as interfering with both mobility and nursing care (see Chapter 12).

Incoordination and Tremor (Cerebellar Features)

As mentioned previously, cerebellar deficits in MS can produce one of the most disabling forms of the disease. Cerebellar intention tremor is usually related to lesions in the cerebellar outflow pathways. Cerebellar manifestations include intention tremor, titubation, gait ataxia, and cerebellar dysarthria. Occasionally an action tremor can be superimposed on the intention tremor. The intention tremor can be so intense that it appears even with "intent to move," therefore occurring at apparent rest (rubral tremor). Examination of such patients must involve complete relaxation (usually in the supine position) to reduce the physiological heightening of motor reactions brought on by the intent to move and to provide stability for movement. The characteristic intention tremor seen in MS is that of an oscillating tremor at 5 to 7 Hz that moves in a plane perpendicular to the direction of intended movement.

Associated with the intention tremor is a characteristic clumsiness of movement that is made evident by the demonstration of irregularities in rapid alternating movements. The Gordon Holmes[95] characteristics of cerebellar deficits, such as errors in rate, range, direction, and force of movement, are distinctive of these patients. However, in a complex disorder such as MS, clumsiness in movement cannot always be taken as an indication of a cerebellar lesion. To ascribe clumsiness in rapid alternating movements to a cerebellar lesion, the physician must ensure that spasticity, pyramidal motor involvement, and proprioception in that limb are not involved.

Movement Disorders (Extrapyramidal Features)

Occasionally some patients with typical MS can develop parkinsonian features. This manifestation probably reflects the presence of MS lesions in the basal ganglia and their connections. However, the combination of MS and parkinsonian features may also be due to the coincidental occurrence of two common neurological diseases. A patient who sequentially developed MS, parkinsonism, and dementia at autopsy had MS, idiopathic Parkinson's disease, and Alzheimer's disease (K. Berry, personal communication 1989). Rarely, patients with MS develop movements that are characteristic of hemiballismus, dystonia chorea, or choreoathetosis (see Chapter 4). In such cases, the movements are probably due to the specific anatomical location of new MS lesions.

Paty and Ebers have seen a patient with MS who developed hemiballismus during an acute relapse. The movement disorder only lasted 36 hours in its complete form. However, she continued to have minor spontaneous movements for 2 months. An MRI scan taken at the time showed extensive lesions in the basal ganglia area. She also had many other lesions disseminated throughout the brain stem and cerebral hemispheres characteristic of MS.

Muscle Wasting (Amyotrophy)

Amyotrophy has been considered an unusual finding in MS (see Chapter 4).[71] However, autopsy studies have shown that muscle wasting is quite common. There are three common mechanisms involved in muscle wasting in MS. The most common cause is the atrophy of disuse, which can be severe in patients with advanced corticospinal disease. However, trauma to peripheral nerves due to poor posture, or associated with the posture of patients confined to a wheelchair, must be excluded. Specifically, bilateral ulnar nerve palsies are common in patients who are confined to a wheelchair or bed, and this finding is not unique to MS. Patients with paraplegia and distal hand weakness commonly use their elbows to turn in bed or to transfer.

Several cases of syringomyelia have been reported, which might explain a few cases of amyotrophy,[143,207] although the association is probably coincidental. In addition, there are some situations in which lesions in the lower motor neuron pathways of the cord cause axonal loss and subsequent denervation of muscle. This phenomenon probably explains most of the instances in which amyotrophic lateral sclerosis (ALS)–like syndromes are seen in MS. For example, wasting in the hand is not rare in MS, and occasionally hand wasting can be severe. Paty and Ebers have seen (once) the coincidental occurrence of MS and ALS, but most amyotrophy in MS is probably caused by MS lesions involving the outflow fibers of the anterior horn cells. Another possibility is that axonal loss in MS occurs secondarily to long-standing demyelination. It is commonly observed that chronic demyelinated MS lesions have loss of axons. The mechanism for the loss of axons is unknown.

PERIPHERAL NEUROPATHY

Several cases have been documented of pathologically proven co-occurrence of MS and various peripheral neuropathies.[195,221,304] Most of this co-occurrence is probably due to chance association, but the literature suggests that subtle involvement of peripheral nerves may be common.[152,304] Electrophysiological studies[61] also show that subtle peripheral nerve abnormalities exist in MS. In addition, several publications have recently described the coexistence of multiple CNS lesions on MRI studies of patients with chronic demyelinating polyneuropathy. However, clinicians must be careful that they are not dealing with age-associated MRI changes in the white matter. Waxman[290] has reviewed the subject of peripheral nerve abnormalities in MS. Table 5–12 lists a number of publications that have described peripheral nerve involvement.

Table 5–12. **REPORTS OF PERIPHERAL NERVE INVOLVEMENT, AMYOTROPHY, AND MYOKYMIA IN MULTIPLE SCLEROSIS**

Year	Senior Author	Report Summary
1934	Davison[52]	Seventeen of 110 patients with MS had muscle atrophy.
		Twelve of 20 autopsied patients with MS had atrophy and corresponding sclerosis of neurons.
1958	Wartenberg[286]	PN abnormalities were frequent; possible association with polyneuritis.
1958	Hasson[90]	Twelve of 20 autopsied cases of MS had peripheral demyelination (6 severe, probably due to malnutrition).
1967	Keuter[115]	Possible overlap between polyneuritis and MS in three cases.
1961	Miglietta[152]	Three of 54 cases had PN (2 probably due to pressure).
1961	Andermann[4]	Four patients with MS had facial myokymia.
1969	Gutmann[88]	Two patients with MS had facial myokymia.
1971	Ginzburg[82]	EMG in 21 patients with MS failed to find a correlation between nerve conduction and muscle strength.
1977	Schoene[237]	Onion bulb neuropathy was found in three autopsy cases of MS (seven other literature cases found).
1977	Pollock[195]	Eight of 10 patients with MS teased fiber studies of sural nerve biopsy had abnormal fibers.
1978	Hopf[97]	In 36 patients with MS, nerve conduction velocity was normal, but many had a prolonged sensory relative refractory period.
1979	Forrester[73]	Two patients with inflammatory polyneuritis subsequently developed MS.
1979	Weir[296]	Six of 15 patients with MS had abnormal neuromuscular transmission on EMG jitter studies; 2/6 had coexisting peripheral neuropathy.
1980	Noseworthy[177]	One MS case demonstrated an L5 motor radiculopathy.
1980	Weir[297]	Motor unit abnormalities were found in many MS patients.
1981	Lassmann[127]	Both PNS and CNS inflammatory demyelination were found in one autopsy case of acute MS.
1982	Eisen[62]	Seventeen of 40 patients with MS did not show super normality after a supramaximal conditioning shock of nerve, suggesting a PN abnormality.
1983	Fisher[71]	Nine patients with MS demonstrated hand atrophy without anterior horn cell or axonal abnormalities on EMG. Atrophy was not thought to be due to denervation, but possibly due to relative disuse.
1987	Sanders[330]	One patient with MS developed acute Guillain-Barré syndrome.
1987	Drake[59]	One patient with MS developed severe signs of denervation in the legs.
1990	Galer[77]	Headache and oculomotor palsy were found at the onset of MS.
1990	Newman[172]	Isolated pupil-sparing oculomotor palsy was found at the onset of MS.

AUTONOMIC DISTURBANCES

Bladder Problems

Perhaps 3 percent of patients will begin with isolated bladder symptoms.[21] The most common symptoms are those of urgency and frequency, sometimes with hesitancy as well. These symptoms suggest a small-volume, excessively contractile bladder in which there is some dyssynergia between the uninhibited muscle in the bladder wall and relaxation of the sphincter. In addition, a number of patients will also be found to have urinary tract infection, which can complicate the picture considerably. If the spastic element of bladder function overrides the problem with spasticity of the functional internal sphincter, incontinence will develop. In addition, if urinary tract infection becomes recurrent, a small spastic bladder can develop into a large-volume atonic bladder. A large-volume bladder will usually have an associated problem with incomplete emptying. The measurement of postvoiding residual urine is helpful in determining the type of bladder disturbance (most often a combination of uninhibited contraction and failure to empty). It has important consequences for eradication of infection, prevention of infection, and selection of pharmacological agents. Urodynamic assessment can be helpful, although symptomatic history and assessment of residual urine are often sufficient. Patients with large, poorly emptying bladders usually respond well to intermittent catheterization, the preferred method of long-term therapy. (See Chapter 12 for the recommended approach to evaluation and treatment of bladder disturbances.)

Bowel Problems

A recent survey of 280 patients with MS[94] showed that 43 percent had constipation. The constipation was not distinctly different from that seen in other diseases known to cause a generalized decrease in functional mobility. The severity of constipation varied in proportion to the severity of the MS. Fecal incontinence occurred at least once in 51 percent of patients and once per week or more frequently in 25 percent. Only 27 of the 142 incontinent patients were heavy laxative users. The overall prevalence of bowel dysfunction was 68 percent. All of these rates were much higher than those seen in control subjects.

A few patients with MS have been found to have malabsorption.[65] Incontinence and frequent diarrhea could indicate that a bowel disturbance has developed.[256] Such patients should be evaluated for specific gastrointestinal diagnoses, and MS should not be assumed to be the cause of the incontinence. However, Caruana and colleagues[41] looked at anorectal sensory and motor function in 22 patients with MS, 11 with fecal incontinence. They found that patients with MS tended to have a high threshold for rectal sensation and for phasic external sphincter contraction. Patients with MS who experience incontinence also had decreased voluntary and sphincter pressures. They concluded that impaired function of the external sphincter, decreased volumes of rectal distension to inhibit the internal sphincter, and increased threshold for conscious rectal sensation all may contribute to fecal incontinence in MS. Patients severely disabled by MS can develop fecal impaction and then have subsequent bowel incontinence around the impaction. This problem is usually easily identified by rectal examination and can be treated by digital breakup of the impaction.

Sexual Dysfunction

There is a high degree of correlation between sexual dysfunction and urinary dysfunction in MS.[132,133,258,265,266,278] That correlation is probably due to a combination of common physiology and concerns of hygiene. In addition, chronic illness and the related depression, stress, and fatigue can have an enormous effect on sexual function. The interplay between neurological and psychological dysfunction makes the evaluation of sexual problems in patients with disabling MS quite difficult. Sexual dysfunction in males usually has an organic component, but psychosocial factors are important. The prevalence is 80 percent in males and 33 percent in females and can be the onset symptom.[102] Valleroy and Kraft[277] surveyed 217 patients with MS and found sexual dysfunction in 56 percent of the females and 75 percent of the males. Females had decreased libido, decreased frequency of orgasm, fatigue, decreased sensation, and decreased arousal. Males had erectile dysfunction, decreased sensation, fatigue, decreased libido, and orgasmic dysfunction. Minderhoud and colleagues[159] found no correlation between sexual dysfunction and motor abnormalities, but they did find a correlation with bladder and bowel dysfunction.

Kirkeby and colleagues[118] investigated 29 males with erectile dysfunction with MS and found 3 to have psychogenic causes. Pudendal evoked potentials were the most discriminating test. Nocturnal erectile activity suggests at least some neurogenic function remaining.

The prognosis for neurogenic erectile dysfunction is probably poor, and male patients should be informed of this fact, after appropriate investigation for treatable causes. However, as in spinal cord injury, erectile function is not the only factor necessary for a satisfactory sexual relationship. Therefore, the entire social and emotional picture must be taken into consideration when trying to help create a meaningful sexual relationship in spite of irreversible dysfunctions such as decreased genital sensation and poor or absent penile erection.

Szasz and colleagues[266] reviewed sexual dysfunction in MS and concluded it was a complex issue with psychogenic and neurogenic components. The first step in evaluation is to determine whether sexual dysfunction is actually present. Areas such as sexual responsiveness, the motor ability for the sex act, including arm and limb mobility, adequacy of bowel and bladder control, genital hygiene, any concerns about fertility and birth control, the general degree of sexual interest, concerns about one's sexual partner, and the historical background of sexual perspectives and expectations in the individual need to be explored. In addition to a neurological examination, the physician must perform a physical examination of such a patient, requiring detailed knowledge of limb mobility, genital hygiene, sensory responses in the genital area, and voluntary control of urinary and anal sphincters. Use of a sexual function scale has been suggested to identify the degree of sexual dysfunction and degree of concern about that dysfunction.[265] Specialty services are now available in most centers for the investigation of sexual dysfunctions. In addition, a number of physiological tests are available for the evaluation of spinal cord function appropriate to sexual dysfunction.

Even though impotence, decreased libido, and other sexual disturbances are unusual at the outset of MS (5 percent), they can eventually be seen in more than half of the patients, more so in males than in females.[22a] Decreased sensation in the genital area can be a major factor in producing both decreased libido and decreased ability to perform in both sexes. In males, decreased ability to maintain an erection and the absence of ejaculation can become major problems. In females, decreased lubrication in the vaginal area can be a problem.

Because of the complex relationship between neurological dysfunction, psychological and cognitive dysfunction, and psychological reaction to disability, the evaluation of sexual disturbances in MS is difficult. Many patients will not complain of sexual disturbance, but when asked specifically, they will admit that sexual dysfunction is indeed a major problem. In this case, evaluation by an experienced sexual medicine unit that is aware of how to deal with neurologically impaired patients is important. Paty and Ebers' experience would suggest that about half of the patients with early MS and sexual dysfunction can be helped by a full evaluation and treatment by a sexual medicine unit. Many such patients have been found to have functional sexual problems not directly due to MS.[266] (Also see Chapter 12 for discussion of investigation and treatment.)

Nonsphincteric Autonomic Problems

Even though surveys of autonomic abnormalities in MS have found that gross disturbances such as postural hypotension are unusual, subtle autonomic changes are common.[111,166,171] For example, it is common to have "coldness" and blue (cyanotic) or blue-orange mottling in paretic limbs, especially the legs. Paroxysmal atrial fibrillation,[190,239] hypothermia,[262] orthostatic hypotension,[7] extreme exercise-induced tachycardia, and breathlessness have also been reported.[40] Noronha and his colleagues[176] studied sweating responses in MS.[278] They found 25 of 60 patients (42 percent) to have abnormal sweat responses. Reder and colleagues found adrenal size to be increased in MS.[215a] Two patients actually had anhidrosis, and four were found to have asymptomatic postural hypotension. The autonomic abnormalities were more likely to be seen in severely disabled patients. The authors concluded that the findings were due to lesions in the descending autonomic pathways in the brain stem or spinal cord. Vita and colleagues[281] found that cardiovascular autonomic abnormalities were likely due to spinal or brain stem lesions.

Yokota and colleagues[303] studied 28 patients with definite MS. They found the sympathetic skin responses (SSR) to be abnormal in 75 percent. Not only did they show that the sympathetic nervous system could be abnormal in MS, but they suggested that SSR might be used as a diagnostic test.

In a number of cardiovascular studies involving 22 patients with MS and 20 control subjects, Sterman and colleagues[259] found that half the patients with MS had abnormalities on two or more tests, but none were symptomatic. One case of cardiac necrosis occurred in association with an MS lesion of the medulla.[214]

Anema and associates[7] looked at blood pressure and cardiovascular control in 34 patients with CDMS and 63 healthy control subjects. They found the following abnormalities in patients with MS: 13 percent had postural hypotension, 28 percent had an abnormal heart rate (HR) response to standing, 36 percent had an abnormal HR after deep breathing, and 53 percent had at least one abnormality. No correlation was found between these abnormalities and other clinical features of MS.

Saito and colleagues[229] did a sural nerve biopsy on a 35-year-old woman with MS in whom deficits in sympathetic functions were present and found degeneration of both myelinated and unmyelinated fibers in the sural nerve.

Cartlidge[40] found that decreased sweating correlated with impotence in males. Pentland and Ewing[190] found at least one abnormal finding in 37 of 50 patients (70 percent) using HR responses to Valsalva's manuever, deep breathing or standing, along with blood pressure responses to standing and sustained hand grip. These autonomic abnormalities are different from those seen in diabetic patients. The complex involvement of the CNS by MS will probably make the elucidation of the exact mechanisms difficult. However, ample evidence has accumulated that autonomic function is frequently disturbed in MS. One recent report has claimed to find decreased SSRs in patients with chronic progressive disease.[111] The same group found increased numbers of beta-adrenergic receptors on the lymphocytes of the same group of patients, perhaps due to a phenomenon similar to denervation hypersensitivity.

In addition, we have personally seen neurogenic pulmonary edema (NPE) in four cases. In one autopsied case, lesions were found in the floor of the fourth ventricle,[57] encompassing sites in which acute lesions have produced NPE in experimental animals. Another recent case has been reported of pulmonary edema with gadolinium-enhanced MRI confirmation of an acute medullary lesion.[251]

HYPOTHERMIA, INAPPROPRIATE ANTIDIURETIC HORMONE SECRETION, COMA, AND FEVER

Chronic hypothermia has been reported by Sullivan and colleagues.[262] We have seen six cases with recurrent hypothermia, some of which were severe enough to produce obtundation or coma. Many of these episodes occurred in the setting of a urinary or other infection. The patients have responded to rewarming and appropriate antibiotic therapy. MRI scans showed hypothalamic lesions in two patients, but in four (G. C. Ebers, 1990), the anticipated bilateral posterior hypothalamic lesions were not seen. Electrolyte disturbances and drop in hemoglobin levels can also be seen during these episodes.

Inappropriate antidiuretic hormone secretion has been reported, even though we have not recognized it where MS was the only reasonable cause. Recurrent episodes of coma and fever have also been reported by Castaigne and colleagues.[42]

MONITORING DISEASE ACTIVITY

Because the degree of disease activity in MS is greater than that detected clinically and because physiological factors may result in ambiguity in interpreting clinical symptoms, objective measures of disease activity are needed.[61] Some of the methods in current use are listed in Table 5–13 (see also Chapter 12).

Evoked Potentials

Just as with MRI studies, studies of EP abnormalities and changes have not shown robust correlation with clinical findings[61] (see Chapter 4). However, asymptomatic as well as clinically correlated changes have been seen. Serial EP studies have shown that prolongation of EP latencies can be interspersed with stable periods. In a few instances, documented decreases in latency have been reported, usually after an acute episode of clinical or EP deterioration. Nuwer and his colleagues[179] used annual EPs in a clinical trial and found a statistically significant difference between the degree of stabilization seen in one treatment arm as compared with the other treatment arm or the placebo arm of the trial. Clinical evaluations in that same trial showed a trend in the same direction of a treatment effect, but none of the differences reached statistical significance. Apparently EPs are of limited value in assessing disease activity, but more must be learned about the natural history of EP changes over time. The fact that EP changes do not correlate well with clinical changes should not impair their use or study for monitoring the course of MS. They are telling us something different from the clinical evaluation.

Cerebrospinal Fluid

Even though CSF changes (most specifically OB) are important in the diagnosis of MS, few CSF findings are useful to monitor during the course of disease. CSF cell levels are probably a sign of active inflammation, but they have little correlation with clinical findings and have no impact on outcome. IgG levels may increase slightly over the years, but the OB pattern is remarkably stable over time. Some authors have suggested that CSF MBP levels fluctuate in proportion to disease activity.[47a,283a] Warren and Catz[283] claimed that antibody to MBP also fluctuates with disease activity. However, none of these changes has been proved to be clinically useful. It is not necessary to sample CSF routinely during the course of the disease. CSF MBP levels appear to increase at times of clinical activity.[298] TNF-α has been found to be elevated in the CSF of patients with CPMS.[240] Glial fibrillary acidic protein is also known to be elevated in some patients with MS.[222] This material may provide a marker for active gliosis.

Magnetic Resonance Imaging

The correlation between neurological and MRI findings has not been a robust one; however, Truyen and colleagues[272] have obtained a reasonable correlation coefficient ($rr = 0.66$) by using a standardized MRI protocol including sagittal views. The lack of correlation between clinical and MRI findings is reminiscent of the classic lack of correlation between the clinical story and the pathology.[138,169] (See Chapters 9 and 12 for detailed discussions of the evolution and meaning of MRI dynamics in MS.)

Recent serial studies with MRI[18,186] have shown that the rate of development of new lesions in the cerebral hemispheres is much greater than the rate of development of new symptoms. Figure 5–2 illustrates an evolving lesion on MRI in a serial study of a patient with relapsing disease.[300] Figure 5–3 shows a series of scans on a patient with SPMS with an evolving lesion. The appearance and evolution of large new

Table 5–13. **METHODS OF MONITORING DISEASE ACTIVITY (See Chapters 9 and 12 for Further Discussion)**

A. Clinical	1. Relapses: number, duration, severity
	2. Recovery from relapses
	3. Impairment scoring: EDSS, etc.
	4. Minimal Record of Disability, activities of daily living, quality of life measures
B. Imaging	1. Radionucleide brain scan (poor)
	2. CT (not sensitive)
	3. MRI (very sensitive)
	4. Enhanced MRI (Gd) (even more sensitive)
C. Physiological	1. Evoked potentials
D. Blood measures	1. Number of cells:
	a. Lymphocytes
	b. T cells
	c. T cell subsets
	d. NK cells
	2. Suppressor activity
	3. Lymphocyte proliferation
	4. Cytotoxicity
	5. Lymphokines
	6. Cortisol
	7. Neopterin
E. Spinal fluid measures	1. Cells (as above)
	2. Myelin basic protein (MBP)
	3. Antibody to MBP
	4. Immunoglobulins
	5. Enzymes
	6. Oligoclonal banding (does not change after becoming positive)
	7. Tumor necrosis factor
	8. Glial fibrillary acidic protein
F. Tissue breakdown products (blood, urine)	1. Enzymes
	2. MBP-like substances and peptides
	3. Immune complexes
	4. Gal C (galactocerebroside)
	5. Prostaglandin release

CT = computed tomography; EDSS = Extended Disability Status Scale; Gd = gadolinium; MRI = magnetic resonance imaging; NK = natural killer.

MRI lesions has followed a typical time course.[299,300] Significant new lesions can develop within a 2-week period, gradually increase in size over the following 4 weeks, and then gradually diminish in size over the next 6 to 8 weeks, closely paralleling the duration of most attacks. Other activity signs, such as new lesions, enhancement, or significant changes in size in previously stable lesions can evolve in less than 1 month. The reader should note that most of the new and dynamic MRI changes seen on systematic serial studies have been asymptomatic. Patients with SPMS tend to have more in the way of periventricular lesions than do patients with RRMS. The heavy load of disease in some of these patients can make it difficult to follow the course of new lesions in the periventricular region. In a follow-up of 49 CT-enhancing lesions over 20 months using serial MRI, Koopmans and his colleagues[120a] showed that 59 percent of lesions became smaller over time, 25 percent continued actively changing in size, and 16 percent went on to become confluent with neighboring lesions. One-half of the MRI scans that showed increasing activity also revealed other lesions to be simultaneously decreasing in size.

In three consecutive serial MRI studies without the use of gadolinium enhancement (each 6 months in duration in separate groups of patients) conducted at UBC, there were 213 follow-up MRI encounters.

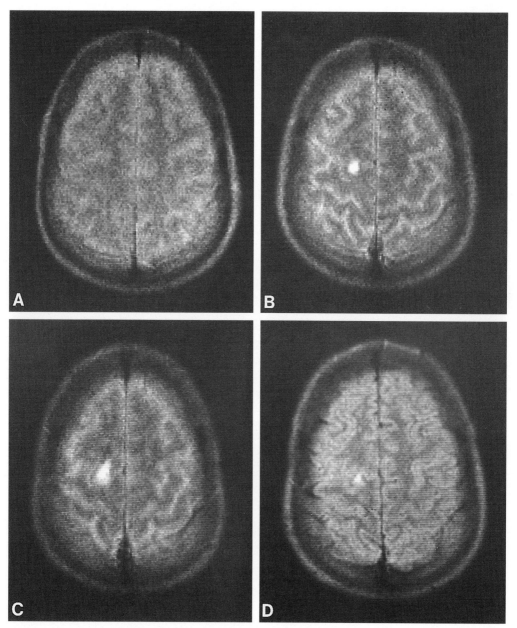

Figure 5–2. This series of MRI images shows the evolution of a single hemispheric lesion in a relapsing-remitting patient scanned once every 2 weeks. The patient was asymptomatic during the time of the lesion evolution. (Courtesy of E. W. Willoughby and colleagues and Annals of Neurology 25:43–49; 1989.[300])

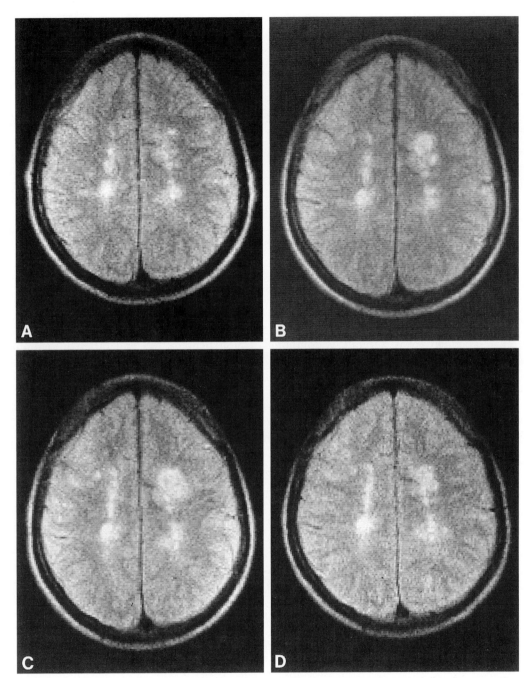

Figure 5–3. This series of MR images was taken once every 2 weeks, showing the evolution of a large, new periventricular lesion in a patient with relapsing-progressive disease. The patient reported an upper respiratory infection 2 weeks before the appearance of the new lesion and then reported excessive fatigue while the lesion was present. There were no changes on the neurological examination during the time of lesion evolution. (Courtesy of R. A. Koopmans and Annals of Neurology 26:248–256, 1989.[120a])

In 79 (37 percent) of these MRI follow-up encounters there was evidence for increasing disease activity. Increasing disease activity was defined as either the development of new lesions, significant increases in size of old lesions, or the reappearance of previously seen lesions that had disappeared. A significant increase in size generally meant an increase in area of at least 70 percent in small lesions (less than 1-cm diameter) or a 10 percent increase in area in large lesions (greater than 1-cm diameter). A lesion that was continuously increasing in size over several scans was counted only once as evidence of increasing disease activity.

Several investigators[113,114,155,255,269] have used a serial MRI method of evaluating patients that uses routine gadolinium enhancement in addition to standard T_2-weighted sequences. Enhancement was seen in 80 percent of new lesions and was occasionally observed before seeing the standard lesion on T_2-weighted scans. Overall, gadolinium enhancement added 150 percent to the scanning time and about 20 percent to the amount of activity information derived.

Other investigators [89,255] have done serial gadolinium-enhanced MRI studies on patients with RRMS and have found that the MRI-detected activity was much higher than clinical activity. Even though the MRI activity was much more constant than clinical signs of activity, the MRI activity tended to come in "bursts," some of which were quite prolonged.

Based on those experiences, it is reasonable to propose that systematic, carefully done, frequent MRI studies will identify much more evidence for disease activity than will clinical studies alone.[154] The MRI rate of development of increasing activity can be at least six times the clinical relapse rate. The new lesions rarely, if ever, completely disappear on high-resolution scanning, even though they routinely become much smaller. These and other studies have made it clear that the rate of the pathological process in MS is substantially greater than can be detected clinically.

The location of the new lesions seen on MRI is variable. The new lesions can be separated in location between those that are periventricular, midcentral white matter, or in the peripheral white matter at the gray-white junction. The pathological process

occurring in these rapidly evolving MRI lesions is unknown. Demyelination could be a late development in these lesions, perhaps only after multiple episodes of inflammation.[186] The peripherally located lesions seem to become less apparent with time.

The predominant MRI lesion seen in patients with CPMS is the chronic periventricular one.[120] Thompson and his colleagues[268] have done several MRI studies that will be very helpful in separating out the various clinical categories of MS. They have found the MRI lesion activity rate to be lowest in patients with primary CP, at a midrange in "benign patients,"[117] and highest in the standard patients with RRMS and SPMS. MRI can be used to monitor clinical trials.[187]

ASSOCIATED DISEASES

Some investigators[56] have found an association between MS and other autoimmune diseases. Lo and Feasby[136] previously reported on a patient who apparently had MS, MG, Graves' disease, and most recently, rheumatoid arthritis. Paty and Ebers also have experience with five patients with both MS and MG, seven patients with MS and lupus, and many patients with both MS and bipolar disease.

Brashear and Pascuzzi[32] have reported on a 19-year-old woman with both Takayasu's arteritis and MS. The authors speculated on an immunopathogenic link between the two diseases.

Cancer does not seem to be increased in MS.[158] The occasional patient with MS will have inflammatory bowel disease, although these two diseases do have similar ethnic or geographic predilections (A.D. Sadovnick, personal communication 1991). The frequency of rheumatic diseases, such as rheumatoid arthritis, appears to be as expected by chance or decreased in our patients with MS, rather than increased (E. Willoughby, personal communication 1992).

Occasionally one encounters narcolepsy in the same patient or in family members. Narcolepsy and MS have the same HLA (human leukocyte antigen) association so it should not come as a surprise that they can coexist in patients, families, or both.

Uveitis is frequently seen in many autoimmune diseases, including MS. Uveitis can be found in approximately 5 percent of patients with MS. Paty and Ebers certainly recognize its concurrence, but whether it is an associated disease or purely a manifestation of MS is unknown.[16,273] (See Chapter 7.)

Paty and Ebers have seen several examples of pars planetis (PP) in MS.[174] We have been able to confirm the occurrence of oligoclonal bands in three patients with PP and normal MRI scans. Another study found that 10 percent of patients with juvenile diabetes have another autoimmune disorder.[43] However, a careful study by Baker and associates[11] found no increase in other autoimmune disorders with MS, although the study was retrospective (see previous discussion and Chapter 6).

CAUSES OF DEATH

A small number of patients die within the first few years of the disease.[128] Some of those patients have a very malignant form of MS with severe progression to helplessness. Others commit suicide.[226] Long-term survival studies[227] have shown that, excluding acute malignant MS, the mean survival is 35 to 40 years. Bronnum-Hansen and colleagues[36] looked at survival in patients from Denmark diagnosed since 1948. They found the median survival in men to be 28 years (cf. 40 years in the population) and 33 years in women (cf. 46 years in the population) (see Table 5–14). (A detailed discussion of prognosis and causes of death is found in Chapter 6; see, in particular, Tables 6–8 and 6–9.)

EFFECT OF MULTIPLE SCLEROSIS ON THE PATIENT AND FAMILY

Multiple sclerosis has a major impact on the quality of life of the patient and the patient's family.[191a,263] It is a great psychological burden to deal with an unpredictable, incurable, and potentially disabling disease. Less than 50 percent of patients function as wage earners or homemakers after 10 years of disease. In reviewing the factors that influence employment, Gronning and colleagues[87] found that progressive disease, heavy physical work, and onset after age 30 years were associated with early underemployment. Fifty-one percent of their patients were unemployed before the usual retirement age. Women had a significantly longer employment record than did men. Cognitive impairment is more important than motor impairment in determining employability.[210]

LaRocca and his colleagues[126] also looked at employment factors. They found that the causes cited for unemployment were 27 percent physical limitations, 14 percent fatigue, 11 percent pregnancy, 7 percent visual decline, 3 percent the employer's negative attitude, and 22 percent other reasons. Forty percent of the unemployed wanted new employment. Patients with higher levels of education remained employed longest.

Jackson and colleagues[103] also looked at occupational patterns in 210 patients with MS surveyed by questionnaire. Ninety-seven percent had been employed at one time, but only 24 percent were employed at the time of the survey. The patients identified fatigue and weakness as the major factors that led to unemployment. Inaccessible environments were also an important factor.

With the spectrum of disability and underemployment to face, not surprisingly many patients with MS become depressed. In addition, the vagueness and evanescent nature of many symptoms makes psychological adaptation difficult. The process of

Table 5–14. MAJOR CAUSES OF DEATH IN 119 PATIENTS WHO DIED OF NON–MULTIPLE SCLEROSIS DIRECTLY RELATED CAUSES

Cause of Deaths	Number	Percentage of Total
Suicide	18	15
Cancer	19	16
Heart Attacks	13	11
Stroke	7	6

Source: Sadovnick AD, Eisen KA, Ebers GC, and Paty DW. Cause of death in patients attending multiple sclerosis clinics. Neurology 41(8):1193–1196, 1991, by permission of Little, Brown and Company (Inc).[226]

adapting to MS might be compared with trying to stand on quicksand.

Standard coping mechanisms might not work in MS. For example, denial, which works well in cancer, usually works in MS only as long as remission persists. When relapses or steady worsening occurs, the denial strategy, which can be sustained for only so long, is shattered. If a person has used denial over several years and has not prepared for the possibility of eventual disability, adjustment becomes much more difficult.

Some patients, probably because of premorbid personality, respond to the diagnosis of MS with a realistic acceptance and an ability to discuss the disease and its possible prognosis in a frank manner. Many of these same people can also create an environment characterized by a positive attitude. They can focus on those things that they can do well and do not dwell on and continually grieve for those things that they cannot continue to do. As one might expect, family support mechanisms can usually persist for such patients. However, if the patient becomes introverted and suspicious and insists on sharing the impact of the disease in a maximum way with those closest to them, manifested by a negative attitude, the family disruption can be major.

Major work adjustments must also be made. Because of potential loss of benefits and insurability, many patients hide their diagnosis until their disability becomes obvious. Waiting that long to discuss their disease with an employer may not be a good idea. For example, if workplace adaptations must be made to accommodate the fatigue and disability, it would be better to bring the employer into the picture early in the course of the disease.

The divorce rate in MS is high, although one large survey found it no higher than the high rate in the general population. As noted above, the premorbid personality is likely to be the best indicator of how well a patient will adjust to MS.

Support and educational groups for patients can help in establishing an interactive pattern by providing emotional support and by allowing the sharing of experiences. Education of the family is also vitally important. One must be careful, however, to avoid situations in which too much reality testing

enhances anxiety. Assistance with housing, transportation, and vocational placement and training can keep patients active in the community for a long time. Also, if the family remains enthusiastic and energetic, patients can be kept at home much longer than otherwise expected.

The provision of facilities focused on the long-term care of the younger disabled population in our society is lacking. Long-term care facilities usually focus on the major group of elderly patients and overlook the needs of the less common disabled young adult. A major advance, however, is that some institutions and organizations are providing daycare for the long-term care patient, specific units for the younger disabled and swing beds for relieving stress and fatigue to caregivers.

IMPACT ON SOCIETY

Swingler and Compston[263] reviewed the morbidity of MS in a cohort of 301 patients in South Wales. They found that MS had a major impact on health care resources. Inman[101] estimated that the average annual expenditure for medical treatment of men with MS in 1983 US dollars was between $282 for nondisabled men and $975 for severely disabled men. The costs for women were $635 to $2766, respectively. The differences in costs between men and women are because spouses of male patients frequently provide direct care, whereas male spouses of female patients usually remain in the workplace and hire needed services. Swingler and Compston[263] emphasized that MS has a major impact on society mostly because of chronic morbidity and decreased quality of life, rather than high mortality. Jönsson[108a] calculated the economic cost of MS in Sweden and found that the major currency costs were for short and long term hospital stays. The indirect costs are much greater than the direct costs (Tretiak, 1996 personal communication—The Canadian Burden of Illness Study, Montreal).

Multiple sclerosis causes an average loss of earning power of up to 90 percent in the severely disabled category, most strikingly in male patients. The aggregate lifetime costs of MS are of the same magnitude as are the economic costs of the major "killer" diseases of middle age, such as myocardial infarction. Inman estimated the total cost to US society of the current MS population in terms of medical care and lost wages at $29 billion!

REFERENCES

1. Abramsky O: Pregnancy and multiple sclerosis. Ann Neurol 36(suppl):38–41, 1994.
2. Achiron A, Ziv I, Djaldetti R, Goldberg H, Kuritzky A, and Melamed E: Aphasia in multiple sclerosis: Clinical and radiologic correlations. Neurology 42:2195–2197, 1992.
3. Amato MP, Ponziani G, Pracucci G, Bracco L, and Amaducci L: The pattern of cognitive dysfunction in MS over a 4-year follow-up. 10th Congress of the European Committee for Treatment and Research in Multiple Sclerosis, Athens, Greece (not published) Book of Abstracts, 1994, p 88.
4. Andermann F, Cosgrove JBR, Lloyd-Smith DL, Gloor P, and McNaughton FL: Facial myokymia in multiple sclerosis. Brain 84:31–44, 1961.
5. Andermann F, Cosgrove JB, Lloyd-Smith DL, and Walters AM: Paroxysmal dysarthria and ataxia in multiple sclerosis. A report of two unusual cases. Neurology 9:211–216, 1959.
6. Andersen E, Isager H, and Hyllested K: Risk factors in multiple sclerosis: Tuberculin reactivity, age at measles infection, tonsillectomy and appendectomy. Acta Neurol Scand 63:131–135, 1981.
7. Anema JR, Heijenbrok MW, Faes TJ, Heimans JJ, Lanting P, and Polman CH: Cardiovascular autonomic function in multiple sclerosis. J Neurol Sci 104:129–134, 1991.
8. Ansari KA: Olfaction in multiple sclerosis, with a note on the discrepancy between optic and olfactory involvement. Eur Neurol 14:138–145, 1976.
9. Arnett PA, Rao SM, Bernardin L, Grafman J, Yetkin FZ, and Lobeck L: Relationship between frontal lobe lesions and Wisconsin Card Sorting Test performance in patients with multiple sclerosis. Neurology 44(3 pt 1):420–425, 1994.
9a. Arnett PA, Rao SM, Hussain M, Swanson SJ, Hammeke TA: Conduction aphasia in multiple sclerosis: A case report with MRI findings. Neurology 47:576–578, 1996.
10. Babinski J, and Dubois R: Douleurs à forme de décharge électrique, consécutive aux tramatismes de la nuque. Presse Méd 26:64, 1918.
11. Baker HWG, Balla JI, Burger HG, Ebling P, and MacKay IR: Multiple sclerosis and autoimmune diseases. Aus NZ J Med 3:256–260, 1972.
12. Bamford CR, Sibley WA, and Laguna JF: Swine influenza vaccination in patients with multiple sclerosis. Arch Neurol 35:242–243, 1978.
13. Bamford CR, Sibley WA, and Thies C: Seasonal variation of multiple sclerosis exacerbations in Arizona. Neurology 33:697–701, 1983.
14. Bamford CR, Sibley WA, Thies C, Laguna JF, Smith MS, and Clark K: Trauma as an etiologic and aggravating factor in multiple sclerosis. Neurology 31:1229–1234, 1981.
15. Bamford CR, Smith MS, and Sibley WA: Horner's syndrome, an unusual manifestation of multiple sclerosis. Can J Neurol Sci 7:65–66, 1980.
16. Bammer HG, Hofmann A, and Zick R: Aderhautentzündungen bei multipler sklerose und die sogenannte uveoencephalomeningitis. Deutsche Seitschrift für Nervenheilkunde 187:300–316, 1965.
17. Barratt HJ, Miller DH, Rudge P, et al: The site of the lesion causing deafness in multiple sclerosis. Scand Audiol 17:67–71, 1988.
18. Baum K, Nehrig C, Schörner W, and Girke W: Long-term follow-up of MS: Disease activity detected clinically and by MRI. Acta Neurol Scand 82:191–196, 1990.
19. Beatty PA, and Gange JJ: Neuropsychological aspects of multiple sclerosis. J Nerv Ment Dis 164:42–50, 1977.
20. Bejar JM, and Ziegler DK: Onset of multiple sclerosis in a 24-month-old child. Arch Neurol 41:881–882, 1984.
21. Bemelmans BL, Hommes OR, Van Kerrebroeck PE, Lemmens WA, Doesburg WH, and Debruyne FM: Evidence for early lower urinary tract dysfunction in clinically silent multiple sclerosis. J Urol 145:1219–1224, 1991.
22. Berr C, Puel J, Clanet M, Ruidavets JB, Mas JL, and Alperovitch A: Risk factors in multiple sclerosis: A population-based case-control study in Hautes-Pyrénées, France. Acta Neurol Scand 80:46–50, 1989.
22a. Betts CD, Jones SJ, Fowler CG, Fowler CJ: Erectile dysfunction in multiple sclerosis: Associated neurological and neurophysiological deficits, and treatment of the condition. Brain 117:1303–1310, 1994.
23. Birk K, Ford C, Smeltzer S, Ryan D, Miller R, and Rudick RA: The clinical course of multiple sclerosis during pregnancy and the puerperium. Arch Neurol 47:738–742, 1990.
24. Birk K, and Rudick RA: Pregnancy and multiple sclerosis. Arch Neurol 43:719–726, 1986.
25. Bocock N: Report on study of pain associated with multiple sclerosis. UK MS Society Survey on Pain in MS, London, UK, 1984.
26. Boné G, Ladurner G, Dinkhauser L, and Mader I: Cognitive disturbances and magnetic resonance imaging findings in multiple sclerosis. J Neuroimaging 3:169–172, 1993.
27. Bostock H, and Sears TA: The internodal axon membrane: Electrical excitability and continuous conduction in segmental demyelination. J Physiol (Lond) 280:273–301, 1978.
28. Boucher RM, and Hendrix RA: The otolaryngic manifestations of multiple sclerosis. Ear Nose Throat J 70:231–233, 1991.
29. Boyle EA, Clark CM, Klonoff H, Paty DW, and Oger JJF: Empirical support for psychological profiles observed in multiple sclerosis. Arch Neurol 48:1150–1154, 1991.
30. Brainin M, Goldenberg G, Ahlers C, Reisner T, Neuhold A, and Deecke L: Structural brain correlates of anterograde memory deficits in multiple sclerosis. J Neurol 235:362–365, 1988.

31. Bramwell B: The prognosis of disseminated sclerosis: Duration in 200 cases of disseminated sclerosis. Edinburgh Medical Journal 18:16–23, 1917.

32. Brashear A, and Pascuzzi RM: Takayasu's arthritis and multiple sclerosis. J Neuroimaging 2:36–38, 1992.

33. Bray PF, Bloomer LC, Salmon VC, Bagley MH, and Larsen PD: Epstein-Barr virus infection and antibody synthesis in patients with multiple sclerosis. Arch Neurol 40:406–408, 1983.

34. Bray PF, Culp KW, McFarlin DE, Panitch HS, Torkelson RD, and Schlight JP: Demyelinating disease after neurologically complicated primary Epstein-Barr virus infection. Neurology 42:278– 282, 1992.

35. Brisman R: Bilateral trigeminal neuralgia. J Neurosurg 67:44–48, 1987.

36. Bronnum-Hansen H, Koch-Henriksen N, and Hyllested K: Survival of patients with multiple sclerosis in Denmark: A nationwide, long-term epidemiologic survey. Neurology 44:1901–1907, 1994.

37. Brown P: Pathophysiology of spasticity (editorial and review). J Neurol Neurosurg Psychiatry 57: 773–777, 1994.

38. Camenga DL, Johnson KP, Alter M, et al: Systemic recombinant alpha-2 interferon therapy in relapsing multiple sclerosis. Arch Neurol 43: 1239–1246, 1986.

39. Carroll M, Gates R, and Roldan F: Memory impairment in multiple sclerosis. Neuropsychologia 22:297–302, 1984.

40. Cartlidge NE: Autonomic function in multiple sclerosis. Brain 95:661–664, 1972.

41. Caruana BJ, Wald A, Hinds JP, and Eidelman BH: Anorectal sensory and motor function in neurogenic fecal incontinence: Comparison between multiple sclerosis and diabetes mellitus. Gastroenterology 100:465–470, 1991.

42. Castaigne P, Escourolle R, Laplane D, and Augustin P: Comas transitoires ave hyerthermie au cours de la scléose en plaques. Rev Neurol 114: 147–150, 1966.

43. Castaño L, and Eisenbarth GS: Type-I Diabetes: A chronic autommune disease of human, mouse, and rat. Annu Rev Immunol 8:647–679, 1990.

44. Catalanotto FA, Dore-Duffy P, Donaldson JO, Testa M, Peterson M, and Ostrom KM: Quality-specific taste changes in multiple sclerosis. Ann Neurol 16:611–615, 1984.

45. Chrousos GP, Wilder RL, and Gold PW: The stress response and the regulation of inflammatory disease. Ann Int Med 117:854–866, 1992.

46. Clark CM, Fleming JA, Li DKB, Oger JJF, Klonoff H, and Paty DW: Sleep disturbance, depression, and lesion site in patients with multiple sclerosis. Arch Neurol 49:641–643, 1992.

47. Clifford DB, and Trotter JL: Pain in multiple sclerosis. Arch Neurol 41:1270–1272, 1984.

47a. Cotten SR, Brooks BR, Jubelt B, Herndon RM and McKhann G: Myelin basic protein in cerebrospinal fluid—index of active demyelination. In: J.H. Wood (Ed.) Neurobiology of Cerebrospinal Fluid, Vol 1. New York. Plenum Press 487– 494, 1980.

48. Confavreux C, Aimard G, and Devic M: Course and prognosis of multiple sclerosis assessed by the computerized data processing of 349 patients. Brain 103:281–300, 1980.

49. Coyle PK, Krupp LB, Mohr K, Doscher C, and Mehta PD: Immune activation markers in neurological patients with symptomatic chronic fatigue. Ann Neurol 30:306, 1991.

50. Dalos NP, Rabins PV, Brooks BR, and O'Donnell P: Disease activity and emotional state in multiple sclerosis. Ann Neurol 13(5):573–577, 1983.

51. Davis FA, Stefoski D, and Rush J: Orally administered 4-aminopyridine improves clinical signs in multiple sclerosis. Ann Neurol 27:186–192, 1990.

52. Davison C, Goodhart SP, and Lander J: Multiple sclerosis and amyotrophies. Arch Neurol 31: 270– 289, 1934.

53. Day TJ, Fisher AG, and Mastaglia FL: Alexia with agraphia in multiple sclerosis. J Neurol Sci 78: 343–348, 1987.

54. D'Costa DF, Vania AK, and Millac PA: Multiple sclerosis associated with trismus. Postgrad Med J 66:853–854, 1990.

55. De Castro P, Carreno M, and Iriarte J: Fatigue in oligosymptomatic patients in multiple sclerosis. 10th Congress of the European Committee for Treatment and Research in Multiple Sclerosis, Book of Abstracts, Athens, Greece (not published) 1994, p 114.

56. De Keyser J: Autoimmunity in multiple sclerosis. Neurology 38:371–374, 1988.

57. D'Hooghe MB, and Ebers GC: HLA in genetic susceptiblity of multiple sclerosis: A recessive effect and the role of other genes. Neurology 39(suppl 1):368, 1989.

58. DiMario FJ Jr, and Berman PH: Multiple sclerosis presenting at 4 years of age: Clinical and MRI correlations. Clin Pediatr 27:32–37, 1988.

59. Drake ME: Peripheral neuropathy in multiple sclerosis. Journal of the National Medical Association 79:672–673, 1987.

60. Duquette P, Murray TJ, Pleines J, et al: Multiple sclerosis in childhood: Clinical profile in 125 patients. J Pediatr 111:359–363, 1987.

61. Eisen AA, and Odusote K: Central and peripheral conduction times in multiple sclerosis. Electroencephalogry Clin Neurophysiol 48:253–265, 1980.

62. Eisen A, Paty D, and Hoirch M: Altered supernormality in multiple sclerosis peripheral nerve. Muscle and Nerve 5:411–414, 1982.

63. Ekbom KA, Westerberg CE, and Osterman PO: Focal sensory-motor seizures of spinal origin. Lancet Vol I:67, 1968.

64. Elbol P, and Work K: Retinal nerve fiber layer in multiple sclerosis. Acta Ophthalmol Scand 68: 481–486, 1990.

65. Fantelli FJ, Mitsumoto H, and Sebek BA: Multiple sclerosis and malabsorption. The Lancet (8072) 1039–1040, 1978.

66. Feinstein A, Ron M, and Thompson AJ: A serial study of psychometric and magnetic resonance imaging changes in multiple sclerosis. Brain 116:569–602, 1993.

67. Ferini-Strambi L, Fillipi M, Martinelli V, et al: Nocturnal sleep in multiple sclerosis: Correla-

tions with clinical and brain magnetic resonance imaging findings. J Neurol Sci 125:194–197, 1994.

68. Field EJ, and Foster JB: Periphlebitis retinae and multiple sclerosis. J Neurol Neurosurg Psychiatry 25:269–270, 1962.

69. Firth D: The Case of Augustus D'Este. Cambridge University Press, Cambridge, 1948.

70. Fischer C, Mauguière F, Ibanez V, Confavreux C, and Chazot G: The acute deafness of definite multiple sclerosis: BAEP patterns. Electroencephalogr Clin Neurophysiol 61:7–15, 1985.

71. Fisher M, Long RR, and Drachman DA: Hand muscle atrophy in multiple sclerosis. Arch Neurol 40:811–815, 1983.

72. Fisk JD, Pontefract A, Rivto PG, Archibald CJ, and Murray TJ: The impact of fatigue on patients with multiple sclerosis. Can J Neurol Sci 21:9–14, 1994.

73. Forrester C, and Lascelles RG: Association between polyneuritis and multiple sclerosis. J Neurol Neurosurg Psychiatry 42:864–866, 1979.

74. Frederiksen JL, Larsson HB, Nordenbo AM, and Seedorff HH: Plaques causing hemianopsia or quadrantanopsia in multiple sclerosis identified by MRI and VEP. Acta Ophthalmol Scand Suppl 69:169–177, 1991.

75. Frith JA, and McLeod JG: Pregnancy and multiple sclerosis. J Neurol Neurosurg Psychiatry 51:495–498, 1988.

76. Furman JMR, Durrant JD, and Hirsch WL: Eighth nerve signs in a case of multiple sclerosis. Am J Otolaryngol 10:376–381, 1989.

77. Galer BS, Lipton RB, Weinstein S, Bello L, and Solomon S: Apoplectic headache and oculomotor nerve palsy: An unusual presentation of multiple sclerosis. Neurology 40:1465–1466, 1990.

78. Gall JC, Hayles AB, Siekert RG, and Haddow MK: Multiple sclerosis in children: A clinical study of 40 cases with onset in childhood. Pediatrics 21:703–709, 1958.

79. Gasperini C, Pozzilli C, and Bernardi S: Irreversible total blindness in multiple sclerosis letter. Ital J Neurol Sci 12:329, 1991.

80. Ghezzi A, and Caputo D: Pregnancy: A factor infuencing the course of multiple sclerosis? Eur Neurol 20:115–117, 1981.

81. Gilbert IJ, and Sadler M: Unsuspected multiple sclerosis. Arch Neurol 40:533, 1983.

82. Ginzburg M, Lee M, and Ginzburg J: Correlation between muscle strength and peripheral nerve conduction in multiple sclerosis. Electromyography 11:5:491–513, 1971.

83. Goodkin DE, Hertsgaard D, and Rudick RA: Exacerbation rates and adherence to disease type in a prospectively followed-up population with multiple sclerosis: Implications for clinical trials. Arch Neurol 46:1107–1112, 1989.

84. Graff-Radford NR, and Rizzo M: Neglect in a patient with multiple sclerosis. Eur Neurol 26:100–103, 1987.

85. Grant I, Brown GW, Harris T, McDonald WI, Patterson T, and Trimble MR: Severely threatening events and marked life difficulties preceding onset or exacerbation of multiple sclerosis. J Neurol Neurosurg Psychiatry 52:8–13, 1989.

86. Grant I, McDonald WI, Trimble MR, Smith E, and Reed R: Deficient learning and memory in early and middle phases of multiple sclerosis. J Neurol Neurosurg Psychiatry 47:250–255, 1984.

87. Gronning M, Hannisdal E, and Mellgren SI: Multivariate analyses of factors associated with unemployment in people with multiple sclerosis. J Neurol Neurosurg Psychiatry 53:388–390, 1990.

87a. Guthrie TC, Nelson DA: Influence of temperature changes on multiple sclerosis: critical review of mechanisms and research potential. (Review article) Journal of the Neurological Sciences 129:1–8, 1995.

88. Gutmann L, Thompson HG Jr, and Martin JD: Transient facial myokymia: An uncommon manifestation of multiple sclerosis. JAMA 209(3): 389– 391, 1969.

89. Harris JO, Frank JA, Patronas N, McFarlin DE, and McFarland HF: Serial gadolinium-enhanced magnetic resonance imaging scans in patients with early, relapsing-remitting multiple sclerosis: Implications for clinical trials and natural history. Ann Neurol 29:548–555, 1991.

90. Hasson J, Terry RD, and Zimmerman HM: Peripheral neuropathy in multiple sclerosis. Neurology 8:503–510, 1958.

91. Herrera WG: Vestibular and other balance disorders in multiple sclerosis: Differential diagnosis of disequilibrium and topognostic localization. In Arenberg IK, and Smith DB (eds): Diagnostic Neurotology: Neurologic Clinics, Vol 8. 1990, pp 407–420. W.B. Saunders, Philadelphia.

92. Herroelen L, de Keyser J, and Ebinger G: Central-nervous-system demyelination after immunization with recombinant hepatitis B vaccine. Lancet 338:1174–1175, 1991.

93. Hess DC, and Sethi KD: Epilepsia partialis continua in multiple sclerosis. Int J Neurosci 50: 109–111, 1990.

94. Hinds JP, Eidelman BH, and Wald A: Prevalence of bowel dysfunction in multiple sclerosis: A population survey. Gastroenterology 98:1538–1542, 1990.

95. Holmes G: Introduction to Clinical Neurology. Livingstone, Edinburgh, 1946.

96. Honig LS, Wasserstein PH, and Adornato BT: Tonic spasms in multiple sclerosis. Anatomic basis and treatment. West J Med 154:723–726, 1991.

97. Hopf HC, and Eysholdt M: Impaired refractory periods of peripheral sensory nerves in multiple sclerosis. Ann Neurol 4:499–501, 1978.

98. Howard RS, Wiles CM, Hirsch NP, Loh L, Spencer GT, and Newsom-Davis J: Respiratory involvement in multiple sclerosis. Brain 115: 479–494, 1992.

99. Huber PW: Galileo's Revenge: Junk Science in the Courtroom. Basic Books, New York, 1991.

100. Huber SJ, Bornstein RA, Rammohan KW, Christy JA, Chakeres DW, and McGhee RB: Magnetic resonance imaging correlates of neuropsychological impairment in multiple sclerosis. J Neuropsychiatry Clin Neurosci 4:152–158, 1992.

101. Inman RP: Disability indices, the economic costs of illness, and social insurance: The case of multiple sclerosis. Symposium on MRD. Acta Neurol Scand Suppl 70:46–55, 1984.

102. Ivers RR, and Goldstein NP: Multiple sclerosis: A current appraisal of symptoms and signs. Proc Mayo Clin 38:457, 1963.

103. Jackson MF, Quaal C, and Reeves MA: Effects of multiple sclerosis on occupational and career patterns. Axone 13:20–22, 1991.

104. Jellinek EH: Trauma and multiple sclerosis (editorial). Lancet 343:1053–1054, 1994.

105. Jensen K, Knudsen L, Stenager E, and Grant I (eds): Mental Disorders and Cognitive Deficits in Multiple Sclerosis. John Libbey, 1989.

106. Jensen TS, Rasmussen P, and Reske-Nielsen E: Association of trigeminal neuralgia with multiple sclerosis: Clinical and pathological features. Acta Neurol Scand 65:182–189, 1982.

107. Joffe RT, Lippert GP, Gray TA, et al: Mood disorder and multiple sclerosis. Arch Neurol 44:376–378, 1987.

108. Johnson MD, Lavin P, and Whetsell WO Jr: Fulminant monophasic multiple sclerosis, Marburg's type. J Neurol Neurosurg Psychiatry 53:918–921, 1990.

108a. Jönsson B: The Economic Cost of Multiple Sclerosis in Sweden. EFI Research paper Nr 6551, Mars 1995.

109. Kahana E, Leibowitz U, and Alter M: Cerebral multiple sclerosis. Neurology 21:1179–1185, 1971.

110. Kaji R, Happel L, and Sumner AJ: Effect of digitalis on clinical symptoms and conduction variables in patients with multiple sclerosis. Ann Neurol 28:582–584, 1990.

111. Karaszewski JW, Reder AT, Maselli R, Brown M, and Arnason BGW: Sympathetic skin reponses are decreased and lymphocyte beta-adrenergic receptors are increased in progressive multiple sclerosis. Ann Neurol 27:366–372, 1990.

112. Kelly RE: Clinical aspects of multiple sclerosis. In Vinken P, Bruyn G, Klawans H (eds): Handbook of Clinical Neurology. Elsevier, Amsterdam, 1985, pp 49–78.

113. Kermode AG, Thompson AJ, Tofts PS, et al: Breakdown of the blood brain barrier precedes symptoms and other MRI signs of new lesions in multiple sclerosis: Pathogenic and clinical implications. Brain 113:1477–1489, 1990(a).

114. Kermode AG, Tofts PS, Thompson AJ, et al: Heterogeneity of blood-brain barrier changes in multiple sclerosis: An MRI study with gadolinium-DTPA enhancement. Neurology 40:229–235, 1990(b).

115. Keuter EJW: Polyneuritis and multiple sclerosis. Psychiatria, Neurologia, Neurochirogia 70:271–279, 1967.

116. Khansari DN, Murgo AJ, and Faith RE: Effects of stress on the immune system. Immunol Today 11:5:170–175, 1990.

117. Kidd D, Thompson AJ, Kendall BE, Miller DH, and McDonald WI: Benign form of multiple sclerosis: MRI evidence for less frequent and less inflammatory disease activity. J Neurol Neurosurg Psychiatry 57:1070–1072, 1994.

118. Kirkeby, HJ, Poulsen EV, Petersen, T Doruf, J: Erectile dysfunction in multiple sclerosis. Neurology 38:1366–1371, 1988.

119. Klonoff H, Clark C, Oger JJF, Paty DW, and Li DKB: Neuropsychological performance in patients with mild multiple sclerosis. J Nerv Ment Dis 179:127–131, 1991.

120. Koopmans RA, Li DKB, Grochowski E, Cutler PJ, and Paty DW: Benign versus chronic progressive multiple sclerosis: magnetic resonance imaging features. Ann Neurol 25:74–81, 1989.

120a. Koopmans RA, Li DKB, Oger JJF, et al: Chronic progressive multiple sclerosis: serial magnetic resonance brain imaging over six months. Ann Neurol 26:248–256, 1989.

121. Korn-Lubetzki I, Kahana E, Cooper G, and Abramsky O: Activity of multiple sclerosis during pregnancy and puerperium. Ann Neurol 16:229– 231, 1984.

122. Krupp LB, Sliwinski M, Masur DM, Friedberg F, and Coyle PK: Cognitive functioning and depression in patients with chronic fatigue syndrome and multiple sclerosis. Arch Neurol 51:705–710, 1994.

123. Kujala P, Portin R, Revonsuo A, and Ruutiainen J: Automatic and controlled information processing in multiple sclerosis. Brain 117:1115–1126, 1994.

123a. Kujala P, Portin R, Ruutiainen J: Language functions in incipient cognitive decline in multiple sclerosis. Journal of the Neurological Sciences 141:79–86, 1996.

123b. Kurland LT, Rodriguez M, O'Brien PC, Sibley WA: Trauma and MS. (Letter to the Editor). Neurology 44:1362–1363, 1994.

124. Kurtzke JF: Clinical manifestation of multiple sclerosis. In Vinken PJ, Bruyn GW (eds): Handbook of Clinical Neurology. Elsevier North-Holland, Amsterdam, 1970, pp 161–216.

125. Langmuir AD: Guillain-Barré syndrome. The swine influenza virus vaccine incident in the United States of America, 1976–77: Preliminary communication. JR Soc Med 72:660–669, 1979.

126. LaRocca NG, Kalb R, Scheinberg LC, and Kendall P: Factors associated with unemployment of patients with multiple sclerosis. Journal of Chronic Diseases 38:203–210, 1985.

127. Lassman H, Budka H, and Schnaberth G: Inflammatory demyelinating polyradiculitis in a patient with multiple sclerosis. Arch Neurol 38:99–102, 1981.

127a. Lauer K: Physical trauma and multiple sclerosis. (Correspondence). Neurology 44:1360–1362, 1994.

128. Leibowitz U, Kahana E, Jacobson SG, and Alter M: The cause of death in multiple sclerosis. In Leibowitz U (ed): Progress in Multiple Sclerosis. Academic Press, New York, 1972.

129. Lepore FE: The origin of pain in optic neuritis. Determinants of pain in 101 eyes with optic neuritis. Arch Neurol 48:748–749, 1991.

130. L'hermitte J, Bollak, and Nicholas M: Les douleurs a type de decharge electrique consecutives a la flexion cephalique dans la sclerose en plaques. Rev Neurol 42:56–62, 1924.

130a. Libenson MH, Stafstrom CE, Rosman NP: Tonic "seizures" in a patient with brainstem demyelination: MRI study of brain and spinal cord. Pediatr Neurol 11:258–262, 1994.

131. Lightman S, McDonald WI, Bird AC, Francis DA, Hoskins A, Batchelor JR, et al: Retinal ve-

nous sheathing in optic neuritis: Its significance for the pathogenesis of multiple sclerosis. Brain 110:405–414, 1987.

132. Lilius HG, Valtonen EJ, and Wirkström J: Sexual problems in patients suffering from multiple sclerosis. J Chron Dis 29:643–647, 1976(a).

133. Lilius HG, Valtonen EJ, and Wirkström J: Sexual problems in patients suffering from multiple sclerosis. Scand J Soc Med 4:41–44, 1976(b).

134. Litvan I, Grafman J, and Vendrell P: Multiple memory deficits in patients with multiple sclerosis: Exploring the working memory system. Arch Neurol 45:607–610, 1988.

135. Litvan I, Grafman J, Vendrell P, and Martinez JM: Slowed information processing in multiple sclerosis. Arch Neurol 45:281–285, 1988.

136. Lo R, and Feasby TE: Multiple sclerosis and autoimmune diseases. Neurology 33:97–98, 1983.

136a. Lublin FD, Reingold SC: Defining the clinical course of multiple sclerosis: Results of an international survey. (Views and Reviews). Neurology 46:907–911, 1996.

137. Ludwin SK: An autoradiographic study of cellular proliferation in remyelination of the central nervous system. Am J Pathol 95:683–690, 1979.

138. Lumsden CE: Fundamental problems in the pathology of multiple sclerosis and allied demyelinating diseases. Br Med J 1:1035–1043, 1951.

139. MacFadyen DJ, Drance SM, Douglas GR, Airaksinen PJ, Mawson DK, and Paty DW: The retinal nerve fiber layer, neuroretinal rim area, and visual evoked potentials in MS. Neurology 38:1353–1358, 1988.

140. Mahler ME: Behavioral manifestations associated with multiple sclerosis. Psychiatr Clin North Am 15:425–438, 1992.

141. Maimone D, Reder AT, Finocchiaro F, and Recupero E: Internal capsule plaque and tonic spasms in multiple sclerosis. Arch Neurol 48:427–429, 1991.

142. Martyn CN, and Colquhoun I: Radiological evidence of sinus infection in patients with multiple sclerosis. J Neurol Neurosurg Psychiatry 54:925–926, 1991.

143. Masur H, and Oberwittler C: MS and syringomyelia (letter to the editor). Neurology 42:464–592, 1992.

144. Mayeux R, and Benson DF: Phantom limb and multiple sclerosis. Neurology 29:724–726, 1979.

145. McAlpine D: The benign form of multiple sclerosis: A study based on 241 cases seen within three years of onset and followed up until the tenth year or more of the disease. Brain 84:186–203, 1961.

146. McAlpine D, and Compston ND: Some aspects of the natural history of disseminated sclerosis. Quarterly Journal of Medicine 21(82):135–167, 1952.

147. McAlpine D, Compston ND, and Lumsden CE: Multiple Sclerosis. Livingstone, Edinburgh, 1955.

148. McAlpine D, Lumsden CE, and Acheson ED: Multiple Sclerosis: A Reappraisal. Churchill Livingstone, Edinburgh, 1972.

149. McDonald WI: Pathophysiology in multiple sclerosis. Brain 97:179–196, 1974.

150. McDonald WI: Pain around the eye: Inflammatory and neoplastic causes. Transactions of the Ophthalmological Society of the United Kingdom. (pt 2):260–262, 1980.

151. McDonald WI: Demyelinating diseases of the optic nerve. Neurology and Neurosurgery 2:179–182, 1989.

152. Miglietta O, and Lowenthal M: A study of peripheral nerve involvement in fifty-four patients with multiple sclerosis. Archives of Physical Medicines and Rehabilitation 42:573–578, 1961.

153. Millar JHD, Allison RS, Cheesman EA, and Merrett JD: Pregnancy as a factor influencing relapse in disseminated sclerosis. Brain 82:417–426, 1959.

154. Miller DH, Barkhof F, Berry I, Kappos L, Scotti G, and Thompson AJ: Magnetic resonance imaging in monitoring the treatment of multiple sclerosis: Concerted action guidelines. J Neurol Neurosurg Psychiatry 54:683–688, 1991.

155. Miller DH, Rudge P, Johnson G, et al: Serial gadolinium enhanced magnetic resonance imaging in multiple sclerosis. Brain 111:927–939, 1988.

156. Miller H, Cendrowski W, and Schapira K: Multiple sclerosis and vaccination. BMJ 2:210–213, 1967.

157. Miller H, and Durh MD: Trauma and multiple sclerosis. The Lancet 1:848–850, 1964.

158. Miller H, Kneller RW, Boice JD, and Olsen JH: Cancer incidence following hospitalization for multiple sclerosis in Denmark. Acta Neurol Scand 84:214–220, 1991.

159. Minderhoud JM, Leemhuis JG, Kremer J, Laban E, and Smits PML: Sexual disturbances arising from multiple sclerosis. Acta Neurol Scand 70:229–306, 1984.

160. Miró J, Carcia-Moncó C, Leno C, and Berciano J: Clinical Note. Pelvic pain: An undescribed paroxysmal manifestation of multiple sclerosis. Pain 32:73–75, 1988.

161. Mitchell DR, Swirsky-Sacchetti T, Knobler RL, et al: Correlation of mood state with cerebral MRI and severity of illness in patients with MS. Neurology 41:145, 1991.

162. Moller A, Wiedemann G, Rohde U, Backmund H, and Sonntag A: Correlates of cognitive impairment and depressive mood disorder in multiple sclerosis. Acta Psychiatr Scand 89:117–121, 1994.

163. Montalban J, Fernandez AL, Duran I, Tintoré M, Galan I, and Acarin N: Antiganglioside antibodies en sera of MS patients (abstract). J Neurol 241(suppl 1):S73, 1994.

164. Moulin DE: Pain in multiple sclerosis. Neurol Clin 7(2):321–331, 1989.

165. Moxon W: Eight cases of insular sclerosis of the brain and spinal cord. Guys Hospital Reports, London 20:437–478, 1875.

166. Mutani R, Clemente S, Lamberti A, and Monaco F: Assessment of autonomic disturbances in multiple sclerosis by measurement of heart rate responses to deep breathing and to standing. Ital J Neurol Sci 2:111–114, 1982.

167. Myers LW, Ellison GW, Lucia M, et al: Swine influenza virus vaccination in patients with multiple sclerosis. J Infect Dis 136:5546–5554, 1977.

168. Namerow NS: A discussion concerning physical trauma in multiple sclerosis. Bulletin LA Neurological Societies 32:117–124, 1969.

169. Namerow NS, and Thompson LR: Plaques, symptoms and the remitting course of multiple sclerosis. Neurology 19:765–774, 1969.

170. Nelson LM, Franklin GM, Jones MC, and the Multiple Sclerosis Study Group: Risk of multiple sclerosis exacerbation during pregnancy and breast-feeding. JAMA 359(23):3441–3443, 1988.

171. Neubauer B, and Gundersen HJG: Analysis of heart 41:417–419, 1978.

172. Newman NJ, and Lessell S: Isolated pupil-sparing third-nerve palsy as the presenting sign of multiple sclerosis. Arch Neurol 47:817–818, 1990.

173. Newton MR, Barrett G, Callanan MM, and Towell AD: Cognitive event-related potentials in multiple sclerosis. Brain 112:1637–1660, 1989.

174. Nissenblatt MJ, Masciulli L, Yarian DL, and Duvoisin R: Pars planitis: A demyelinating disease? Archives of Ophthalmology 99(4):697, 1981.

175. Noffsinger D, Olsen WO, Carhart R, Hart CW, and Sahgal V: Auditory and vestibular aberrations in multiple sclerosis. Acta Oto-Laryngolouila Supplement 303:1–63, 1972.

176. Noronha MJ, Vas CJ, and Aziz H: Autonomic dysfunction (sweating responses) in multiple sclerosis. J Neurol Neurosurg Psychiatry 31:19–22, 1968.

177. Noseworthy JH, and Heffernan LPM: Motor radiculopathy: An unusual presentation of multiple sclerosis. Can J Neurol Sci 1(3):207–209, 1980.

178. Noseworthy JH, Paty DW, Wonnacott T, Feasby TE, and Ebers GC: MS after age 50. Neurology 33:1537–1544, 1983.

179. Nuwer MR, Packwood JW, Myers LW, and Ellison GW: Evoked potentials predict the clinical changes in a multiple sclerosis drug study. Neurology 37:1754–1761, 1987.

180. Olerup O, Hillert J, Fredrikson S, et al: Primarily chronic progressive and relapsing/remitting multiple sclerosis: Two immunogenetically distinct disease entities. Proc Natl Acad Sci USA 86:7113–7117, 1989.

181. Oppenheim H: Textbook of Nervous Diseases for Physicians and Students. O Schulze & Co, Edinburgh, 1911.

182. Optic Neuritis Study Group: The clinical profile of optic neuritis: Experience of the Optic Neuritis Treatment Trial. Arch Ophthalmol 109:1673–1678, 1991.

183. Osterman PO: Paroxysmal itching in multiple sclerosis. Int J Dermatol 18:626–627, 1979.

184. Parker HL: Trigeminal neuralgic pain associated with multiple sclerosis. Brain 51:46–62, 1928.

185. Parsons OA, Stewart KD, and Arenberg D: Impairment of abstracting ability in multiple sclerosis. J Nerv Ment Dis 125:221–225, 1957.

186. Paty DW: Magnetic resonance imaging in the assessment of disease activity in multiple sclerosis. Can J Neurol Sci 15:266–272, 1988.

187. Paty DW, Li DKB, the UBC MS/MRI Study Group, and the IFNB Multiple Sclerosis Study Group: Interferon beta-1b is effective in relapsing-remitting multiple sclerosis. 2. MRI analysis of results of a multicenter, randomized, double-blind, placebo-controlled trial. Neurology 43: 662–667, 1993.

188. Paty DW, Oger JJF, Kastrukoff LF, et al: MRI in the diagnosis of MS: A prospective study with comparison of clinical evaluation, evoked potentials, oligoclonal banding and CT. Neurology 38:180–185, 1988.

189. Patzold U, and Pocklington PR: Course of multiple sclerosis: First results of a prospective study carried out of 102 MS patients from 1976–1980. Acta Neurol Scand 65:248–266, 1982.

190. Pentland B, and Ewing DJ: Cardiovascular reflexes in multiple sclerosis. Eur Neurol 26:46–50, 1987.

191. Perniola T, Russo MG, Margari L, Butiglione M, and Simone IL: Multiple sclerosis in childhood: Longitudinal study in 14 cases. Acta Neurol (Napoli) 13:236–248, 1991.

191a. Petajan JH, Gappmaier E, White AT, Spencer MK, Mino L, Hicks RW: Impact of aerobic training on fitness and quality of life in multiple sclerosis. Ann Neurol 39:432–441, 1996.

192. Peyser JM, Edwards KR, Poser CM, and Filskov SB: Cognitive function in patients with multiple sclerosis. Arch Neurol 37:577–579, 1980.

193. Peyser JM, Rao SM, LaRocca NG, and Kaplan E: Guidelines for neuropsychological research in multiple sclerosis. Arch Neurol 47:94–97, 1990.

194. Poirier G, Montplaisir J, Dumont M, et al: Clinical and sleep laboratory study of narcoleptic symptoms in multiple sclerosis. Neurology 37: 693–695, 1987.

195. Pollock M, Calder C, and Allpress S: Peripheral nerve abnormality in multiple sclerosis. Ann Neurol 2:41–48, 1977.

196. Portenoy RK, Yang K, and Thorton D: Chronic intractable pain: An atypical presentation of multiple sclerosis. J Neurol 235:226–228, 1988.

197. Poser CM: Trauma and multiple sclerosis: A hypothesis. J Neurol 234:155–159, 1987.

198. Poser CM: Multiple sclerosis. Observations and reflections: A personal memoir. J Neurol Sci 107:127–140, 1992.

198a. Poser CM: Letter to the editor. Neurology 44:1360–1362, 1994.

199. Poser S: Multiple Sclerosis: An Analysis of 812 Cases by Means of Electronic Data Processing. Springer-Verlag, New York, 1978.

200. Poser S, and Poser W: Multiple sclerosis and gestation. Neurology 33:1422–1427, 1983.

201. Povlishock JT, Becker DP, Sullivan HG, and Miller JD: Vascular permeability alterations to horseradish peroxidase in experimental brain injury. Brain Res 153:223–229, 1978.

202. Pozzilli C, Bastianello S, Padovani A, et al: Anterior corpus callosum atrophy and verbal fluency in multiple sclerosis. Cortex 27:441–445, 1991.

203. Pozzilli C, Fieschi C, Perani D, Paulesu E, and Comi G: Relationship between corpus callosum atrophy and cerebral metabolic assymmetries in multiple sclerosis. J Neurol Sci 112:51–57, 1992.

204. Pozzilli C, Grasso MG, Bastianello S, et al: Structural brain correlates of neurologic abnormalities in multiple sclerosis. Eur Neurol 32:228–230, 1992.

205. Prineas JW: The neuropathology of multiple sclerosis. In Koetsier J (ed): Handbook of Clinical Neurology. Elsevier, Amsterdam, 1985, pp 213–257.

206. Quine DB, Regan D, Beverley KI, and Murray TJ:

Patients with multiple sclerosis experience hearing loss specifically for shifts of tone frequency. Arch Neurol 41:506–508, 1984.

207. Ransohoff RM, Whitman GJ, and Weinstein MA: Noncommunication syringomyelia in multiple sclerosis: Detection by magnetic resonance imaging. Neurology 40:718–721, 1990.

208. Rao SM: Neuropsychology of multiple sclerosis: A critical review. J Clin Exp Neuropsychol 8:503–542, 1986.

209. Rao SM: Neurobehavioral Aspects of Multiple Sclerosis. Oxford University Press, New York, 1990.

210. Rao SM, Leo GJ, Ellington L, Nauertz T, Bernardin L, and Unverzagt F: Cognitive dysfunction in multiple sclerosis. 2. Impact on employment and social functioning. Neurology 41:692–696, 1991.

211. Rao SM, Leo GJ, and St Aubin-Faubert P: On the nature of memory disturbance in multiple sclerosis. J Clin Exp Neuropsychol 11:699–712, 1989.

212. Rasminsky M: The effects of temperature on conduction in demyelinated single nerve fibers. Arch Neurol 28:287–292, 1973.

213. Rasminsky M, and Sears TA: Internodal conduction in undissected demyelinated nerve fibres. J Physiol 227:323–350, 1972.

214. Raza-Ahmad A, Sangalang V, Klassen GA, and McCormick CW: Focal myocardial necrosis associated with multiple sclerosis of the medulla. Am J Cardiol 68:1542–1544, 1991.

215. Remick RA, Sadovnick AD, Allen JM, Swartz E, Yee IML, and Paty DW: Mood disorders and multiple sclerosis (abstract). Canadian Psychiatric Association Annual Meeting, Ottawa, 1994.

215a. Revesz T, Kidd D, Thompson AJ, Barnard RO, McDonald WI: A comparison of the pathology of primary and secondary progressive multiple sclerosis. Brain 117:759–765, 1994.

216. Ritchie JM, and Rogart RB: Density of sodium channels in mammalian myelinated nerve fibers and nature of the axonal membrane under the myelinated nerve impulses from the myelinized part of the axon into the nonmyelinated terminal. Proc Nat Acad Sci USA 74:211–215, 1977.

217. Rolak LA, and Brown S: Headaches and multiple sclerosis: A clinical study and review of the literature. J Neurol 237:300–302, 1990.

218. Ron MA, Callanan MM, and Warrington EK: Cognitive abnormalities in multiple sclerosis: A psychometric and MRI study. Psychol Med 21:59–68, 1991.

219. Ron MA, and Feinstein A: Multiple sclerosis and the mind (editorial). J Neurol Neurosurg Psychiatry 55:1–3, 1992.

220. Rose AS, Kuzma JW, Kurtzke JF, Namerow NS, Sibley WA, and Tourtellotte WW: Cooperative study in the evaluation of therapy in multiple sclerosis: H vs. placebo. Neurology 20:1–59, 1970.

221. Rosenberg NL, and Bourdette D: Hypertrophic neuropathy and multiple sclerosis. Neurology 33:1361–1364, 1983.

222. Rosengren LE, Lycke J, and Andersen O: Glial fibrillary acidic protein in CFS of multiple sclerosis patients: Relation to neurological deficit. Journal of the Neurological Sciences 133(1-2): 61–65, Nov. 1995.

223. Ruchkin DS, Grafman J, Krauss GL, Johnson R Jr, Canoune H, and Ritter W: Event-related brain potential evidence for a verbal working memory deficit in multiple sclerosis. Brain 117(pt 2): 289–305, 1994.

224. Rucker CW: Retinopathy of multiple sclerosis. Trans Am Ophthalmol Soc 45:564–570, 1947.

225. Rushton JG, and Olafson RA: Trigeminal neuralgia associated with multiple sclerosis. Arch Neurol 13:383–384, 1965.

226. Sadovnick AD, Eisen K, Ebers GC, and Paty DW: Cause of death in patients attending multiple sclerosis clinics. Neurology 41:1193–1196, 1991.

227. Sadovnick AD, Ebers GC, Wilson RW, and Paty DW: Life expectancy in patients attending multiple sclerosis clinics. Neurology 42:991–994, 1992.

228. Sadovnick AD, Eisen K, Hashimoto SA, Farquhar R, Yee IML, Hooge J, Kastrukoff L, et al.: Pregnancy and multiple sclerosis: A prospective study. Arch Neurol 51:1120–1124, 1994.

229. Saito H, Kobayashi K, Mochizuki H, and Ishii T: Axonal degeneration of the peripheral nerves and postganglionic anhidrosis in a patient with multiple sclerosis. Tohoku J Exp Med 162:279–291, 1990.

230. Sanders EACM, and Lee KD: Acute Guillain-Barré syndrome in multiple sclerosis. J Neurol 234:128, 1987.

231. Sandroni P, Walker C, and Starr A: 'Fatigue' in patients with multiple sclerosis: Motor pathway conduction and event-related potentials. Arch Neurol 49:517–524, 1992.

232. Sandyk R: Coexisting bipolar affective disorder and multiple sclerosis: The role of the pineal gland (letter). Int J Neurosci 59:267–270, 1991.

233. Schapira K: The seasonal incidence of onset and exacerbations in multiple sclerosis. J Neurol Neurosurg Psychiatry 22:285–286, 1959.

234. Schapira K, Poskanzer DC, Newell DJ, and Miller HD: Marriage, pregnancy and multiple sclerosis. Brain 89:419–428, 1966.

235. Schauf CL, and Davis FA: Impulse conduction in multiple sclerosis: A theoretical basis for modification by temperature and pharmacological agents. J Neurol Neurosurg Psychiatry 37:152–161, 1974.

236. Schiffer RB, Rudick RA, and Herndon RM: Psychological aspects of multiple sclerosis. New York State Journal of Medicine 83(3):312–316, 1983.

237. Schoene WC, Carpenter S, Behan PO, and Geschwind N: 'Onion bulb' formations in the central and peripheral nervous sustem in association with multiple sclerosis and hypertrophic polyneuropathy. Brain 100:755–773, 1977.

238. Schumacher GA, Beebe G, Kibler RF, et al: Problems of experimental trials of therapy in multiple sclerosis: Report by the panel on the evaluation of experimental trials of therapy in multiple sclerosis. Ann NY Acad Med 122:552–568, 1965.

239. Senaratne MPJ, Carroll D, Warren KG, and Kappagoda T: Evidence for cardiovascular autonomic nerve dysfunction in multiple sclerosis. J Neurol Neurosurg Psychiatry 47:947–952, 1984.

240. Sharief MK, and Hentges R: Association between tumor necrosis factor-alpha and disease

progression in patients with multiple sclerosis. N Engl J Med 325:467–472, 1991.

241. Sharpe JA, and Sanders MD: Atrophy of myelinated nerve fibers in the retina in optic neuritis. Br J Ophthalmol 59:229–232, 1975.

242. Shaw CM, and Alvord EC: Multiple sclerosis beginning in infancy. J Child Neurol 2:252–256, 1987.

243. Shibasaki H, and Kuroiwa Y: Painful tonic seizure in multiple sclerosis. Arch Neurol 30:47–51, 1974.

244. Sibley WA: Therapeutic Claims in Multiple Sclerosis. Demos Publications, New York, 1988.

245. Sibley WA: Physical trauma and multiple sclerosis (editorial, comment, and review). Neurology 43:1871–1874, 1993.

246. Sibley WA, Bamford CR, and Clark K: Clinical viral infections and multiple sclerosis. The Lancet 1:1313–1315, 1985.

247. Sibley WA, Bamford CR, Clark K, Smith MS, and Laguna JF: A prospective study of physical trauma and multiple sclerosis. J Neurol Neurosurg Psychiatry 54:584–589, 1991.

248. Sibley WA, and Foley JM: Infection and immunization in multiple sclerosis. Ann NY Acad Sci 122:457–468, 1965.

249. Sibley WA, and Paty DW: A comparison of multiple sclerosis in Arizona (USA) and Ontario (Canada) preliminary report. Acta Neurol Scand 64 (suppl 87):60-65, 1981.

250. Siemkowicz E: Multiple sclerosis and surgery. Anaesthesia 31:1211–1216, 1976.

251. Simon RP, Gean-Marton AD, and Sander JE: Medullary lesion inducing pulmonary edema: A magnetic resonance imaging study. Ann Neurol 30:727–730, 1991.

252. Siva A, Radhakrishnan K, Kurland LT, O'Brien PC, Swanson JW, and Rodriguez M: Trauma and multiple sclerosis: A population-based cohort study from Olmsted County, Minnesota. Neurology 43:1878–1882, 1993.

253. Slamovits TL, Rosen CE, Cheng KP, and Striph GG: Visual recovery in patients with optic neuritis and visual loss to no light perception. Am J Ophthalmol 111:209–214, 1991.

254. Smith KJ, Blakemore WF, and McDonald WI: Central remyelination restores secure conduction. Nature 280:395–396, 1979.

255. Smith ME, Stone LA, Albert PS, et al: Clinical worsening in multiple sclerosis is associated with increased frequency and area of gadopentetate dimeglumine-enhancing magnetic resonance imaging lesions. Ann Neurol 33:480–489, 1993.

256. Sorensen M, Lorentzen M, Petersen J, and Christiansen J: Anorectal dysfunction in patients with urologic disturbance due to multiple sclerosis. Dis Colon Rectum 34:136–139, 1991.

257. Stenager E, Knudsen L, and Jensen K: Acute and chronic pain syndromes in multiple sclerosis. Acta Neurol Scand 84:197–200, 1991.

258. Stenager E, Stenager EN, and Jensen K: Sexual aspects of multiple sclerosis. Semin Neurol 12:120–124, 1992.

259. Sterman AB, Coyle PK, Panasci DJ, and Grimson R: Disseminated abnormalities of cardiovascular autonomic functions in multiple sclerosis. Neurology 35:1665–1668, 1985.

260. Sternberg EM (moderator), Chrousos GP, Wilder RL, and Gold PW (discussants): The stress response and the regulation of inflammatory disease. NIH Conference. Ann Int Med 117:854–866, 1992.

261. Studney D, Lublin F, Marcucci L, et al: MS COSTAR: A computerized record for use in clinical research in multiple sclerosis. J of Neurological Rehabilitation 7(3–4):145–152, 1993.

262. Sullivan F, Hutchinson M, Bahandeka S, and Moore RE: Chronic hypothermia in multiple sclerosis. J Neurol Neurosurg Psychiatry 50:813–815, 1987.

263. Swingler RJ, and Compston DAS: The morbidity of multiple sclerosis. QJM 83:325–337, 1992.

264. Swirsky-Sacchetti T, Mitchell D, Knobler RL, et al: Analysis and correlation of neuropsychological deficits with structural brain lesions in patients with multiple sclerosis. Neurology (suppl 1) 41:145, 1991.

265. Szasz G, Paty DW, Lawton-Speert S, and Eisen KA: A sexual functioning scale in multiple sclerosis. Acta Neurol Scand 70(suppl 101):37–43, 1984.

266. Szasz G, Paty DW, and Maurice WL: Sexual dysfunctions in multiple sclerosis. Ann NY Acad Sci 436:443–452, 1984.

267. Thompson AJ, Hutchinson M, Brazil J, Feighery C, and Martin EA: A clinical and laboratory study of benign multiple sclerosis. QJM 58:69–80, 1986.

268. Thompson AJ, Kermode AG, Wicks DAG, et al: Major differences in the dynamics of primary and secondary progressive multiple sclerosis. Ann Neurol 29:53–62, 1991.

269. Thompson AJ, Youl B, Feinstein A, et al: Serial enhanced MRI in early relapsing/remitting and benign multiple sclerosis. Neurology (suppl 1) 41:169, 1991.

270. Thompson DS, Nelson LM, Burns A, Burks JS, and Franklin GM: The effects of pregnancy in multiple sclerosis: A retrospective study. Neurology 36:1097–1099, 1986.

271. Truyen L, Barkhof F, Frequin STF, Polman CH, Hommes O, and Valk J: A case-control study of epilepsy in multiple sclerosis using magnetic resonance imaging: Implications for treatment trials with 4-aminopyridine. 10th Congress of the European Committee for Treatment and Research in Multiple Sclerosis, Book of Abstracts, Athens, Greece (not published), 1994, p 38.

272. Truyen L, Gheuens J, Van de Vyver FL, Parizel PM, Peersman GV, and Martin JJ: Improved correlation of magnetic resonance imaging (MRI) with clinical status in multiple sclerosis (MS) by use of an extensive standardized imaging-protocol. J Neurol Sci 96:173–182, 1990.

273. Tschabitscher H: Die klinischen und experimentallen forschungen bie der multiplen sklerose. Wiener Zeitschrift für Nervenheilkunde 14:381– 436, 1958.

274. Uhthoff W: Untersuchungen uber bei multiplen Herdsklerose vorkommenden Augenstorungen. Archiv Fur Psychiatrie und Nervenkrankheiten 21:55–116, 303–410, 1890.

275. Uitti RJ, and Rajput AH: Multiple sclerosis pre-

senting as isolated oculomotor nerve palsy. Can J Neurol Sci 13:270–272, 1986.

276. Uitti RJ, and Rajput AH: Headache, third nerve palsy, and MS. Neurology 41:331, 1991.

277. Valleroy ML, and Kraft GH: Sexual dysfunction in multiple sclerosis. Arch Phys Med Rehab 65:125–128, 1984.

278. Vas CJ: Sexual impotence and some autonomic disturbances in men with multiple sclerosis. Acta Neurol Scand 45:166–182, 1969.

278a. Vercoulen JHMM, Hommes OR, Swanink CMA, et al: The measurement of fatigue in patients with multiple sclerosis: A multidimensional comparison with patients with chronic fatigue syndrome and healthy subjects. Arch Neurol 53:642–649, 1996.

279. Vermote R, Ketelaer P, and Carton H: Pain in multiple sclerosis patients: A prospective study using the McGill pain questionnaire. Clin Neurol Neurosurg 88:87-93, 1986.

280. Visintainer PF, Lauer K, and Poser CM: Physical trauma and multiple sclerosis. (letters to editor). Neurology 44:1360–1362, 1994.

281. Vita G, Fazio MC, Milone S, Blandino A, Salvi L, and Messina C: Cardiovascular autonomic dysfunction in multiple sclerosis is likely related to brainstem lesions. J Neurol Sci 120:82–86, 1993.

282. Warnell P: The pain experience of a multiple sclerosis population: A descriptive study. Axone 13:26–28, 1991.

283. Warren KG, and Catz I: A correlation between cerebrospinal fluid myelin basic protein and anti-myelin basic protein in multiple sclerosis patients. Ann Neurol 21:183–189, 1987.

283a. Warren KG, Catz I and McPherson TA: CSF myelin basic protein levels in acute optic neuritis and multiple sclerosis. Can. J. Neurol Sci 10:235–238, 1983.

284. Warren S, Greenhill S, and Warren KG: Emotional stress and the development of multiple sclerosis: Case-control evidence of a relationship. Journal of Chronic Diseases 35:821–831, 1982.

285. Warren S, Warren KG, and Cockerill R: Emotional stress and coping in multiple sclerosis (MS) exacerbations. J Psychosom Res 35:37–47, 1991.

286. Wartenberg R: Neuritis and multiple sclerosis: Neuritis, Sensory Neuritis, Neuralgia, vol 32. Oxford University Press, New York, 1958, pp 296–305.

287. Waxman SG: Biophysical mechanisms of impulse conduction in demyelinated axons. In Waxman SG (ed): Advances in Neurology: Functional Recovery in Neurological Disease. Raven Press, New York, 1988, pp 185–221.

288. Waxman SG: Clinical course and electrophysiology of multiple sclerosis. In Waxman SG (ed): Advances in Neurology: Functional Recovery in Neurological Disease. Raven Press, New York, 1988, pp 157–184.

289. Waxman SG: Clinicopathological correlations in multiple sclerosis and related diseases. In Waxman SG, and Ritchie JM (eds): Demyelinating Disease: Basic and Clinical Electrophysiology. Raven Press, New York, 1981, pp 169–182.

290. Waxman SG: Peripheral nerve abnormalities in multiple sclerosis (editorial). Muscle Nerve 16:1–5, 1993.

291. Waxman SG, and Geschwind N: Major morbidity related to hyperthermia in multiple sclerosis. Ann Neurol 13:348, 1983.

292. Weinshenker BG, Bass B, Rice GPA, et al: The natural history of multiple sclerosis: A geographically based study. I. Clinical course and disability. Brain 112:133–146, 1989.

293. Weinshenker BG, and Ebers GC: The natural history of multiple sclerosis. Can J Neurol Sci 14:255–261, 1987.

294. Weinshenker BG, Gilbert JJ, and Ebers GC: Some clinical and pathologic observations on chronic myelopathy: A variant of multiple sclerosis. J Neurol Neurosurg Psychiatry 53:146–149, 1990.

295. Weinshenker BG, Hader W, Carriere W, Baskerville J, and Ebers GC: The influence of pregnancy on disability from multiple sclerosis: A population-based study in Middlesex County, Ontario. Neurology 39:1438–1440, 1989.

296. Weir AI, Hansen S, and Ballantyne JP: Single fibre electromyographic jitter in multiple sclerosis. J Neurol Neurosurg Psychiatry 42:1146–1150, 1979.

297. Weir AI, Hansen S, and Ballantyne JP: Motor unit potential abnormalities in multiple sclerosis: Further evidence for a peripheral nervous system defect. J Neurol Neurosurg Psychiatry 43:999–1004, 1980.

298. Whitaker JN: The presence of immunoreactive myelin basic protein peptide in urine of persons with multiple sclerosis. Ann Neurol 22:648–655, 1987.

299. Willoughby EW, Grochowski E, Li DKB, Oger JJF, Kastrukoff LF, and Paty DW: A prospective study of MRI scanning in multiple sclerosis. Neurology (suppl 1) 37:231, 1987.

300. Willoughby EW, Grochowski E, Li DKB, Oger JJF, Kastrukoff LF, and Paty DW: Serial magnetic resonance scanning in multiple sclerosis: A second prospective study in relapsing patients. Ann Neurol 25:43–49, 1989.

301. Worthington J, Jones R, Crawford M, and Forti A: Pregnancy and multiple sclerosis: A 3-year prospective study. J Neurol 241:228–233, 1994.

302. Wuthrich R, and Rieder HP: The seasonal incidence of multiple sclerosis in Switzerland. Eur Neurol 3:257–264, 1970.

303. Yokota T, Matsunaga T, Okiyama R, et al: Sympathetic skin response in patients with multiple sclerosis compared with patients with spinal cord transection and normal controls. Brain 114 (pt 3):1381–1394, 1991.

304. Zee PC, Cohen BA, Walczak T, and Jubelt B: Peripheral nervous system involvement in multiple sclerosis. Neurology 41:457–460, 1991.

CHAPTER 6

NATURAL HISTORY STUDIES AND APPLICATIONS TO CLINICAL TRIALS

George C. Ebers, MD
Donald W. Paty, MD

Despite many years of study, knowledge of the natural history of MS continues to be refined and modified.[43,76,78,79,95–98] The diagnostic uncertainties, a poorly defined biologic age of onset, and wide variation in both age of clinical onset and severity have been among the confounding factors. Until recently, disagreement about outcome, its measurement, and the factors that influence it have left the impression that MS is largely, if not entirely, unpredictable. This perception is shared with many other chronic putatively autoimmune disorders that also have wide variation in age of onset and severity.

Outcome is often paramount in the minds of the newly diagnosed patients and their families. Self-perception of prognosis is often heavily influenced by prior exposure to MS. If such exposure is limited to a bedridden neighbor or to the wheelchair-bound patients seen in promotional literature, expectations are often unnecessarily gloomy. Young patients contemplating career choices or families often want more information than vague statements about unpredictability, or testimonials about individual patients with extraordinarily benign outcomes. For the practicing neurologist, the identification of factors that influence prognosis has considerable practical value in the assessment of risk to benefit ratios for putatively effective therapies.[25] Finally, the efficient, ethical conduct of clinical trials demands a thorough knowledge and understanding of the natural history to avoid the oft-repeated errors that have made the results of many MS clinical trials inconclusive or erroneous.[61] In particular, when potentially toxic therapies are being tested, investigators have a responsibility to shorten the duration of exposure to the minimum required to reach an unequivocal result. This principle is particularly relevant when it is recalled that no therapy has yet been identified that alters the long-term natural history of the disease.

In this chapter, the current understanding of natural history in MS is reviewed, with emphasis on recent population-based studies, which have served to increase our confidence in the validity of prognostic indicators. In addition, some of the natural history data are applied to the interpretation of completed trials, illustrating the potential usefulness of this approach in putting trial results in a more general and practical context.

THE IDEAL STUDY

The characteristics of the ideal study of natural history have been described by Sackett and colleagues.[85] First, a population-based sample of patients ascertained near the onset of disease (inception cohort) is identified. Then longitudinal outcome data are gathered over a duration of follow-up appropriate to the course of the disease.

Several practical constraints make attainment of this ideal difficult in MS. One problem is difficulty in identifying patients at biologic onset of MS. This is epitomized by the many patients found to have the disease incidentally on autopsy.[18,22,49] It is also difficult to maintain longitudinal follow-up of adequate sample sizes and to avoid bias toward the more severe cases that characterize tertiary referral centers. Benign cases are well known.[2] An additional constraint is imposed by the lack of concordance of the most commonly used outcome measures of disability with biologic activity being demonstrated pathologically, by MRI, or by both methods. Finally, it is no longer easy to identify cohorts of patients who have not received various forms of therapy, a confounding factor often self-selected by performance on one or another outcome measure. All studies to date, including our own, define the "unnatural" history of MS inversely proportionate to the ability to conform with these ideal requirements.

Table 6–1 summarizes the major outcome studies in MS and lists the important characteristics of each. It is clear that considerable heterogeneity exists among these studies, with wide variation in methods of ascertainment and duration of longitudinal follow-up (summarized in Table 6–2). Early studies were largely clinic-based and included mixtures of inpatients and outpatients,[52,58] with a bias toward patients with rapid disease progression, especially evident in hospital-based data.[77]

Sample Size and Ascertainment

The ideal sample size is unknown; however, given the considerable variation in both clinical phenotype and outcome, few authors have hazarded conclusions on samples of less than 200 patients. The recognition that the method of ascertainment is an important determinant of outcome is illustrated in the excellent systematic study by Poser and colleagues.[77] A strong bias toward more severe disability in a hospital-based series as compared with a community-based one was clearly shown. Because many patients seek medical evaluation

Table 6–1. STUDIES OF OUTCOME IN MULTIPLE SCLEROSIS: POPULATION SIZE AND PATIENT ASCERTAINMENT

SENIOR AUTHOR	YEAR	LOCATION	POPULATION SIZE	DIAGNOSTIC CERTAINTY	ASCERTAINMENT H	ASCERTAINMENT C	ASCERTAINMENT P	GEOGRAPHICALLY BASED*	MEAN O–A
Runmarker[84]	1993	Goteborg, Sweden	308	DP	—	—	+	+	NR
Miller[53]	1992	Wellington, New Zealand	245	DPP	+	+	+	+	NR
Phadke[74]	1990	Scotland	1055	DPP	+	+	+	+	NR
Goodkin[27†]	1989	North Dakota	425	DP	+	+	—	—	NR
Thompson[92]	1986	Dublin	290	DP	+	+	—	—	NR
Visscher[94]	1984	Los Angeles County; King and Pierce counties, Wash.	941	—	—	—	—	—	—
Detels[14]	1982	Los Angeles County; King and Pierce counties, Wash.	886	DP	—	—	+	+	<10
Clark[10]	1982	Los Angeles County; King and Pierce counties, Wash.	834	—	—	—	—	—	—
Verjans[93]	1983	Belgium	200	D	—	+	—	—	NR
Patzold[72]	1982	Hanover, Germany	102	NR	—	+	—	—	3‡
Poser[77]	1982	Gottigen, Germany	2058	DPP	+(1837)	+(221)	—	+(221)	NR
Broman[5]	1981	Gothenburg, Sweden	312	DPP	—	+	—	+	NR
Confavreux[11]	1980	Lyon, France	349	DPP	—	+	—	+	NR
Kurtzke[43]	1977	United States	527	DP	—	—	+ (army discharges)	—	3‡
Percy[73]	1971	Rochester, Minn.	67	CP		+		—	NR
Gudmundsson[28]	1971	Iceland	104	DPP		+	—	+	12
Fog[21]	1970	Copenhagen, Denmark	73	D		+	—	—	NR
Leibowitz[46]	1970	Israel	266	DPP		—	+	+	11.5
Panelius[67]	1969	Turku District, Finland	146	DP		—	+	+	5
McAlpine[51]	1961	London, England	247	—	+	+	—	—	<3
McAlpine[52]	1952	London, England	675	—	+	+	—	—	NR

Source: Adapted from Weinshenker and Ebers,[99] p 256.

*According to author; supported or unsupported, most cases in the area surveyed were identified.

†The dropout rate was 62% in 2.5 yr mean follow-up.

‡Estimate is based on available data.

C = clinic; D = clinically definite; DP = clinically definite and probable; DPP = clinically definite, probable and possible; H = hospital; NR = not recorded; O–A = onset to ascertainment (time in years); P = prevalence survey; + = yes.

Table 6–2. **PATIENT FOLLOW-UP**

SENIOR AUTHOR	TYPE OF STUDY			YEARS OF FOLLOW-UP (MEAN)	YEARS OF DISEASE (MEAN)*
	P	L	CS		
Runmarker[84]	+	+	+	25+	25+
Miller[53]	—	+	+	15	15
Phadke[74]	—	+	+	—	—
Goodkin[27]	+	+	—	2.6	—
Thompson[92]	—	—	+	—	11.4
Visscher[94] Detels[14] Clark[10]	+	—	—	10	—
Verjans[93]	—	—	+	—	—
Patzold[72]	+	—	—	3.5	—
Poser[77]					
Epidemiological	—	+	—	—	12.1
Hospital	—	—	+	—	10.5
Broman[5]	—	+	—	—	—
Confavreux[11]	—	+	—	9	—
Kurtzke[43]	—	—	+(multiple points)	—	—
Percy[73]	—	+		—	—
Gudmundsson[28]	+	—		—	24
Fog[21]	+	—		10*	20†
Leibowitz[46]	—	+		—	11.5
Panelius[67]	—	+		—	—
McAlpine[51]	+	—		—	—
McAlpine[52]	—	+		—	—

Source: Adapted from Weinshenker and Ebers,[99] p 257.
*Duration shown is that at the conclusion of follow-up in prospective and longitudinal studies.
†Estimate is based on available data.
CS = cross-sectional; L = longitudinal; P = prospective; + = yes; — = not applicable or available.

some years after clinical symptoms begin, it seems that a true inception cohort is impossible.

Two strategies that can help to minimize ascertainment bias are:

1. Separately evaluating patients seen at onset, and
2. Confining analysis to population-based samples from communities subjected to formal prevalence studies.

The first approach has been used by McAlpine and Compston[52] and Kurtzke and colleagues,[43] among others, and the second approach by a number of investigators, including Visscher and colleagues[94] in the United States; Confavreux and colleagues[11] in Lyon, France; Leibowitz and colleagues[46,47] in Israel; and Gudmundsson[28] in Iceland. However, some of these studies have included patients treated with immunosuppressive drugs.[11,72] Both approaches characterize recent studies from Canada.[16,96–98]

Follow-up

The unattainable ideal for follow-up is from onset of MS to death. In practice, even in studies that use prospectively collected samples,[14,72,94] one finds heterogeneity in duration of illness and in disability at entry. Cross-sectional studies are not easily interpreted because outcome measures are likely to be unstable or reversible. This problem is well exemplified in Kurtzke and colleagues' study,[43] which found that of 34 patients with *severe* disability at diagnosis, 11.8 percent had only *mild* disability at 10 years and 32.4 percent had *moderate* disability at 10 years. Accordingly, more than 40 percent of patients were actually better 10 years later than they had been when they were first surveyed. This finding clearly implies that the initial evaluation did not take place at a time when disability had stabilized or was irreversible. Again, the characteristics of a hospital-derived sample are evident. Maximum improvement after an acute exacerbation resulting in hospitalization is rarely achieved at discharge. A minimum duration of follow-up of at least a decade would be required for significant disability to occur in at least 50 percent of patients. Relatively few studies, however, have been able to follow patients for this duration. One recent report describing "natural history" had a mean follow-up of 2.6 years[26]—less than the duration of many clinical trials.

Clinical Outcome Measures

The standard for measuring outcome in most studies has been the Kurtzke Disability Status Scale (DSS),[40] or the Expanded Disability Status Scale (EDSS).[41] Although meant to be a measure of impairment, it is primarily a mobility scale and is insensitive to other forms of major impairment, such as blindness or dementia. The cross-sectional distribution of EDSS scores clearly does not follow a normal Gaussian distribution as initially claimed.[40] This is shown in data from both the Vancouver clinic (see Chapter 12) and the London clinic (Table 6–3). The two data sets are remarkably similar and show a biphasic (Bactrian) distribution of EDSS scores with a "valley" for Kurtzke disability levels 4 and 5.

Despite these drawbacks, the EDSS is clinically relevant, familiar, and has useful sensitivity. Furthermore, as a nonlinear (ordinal) scale, changes appear to reliably reflect biologic activity and meaningful progression. From the standpoint of clinical trials, progress by one level on this scale is

Table 6–3. CROSS-SECTION OF DISABILITY AT FINAL REVIEW

DSS Level	No. (%) of Patients at DSS Level*
1	182 (17)
2	156 (14)
3	123 (11)
4	71 (6)
5	31 (3)
6	205 (19)
7	203 (18)
8	88 (8)
9	23 (2)
10	16 (1)
Data unavailable	1
Total	1099

Source: From Weinshenker et al,[95] p 139.
*These data are derived from the total population surveyed at the MS Clinic, London, Ontario, 1984.
DSS = Disability Status Scale (Kurtzke).

clearly not equivalent at different levels on the scale. This concept poses potential difficulties for trials that include patients at several different levels, because a randomization process may not distribute equal numbers of patients at different DSS levels. Comparing changes in mean DSS levels, as has been done in many clinical trials, is accordingly hazardous. In this discussion, the term *disability* is used in referring to the DSS, which represents a mixed impairment and disability measurement.

Several studies have evaluated the degree of interrater and intrapatient variability[24,60,64] using this scale, a major factor in its continued use. Even though this variability is not uniform throughout the scale, with practice, the EDSS scale is acceptable. Although the variability is greater than many would have expected, some of this variability derives from the subjects' motivation and performance, a factor over which the investigator has relatively little control. Clinical observation of performance (observed EDSS) is strongly preferred to patient testimonial.

Other clinical measures have been designed for clinical trials, although their use has been irregular. Some scales have been designed and first used by investigators in their own specific trials.[12,32] The ambulation index,[32] for example, while appropriately focusing on direct observation of the core component of the EDSS, can be overly sensitive and needs further validation of variability. It was used as a measure for a major trial in concert with the Kurtzke scale. Reassuringly, both these scales gave results that were highly concordant. Although one might intuit that a scoring system based on the neurological examination would be the most sensitive and reproducible measure, this has not yet been demonstrated. In one trial, the standard neurological examination score[83] had disappointingly high examiner variability.[30] Substantial changes on the scale occurred between examiners and between scores by the same examiner in the absence of symptomatic changes. There appears to be little biologic meaning to point intervals on this scale, but undoubtedly it does measure some real deficits that have little impact on the EDSS scale. Despite its drawbacks,[102] the EDSS or DSS has not yet been replaced. The authors strongly believe that the maximum usefulness derived from the DSS or EDSS is obtained when it is based on observed performance, as intended by Kurtzke, because it relies so heavily on ambulation.

Laboratory Indicators of Outcome

Relatively little information is available on the correlation of specific laboratory abnormalities with subsequent prognosis, at least in terms of disability. However, relevant information about the likelihood of conversion from monosymptomatic demyelination to MS has come from both cerebrospinal fluid (CSF) and MRI studies and is bolstering early hopes for the use of this technique as an outcome measure.[70] Patients with monosymptomatic demyelination who have normal CSF studies appear to be much less likely to develop disseminated disease in the short and intermediate term.[57] Similar data are available for normal versus abnormal MRI scans in monosymptomatic disease.[54,71] For patients with clinically definite MS, serial MRI studies have given a measure of disease activity and extent.[38] However, the duration of follow-

up in these patients has been too short to determine reliably the prognostic value of MRI measurements. The University of British Columbia (UBC) group examined outcome in a follow-up of 24 patients who had been studied with serial MRI scans.[69] Seven of the patients deteriorated at follow-up, and the mean MRI activity rate in these patients was triple the rate of the 17 patients who remained clinically stable. Unfortunately, the number of patients was relatively small and the period of follow-up short (less than 2 years), so that the differences were not statistically significant.

Similar natural history information on the evolution of MRI findings in untreated MS has been accumulated.[100] It is clear from the UBC and other studies* that the appearance of new lesions on serial MRI scans is increased severalfold over those surmised from clinical exacerbations. The frequency of MRI lesions, however, depends on the clinical phenotype, with the most frequent accumulation of new lesions appearing in patients with relapsing progressive disease, followed by those with relapsing-remitting disease. MRI activity in patients with primarily chronic progressive disease is quite infrequent.[53]

Little information is available correlating the numbers, size, and location of lesions at presentation with subsequent outcome. Further studies are necessary to see how these findings can predict subsequent disability. The degree of correlation between MRI abnormality and disability as measured by the EDSS scale is relatively modest, at least for cross-sectional data. The lack of a one-to-one correlation between MRI and clinical measures may be, in part, due to the lack of sensitivity of the clinical measures (see Chapter 12 for a full discussion).

If a CSF immunoglobulin abnormality (IgG level or the presence of oligoclonal bands) is present, the degree of abnormality seems not to have a major influence on prognosis.[98] However, even if "possible" cases are excluded,[57] our own data suggest that patients without CSF oligoclonal bands have a more benign outcome, in accordance with the report by Stendahl-Brodin

---

*References 23, 31, 33, 37, 38, 39, 68, 92, 101.

and colleagues.[90] On the other hand, follow-up of patients with extremely high IgG levels has indicated an outcome no worse than average.[89] It must be recalled, however, that studies of the natural history of MS have generally excluded monosymptomatic cases because they do not fulfill the criteria for MS.

TEMPORAL COURSE OF MULTIPLE SCLEROSIS

Attack or Relapse Rate

The defining requirements for relapse have been outlined[88] and have proved in practice to be helpful. Numerous investigators have studied defined relapse rates, and they have been commonly used as outcome measures for therapeutic trials. As with disability measures, considerable variation has been reported in attack frequencies (Table 6–4), despite agreement on the definition of an attack. This disparity encompasses an entire order of magnitude! These data are not entirely irreconcilable, however. It seems clear that attack rate varies with age, being higher in the younger patient and, further, it appears to vary inversely with duration of disease.[45] It seems to be largely independent of the progressive or stable nature of the clinical course. Attack rates

determined prospectively are higher than those determined retrospectively. Ideally, the former should be the rate used in determining pretrial attack rate as well as for calculating sample size, because the attack rate during a clinical trial will be a prospectively determined number. Although exacerbations are often temporarily disabling and, when recovery is incomplete, do contribute to cumulative disability, it is clear that unremitting deficit is the more important outcome measurement in the long term. A therapy that abolishes exacerbations but has no influence on progressive disability would have only modest attraction unless it was innocuous.

Disability

Although many studies have examined the cross-sectional distribution of disability at a given point in time, surprisingly little information is available on the rate of accumulation of functional disability (EDSS) in MS. Virtually no data are available on the rate of progression of disability dating from the onset of progressive disease, although this onset has generally been considered a more deleterious development in the illness. The few studies that have examined the rate of accumulation of functional dis-

Table 6–4. **ATTACK RATE IN MULTIPLE SCLEROSIS (Per Person-Year)**

SENIOR AUTHOR	YEAR	YEARS FROM ONSET				AVERAGE
		1	2	5	10	
Patzold[72]	1982					
Prospective		1.8	1.3	1.0	0.9	1.1
Retrospective		1.8	1.2	0.8	0.5	—
Gudmundsson[27]	1971	—	—	—	—	0.14
Fog[21]	1970					
Prospective		—	—	—	—	0.56
Retrospective		—	—	—	—	0.35
Leibowitz[46,47]	1964, 1970					0.39
						(First 5 yr)
Panelius[67]	1969	—	—	—	—	0.26
McAlpine[52]	1952	1.23	0.42	0.35	0.30	0.39

Source: From Weinshenker and Ebers,[99] p 258, with permission.

Table 6–5. **DISABILITY IN MULTIPLE SCLEROSIS AS A FUNCTION OF DURATION***

| | PERCENTAGE OF PATIENTS AT OR BEYOND | | | | | | | | | |
| | DSS 3 (MODERATE DISABILITY) | DSS 6 (ASSISTANCE REQUIRED FOR WALKING) | | | | | DSS 8 (BEDRIDDEN) | | | |
YEARS FROM ONSET	K[†]	C[†]	K[†]	P	M	R	C[†]	K[†]	P	M
5	82	8	25	42	18	13	8	4	<1	
10	77	25	37	68	32	34	17	9	<1	
15	82	40	46	76	32	46	29	14	<1	

Source: From Weinshenker and Ebers,[99] p 258, with permission.

*Data are based on equivalents of the Kurtzke Disability Status Scale (DSS) score according to the conversion scheme of Detels.

†Deaths due to MS (DSS 10) are included.

C = Confavreux;[11] K = Kurtzke;[43] M = McAlpine;[52] P = Panelius;[67] R = Runmarker.[84]

ability in MS are summarized in Table 6–5.[99] The fact that different scales were used in these studies accounts in part for the disparity in outcomes, although ascertainment bias, as always, was probably more influential on outcome than were other variations in methodology. All the series[11,44,52,80] suggest that approximately 50 percent of patients with MS are still able to ambulate independently after 15 years of disease. Results from a more recent study are consistent with this finding.[53]

There are disadvantages to measuring the rate of development of disability as a function of the DSS points accumulated per year of disease. Many of these have been repeatedly emphasized and relate to the nature of the scale, its nonlinearity, and the non-Gaussian distribution found in defined populations. Mean EDSS is somewhat more precise than listing one's five favorite colors and trying to take the mean of them. However, emphasizing the ordinal nature of both these rankings, we prefer to use the median time taken to reach specific levels of the EDSS, as it is simpler and more readily conveyed to patients. For example, it could be said that "at 15 years the chances are 50/50 of being able to walk unaided." Finally, this measure has direct relevance to the planning and execution of clinical trials and allows specification of endpoints on the Kurtzke scale itself (see following discussion).

Survival

Early workers in MS found a very high mortality rate. Two hundred fatal cases from Edinburgh had a mean duration of illness of 12 years.[4] Recent studies paint a less gloomy picture; however, one limitation of many of these studies is the ascertainment bias discussed earlier in relation to disability. Table 6–6 includes those survival studies in MS that have employed actuarial analysis. In these studies, survival has only modestly been influenced by MS, with some 75 percent of patients surviving 25 years. Clearly, short-term survival is very high, and there is little influence of MS on survival until at least 15 years have passed. In Broman's careful population-based study, patients with MS for 20 years had 85 percent of the expected survival. Our own population-based results from Vancouver and London are similar. The reduction in survival was roughly equivalent to that associated with the smoking of more than one package of cigarettes per day.[86] Table 6–7 provides lifetable data from these two populations expressed as years remaining of life expectancy. In this table, comparison with a control group of the insured general population is possible with the inclusion and exclusion of suicide. Survival in the insured general population is significantly better than in the total population.[86] It is hoped that these data will make it easier

Table 6–6. SURVIVAL IN MULTIPLE SCLEROSIS DETERMINED BY ACTUARIAL ANALYSIS

SENIOR AUTHOR	YEAR	YEARS AFTER ONSET: PERCENTAGE OF PATIENTS SURVIVING					
		5	10	15	20	25	30
Runmarker[84]	1993	100	98	95	90	85	—
Miller[53]	1992	—	—	95	87	72	58
Poser[78]	1989	100	96	87	79	63	60
Riise[81]	1988	94	87	79	65	52	48
Broman[5]	1981	99	96	90	85	75	—
Confavreux[11]	1980	99	96	88	—	—	—
Percy[73]	1971	99	98	90	80	74	—
Kurtzke[42]	1969	96	90	83	74	66	—
Kurtzke[44] (corrected for non-MS-related deaths)	1970	98	91	85	79	75	

Source: Updated from Weinshenker and Ebers,[99] p 257.

Table 6–7. LIFETABLE ANALYSES BY SEX

AGE	LIFE EXPECTANCY (EXPRESSED AS YEARS REMAINING)		
	INSURED POPULATION	MS POPULATION (SUICIDE EXCLUDED)	MS POPULATION (SUICIDE INCLUDED)
FEMALES			
10	69.47	63.24	62.07
20	59.70	53.61	52.47
30	50.00	44.09	42.99
40	40.40	34.71	33.66
50	31.18	25.89	24.94
60	22.48	17.78	16.96
70	14.79	10.97	10.33
80	8.43	5.62	5.18
90	4.45	2.63	2.36
100	1.72	0.82	0.50
MALES			
10	63.88	57.08	55.81
20	54.33	47.78	46.58
30	45.01	38.85	37.74
40	35.57	29.70	28.66
50	26.53	21.11	20.16
60	18.47	13.79	13.00
70	11.90	8.23	7.64
80	7.01	4.45	4.06
90	3.84	2.19	1.95
100	0.50	0.50	0.50

Source: From Sadovnick et al,[86] p 993, with permission.

Table 6–8. **PROFILE OF PATIENTS WITH MULTIPLE SCLEROSIS (N = 3126) ACCORDING TO CAUSE OF DEATH (FROM LONDON AND VANCOUVER, CANADA)**

	Male:Female Ratio	Mean EDSS	Mean age of Death (yr)	Mean Duration of MS (yr)
Complications of MS	1:1.1	8.0*	51.0	16.3
Suicide	1:1.2	4.6*	44.0*	12.9*
Malignancy	1:0.9	5.1	58.5	22.8
Acute myocardial infarct	1:1.2	5.1	60.0	22.1
Stroke	1:0.8	6.6	63.5	23.8

Source: From Sadovnick et al,[87] p 1194, with permission.
*($P<.05$ for all the pairwise comparisons within the column.

for patients with MS to obtain life insurance.

Table 6–8 presents the causes of death in two large MS clinics by cause, disability, age at death, and disease duration. Table 6–9 shows the age-specific percentages of deaths by cause in the MS and general populations of British Columbia.[87] The cause of death in some 50 percent of patients with MS is due to some complication of MS, commonly pneumonia or urinary sepsis. In the other half, it is attributable to the common causes of death in the general population, with a substantial minority of patients being victims of suicide. The suicide rate in patients with MS is increased fourfold over the general age-adjusted population, but rates as high as 7.5-fold have been reported in one prospective study.[87] When suicide occurs at a young age, it entails a major impact on overall mortality ratios for this disease. It could also be argued that when suicide occurs in a patient with MS, it should be considered a complication of the disease. A lack of social support systems is an important predictor of suicide.

Table 6–9. **COMPARISON OF RELATIVE PROPORTIONS OF DEATH BY CAUSE AMONG PATIENTS WITH MULTIPLE SCLEROSIS AND THE AGE-MATCHED BRITISH COLUMBIA POPULATION***

	MS DEATHS (N = 119)		BRITISH COLUMBIA DEATHS (N = 21,113)[†]		COMPARISON OF PROPORTIONS FOR MS POPULATION AND THE BRITISH COLUMBIA AGE-MATCHED POPULATION
	No.	Proportion	No.	Proportion	
Suicide	18	0.15	452	0.02	7.50×[‡]
Malignancy	19	0.16	5121	0.24	0.67×[¶]
Acute myocardial infarct	13	0.11	2423	0.11	1.00×
Stroke	7	0.06	1011	0.05	1.20×

Source: From Sadovnick et al,[87] p 1195, with permission.
*Note that these are not mortality rates but rather relative frequencies (proportions) of death by cause among those with known cause.
†Data are from Province of British Columbia, Ministry of Health, Division of Vital Statistics, Annual Report, 1987.
‡The proportion of deaths due to suicide in the MS population is significantly greater (7.5×; $P<.01$) than that for the age-matched British Columbia population.
¶The proportion of deaths due to malignancy in the MS population is significantly lower (0.67×; $P<.01$) than that for the age-matched British Columbia population.

PARAMETERS PREDICTIVE OF OUTCOME

Demographic and Clinical Features

Several studies have evaluated the influence of demographic features and clinical presentation on outcome. The major studies are summarized in Table 6–10 by sex, age at onset, and initial signs and symptoms. These factors are not independent of one another. For example, older patients commonly have progressive motor disability and vice versa. There has been some consensus but not unanimity that outcome is adversely effected by male gender and by early pyramidal and/or cerebellar symptoms or findings. Optic neuritis or sensory

Table 6–10. **CLINICAL AND DEMOGRAPHIC PREDICTIVE FACTORS***

Senior Author	Year	Relatively Favorable	No Influence	Relatively Unfavorable
		SEX		
Runmarker[84]	1993	Female	—	Male
Thompson[92]	1986	—	+	—
Visscher[94]	1984	—	+	—
Detels[14]	1982	Female	—	Male
Verjans[93]	1983	—	+	—
Confavreux[11]	1980	—	+	—
Leibowitz[46]	1970	Male	—	Female
Panelius[67]	1969	Female	—	Male
McAlpine[52]	1952	Female	—	Male
		AGE AT ONSET (YEARS)		
Runmarker[84]	1993	Young age	—	Older age
Thompson[92]	1986	Young age	—	—
Visscher[94]	1984	<40	—	>40
Verjans[93]	1983	<31	—	>31
Poser[77]	1982	<39	<20 vs 20–29 vs 30–39	>39
Kurtzke[43]	1977	—	+	—
Gudmundsson[28]	1971	—	+	—
Leibowitz[46]	1970	<40	—	>40
McAlpine[51]	1961	—	+	—
		INITIAL SIGNS/SYMPTOMS		
Runmarker[84]	1993	Attack onset	—	Progressive onset
Thompson[92]	1986	—	—	Motor
Visscher[94]	1984	ON, sensory	—	Motor, incoordination
Poser[77]	1982	ON	—	—
Confavreux[11]	1980	—	+	—
Kurtzke[43]	1977	—	BS, sensory, sphincter	Motor, cerebellar
Leibowitz[46]	1970	Motor, sensory	ON	Cerebellar
Fog[21]	1970	—	+	—
Gudmundsson[28]	1971	—	ON	Motor, motor + sensory
McAlpine[51]	1961	ON, BS, sensory	—	Pyramidal, cerebellar

Source: Updated from Weinshenker and Ebers,[99] p 259.
*According to authors' conclusions.
BS = brain stem; ON = optic neuritis.

onset appears to predict a more favorable outcome. Table 6–11 lists factors that find some general agreement or factors for which there is consensus among researchers which is supported by the population-based studies emphasized in this chapter. Many of these factors have long been recognized.[1]

Early Clinical Course

The identification of demographic and onset features that influence outcome is of potential value because this information is available early in the course of disease. Although there is general agreement that progressively worsening disease or disability is unfavorable, this observation is to some extent retrospective. An important observation was made by Kurtzke and colleagues,[43] who demonstrated that early disability predicted a more rapid than usual deterioration. He demonstrated that only 7 percent of those with mild disability at 5 years of onset were severely disabled at 10 years, and only 11.4 percent were severely disabled at 15 years. Because 37 and 46 percent of patients with durations of 10 and 15 years, respectively, in Kurtzke and colleagues' series had progressed to DSS 6 or beyond, this finding provided a significant refinement in prognosis for the 20 percent of patients with mild disability at 5 years. However, a moderate disability, which affected more than 50 percent of his cases at 5 years, was of no more predictive value than the inferences made from the entire group.

The influence of attack rate early in the disease on outcome has been less clear. Some studies have reported a correlation of attack rate and outcome, while others have not.[21,51,72] Late onset seems related to more rapid progression,[9,65] but also, by definition, to a longer disease-free period before onset. Childhood onset is more benign for progression but leads to disability at a younger age.[17]

Genes and Outcome

In all likelihood, genes influence the age of onset, because the intraclass correlation for the age of onset of concordant monozygotic twins is greater than that for concordant sibling pairs.[7] However, data to date have not provided a consistent association between any specific genetic factor and disease outcome. In some studies, HLA-B7 or DR2 has been associated with a worse than average prognosis, whereas in others, the opposite has held true.[13,16,19,34,50,80] It has been suggested that DNA polymorphisms in MHC class II antigens are associated with progressive disease, a feature known to correlate with a worse than average prognosis.[66] This finding has not been confirmed.

Trauma, Stress, and Outcome

There is no good evidence that minor trauma influences outcome. However, a few authors support this concept.[22,75]

Table 6–11. **PROGNOSTIC FACTORS**

Better	Worse
Female	Male
Onset: relapsing-remitting; ON, sensory; complete recovery	Onset: polysymptomatic, motor, incomplete recovery
Decreased age	Increased age
Longer interattack interval	More frequent attacks
Low frequency of attacks in early course	High frequency of attacks in early course
Long time to DSS 3	Short time to DSS 3

DSS = Disability Status Scale; ON = optic neuritis.

Until prospective studies can in some way objectively quantify stress, the commonly held view that stress aggravates the disease will continue to prevail in the absence of hard data. We commonly see patients with MS endure exceptional coincidental stress without appreciable change in their course. Major trauma is uncommon, and our own view is that the course of MS is usually independent of major trauma, including injuries severe enough to produce unconsciousness. However, our experience with many patients does not suggest a difference in outcome between those patients who burn the candle at both ends and those burning it at neither end.

MRI Findings

MRI abnormalities at outset may predict clinical outcome.[20,56] Data from a recent clinical trial also showed modest correlations between baseline and endpoint MRI burden and disability and, even more important, between change in MRI during the study and change in disability measured by the EDSS.[70] MRI studies are addressed in more detail in Chapter 9, but it is clear that the measurement of T_2-weighted signal for area, enlargement, and appearance of new lesions does not detect some of the changes indicative of disability. Spinal cord imaging was expected to show better correlations but did not, although measures of spinal cord atrophy showed the best correlation with disability.

RESULTS OF A GEOGRAPHICALLY BASED STUDY OF NATURAL HISTORY

A series of papers outlining the natural history of MS have reported data derived from the longitudinal follow-up of a population-based sample. In these studies carried out in London, Canada, some of the problems of ascertainment and follow-up discussed earlier have been attenuated, but by no means eliminated. The investigators had a special interest in MS, and the studies were conducted in a geographically restricted area served by a single university center. The data were collected in an MS clinic that, since 1972, has been collecting detailed information on disability based on the regular (annual or more frequent) visits of clinic patients regardless of disease activity. These data were collected in such a

Table 6–12. **CHARACTERISTICS OF PATIENT SUBGROUPS IN THE LONDON (ONTARIO) POPULATION**

Characteristic	Total Clinic Population	Middlesex County Subgroup	Seen-at-Onset Subgroup
No. of patients	1099	196	197
Males	377	63	62
Females	722	133	135
Sex ratio (M/F)	0.52	0.47	0.46
Diagnostic certainty			
Probable	916 (83.3%)	176 (89.8%)	162 (82.2%)
Possible	183 (16.4%)	20 (10.2%)	35 (17.7%)
Disease Duration			
Mean (years ± SE)	11.9 ± 0.3	13.0 ± 0.6	4.2 ± 0.2
Median (years)	10	12	3
Age at onset			
Mean (years ± SE)	30.5 ± 0.3	28.0 ± 0.6	29.9 ± 0.7
Median (years)	29	26	28

Source: From Weinshenker,[95] p 136, with permission.

Table 6–13. **CLINICAL COURSE AT ONSET OF DISEASE**

Course	Total Population	Middlesex County Subgroup	Seen-at-Onset Subgroup
Relapsing-remitting	722 (65.8%)	138 (70.4%)	166 (84.7%)
Relapsing progressive	162 (14.8%)	35 (17.9%)	14 (7.1%)
Chronically progressive	205 (18.7%)	23 (11.7%)	15 (7.7%)
Data unavailable	10 (0.9%)	0	2 (1.0%)
Total	1099	196	197

Source: Adapted from Weinshenker et al,[95] p 137, with permission.

way that studies could be made on factors influencing outcome. A formal prevalence study was carried out in the area just before the study, and it demonstrated near complete ascertainment of the subgroup of local patients.[29] This method permitted a comparison of the local subgroup to the overall clinic population, allowing internal control for the validity of subsequent demographic, clinical, and prognostic data. The criticism that this population was largely institutionalized has no basis.[55,95]

Much of the remainder of this chapter details the results of natural history studies in this London population, whose demographic and clinical features are outlined in Table 6–12. The total clinic population (TP) consists of two subgroups: MC (the Middlesex County, Ontario, population, representing a geographic area defined by a formal prevalence study) and SO (the seen-at-onset subgroup). The shorter disease duration in the SO group reflects the exclusion of cases with long antecedent clinical symptoms. Put another way, this subgroup is restricted to patients who have developed dissemination in the comparatively short period of follow-up.

The type of clinical course (Table 6–13) was divided into relapsing-remitting MS (RRMS) or progressive from onset, the latter with relapsing progressive MS (RPMS) or without chronic progressive (CPMS) superimposed acute episodes of worsening. Progressive disease was defined as continuing deterioration without remission, regardless of the rate of worsening. The SO subgroup, by definition, almost completely excluded cases progressive from onset.

The frequency of conversion from remitting to progressive disease as a function of 5-year intervals in age is presented in Table 6–14. The relative age specificity of a progressive course from onset is seen in Table 6–15. With onset before the fourth decade, some 20 percent of the total population was progressive from onset, but this rose to almost 75 percent in those developing their

Table 6–14. **FREQUENCY OF CONVERSION FROM REMITTING TO PROGRESSIVE MULTIPLE SCLEROSIS**

| Duration of MS at Final Review (yr) | PATIENTS WITH REMITTING DISEASE AT ONSET WHO CONVERT TO PROGRESSIVE MS | | |
	Total Population	Middlesex County Subgroup	Seen-at-Onset Subgroup
1–5	231 (12.1%)	34 (8.8%)	126 (10.3%)
6–10	179 (41.3%)	34 (29.4%)	33 (42.4%)
11–15	118 (57.6%)	26 (53.8%)	7 (28.6%)
16–25	131 (65.6%)	33 (72.7%)	0
26+	63 (88.9%)	11 (90.0%)	0
Total	722	138	166

Source: Adapted from Weinshenker et al,[95] p 137.

Table 6–15. **PROGRESSIVE MULTIPLE SCLEROSIS FROM ONSET ACCORDING TO AGE**

Age at Onset (yr)	PATIENTS PROGRESSIVE AT ONSET		
	Total Population	Middlesex County Subgroup	Seen-at-Onset Subgroup
<20	131 (17.6%)	23 (13.0%)	21 (14.3%)
20–29	435 (19.1%)	84 (17.9%)	105 (8.6%)
30–39	310 (37.7%)	54 (37.0%)	48 (14.6%)
40–49	173 (63.0%)	27 (63.0%)	19 (36.8%)
>49	47 (74.5%)	8 (37.5%)	3 (100%)
Data unavailable	3	0	1
Total	1099	196	197

Source: Adapted from Weinshenker et al,[95] p 138.

initial symptoms in the sixth decade of life or later. The older-onset subgroup accounts for some 4.3 percent of all patients, although twice that many may have their initial neurological presentation in this period.[65] It is of interest that the age of conversion to a progressive course in patients who initially had RRMS tended to parallel the age at which the initial onset was usually chronic progressive. These observations imply that some maturational or aging process determines the progressive phenotype, as first pointed out by Minderhoud and colleagues.[55]

Disability

CROSS-SECTIONAL ANALYSIS

In evaluating a cross-sectional distribution of disability in these population samples, it should be remembered that the population is probably not yet at equilibrium with entry incidence matching death

incidence (age corrected). In fact, we are not even confident that the incidence is static. Nevertheless, the distribution of DSS scores is quite instructive and unlikely to be materially altered in general distribution when this equilibrium is reached. Table 6–3 documents and enumerates the cross-sectional distribution of patients on the EDSS scale and also demonstrates the absence of a normal distribution. These findings are clearly indicative of the differing length of time spent at each level in the scale (see following). More patients were at the DSS 3 level than DSS 4 and 5 combined, and almost twice as many were at DSS 6 than at DSS 3, 4, and 5 combined.

LONGITUDINAL ANALYSIS

The median time to reach given levels of the DSS scale was used for the three subgroups because of the nature of the scale itself. The median time to reach DSS 3 (mild disability) and 6 (aids required for walking) is given in Table 6–16. For the TP,

Table 6–16. **TIME (YEARS) FROM ONSET OF MULTIPLE SCLEROSIS TO REACH SELECTED LEVELS OF DISABILITY (MEDIAN ± SE)**

Level of Disability	Total Clinic Population	Seen-at-Onset Subgroup
DSS 3	7.69 ± 0.42	6.28 ± 0.34
DSS 6	14.97 ± 0.31	9.42 ± 0.44

Source: From Weinshenker et al,[95] p 139, with permission.
DSS = Disability Status Scale (Kurtzke).

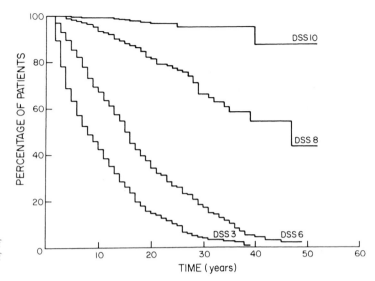

Figure 6–1. Actuarial analysis of disability with time from onset of MS in the total population.

50 percent of patients were walking without aids at 15 years from onset. An actuarial analysis of disability from onset of MS for the total population is shown in Figures 6–1 and 6–2. The number of patients having reached DSS 8 and 10 is small, and these data should not be considered as well established. On the other hand, the times to DSS 3 and 6 have relatively narrow confidence intervals and are based on the analysis of large numbers of cases (data not shown).

This data set also allowed the longitudinal analysis of disability from onset of pro-

gressive MS. These data support the widely held belief that the onset of a progressive phase yields a poor outcome (Figures 6–3 through 6–5).

The median time to reach selected levels of disability from the onset of progressive MS for the TP and MC groups is given in Table 6–17. The more rapid progression in the SO group is largely a definitional artifact. Patients with a mild-onset attack and a long interattack interval (therefore a longer time to fulfill criteria for diagnosis) are necessarily excluded from the SO population, but are much more likely to be in-

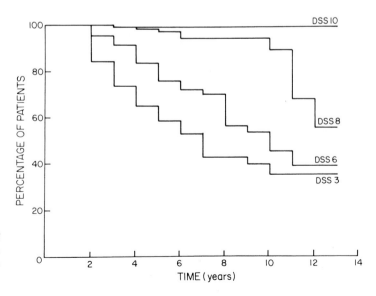

Figure 6–2. Actuarial analysis of disability with time from onset of MS in the "seen-at-onset" subgroup.

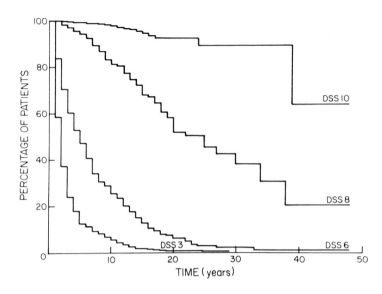

Figure 6–3. Time from onset of progressive MS to disability levels in the total population.

cluded in the TP group, in which duration of follow-up was considerably longer. It has been well recognized that progressive disease early after an initially relapsing-remitting course is associated with a poor outcome. Table 6–17 demonstrates this for the TP and MC groups. Recalling the problem of defining progression in terms of Kurtzke points per year of disease, we found the mean rate of change was 0.53 ± 0.02 DSS points per year for the total population, with a median change of 0.4 DSS per year.

The frequency distribution for progression rates in the first 5 years is seen in Figure 6–6. These data are discussed later in relationship to clinical trials.

It is interesting to note from this frequency distribution that only a quarter of the patients in this population worsened at the rate of 1 or more Kurtzke points per year. These natural history data have immediate relevance for the analysis and interpretation of results from uncontrolled clinical trials.

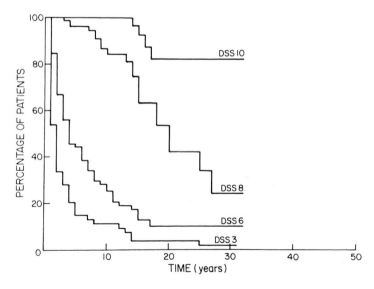

Figure 6–4. Time from onset of progressive MS to disability levels in the Middlesex County subgroup.

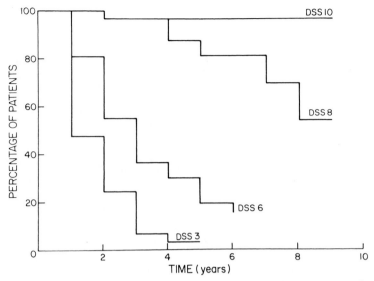

Figure 6–5. Time from onset of progressive MS to disability levels in the "seen-at-onset" subgroup.

Predictive Value of the Early Clinical Course

It would be advantageous to predict outcome from factors available early in the course of MS, particularly for therapeutic decisions.[82] Attempts have been made to correlate long-term prognosis with the early clinical course in the London population. Specifically, three parameters were examined:

1. Attack rate
2. First interattack interval
3. Rate at which disability develops in the early years of the disease

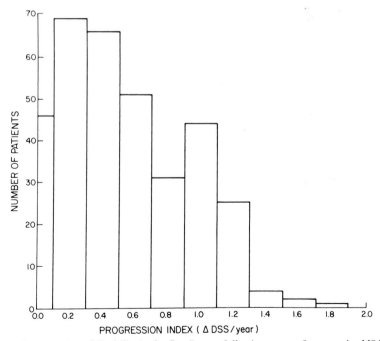

Figure 6–6. Rate of progression of disability in the first 5 years following onset of progressive MS in 339 patients.

Table 6–17. **MEDIAN TIME (YEARS) FROM ONSET OF PROGRESSIVE MULTIPLE SCLEROSIS TO REACH SELECTED LEVELS OF DISABILITY (MEDIAN ± SE)**

Level of Disability	Total Clinic Population	Middlesex County Subgroup
DSS 3	1.40 ± 0.11	1.20 ± 0.33
DSS 6	4.51 ± 0.38	3.58 ± 0.52
DSS 8	24.08 ± 0.44	19.32 ± 0.46
DSS 10	—	—

Source: From Weinshenker et al,[95] p 142, with permission.
DSS = Disability Status Scale (Kurtzke).

For the outcome measure of time to DSS 6, a correlation was found with each of these three parameters. Thus, attack rate in the first year of disease, the first interattack interval, and the rate of development of early disability (time to DSS 3) are all of predictive value.[96] Figure 6–7 plots time from onset to reach DSS 6 against the distribution of attacks in the first two years. Table 6–18 shows the observed distributions of these three variables in the TP of patients studied (chronic progressive cases are necessarily excluded).

Table 6–19 gives the attack frequency in the first and second year after onset for both the TP and the SO groups. Even in the SO subgroup, the attack rate exceeds one per year in only approximately 40 percent of patients; only 4 percent of the TP had five or more attacks in 2 years, and perhaps less than half of those would have three or more attacks per year.

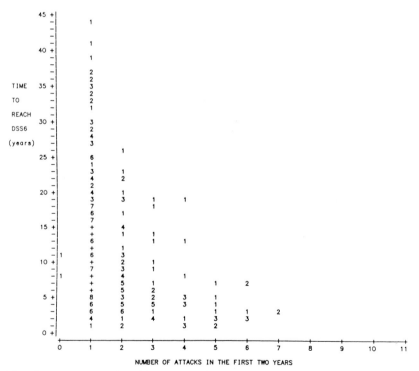

Figure 6–7. Time from onset to reach DSS 6 versus number of attacks in first 2 years after onset (+ = more than 10 observations at this point).

Table 6–18. **STRATIFICATION OF PATIENTS**

Criteria	Subgroup	Defining Measurement	No. of Patients
	TOTAL POPULATION		
Number of attacks in first 2 yr*	Low	0–1	452
	Intermediate	2–4	244
	High	≥5	34
First interattack interval (yr)*	Short	0–2	425
	Intermediate	3–5	153
	Long	≥6	174
Time to reach DSS 3 (yr)*	Short	0–2	209
	Intermediate	3–7	239
	Long	≥8	226
	SEEN-AT-ONSET SUBGROUP		
Number of attacks in first 2 yr*	Low	0–2	77
	Intermediate	3–4	35
	High	≥5	16
First interattack interval (yr)*	Short	0–1	109
	Long	≥2	39
Time to reach DSS 3 (yr)*	Short	0–2	44
	Long	≥3	27

Source: From Weinshenker et al,[96] p 1421, with permission.
*Patients with chronically progressive MS from onset were excluded.
DSS = Disability Status Scale (Kurtzke).

The mean attack rate in the first year is 1.57 ± 0.05 in the TP group, whereas in the SO group, it is 1.80 ± 0.1. Of particular interest is the remarkable drop in attack rate in both groups in the second year. Although it can be argued that this is in part artifactual and that the onset bout should be excluded because it is required by definition, the comparison of years 1 and 2 has practical clinical significance. Patients selected for relapse prevention trials have met the relapse frequency criteria, which

Table 6–19. **ATTACK FREQUENCY (MEAN ± SEM)**

	Total Population (n)	Seen-at-Onset Subgroup (n)
First Year after Onset		
RR	1.57 ± 0.05 (358)	1.80 ± 0.10 (119)
RR to P	1.28 ± 0.05 (272)	2.08 ± 0.22 (25)
RP	1.42 ± 0.06 (132)	2.33 ± 0.37 (9)
Second Year after Onset		
RR	0.35 ± 0.04 (322)	0.55 ± 0.08 (99)
RR to P	0.40 ± 0.06 (255)	1.08 ± 0.22 (24)
RP	0.48 ± 0.07 (119)	1.43 ± 0.37 (7)

Source: From Weinshenker et al,[96] p 1421, with permission.
n = number of patients with available data; RR = relapsing-remitting; RP = progressive from onset with superimposed attacks; RR to P = remitting and subsequently progressive.

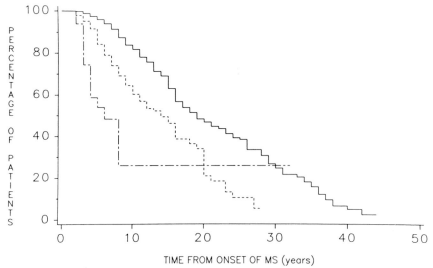

Figure 6–8. Actuarial analysis of disability in the total population of patients not having reached DSS 6 with low (—), intermediate (– –), and high (– – –) attack rate in the first 2 years with time from onset (*P*<.0001).

typically depended on the frequency of relapse in the previous year. These results clearly demonstrate at least one reason why patients do not maintain their pretrial attack rates. This phenomenon can be termed the *regression to the mean*. Patients selected for more than average disease activity in the previous year infrequently maintain this level of disease activity. A second factor is a true drop in the attack frequency, even if the onset bout is included. This phenomenon is not apparent in the relapsing progressive and chronic progressive groups, either in the TP or SO groups, indicating that this change may in fact be associated with a worse than average prognosis.

The actuarial analysis of disability using time to DSS 6 for the three attack rate subgroups in the total population is seen in

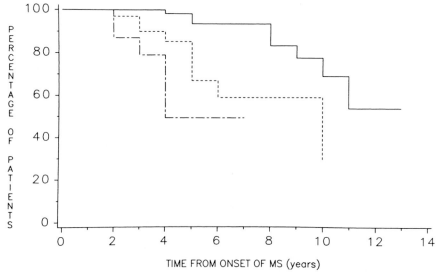

Figure 6–9. Actuarial analysis of disability in the "seen-at-onset" subgroup of patients not having reached DSS 6 with low (—), intermediate (– –), and high (– – –) attack rate in the first 2 years with time from onset (*P*<.0001).

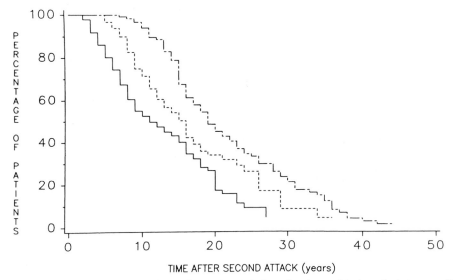

Figure 6–10. Actuarial analysis of disability in the total population of patients with short (—), intermediate (– –), and long (– – –) first interattack interval, with time after second attack ($P < .0001$).

Figures 6–8 and 6–9, with the difference between groups being highly significant. Not surprisingly, similar data are found for the first interattack interval (Figs. 6–10 and 6–11).

Figures 6–12 and 6–13 show the actuarial analysis of disability according to short, intermediate, and long times to reach DSS 3.

Clearly, the time to DSS 6 is predicted by time to DSS 3, but the correlation is weaker than might be expected. In summary, the early course was of predictive value: high attack frequency in the first year, short interattack interval, and short time to mild disability are all negative prognostic indicators.

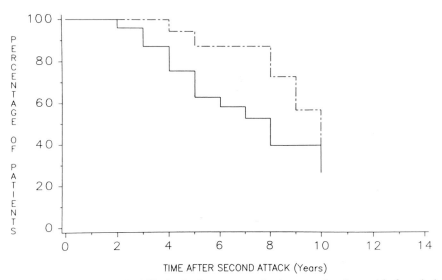

Figure 6–11. Actuarial analysis of disability in the "seen-at-onset" subgroup of patients with short (—) and long (– – –) first interattack interval, with time after second attack ($P < .09$).

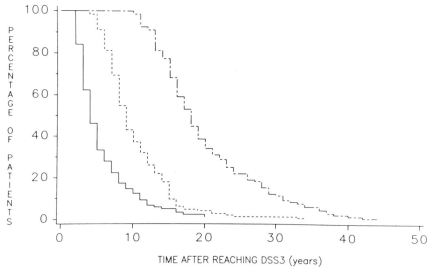

Figure 6–12. Actuarial analysis of disability in the total population of patients with short (—), intermediate (– –), and long (– – –) time to DSS 3, with time after reaching DSS 3 (*P*<.0001).

Factors Influencing Outcome: Multivariate Analysis and Hierarchical Significance

Several studies have shown an influence of a variety of clinical demographic and laboratory measures on outcome as measured by disability (see Table 6–11 for a list of these factors based on consensus). However, these studies examined the question of prognosis from the standpoint of individual influences, not considering that a number of those factors usually combine to contribute to prognosis. For example, age of onset and progressive course are each strongly associated, yet they are listed separately in the table. The

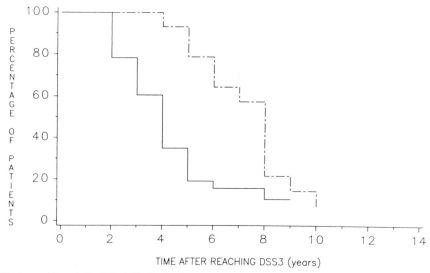

Figure 6–13. Actuarial analysis of disability in the "seen-at-onset" subgroup of patients with short (—) and long (– – –) time to DSS 3, with time after reaching DSS 3 (*P*<.0001).

most efficient application of natural history information for management of clinical trials would be to know the independent contribution from each prognostic variable, preferably in sequential fashion, so that information as it becomes available could be added to improve the prognostic accuracy.

With this thought in mind, we have analyzed our own natural history information in a hierarchical way. In this context, *hierarchical* refers to the sequence in which data on the variables in Table 6–20 would become available in the evaluation and follow-up of patients with MS. Initially, we considered demographic data followed by initial symptoms, type of clinical course, neurological system involvement, and finally, details of the early clinical course of disease. Actuarial analyses (failure to reach DSS 6) were carried out for identified prognostic variables and individual correlation coefficients are given. These data are summarized in Table 6–20 and are more or less self-explanatory. Negative correlation coefficients indicate an adverse effect on prognosis, whereas positive coefficients are desirable characteristics. Each sequential test then controls the variables that were found to be significant as indicated in the table. For example, in going from level B (initial symptoms) to level C (laboratory results), motor symptoms (insidious), ataxia, balance disturbance, or all three are controlled. Each sequential test can then control the variables previously found to be significant. This technique probably accounts for a few of the surprises. For example, the influence of pyramidal involvement, which is clearly a major influence on the ambulation-weighted DSS, appears to be in large part accounted for by preceding variables because of coassociation and because of its high prevalence at the "last evaluation" used for calculating the influence of system involvement at level E.

Because studies of the effect of major histocompatibility complex (MHC) antigens on prognosis have been controversial, we note that this study showed a modest deleterious effect of MHC-DR2 antigen and of oligoclonal bands, but neither effect reached statistical significance, with correlates of -0.27 ($P = 0.07$) and -0.22 ($P = 0.08$).

Applications to Planning and Interpretation of Clinical Therapeutic Trials

The data from natural history studies have a number of practical applications. If clinical efficacy is the endpoint, it would rarely, if ever, be appropriate to conduct short-term trials in MS without a randomized placebo-controlled design. Recently, this rule has arguably been softened by the emergence of therapies reducing relapse rate. However, the concept, in part, reflects the knowledge that the rate of deterioration in the short term for most patients is relatively slow, and for therapies aimed at retarding progression, the demonstration of efficacy depends largely on the deterioration of the control group. This requirement will hold true until a therapy that is proved to be effective in delaying progression must be given to the control group as the "best medical therapy." In the meantime, data from studies of natural history can serve as a form of historical control. More important, however, these data provide information that can be used to identify the number of patients required to show a given therapeutic effect when the duration of the trial and the power to detect a significant result are specified. Finally, and most important, for patients themselves, the data give relatively accurate information on the duration-specific probability of disability.

CONTROL GROUP OUTCOMES IN PROGRESSIVE AND RELAPSING PATIENTS

Unquestionably variation in the outcome in placebo-treated or untreated groups of patients in randomized clinical therapeutic trials in MS can confound the interpretation of such studies. Unduly pessimistic expectations for the outcome of chronically progressive MS in the short term have plagued trial design and interpretation. Clearly, an insufficient appreciation of the natural history of MS can lead to suboptimal design of trials, so that the rate of deterioration in the control group may be too low to permit identification of a clinically

Table 6–20. **HIERARCHICAL TESTS OF SIGNIFICANCE OF PROGNOSTIC VARIABLES**

Variable	Coefficient	*P* value
DEMOGRAPHIC CHARACTERISTICS		
Age at onset	−0.030	<.001
Male sex	−0.175	.004
Seen at onset of MS	−0.499	<.001
INITIAL SYMPTOMS (CONTROLLING FOR AGE AT ONSET, SEEN AT ONSET, AND SEX)		
Optic neuritis	0.182	.03
Sensory	0.035	.55
Motor (acute)	0.182	.18
Motor (insidious)	−0.204	.01
Limb ataxia and/or impairment of balance	−0.287	<.001
Diplopia and/or vertigo	0.028	.75
LABORATORY RESULTS (CONTROLLING FOR AGE AT ONSET, SEX, MOTOR [INSIDIOUS], ATAXIA AND/OR BALANCE, AND SEEN AT ONSET)		
Oligoclonal bands detected	−0.220	.08
CSF cells >10/mm^3	−0.051	.72
DR2+	−0.267	.07
DR3+	−0.027	.89
Neither DR2+ or DR3+	−0.057	.88
CLINICAL COURSE (CONTROLLING FOR AGE AT ONSET, SEX, MOTOR [INSIDIOUS], ATAXIA AND/OR BALANCE, AND SEEN AT ONSET)		
Remitting at onset	0.650	<.001
SYSTEMS INVOLVED AT LAST VISIT (CONTROLLING FOR AGE AT ONSET, SEX, MOTOR [INSIDIOUS], ATAXIA AND/OR BALANCE, AND SEEN AT ONSET)		
Visual	−0.006	.94
Brain stem	−0.210	<.001
Pyramidal	−0.149	.09
Cerebellar	−0.416	<.001
Cerebral	−0.400	<.001
EARLY CLINICAL COURSE (CONTROLLING FOR AGE AT ONSET, SEX, MOTOR [INSIDIOUS], ATAXIA AND/OR BALANCE, AND SEEN AT ONSET)		
Number of attacks in first 2 yr	−0.103	<.001
Interval between first 2 attacks	0.039	<.001
DSS at 2 yr	−0.415	<.001
DSS at 5 yr	−0.340	<.001

Source: From Weinshenker et al,[97] p 1048, with permission.
CSF = cerebrospinal fluid; DSS = Disability Status Scale (Kurtzke).

relevant treatment effect. Several examples can be found in MS trials carried out in the past few years.

Patients are often selected for trials based on a single criterion, usually a threshold change in disability score over the previous year. This observation has often carried the inherent assumption that disability will continue to progress at approximately the same rate over the ensuing years without effective medical intervention and, furthermore, that progression from any level to the next on the DSS is taken to be equivalent. This assumption is usually erroneous and a striking tendency of patients to regress towards a mean rate of progression of disability has now been seen in many clinical trials. It has been suggested that this phenomenon results from a placebo effect. This view is at best a partial explanation because the effect was of similar, if not identical, magnitude in a "natural history mock trial"[98] based on the data from London, Ontario, natural history studies. Using a variety of entry criteria, including those used in a number of recent clinical trials (rate of Kurtzke level deterioration in previous 1 to 5 years), patients were selected from the natural history files, and their subsequent outcome was examined as if they had been in a clinical trial. The rate of stabilization in this imaginary mock trial in the absence of any trial participation or therapy closely resembled that documented in the control group taken from several recent clinical trials of specific therapy in MS.[26,98] In conclusion, the degree of MS activity observable over the short term is by no means a fundamental characteristic of the individual. Regression to the mean is the major factor influencing the "better than expected" performance of patients in clinical trials where the entry criterion has demanded worse than average progression in the immediate pretrial period.

Similarly, clinical trials designed to reduce the attack frequency often do not take into account three factors:

1. The attack rate diminishes over time.
2. It is to some extent age specific.
3. It also demonstrates regression to the mean.

Clearly, on average, patients with a high attack rate in the previous year tend to have a substantially lower rate during the subsequent year in the absence of any therapy. Attacks can be triggered by randomly occurring, but ubiquitous, events. If so, the patient with an improbably high attack rate one year could be compared with a person who survives being struck by lightning. Neither outcome is likely to reoccur in the subsequent year. Specific examples of the problems encountered in widely publicized trials are discussed below. Several of these trials have led to the treatment of large numbers of patients based on what subsequently were shown to be unconfirmable positive results.

PATIENT SELECTION AND SAMPLE SIZE CALCULATIONS

The data accumulated from natural history studies have practical applications for the design and conduct of clinical trials in MS. First, the data allow computation of the number of patients that would need to be screened to identify patients with specific entry criteria. Such data can be used to predict what their likely subsequent behavior would be in the short term and to closely approximate the numbers of patients required to demonstrate treatment effects of specified magnitude with a preset power. These data can also be used to take into account the nonlinearity of the EDSS scale by allowing stratification for EDSS at entry. The problem of calculating sample size in clinical trials has been reviewed in detail.[15]

Table 6–21 gives the number of eligible patients from a population base of 1099 for three different hypothetical entry criteria, which were chosen because they approximate the criteria used in several recent clinical trials of therapy in MS. Patients were considered eligible if they met the criteria at any point during the recorded course of their disease. In this table, for each of the three criteria, we give the percentage of patients who would be expected to deteriorate by one level in the DSS based on entry criteria. For example, for criterion A (i.e., a drop of 1 DSS point in the previous year or 3 points in 5 years), the percentage among this population who would deteriorate by an additional DSS point in the first year

Table 6–21. **OBSERVED PERCENTAGE OF PATIENTS IN TOTAL POPULATION (n = 1099) DETERIORATING BY ONE LEVEL ON THE DISABILITY STATUS SCALE BASED ON ENTRY CRITERIA***

Years after Entry	PERCENTAGE (N) OF PATIENTS		
	Criterion A	Criterion B	Criterion C
0	0 (635)	0 (668)	0 (657)
1	30 (558)	35 (586)	32 (574)
2	46 (465)	48 (474)	43 (468)
3	54 (381)	57 (390)	52 (390)
4	62 (329)	64 (324)	58 (324)
5	70 (284)	69 (271)	67 (276)
6	76 (241)	72 (226)	70 (226)
7	76 (199)	72 (190)	72 (185)
8	79 (165)	74 (154)	74 (142)
9	81 (126)	77 (125)	76 (118)
10	85 (112)	84 (110)	82 (104)

Source: Adapted from Weinshenker et al,[98] p 1060.
*Hypothetical entry criteria:
A = deterioration of 1 point in previous year.
B = deterioration of 1 point in previous 2 yr or 3 points in 10 yr.
C = deterioration of 1 point in previous year and 2 points in the previous 3 yr.
n = number of patients with follow-up data.

Table 6–22. **OBSERVED PERCENTAGE OF PATIENTS IN SEEN-AT-ONSET SUBGROUP DETERIORATING BY ONE LEVEL ON THE DISABILITY STATUS SCALE BASED ON ENTRY CRITERIA***

Years after Entry	PERCENTAGE (N) OF PATIENTS		
	Criterion A	Criterion B	Criterion C
0	0 (60)	0 (60)	0 (59)
1	51 (47)	51 (47)	44 (48)
2	72 (29)	81 (16)	58 (24)
3	84 (19)	80 (10)	64 (14)
4	73 (11)	88 (8)	50 (8)
5	75 (8)	100 (4)	57 (7)
6	83 (6)	100 (1)	75 (4)
7	100 (4)	100 (1)	100 (3)
8	100 (2)	—(0)	—(0)

Source: Adapted from Weinshenker et al,[98] p 1060, with permission.
*Hypothetical entry criteria:
A = deterioration of 1 point in previous year.
B = deterioration of 1 point in previous 2 yr or 3 points in 10 yr.
C = deterioration of 1 point in previous year and 2 points in the previous 3 yr.
n = number of patients with follow-up data.

would be 30 percent; 46 percent at 2 years; and 54 percent at 3 years. Put another way, a stabilization rate of 70 percent would be expected on the basis of natural history alone![98] This stabilization of course would not take into account any placebo effect or the influence of unblinded examiners (see below). Table 6–22 gives the results for the SO population. Table 6–23 summarizes this information for each of the three criteria for nine 1-year intervals after entry into a hypothetical trial. The reader should note that the stabilization rates are remarkably similar. Clearly, the results from the natural history study conform well to the outcome in the placebo arm of most trials on progressive MS.

Table 6–24 gives the number of patients per group (treated and controls) that would be required to demonstrate an increase of 10, 30, and 50 percent in the proportion of patients remaining stable. Further information on clinical trial design is beyond the scope of this chapter but can be readily derived from natural history data.

Nonlinearity of the Disability Status Scale

For many reported MS clinical trials, it has been assumed that deterioration on the DSS scale is a linear function of duration. Overall, mean rates of long-term deterioration have been applied to isolated points on the scale in the expectation that worsening in the short term would approximate the mean. Table 6–25 demonstrates the inaccuracy of this assumption. It gives the time spent at each level of the DSS for patients who reach the next level. It can be readily seen that the mean time spent at different DSS levels can vary almost fourfold, ranging from a low of 1.22 years at DSS 4 to a high of 4.09 at DSS 1. DSS 1, 6, and 7 are particular "sticking points," and the inclusion of patients at DSS 6 will clearly lessen the power of the study to demonstrate an effect because the time spent at this level is disproportionately long (and even longer at DSS 7). The natural history studies used the DSS, but the newer EDSS allows splitting the 6 to 7 interval into two half-points.

Table 6–23. **SURVIVAL ANALYSIS: PERCENTAGE OF PATIENTS WHO HAVE NOT DETERIORATED BY ONE LEVEL ON THE DISABILITY STATUS SCALE BASED ON ENTRY CRITERIA***

	PERCENTAGE OF PATIENTS		
Years after Entry	**Criterion A**	**Criterion B**	**Criterion C**
1	71	67	70
2	54	53	57
3	43	42	45
4	35	33	37
5	27	28	29
6	21	22	23
7	17	20	20
8	14	16	17
9	11	14	15
Median time (yr)	2.3	2.2	2.6

Source: From Weinshenker et al,[98] p 1061, with permission.
***Hypothetical entry criteria:**
A = deterioration of 1 point in previous year.
B = deterioration of 1 point in previous 2 yr or 3 points in 10 yr.
C = deterioration of 1 point in previous year and 2 points in the previous 3 yr.

Table 6–24. **NUMBER OF PATIENTS PER GROUP NECESSARY TO DETECT AN INCREASE OF 0.10, 0.30, OR 0.50 IN THE PROPORTION OF PATIENTS WHO REMAIN STABLE**

Years after Entry	CONTROL RATE	NO. OF PATIENTS*		
		0.10	0.30	0.50
1	0.70	332 (431)	—	—
2	0.55	415 (542)	48 (60)	—
3	0.45	430 (563)	53 (67)	19 (23)
4	0.35	415 (542)	55 (69)	21 (25)
5	0.30	395 (515)	54 (68)	22 (26)
7	0.20	332 (431)	51 (64)	22 (26)
9	0.15	289 (373)	48 (60)	21 (25)

Source: From Weinshenker et al,[98] p 1061, with permission.
*To assure level of significance, alpha equals 0.05, and power, 80% (90%).

Table 6–25. **NUMBER OF YEARS AT EACH LEVEL OF DISABILITY STATUS SCALE FOR PATIENTS WHO REACH THE NEXT LEVEL**

DSS	NO. ENTERING	NO. PROGRESSING		TIME AT DSS (YR)			MEAN TIME PER LEVEL OF DSS		
		n	Percentage	Mean	SEM	Median	Mean	SEM	Median
				TOTAL POPULATION					
1	1037	854	82	4.09	0.19	1	2.78	0.08	2.17
2	829	675	81	2.80	0.14	1.5	2.44	0.07	2.00
3	662	539	82	1.95	0.11	1	2.17	0.06	1.86
4	536	467	88	1.22	0.06	1	2.07	0.06	1.83
5	475	444	94	1.25	0.06	1	2.06	0.06	1.81
6	489	292	60	3.06	0.17	2	2.06	0.07	1.86
7	306	114	37	3.77	0.32	3	1.87	0.10	1.65
8	114	32	28	2.41	0.38	2	1.61	0.17	1.42
9	34	14	41	2.51	0.56	2	1.41	0.27	1.25
10	16	—	—	—	—	—	—	—	—
				SEEN AT ONSET					
1	196	125	64	1.77	0.18	1.0	1.46	0.11	1.00
2	125	72	58	1.29	0.19	0.75	1.04	0.08	0.83
3	71	52	73	0.94	0.17	0.5	0.89	0.07	0.73
4	51	46	90	0.63	0.08	0.5	0.83	0.06	0.71
5	45	44	98	0.75	0.09	0.5	0.80	0.06	0.71
6	44	26	59	1.43	0.24	1.0	0.77	0.08	0.71
7	26	10	38	1.65	0.53	1.0	0.89	0.14	1.00
8	10	4	40	1.31	0.43	1.5	0.66	0.22	0.61
9	4	1	25	0.25	0	0.25	0.20	0	0.20
10	1	—	—	—	—	—	—	—	—

Source: From Weinshenker et al,[98] p 1062, with permission.
DSS = Disability Status Scale (Kurtzke).

Table 6–26. **NUMBER OF YEARS AT EACH GROUPED LEVEL OF DSS* FOR PATIENTS WHO REACH THE NEXT LEVEL**

	NO. ENTERING	NO. PROGRESSING		TIME AT DSS GROUPED LEVEL (YR)		
DSS		n	%	Mean	SEM	Median
1–3	1012	547	54	7.96	0.31	6
4–6	543	271	50	5.10	0.22	4
7–8	308	33	11	5.04	0.62	4
9–10	34	—	—	—	—	—

Source: From Weinshenker et al,[98] p 1063, with permission.
*Modified Disability Status Scale (DSS).

Little enthusiasm has been generated for using patients with DSS levels greater than 7 in clinical trials for obvious reasons, including the fact that prognostic variables are incompletely established.

Table 6–26 groups DSS 1 to 3, 4 to 6, 7 and 8, and 9 and 10 and gives median times at each group level for patients who reach the next level. Intraclass correlations that compare individual patients to the entire group demonstrate substantial within-patient variability in times spent at different DSS levels.

Table 6–25 lists the time spent at each level of the DSS for patients who have reached the next level. The mean and median times conform remarkably well with the cross-sectional frequency distribution of the number of patients at each level in the Kurtzke scale. The relative length of time spent at DSS 1 through 3 and at DSS 6 and 7 should be noted.

APPLICATION OF NATURAL HISTORY DATA TO THE INTERPRETATION OF CLINICAL TRIALS RESULTS

There are few disorders in which the planning, execution, and interpretation of clinical trials is more difficult than in MS. The investigators who carried out the trials discussed in this chapter have invested enormous time, effort, and expense. The problems highlighted reflect largely the difficult nature of this disease. However, as clinical trial investigators ourselves, we believe that many investigators are interested in the completion of the task, rather than in the difficulty of the task. On the other hand, patients are more interested in the results and their applications than in the fine points of methodology. Unfortunately, interpretation of results and methodology are the inseparable elements of clinical trials in MS. We illustrate some of the points being made from the natural history studies discussed previously, using data published on some specific trials.

It is important to understand that ethical MS investigators confront the problems of testing potentially toxic drugs in a variably progressive disease. Because one can predict with certainty the short-term and intermediate-term outlook in any one patient, there is a strong desire to select patients who are the most likely to deteriorate quickly. This not only relates to the necessary justification for the use of toxic therapies, but also to the actual success of the trial in determining efficacy or lack of it for a given drug. Unfortunately for current therapies, it is necessary to demonstrate that patients in the control group deteriorated to demonstrate that those in the treatment group are deriving benefit. For this reason, it has become increasingly desirable to select patients with more than average MS activity. A once-prevailing belief was that the level of activity of the MS in the short time preceding trial entry was a fundamental characteristic of a patient's disease and that this behavior would continue at much the same rate. This assumption is often untrue. A clear understanding of the reason is important both for trial design and interpretation.

This phenomenon may be seen in conflicting results from two studies carried out by the same investigator.[26,27] The first of these was a natural history study (although of shorter duration than many clinical trials) in which the relapse rate was not shown to alter greatly during the period of observation. This finding conflicts to some extent with many other reports, which have shown that the relapse rate diminishes with time. However, this discrepancy could result from the short follow-up and the fact that follow-up ascertainment of the patients may well have occurred because they were having new symptoms. If true, this would tend to homogenize the group under observation and naturally exclude patients who had not come to attention for symptoms. In contrast, in a clinical trial using azathioprine versus placebo, the same investigator noted that the attack rate dropped in both groups. However, he failed to point out that the attack rate was much higher in the trial study than in his own natural history study. Possibly the difference could be accounted for by regression to the mean in the clinical trial group because it was selected for a higher than average exacerbation rate. However, attack rates followed prospectively in one cohort cannot easily be compared with rates obtained retrospectively from another cohort.

Regression to the Mean

RELAPSE RATE

The relapse prevention trial of copolymer I may illustrate the phenomenon of regression to the mean.[3] This study, which was difficult to mask, has been replicated[35] (see Chapter 12). One unusual feature of the first trial was the high pretrial relapse rate. The investigators expressed surprise at the reduction in relapse rate found for the control group, but some change was to be expected (regression to the mean). The relapse frequency in the controls dropped from a mean of 3.9 attacks in the 2-year pretrial period to 2.7 attacks during the 2-year

trial period. In comparing relapse rates from one year to another, one must consider that at least one exacerbation would be necessary for satisfying the criterion for trial entry in a relapse prevention trial. Accordingly, it may be appropriate to omit one of the relapses from the pretrial period because it was required for definition. If this adjustment is made, the number of exacerbations in the placebo group that seemed to favor patients with exceptional relapse rates barely dropped (2.9 per 2-year interval versus 2.7 per 2-year interval). This finding raised the possibility that the relatively high relapse rate in the control group may have accounted for some of the statistical significance of the difference in relapse rate between the two groups (some of the treated group's reduction in relapses could be attributed to regression to the mean). It could be argued that the control group did not show the expected regression to the mean, an outcome that is proportional to the degree of deviation from the mean attack rate in the pretrial period. However, there is no apparent reason for this occurrence.

RATE OF PROGRESSION

Similarly, progressive patients selected for rapid chronic deterioration in the pretrial year also have a striking tendency to regress to the mean. This phenomenon is seen in a number of recent trials, including large multicenter studies of the effect of cyclophosphamide, plasmapheresis, cyclosporine A, and total lymphoid irradiation in chronic progressive MS. The findings from the control groups of these trials closely paralleled predicted stabilization rates from natural history data.[98] Stabilization rates for patients similarly selected for a drop of 1 Kurtzke point in the previous year closely resembled those from the mock natural history trial described earlier in this chapter. Specifically, stabilization rates of 75 to 85 percent at 1 year and of 67 to 72 percent at 2 years were found for patients in the control group of the Canadian cyclophosphamide trial as well as the copolymer I trial in progressive MS. It is difficult to give similar data for the cyclosporine trial[59] because of the large number of dropouts, but the control group's behavior did not appear to be substantially different from that of the other control groups just mentioned. Moreover, these stabilization rates were recorded on patients who had dropped 1 Kurtzke point in the previous year, and we attribute the fact that only about one-quarter of such patients will drop another point in the subsequent year to the phenomenon of regression to the mean.

The Control Group and the Effect of Blinding

CYCLOPHOSPHAMIDE

A large number of patients in parts of Europe and more recently in North America received cyclophosphamide over more than a decade. Results were believed to be promising, and a single retrospectively controlled study that yielded negative findings had little impact in retarding its use.[91]

In 1983, the results of an influential controlled trial in Boston that ascribed remarkable benefits to high-dose intravenous cyclophosphamide were published.[32] This report led to the widespread use of cyclophosphamide in North America. However, this study had a suboptimal design. Both the investigators and the patients were unblinded (the latter necessarily so owing to the nature of the therapy).

Two subsequent controlled trials, one by Likosky and colleagues[48] and a multicenter Canadian trial (Canadian Cooperative Study Group[8]), showed cyclophosphamide to be ineffective. A partial explanation for this spuriously positive result[32] comes from the natural history studies that became available while the Canadian study was in progress. The results of these studies demonstrated that the Boston treated group did little if any better than untreated patients similarly selected. The difference between the treated group and the control group in the study may have been entirely attributable to the exceptionally bad outcome in the Boston control group. Although the control group did as predicted at the time, it remains uncertain why these investigators found an outcome that had been erroneously expected by many neurologists treating patients with MS (the control group in this study did worse than in any previously reported clinical trial in MS). A second explanation has been suggested by the data from the Canadian trial after a comparison of disability scores assigned by the blinded examiner with those assigned by the unblinded examiner. The significant difference found between the scores was such that the use of the unblinded examiner's score would have led to the conclusion that high-dose intravenous cyclophosphamide was effective, although not as effective as plasmapheresis and cyclophosphamide.[62] The influence of blinding cannot be discounted, therefore, as a factor in reproducibility of the Boston study, which used unblinded evaluators.

Finally, no placebo control groups were used in the Boston study, but instead, the control groups received adrenocorticotropic hormone (ACTH), which has generally been considered standard therapy. This was an extraordinary design because patients in the control group would, almost by necessity, have been ACTH failures. It would be highly unlikely that a patient would bypass standard therapy before volunteering for a treatment with substantial toxicity. Accordingly, it is difficult to imagine any placebo effect occurring in a group of unblinded patients receiving therapy they knew had not helped them previously. In fact, the ACTH control group may even have demonstrated a negative placebo effect in response to this previously ineffective therapy, which would explain unusually poor outcome. Remarkably, the rating scores of unblinded examiners in the Canadian trial supported some modest therapeutic effect of plasmapheresis and, to a lesser extent, cyclophosphamide; however, the blinded examiners' scores, on which greater reliance should be placed, demonstrated no benefit. One explanation is that the unblinded examiners in the Canadian trial must have had an unconscious belief or wish that the drug be effective. Although the Boston group has suggested that differences in the treatment protocol were responsible for the differences seen in the two studies, these arguments seem spurious because their treated group did not do better than the Canadian treated group, the

Canadian control group, or the natural history group, all of which had very similar stabilization rates. Rather, it was the Boston controls who did much worse.

We wish we were as sage when these trials were first viewed retrospectively as we are now. We were initially quite impressed by the Boston cyclophosphamide data and carried out the Canadian study because we believed that the magnitude of the benefit was important to establish, given the potential long-term consequences of this drug. Moreover, many of the data from the natural history studies came as somewhat of a surprise. Our own impression, along with others, had been that in progressive cases, the rate of stabilization was much lower than it really turned out to be. We were incorrect in predicting the results of the Canadian trial when forced to do so before the unmasking of the data.[63]

The Canadian Cooperative Study Group's cyclophosphamide trial, initiated to reproduce the remarkable results previously reported,[32] carried some important lessons. Indeed, the failure of this medication to alter the course of progression in MS had already been reported by Likowsky and colleagues, although not published until later.[48] Nevertheless, the design of the Canadian trial has allowed for analysis of the reasons for the inability to replicate the promising results from the Boston study. It is sobering to note that these lessons about MS trials, insofar as they relate to proper controls, blinding, and so forth, illustrate the peril in ignoring the oft-repeated admonitions of those doing trials in MS a generation ago.[6,88]

A final comment concerns the disability outcome measure used. Few investigators carrying on clinical trials in MS can view the Kurtzke disability scale or even the EDSS with great enthusiasm. However, the scale does have some merits. For one, because it has been widely used, there are relatively few problems in interpretation, and more important, no better clinical measure has been designed, validated, or both. The employment in trials of scales for which there had yet to be data on interobserver or intraobserver variability seems potentially hazardous (cf. the Harvard ambulation index and the Troiano scale used in the total lymphoid irradiation study[12]) and makes interpretation less easy.

CYCLOSPORINE

Cyclosporine has been employed in two major clinical trials in MS.[36,59] The larger of these has been the recent American trial, which suggested a small benefit on a secondary outcome measure (time to wheelchair). The high frequency of dropouts raised some concerns about the interpretation of the data. The analysis of dropouts in this paper neatly attributed their actions to either side effects or lack of efficacy. This may appear counterintuitive to investigators who have carried out trials with medications having side effects, because it is well known that patients discontinue therapy on the basis of a combination of side effects and lack of efficacy. There is potential hazard in relegating to the investigator the task of determining a single reason for the high dropout rate. The investigator would have to be as objective as possible in making this determination, because the shifting into the "side effect" group of even a small number of patients for whom "lack of efficacy" entered into their decision to stop the medication could potentially have a major influence on the interpretation of these outcome measures. Finally, dropouts tend to be the Achilles' heel of progressive trials, and they are especially burdensome when an intention-to-treat analysis is performed. The greater the number of dropouts (time off medication), the more difficult it will be to prove that an effective therapy works.

TOTAL LYMPHOID IRRADIATION

Several issues are raised by the controlled trial of total lymphoid irradiation reported by Cook and colleagues.[12] The treated patients did not appear to do much better than the natural history studies indicate, and the untreated group seemed to do somewhat worse. Both groups appear to have regressed to the mean with the passage of time. If the outcome in the total group is examined (i.e., treated plus control group) they resemble the natural history data. The scale in this trial had not been validated. Although it appears to be a 12-point scale, clearly the scores on the three individual subsections are not at all independent of one another. Confirmation of the study results would help allay these concerns. Finally, although the study is reported as a double-blind study, it must have been difficult to preserve blinding of the patient or examiner with a therapy that produces amenorrhea in 90 percent of treated females and engenders the loss of axillary and pubic hair in at least half the recipients.

SUMMARY

The data from natural history studies are useful in several practical ways. They provide reasonable expectations for patients regarding their long-term outcome. They assist in identifying prognostic factors and in the design of clinical trials. Although more reliance should be placed on a parallel controlled trial, clinical trial results may be checked against natural history data to help place a finding in context. Because of regression to the mean, the behavior of patients during the course of trials often resembles that of the natural history more closely than their own pretrial behavior, especially when patients are selected for unusually active short-term pretrial courses.

REFERENCES

1. Bauer HJ, Firnhaber W, and Winkler W: Prognostic criteria in multiple sclerosis. Ann NY Acad Sci 122:542–551, 1965.
2. Bondeulle M: Les formes benignes de la sclerose en plaques. Presse Med 75:2023–2026, 1967.
3. Bornstein MB, Miller A, Slagle S, et al: A pilot trial of Cop 1 in exacerbating-remitting multiple sclerosis. N Engl J Med 317:408–414, 1987.
4. Bramwell B: The prognosis of disseminated sclerosis: duration in 200 cases of disseminated sclerosis. Edinburgh Med J 18:16–23, 1917.
5. Broman T, Andersen O, and Bergmann L: Clinical studies on multiple sclerosis. 1. Presentation of an incidence material from Gothenburg. Acta Neurol Scand 63:6–33, 1981.
6. Brown JR, Beebe GW, Kurtzke JF, et al: The design of clinical studies to assess therapeutic efficacy in multiple sclerosis. Neurology 29:1–23, 1979.
7. Bulman DE, Sadovnick AD, and Ebers GC: Age of onset in siblings concordant for multiple sclerosis. Brain 114:937–950, 1991.
8. Canadian Cooperative Study Group: The Canadian cooperative trial of cyclophosamide and phosmaphorous in progressive multiple sclerosis. Lancet 337:442–446, 1991.
9. Cazzullo CL, Ghezzi A, Marforia S, and Caputo D: Clinical picture of multiple sclerosis with late onset. Acta Neurol Scand 58:190–196, 1978.
10. Clark VA, Detels R, Visscher BR, Valdiviezo NL, Malmgren RM, and Dudley JP: Factors associated with a malignant or benign course of multiple sclerosis. JAMA 248:856–860, 1982.
11. Confavreux C, Aimard G, and Devic M: Course and prognosis of multiple sclerosis assessed by the computerized data processing of 349 patients. Brain 103:281–300, 1980.
12. Cook SD, Devereux C, Troiano R, et al: Effect of total lymphoid irradiation in chronic progressive multiple sclerosis. Lancet 1:1405–1409, 1987.
13. Dejaegher L, de Bruyere M, Ketelaer P, and Carton H: HLA antigens and prognosis of multiple sclerosis. Part II. J Neur 229:167–174, 1983.
14. Detels R, Clark VA, Valdiviezo NL, Visscher BR, Malmgren RM, and Dudley JP: Factors associated with a rapid course of multiple sclerosis. Arch Neurol 39:337–341, 1982.
15. Donner A: Approaches to sample size estimation in the design of clinical trials: A review. Stat Med 3:199–214, 1984.
16. Duquette P, Decary F, Pleines J, et al: Clinical subgroup of MS in relation to HLA: DR alleles as possible markers of disease progression. Can J Neurol Sci 12(2):106–110, 1985.
17. Duquette P, Murray TJ, Pleines J, et al: Multiple sclerosis in childhood: Clinical profile in 125 patients. J Pediatr 3:359–363, 1987.
18. Engell T: A clinical patho-anatomical study of clinically silent multiple sclerosis. Acta Neurol Scand 79:428–430, 1989.
19. Engell T, Raun NE, Thompson N, et al: HLA-linked and unlinked determinants. 1982.
20. Filippi M, Horsfield MA, Morrissey SP, et al: Quantitative brain MRI lesion load predicts the course of clinically isolated syndromes suggestive of multiple sclerosis. Neurology. 44:635–641, 1994.
21. Fog T, and Linnemann F: The course of multiple sclerosis in 73 cases with computer-designed curves. Acta Neurol Scand Suppl 46:1–175, 1970.
22. Georgi W: Multiple sklerose: Pathologisch-anatomische Befund multipler sklerose bei klinisch nicht diagnostizierten Krankheiten.* Wochenschrift 91:605–607, 1961.
23. Gonzalez-Scarano F, Grossman RI, Galetta S, Atlas SC, and Silberberg DH: Multiple sclerosis disease activity correlates with gadolinium-enhanced magnetic resonance imaging. Ann Neurol 21:300–306, 1987.
24. Goodkin DE: Inter and intra observer variability for grades 1.0–3.5 of the Kurtzke Expanded Disability Status Scale (EDSS). Neurology 41:145, 1991.
25. Goodkin DE: The natural history of multiple sclerosis in treatment of multiple sclerosis. In Rudick R, and Goodkin DS (eds). Springer-Verlag, New York, 1992, pp 17–45.
26. Goodkin DE, Bailly RC, Tewetzew ML, Hertsgaard D, and Beatty WW: The efficacy of azathio-

prine in relapsing-remitting MS. Neurology 41: 20–25, 1991.

27. Goodkin DE, Hertsgaard D, and Rudick RA: Exacerbation rates and adherence to disease type in a prospectively followed-up population with multiple sclerosis: Implications for clinical trials. Arch Neurol 46:1107–1112, 1989.

28. Gudmundsson KR: Clinical studies of multiple sclerosis in Iceland. Acta Neurol Scand 47(suppl 48):1–78, 1971.

29. Hader WJ, Elliot M, and Ebers GC: Epidemiology of multiple sclerosis in London and Middlesex County, Ontario, Canada. Neurology 38:617–621, 1988.

30. Harpur GD, Sure R, Bass BH, et al: A double-blind controlled study of hyperbaric oxygen in chronic stable multiple sclerosis. Neurology 36:988–990, 1986.

31. Harris JO, Frank JA, Patronas N, McFarlin DE, and McFarland HF: Serial gadolinium-enhanced magnetic resonance imaging scans in patients with early, relapsing-remitting multiple sclerosis: Implications for clinical trials and natural history. Ann Neurol 29:548–555, 1991.

32. Hauser SL, Dayson DM, Lehrich JR, et al: Intensive immunosuppression in progressive multiple sclerosis. N Engl J Med 308:173–180, 1983.

33. Isaac C, Li D, Genton M, et al: Multiple sclerosis: A serial study using MRI in relapsing patients. Neurology 38:1511–1515, 1988.

34. Jersild C, Fog T, Hansen GS, Thomsen M, Sveijgaard A, and Dupont B: Histocompatability determinants in multiple sclerosis with special reference to clinical course. Lancet 2:1221–1224, 1973.

35. Johnson KP, Brooks BR, Cohen JA, et al: Copolymer 1 reduces relapse rate and improves disability in relapsing-remitting multiple sclerosis: Results of a phase III multicenter, double-blind, placebo-controlled trial. Neurology 45:1268–1276, 1995.

36. Kappos L: Cyclosporine versus azathioprine in the long-term treatment of multiple sclerosis: Results of the German multicenter study. Ann Neurol 23:56–63, 1988.

37. Koopmans RA, Li DK, Grochowski E, Cutler PJ, and Paty DW: Benign versus chronic progressive multiple sclerosis: Magnetic resonance imaging features. Ann Neurol 25:74–81, 1989.

38. Koopmans RA, Li DK, Oger JJ, et al: Chronic progressive multiple sclerosis: Serial magnetic resonance brain imaging over six months. Ann Neurol 26:248–256, 1989.

39. Koopmans RA, Li DK, Oger J, Mayo J, and Paty DW: The lesion of multiple sclerosis: Imaging of acute and chronic stages. Neurology 39:959–963, 1989.

40. Kurtzke J: On the evolution of disability of multiple sclerosis. Neurology 11:686–694, 1961.

41. Kurtzke JF: Rating neurologic impairment in multiple sclerosis: An expanded disability status scale (EDSS). Neurology 33:1444–1452, 1983.

42. Kurtzke JF, Auth TL, Beebe GW, Kurland LT, Nagler B, and Nefzger MD: Survival in multiple sclerosis: Transactions of the American Neurological Association. 94:134–139, 1969.

43. Kurtzke JF, Beebe GW, Nagler B, Kurland LT, and Auth TL: Studies on the natural history of multiple sclerosis. VIII. Early prognostic features of the later course of the illness. Journal of Chronic Diseases 30:819–830, 1977.

44. Kurtzke JF, Beebe GW, Nagler B, Nefzger MD, Auth TL, and Kurland LT: Studies on the natural history of mulitple sclerosis. V. Long-term survival in young men. Arch Neurol 22:215–225, 1970.

45. L'hermitte F, Marteau R, Gazengel J, Dordain G, and Deloche G: The frequency of relapse in multiple sclerosis: a study based on 245 cases. J Neurol 205:47–59, 1973.

46. Leibowitz U, and Alter M: Clinical factors associated with increased disability in multiple sclerosis. Acta Neurol Scand 46:53–70, 1970.

47. Leibowitz U, Alter M, and Halpern L: Clinical studies of multiple sclerosis in Israel. III. Clinical course and prognosis related to age at onset. Neurology 14:926–932, 1964.

48. Likosky W, Fireman B, Elmore R, et al: Intense immunosuppression in chronic progressive multiple sclerosis: The Kaiser Study. J Neurol Neurosurg Psychiatry 54:1055–1060, 1991.

49. Mackay RP, and Hirano A: Forms of benign multiple sclerosis: Report of two "clinically silent" cases discovered at autopsy. Arch Neurol 17:588–600, 1967.

50. Madigand M, Oger JF, Fauchet R, Sabouraud O, and Genetet B: HLA profiles in multiple sclerosis suggest two forms of disease and the existence of protective haplotypes. J Neurol Sci 53:519–529, 1982.

51. McAlpine D: The benign form of multiple sclerosis: A study based on 241 cases seen within three years of onset and followed up until the tenth year or more of the disease. Brain 84:186–203, 1961.

52. McAlpine D, and Compston N: Some aspects of the natural history of disseminated sclerosis: Incidence, course and prognosis—Factors affecting the onset and course. QJM 21:135–167, 1952.

53. Miller DH, Hornabrook RW, and Purdie G: The natural history of multiple sclerosis: A regional study with some longitudinal data. J Neurol Neurosurg Psychiatry 55:341–346, 1992.

54. Miller DH, Ormerod EC, Rudge P, Kendall BE, Moseley IF, and McDonald WI: The yearly risk of multiple sclerosis following isolated acute syndromes of the brainstem and spinal cord. Ann Neurol 26:635–639, 1989.

55. Minderhoud JM, van der Hoeven JH, and Prange AJA: Course and prognosis of chronic progressive multiple sclerosis. Acta Neurol Scand 78:10–15, 1988.

56. Morrissey SP, Miller DH, Kendall BE, et al: The significance of brain magnetic resonance imaging abnormalities at presentation with clinically isolated syndromes suggestive of multiple sclerosis: A 5-year follow-up study. Brain 116 (pt 1): 135–146, 1993.

57. Moulin D, Paty DW, and Ebers GC: The predictive value of cerebrospinal electrophoresis in "possible" multiple sclerosis. Brain 106:809–816, 1983.

58. Muller R: Studies on disseminated sclerosis with special reference to symptomatology: Course and prognosis. Acta Medica Scandinavica (Supplement) 222:1–214, 1949.

59. Multiple Sclerosis Study Group: Efficacy and toxicity of cyclosporin in chronic progressive multiple sclerosis: A randomized, double-blinded placebo controlled clinical trial. Ann Neurol 27:591–605, 1990.

60. Noseworthy J: Concordance between examining neurologists on multiple sclerosis disability scales in a blinded, prospective clinical trial. Neurology 38:195, 1988.

61. Noseworthy JH, Seland TP, and Ebers GC: Therapeutic trials in multiple sclerosis. Can J Neurol Sci 11:355–362, 1984.

62. Noseworthy JH, Vandervoort MK, Ebers GC, Farquhar R, Yetisir E, and Roberts R: The impact of blinding on the results of a randomized controlled multiple sclerosis clinical trial. Neurology 44(1):16–20, 1994.

63. Noseworthy JH, Vandervoort MK, Hopkins M, and Ebers GC: A referendum on clinical trial research in multiple sclerosis: the opinion of the participants at the Jekyll Island Conference. Neurology 39:977–981, 1989.

64. Noseworthy JH, Vandervoort MK, Wong CJ, and Ebers CB: Interrater variability with the Expanded Disability Status Scale (EDSS) and Functional Systems (FS) in a multiple sclerosis clinical trial: The Canadian Cooperative MS Study Group. Neurology 40:971–975, 1990.

65. Noseworthy J, Paty DW, Wonnacott T, Feasby T, and Ebers GC: Multiple sclerosis after 50. Neurology 33:1537–1544, 1983.

66. Olerup O, and Hillert J: HLA class II-associated genetic susceptibility in multiple sclerosis: a critical evaluation (review). Tissue Antigens 38(1): 1–15, 1991.

67. Panelius M: Studies on epidemiological, clinical and etiological aspects of multiple sclerosis. Acta Neurol Scand Suppl 45:1–82, 1969.

68. Paty DW: Magnetic resonance imaging in the assessment of disease activity in multiple sclerosis. Can J Neurol Sci 15:266–272, 1988.

69. Paty DW: Magnetic resonance imaging in the diagnosis and follow-up of patients with multiple sclerosis. Ital J Neurol Sci. 13(9 suppl 14): 125–131, 1992.

70. Paty DW: Trial measures in multiple sclerosis: The use of magnetic resonance imaging in the evaluation of clinical trials. Neurology 38:82–83, 1988.

71. Paty DW, Oger JJ, Kastrukoff LF, et al: MRI in the diagnosis of MS: A prospective study with comparison of clinical evaluation, evoked potentials, oligoclonal banding and CT. Neurology 38: 180–185, 1988.

72. Patzold U, and Pocklington PR: Course of multiple sclerosis: First results of a prospective study carried out of 102 MS patients from 1976–1980. Acta Neurol Scand 65:248–266, 1982.

73. Percy AK, Nobrega FT, Orazaki H, Glattre E, and Kurland LT: Multiple sclerosis in Rochester, Minnesota: A 60-year appraisal. Arch Neurol 25: 105–111, 1971.

74. Phadke JG: Clinical aspects of multiple sclerosis in north-east Scotland with particular reference to its course and prognosis. Brain 113(pt 6): 1597–1628, 1990.

75. Poser CM: Trauma and multiple sclerosis: An hypothesis. J Neurol 234:155–159, 1987.

76. Poser S: Multiple Sclerosis. An analysis of 812 cases by means of electronic data processing. Springer-Verlag, Berlin, 1978, pp 54–66.

77. Poser S, Bauer HJ, and Poser W: Prognosis of multiple sclerosis: Results from an epidemiological area in Germany. Acta Neurol Scand 65: 347–354, 1982.

78. Poser S, Kurtzke JF, Poser W, and Schlaf G: Survival in multiple sclerosis. J Clin Epidemol 42:159–168, 1989.

79. Poser S, Poser W, Schlaf G, et al: Prognostic factors in multiple sclerosis. Acta Neurol Scand 74:387–392, 1986.

80. Poser S, Ritter G, Bauer HJ, Grosse-Wilde H, Kuwert EK, and Raun NE: HLA-antigens and the prognosis of multiple sclerosis. J Neurol 225: 219–221, 1981.

81. Riise T, Gronning M, Aarli JA, Nyland H, Larsen JP, and Edland A: Prognostic factors for life expectancy in multiple sclerosis analysed by Cox models. J Clin Epidemiol 41:1031–1036, 1988.

82. Riise T, Gronning M, Fernández O, et al: Early prognostic factors for disability in multiple sclerosis: A European multicenter study. Acta Neurol Scand 85:212–218, 1992.

83. Rose AS, Kuzma JW, Kurtzke JF, Namerow N, Sibley WA, and Tourtellotte WW: Cooperative study in the evaluation of therapy in multiple sclerosis: ACTH versus placebo-Final report. Neurology 20:1–59, 1970.

84. Runmarker B, and Andersen O: Prognostic factors in a multiple sclerosis incident cohort with twenty-five years of follow-up. Brain 116:117–134, 1993.

85. Sackett DL, Haynes RB, and Tugwell P: Clinical epidemiology: A basic science for clinical medicine. Boston: Little, Brown, 1985.

86. Sadovnick AD, Ebers GC, Wilson RW, and Paty DW: Life expectancy in patients attending multiple sclerosis clinics. Neurology 42:991–994, 1992.

87. Sadovnick AD, Eisen K, Ebers GC, and Paty DW: Cause of death in patients attending multiple sclerosis clinics. Neurology 41:1193–1196, 1991.

88. Schumacher GA, Beeber G, Kibler RF, et al: Problems of experimental trials of therapy in multiple sclerosis: Report by the panel on the evaluation of experimental trials of therapy in multiple sclerosis. Ann NY Acad Sci 122:552–568, 1965.

89. Stendahl-Brodin L, and Link H: Relation between benign course of multiple sclerosis and low-grade humoral immune response in cerebrospinal fluid. J Neur Neurosurg Psychiatry 43:102–105, 1980.

90. Stendahl-Brodin L, Link H, Moller E, and Norby E: Genetic basis of multiple sclerosis: HLA antigens, disease progression and oligoclonal IgG in CSF. Acta Neurol Scand 59:297–308, 1979.

91. Theys P, Gosseys-Lissoir, Ketelaer P, and Carton H: Short-term intensive cyclophosphamide treatment in multiple sclerosis: a retrospective controlled study. J Neurol 225:119–133, 1981.

92. Thompson AJ, Hutchinson M, Brazil J, Feighery C, and Martin EA: A clinical and laboratory study of benign multiple sclerosis. QJM 58:69–80, 1986.

93. Verjans E, Theys P, Delmotte P, and Carton H: Clinical parameters and intrathecal IgG synthesis as prognostic features in multiple sclerosis. J Neurol 229:155–165, 1983.

94. Visscher BR, Liu KS, Clark VA, Detels R, Malmgren RM, and Dudley JP: Onset symptoms as predictors of mortality and disability in multiple sclerosis. Acta Neurol Scand 70:321–328, 1984.

95. Weinshenker BG, Bass B, Rice GP, et al: The natural history of multiple sclerosis: A geographically based study. I. Clinical course and disability. Brain 112:133–146, 1989.

96. Weinshenker BG, Bass B, Rice GP, et al: The natural history of multiple sclerosis: A geographically based study. II. Predictive value of the early clinical course. Brain 112:1419–1428, 1989.

97. Weinshenker BG, Rice GPA, Noseworthy JH, Carriere W, Baskerville J, and Ebers GC: The natural history of multiple sclerosis: A geographically based study. III. Multivariate analysis of predictive factors and models of outcome. Brain 114:1045–1056, 1991.

98. Weinshenker BG, Rice GPA, Noseworthy JH, Carriere W, Baskerville J, and Ebers GC: The natural history of multiple sclerosis: A geographically based study. IV. Applications to planning and interpretation of clinical therapeutic trials. Brain 114:1057–1067, 1991.

99. Weinshenker BG, and Ebers GC: The natural history of multiple sclerosis. Can J Neurol Sci 14:255–261, 1987.

100. Wiebe S, Lee DH, Karlik SJ, et al: Serial cranial and spinal cord imaging in multiple sclerosis. Ann Neurol 32:643–650, 1992.

101. Willoughby EW, Grochowski E, Li D et al: Serial magnetic resonance scanning in multiple sclerosis: A prospective study in relapsing patients. Ann Neurol 25:43–49, 1989.

102. Willoughby EW, and Paty DW: Scales for rating impairment in multiple sclerosis: A critique. Neurology 38:1793–1798, 1988.

CHAPTER 7

VISUAL SIGNS AND SYMPTOMS

Duncan Anderson, MD
Terry Cox, MD

Most patients with MS have visual symptoms at some point during their illness. In a series of 157 autopsy-proven cases of MS, 85 percent had "ocular disturbance" as a symptom.[114] Many other patients with no symptoms have clinical evidence of ocular dysfunction. In a group of 229 patients with clinically definite MS seen in our clinic, only 26 had normal eye examinations (Table 7–1). A wide variety of clinical neuro-ophthalmologic signs occur in the MS clinic involving many of the neurological systems of interest to the neuro-ophthalmologist, including all levels of the visual sensory system, supranuclear and infranuclear ocular motor pathways, and the pupil. Detection of abnormalities in these systems is usually apparent on careful clinical examination but occasionally may require

229

Table 7-1. CLINICAL FINDINGS AT THE UNIVERSITY OF BRITISH COLUMBIA MULTIPLE SCLEROSIS CLINIC

Clinical Findings	Definite MS	Probable MS	Possible MS	Total
Normal eye examinations	26/229 (11.4%)	18/72 (25.0%)	49/85 (57.6%)	93/386 (24.2%)
Relative afferent pupillary defects	55/229 (24%)	10/72 (13.9%)	4/85 (4.7%)	69/386 (17.9%)
Optic atrophy	161/229 (70.3%)	32/72 (44.4%)	16/85 (18.8%)	209/386 (54.2%)
Retinal venous sheathing	14/229 (6.1%)	4/72 (5.5%)	2/85 (2.4%)	20/386 (5.2%)
Internuclear ophthalmoplegia*	49/226 (21.7%)	4/70 (5.7%)	3/85 (3.5%)	56/381 (14.7%)
Abnormal visual suppression of VOR	61/194 (31.4%)	11/66 (16.7%)	9/79 (11.4%)	81/339 (23.9%)
Gaze-evoked nystagmus	81/229 (35.4%)	15/72 (20.8%)	11/85 (12.9%)	107/386 (27.7%)

*Bilateral involvement in 28/56 (50%).
VOR = vestibulo-ocular response.

special techniques, such as visual evoked potential (VEP) testing or eye movement recording for accurate diagnosis.

The following discussion emphasizes findings that can be detected in the office or at the bedside. Included are summary statistics regarding clinical findings in 386 patients seen by Dr. Cox at the University of British Columbia MS Clinic between February 1, 1985 and April 30, 1987.

OPTIC NEURITIS

Optic neuritis is the most common cause of visual difficulties in MS; 122 of our 386 patients had a history consistent with this diagnosis. Optic neuritis is characterized by acute or subacute visual loss in one eye, usually associated with retrobulbar pain or pain on eye movement, followed by recovery. Visual loss in optic neuritis usually progresses over 3 to 7 days and then gradually improves over weeks to months. Most patients experience haziness or blurring of vision with loss of color perception. Occasionally loss of color vision is the only symptom. Phosphenes (perceptions of flashes of light) sometimes occur in the affected eye and may be induced by eye movements[34] or sounds.[84,106]

Pain occurs in approximately 90 percent of patients[103,112] and is described as aching or as discomfort in and around the eye, occasionally associated with tenderness on palpation of the globe. In approximately 40 percent of cases, pain begins several days before visual loss, but more often, it occurs in association with the visual blurring.[103] Pain is usually made worse with eye movement, particularly in extremes of gaze. Total duration of pain is variable, usually lasting 7 to 10 days, but occasionally lasting weeks.

Uhthoff's symptom, characterized by worsening of vision with exercise, fatigue, stress, or increased body temperature, occurs in approximately one-third of patients after recovery from optic neuritis.[112] Occasionally Uhthoff's symptom occurs without previous acute optic neuritis, and it may be the first evidence of MS. The chapter by MacKarell[87] is an excellent discussion of optic neuritis from the point of view of the patient.

Prognosis for spontaneous recovery of vision in optic neuritis is good. Seventy percent of patients recover 20/20 vision, and 95 percent recover 20/40 or better.[8,112] Nearly all patients will show at least some improvement in visual function after the acute phase, even when the final visual outcome is poor. Optic neuritis recurs within 2 years in 15 to 20 percent of cases, each eye being equally at risk.[9,112] Bilateral simultaneous optic neuritis from demyelination is rare[107] and is more often associated with a postinfectious or postvaccination etiology, especially in children.

Most patients with optic neuritis are between 20 and 50 years old. Perkin and Rose[112] found that 84 percent of their 170 patients fell into this age group. The mean age of patients in the Optic Neuritis Treatment Trial was 32.[103] Kennedy and Carroll[78] reported 30 children with idiopathic optic neuritis; the age range was 4 to 15 years, and 8 of the 30 developed MS. Riikonen and colleagues[119] described 21 children with optic neuritis between ages 4 and 14 years. Bilateral involvement and papillitis were more common in the children than in adults. Nine children with unilateral involvement developed MS.

Not all patients with optic neuritis develop other signs and symptoms of MS. In several prospective studies of patients with isolated optic neuritis (summarized by Cohen and colleagues[25] and Francis[47]), the frequency of development of MS has varied from 17 to 85 percent. The Optic Neuritis Study Group publications[8,9,10,103] reported that 12 percent of cases had clinically definite MS 2 years after an attack of optic neuritis. Only 4 percent of patients with a normal magnetic resonance imaging (MRI) scan developed MS, whereas 30 percent with an abnormal MRI scan did so. Other studies[25,47] suggest a 2-year risk of MS after optic neuritis of approximately 20 percent and a 15-year risk of 45 to 80 percent. It appears that the risk of developing MS after an attack of optic neuritis is approximately 5 to 6 percent per year.[10,25,47,91]

The different percentages may reflect regional differences in study groups, different criteria for diagnosing isolated optic neuritis, and variable length of follow-up. Some investigators have found that the course of

MS tends to be more benign if the presenting event is optic neuritis.[134] Wikström and associates[159] found that isolated optic neuritis was the first evidence of multiple sclerosis in 16.6 percent of 1271 patients with MS, and the optic nerve was involved at the first appearance of the disease in 34.7 percent.

No test or combination of tests has proved completely reliable in predicting the development of MS after acute optic neuritis. Patients who have had recurrent attacks have an increased risk, but female gender is probably not an increased risk factor.[10,79,120] Nikoskelainen and colleagues[100,101] found that abnormalities of cerebrospinal fluid (CSF) protein and cell count were more common in patients with optic neuritis who later developed MS, but a few patients with isolated optic neuritis also had abnormal findings on CSF analysis, and some patients who developed MS had normal findings on CSF analysis. Sandberg-Wollheim[133] obtained similar results, whereas Stendahl-Brodin and Link[151] found a significantly increased risk of developing MS when the patient with optic neuritis had oligoclonal bands in the CSF. Optic neuritis causes an elevation of CSF myelin basic protein in many patients.[158]

A retrospective analysis of 146 patients who presented with isolated optic neuritis[47] found that the HLA antigen, DR3, significantly increased the risk of developing MS, particularly when the antigen HLA-DR2 was also present. Another study[64] found an increased risk of developing MS when HLA-DR2 and B7 tissue types were present. A curious association found in a study by Compston and associates[26] was an increased frequency of progression to MS in patients whose initial attack of optic neuritis occurred in the winter months.

Multimodality evoked potentials detect disseminated central nervous system (CNS) abnormalities in approximately 35 percent of patients[105,135] and MRI in approximately 60 percent of patients with isolated optic neuritis.* These and other studies[10] suggest that the greater the number of the subclinical MRI abnormalities, the greater the likelihood of future development of MS.

---

*References 32, 72–74, 95, 103, 105, 110, 127.

In acute optic neuritis, the computed tomography (CT) scan often shows a diffusely thickened nerve that demonstrates contrast enhancement.[69] After recovery, the CT scan is normal. Using MRI with a surface coil for orbital imaging, Miller and colleagues[94] found plaques in 10 of 14 nerves affected by optic neuritis. The same authors[95] subsequently examined 37 adult patients with recent or old optic neuritis and found MRI signal abnormalities in 84 percent of their symptomatic nerves and 20 percent of their asymptomatic nerves. They found the mean longitudinal extent of the lesion was 1 cm, and slow or poor visual recovery was associated with more extensive lesions within the optic canal. Disk swelling was usually associated with anterior lesions but could also occur with lesions in the canal. They found, however, that VEPs were even more sensitive than MRI in detecting lesions of the optic nerve.

Treatment

Most patients with an isolated attack of optic neuritis have a good visual outcome.[8,9] Patients with recurrent attacks of optic neuritis may eventually develop permanent visual loss and should be evaluated by a competent low vision specialist. Hand magnifiers and magnifying glasses are useful for near tasks. If more magnification is needed, closed-circuit television magnifiers are helpful. For distance tasks, monocular hand-held telescopes are beneficial. These telescopes drastically reduce the visual field and are most useful for spotting street signs, bus numbers, and a lecture hall blackboard or projected material. They are of no value for driving.

Patients with optic nerve disease generally require increased illumination of reading material. However, patients with optic neuritis occasionally complain of visual difficulties under bright lights, especially when reading or writing. These patients can benefit from using tinted lenses in their glasses. Some experimentation may be required to determine the correct lens transmittance. Tagami and colleagues[152] found that their patients required lenses

COLOR PLATE I

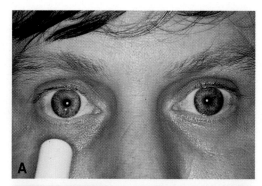

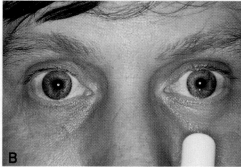

Figure 7–2. Left relative afferent pupil defect in a patient with left optic neuritis. Although both pupils react to light reasonably well, they react less well on left eye stimulation *(B)* than on right eye stimulation *(A)* when the flashlight is swung back and forth between the two eyes.

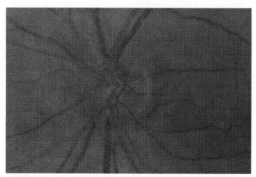

Figure 7–3. Normal hyperopic left disk. Disk is small and crowded with uniform pink color throughout.

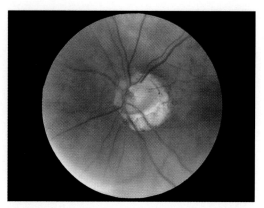

Figure 7–4. Normal myopic left disk. Normal physiological temporal pallor and peripapillary pale crescent.

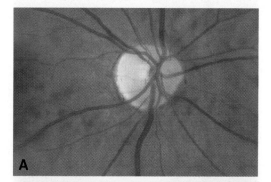

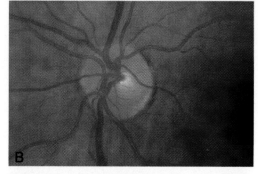

Figure 7–5. *(A)* Pathological right optic atrophy. *(B)* Normal fellow left disk for comparison. Both eyes have 20/20 vision but mild permanent nerve fiber loss has taken place on the right from previous optic neuritis.

COLOR PLATE II

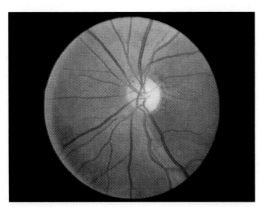

Figure 7–6. Left retinal nerve fiber layer loss. Note large area of loss of normal retinal striations temporal to the disk, which shows some temporal pallor (right side of photo). The nasal disk (left side of photo) is pinker, with normal retinal nerve fiber layer striations.

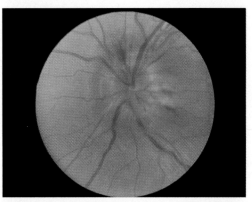

Figure 7–7. Left papillitis. Note swollen disk with blurred margins and multiple disk margin hemorrhages and a few exudates.

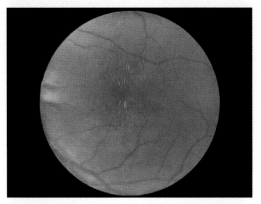

Figure 7–8. Left macular star. Note yellow radiating exudates around macula in the same eye as that in Fig. 7–7.

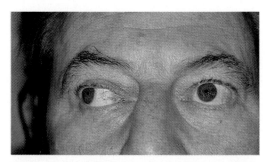

Figure 7–10. Left internuclear ophthalmoplegia. Defective adduction of left eye on right gaze with associated abducting nystagmus of right eye due to left medial longitudinal fasciculus (MLF) lesion.

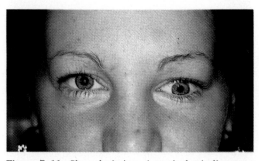

Figure 7–11. Skew deviation. A vertical misalignment of the eyes that does not fit the pattern of an isolated cyclovertical muscle palsy.

COLOR PLATE III

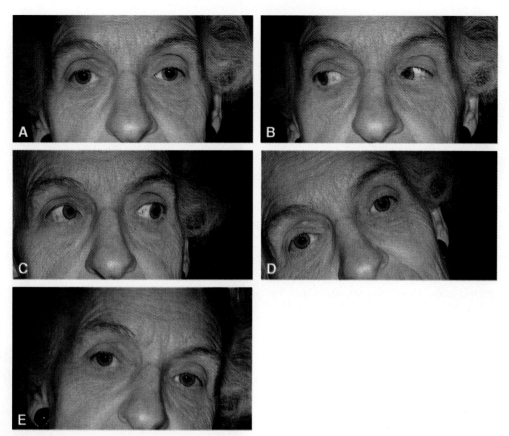

Figure 7–12. Right fourth nerve palsy. Note right hypertropia in the primary position (*A*), which decreases on right gaze (*B*), increases on left gaze (*C*) and right tilt (*D*), and decreases on left tilt (*E*). This deviation was worse in downgaze and the right image was subjectively intorted.

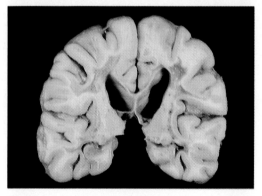

Figure 8–3. Formalin-fixed coronal slice of cerebral hemispheres from a patient with MS. Note the extensive demyelination of the periventricular regions of the lateral ventricles. Focal smaller plaques of demyelination are also evident in the parasagittal white matter.

COLOR PLATE IV

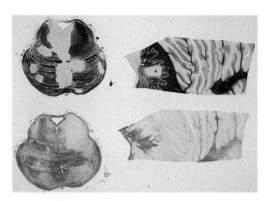

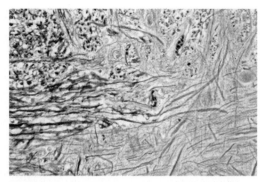

Figure 8–4. Horizontal section of rostral pons (left) and sagittal section through cerebellum and dentate nucleus (right) of a case of MS. The upper half of the figure is stained with Heidenhain stain, which stains myelin dark blue. Note the focal regions of demyelination, which do not respect anatomical boundaries in the pontine tegmentum and basis pontis. A plaque is also evident in the hilum of the dentate nucleus. The lower half shows the Holzer stain, which demonstrates gliosis in the areas of myelin loss. (Courtesy of Dr. G. Mathieson, Memorial University of Newfoundland.)

Figure 8–8. The relatively well demarcated border of a chronic silent MS plaque stained with Luxol fast blue and Bodian stains. The Luxol fast blue stains myelin sheaths blue; the Bodian stain produces dark brown axons. Note the abrupt loss of myelin sheaths, but the relative preservation of axons which have been demyelinated within the lesion (right).

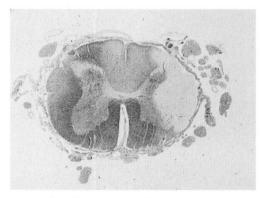

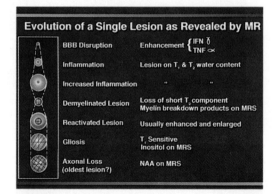

Figure 8–5. Cross-section of lumbar spinal cord stained with Luxol fast blue (LFB)-Cresyl Violet. The LFB stains myelin blue and cresyl violet stains nucleic acids (such as nuclei and neuronal Nissl substance). Note the MS plaque in the right lateral funiculus, which extends into the gray matter. The anterior horn cells are preserved in the lesion. The faint myelin pallor in the posterior columns may be due to loss of fibers from axonal involvement in a more destructive lesion or lesions caudal to this level (wallerian degeneration), or may be a shadow plaque. The same is also true of the myelin pallor of the left lateral corticospinal tract, which could be produced by axonal involvement of this tract by lesion or lesions at more rostral levels. The anatomical localization of these two latter lesions would favor wallerian degeneration and point out that, although many lesions, such as that in the right lateral funiculus, are demyelinative, axonal loss can also occur.

Figure 9–17. Evolution of a single lesion as revealed by magnetic resonance techniques. This cartoon outlines the MR techniques that can help in distinguishing specific pathological changes in the evolution of a single MS lesion.

with a total light transmission ranging from 20 to 55 percent. Yellow ("blue-blocking") lenses may be more useful than other types.

The pain associated with optic neuritis is self-limited and usually requires no treatment. Nonsteroidal anti-inflammatory agents usually provide symptomatic relief. An occasional patient has pain severe enough to consider treatment with a short course of steroids.

The controversy surrounding the use of steroids to treat visual loss[15,31,50, 58,115] in optic neuritis has been significantly reduced with the publication of the results of the Optic Neuritis Treatment Trial.[9] Four hundred and fifty-seven patients with acute optic neuritis were recruited from 15 clinical centers for this randomized, partially blinded, controlled clinical trial comparing the visual outcomes of patients with acute optic neuritis who were treated with either placebo or steroids. The patients were randomly assigned to one of three treatment groups: (1) oral prednisone (1 mg/kg per day for 14 days), (2) IV methylprednisolone (1 g/day for 3 days) followed by oral prednisone (1 mg/kg per day for 11 days), or (3) oral placebo for 14 days. Entry criteria for the study included acute unilateral optic neuritis with visual symptoms for 8 days or less, ages from 18 to 45 years, no previous history of optic neuritis in the affected eye, no evidence of systemic disease other than MS, and no previous treatment of optic neuritis or MS with steroids.

These results showed that the rate of improvement in visual function was more rapid for the intravenous and oral steroid groups than for the placebo group. At 2 years, however, no statistically significant difference in visual function was found in any of the three groups. An unexpected finding was that the oral prednisone–treated group had a greater number of new episodes of optic neuritis in either eye than the placebo- and intravenous ethylprednisolone–treated groups. These results suggest that patients with acute optic neuritis should not be treated with oral prednisone and that unless speed of return of visual function is crucial, treatment with intravenous methylprednisolone is probably not warranted in terms of eventual visual outcome.

A subsequent publication by the Optic Neuritis Study Group[10] found that at 2-year follow-up of the initial cohort of patients, the intravenous steroid–treated group had a lower rate of development of MS than those treated with placebo or oral prednisone. Moreover, this beneficial effect of treatment on the subsequent development of MS was most apparent in patients with abnormal MRI scans at entry into the study. The authors recommended that in patients with acute optic neuritis and other signal abnormalities on MRI scanning, treatment with intravenous methylprednisolone should be considered to reduce the future risk of development of MS even though visual improvement in this group of treated patients was clinically insignificant.

It should be noted that the Optic Neuritis Treatment Trial was designed to evaluate improvement in visual function in three treatment groups, not the rate of development of MS. Therefore, the finding of a reduced rate of development of MS after treatment, though a promising development, should be treated with some caution.

If the patient's vision decreases when oral steroids are tapered, the clinician must reconsider the diagnosis. Several kinds of tumors are steroid sensitive (see following discussion). When the diagnosis is in doubt, treatment with steroids should be deferred. Most patients with optic neuritis will improve without treatment in a few weeks. Because few other optic nerve diseases that cause subacute visual loss improve spontaneously, the natural history helps to make the diagnosis.

Becker and colleagues[13] improved visual function in five patients with MS by lowering serum calcium using oral phosphate. All patients noted paresthesias as their vision improved. The authors concluded that chronic administration of similar agents would not be effective because the parathyroid glands would tend to maintain normal serum calcium levels.

Patients with Uhthoff's symptom should avoid hazardous situations. Examples include riding a bicycle or driving a car without air conditioning on a hot day.

Differential Diagnosis

Most experts reserve the term *optic neuritis* (or *retrobulbar neuritis*) for that group of young to middle-aged patients who have subacute, usually unilateral, visual loss associated with eye movement pain, an afferent pupil defect, and central visual field defects, followed by gradual visual recovery. The vast majority of these patients do not have evidence of anything other than demyelination as the presumed cause of the optic neuritis. A small number have a presumed viral or postviral syndrome.

Diseases occasionally confused with optic neuritis include cytomegalovirus disease, syphilis, sarcoidosis, toxocariasis, toxoplasmosis, systemic lupus erythematosus, and Guillain-Barré syndrome. Optic neuritis may occur in association with chickenpox or infectious mononucleosis, as well as after various types of vaccinations. Most of these diseases have a totally different presentation, time course, and recovery than that seen in demyelinating optic neuritis, although some of the viral and postviral syndromes are similar.

Patients with ischemic optic neuropathy lose vision from infarction of the optic disk. Onset of visual loss is sudden, and spontaneous recovery is rare. The optic disk is pale and edematous in the acute phase, and visual field defects are predominantly related to the disk (arcuate or altitudinal). The presumed causes of ischemic optic neuropathy in young adults include migraine, vasculitis (e.g., lupus), hypertension, and diabetes. In the elderly patient, temporal arteritis must be ruled out.

Leber's optic neuropathy is a familial condition that occurs in young adults, usually men. Subacute visual loss in one eye is followed within weeks to months by visual loss in the other eye. The optic disk is moderately swollen in the acute phase. The characteristic visual field defect is a central or cecocentral scotoma.

Toxic nutritional optic neuropathy usually presents with painless, bilateral, slowly progressive visual loss with central or cecocentral scotomas and initially normal disks that eventually become atrophic. This condition is usually seen in heavy drinkers, smokers, or both, or in those who are severely malnourished.[2] The etiology is felt to be related to vitamin B deficiency. Retinal conditions that can be confused with optic neuritis include central serous choroidopathy, acute macular neuroretinopathy, acute retinal pigment epithelitis, and the multiple evanescent white-dot syndrome. Central serous choroidopathy can mimic optic neuritis: visual loss can be acute, central scotomas are the rule, the subretinal fluid can be difficult to see with the ophthalmoscope, and VEP can be delayed.[62] Patients with central serous choroidopathy usually complain of metamorphopsia, micropsia, or both, and they usually do not have as dense a relative afferent pupillary defect as one usually sees in optic neuritis. The condition affects males more than females.

Compressive optic neuropathy also presents with slowly progressive unilateral or bilateral visual loss with central visual field defects and initially pink disks. Compressive lesions that can cause visual loss include pituitary tumor, craniopharyngioma, meningioma, lymphoma, and aneurysm. Sphenoid sinus mucocele can cause visual loss and eye pain. Many of these tumors are steroid-responsive, thus mimicking optic neuritis. In compressive optic neuropathy, however, visual loss recurs when steroids are discontinued, whereas in optic neuritis vision usually continues to improve. This is another reason to be cautious with the use of steroids in optic neuritis.

The Optic Neuritis Study Group[103] found that of the 457 subjects entered into the Optic Neuritis Treatment Trial, only two cases of compressive optic neuropathy were identified as a result of the MRI scan. One was a pituitary tumor, and the other was an ophthalmic artery aneurysm. This finding shows that a good history and clinical examination in cases of optic neuritis almost always results in the correct diagnosis, and only very rarely will MRI scanning elucidate any other etiology.

Pathological studies have shown that optic nerve demyelination occurs in nearly all patients with MS. Gartner[54] examined 14 eyes from 10 patients with autopsy-proven MS and found optic nerve demyelination in all 14. Ikuta and Zimmerman[71] reported that 68 of 69 autopsied cases of MS had optic nerve demyelination. Ulrich and Groebke-Lorenz[155] found demyelination in 35 of 36 optic nerves in 18 cases of long-standing MS. Only 8 of the 16 patients with adequate clinical histories had a documented clinical attack of acute optic neuritis. The prevalence of optic neuritis in other series of patients with MS varies from 27 to 46.5 percent.[88,111,161]

A significant number of patients with MS suffer progressive demyelination of the optic nerves,[75] usually as a result of recurrent acute attacks and remissions, but occasionally this may take a more chronic progressive course.[75] Sometimes this form of optic neuritis occurs before other clinical symptoms; therefore, arriving at the correct diagnosis may be difficult.[104,122] Slowly progressive optic neuropathy seems to have a poorer visual outcome, but spontaneous improvement can occur.

CHIASMAL NEURITIS

Although the optic chiasm is frequently involved in MS, reports of chiasmal visual field defects are few. Sacks and Melen[130] reported three patients with bitemporal visual field defects caused by MS, and Spector and associates[150] reported six patients with MS who developed such defects subacutely. In two of these nine patients, the onset of visual field loss was associated with retrobulbar pain or pain on eye movement. Two patients had visual loss in one eye associated with a temporal visual field defect in the other eye (junction scotoma); five patients had bitemporal visual field defects with good central vision; and two patients had bilateral central scotomas and bitemporal visual field defects. Pneumoencephalography in one case showed enlargement of the chiasm and nerves, and exploratory craniotomy in another case showed swelling of the chiasm. In three cases, the visual involvement preceded other evidence of the disease. The prognosis was good, with improvement of the visual field defects and central vision in most cases; however, the vision in one patient remained less than 20/200 after onset of visual loss.

RETROCHIASMAL LESIONS

Homonymous hemianopia is a rare occurrence in MS. Chamlin and Davidoff[22] reported four cases and cited three others in the literature, and Vedel-Jensen[156] added two cases and cited 10 more from the literature. Boldt[14] found such defects in 5 of 365 patients; in 4 cases, the lesion was thought to be in the optic tract, and in the other case, a temporal lobe lesion was considered likely. Rosenblatt and associates[123] described two patients with homonymous hemianopia and optic tract lesions. Beck and colleagues[12] described three patients with homonymous hemianopia, with CT evidence of optic radiations involvement in the temporoparietal lobes. The visual field defect improved in all three patients, but only one recovered to normal. We have seen several examples of homonymous hemianopias associated with occipital lesions documented by MRI scans that have cleared in patients with MS.

EXAMINATION OF THE VISUAL SENSORY SYSTEM

Patients with optic neuritis usually seek medical attention in the acute phase; however, the occasional patient demonstrates a history of visual loss that is poorly documented, and the clinician may wish to detect residual optic nerve dysfunction. The evaluation of these two groups of patients is similar, but abnormalities of optic nerve function are less pronounced in the latter group. Another clinical problem is the patient with other neurological signs and symptoms in whom the clinician is seeking evidence of subclinical optic nerve demyelination. Again, the same tests for optic nerve dysfunction are required; abnormalities are similar to those in the group of patients with recovered optic neuritis.

Visual Acuity

Acuity should be tested with the patient's best refractive correction in place. Looking through a pinhole will improve the visual acuity of many patients with refractive errors, but a good refraction is preferable. Each patient should be tested with standardized room and eye chart illumination.

The usual tests of visual acuity are relatively insensitive indicators of optic nerve dysfunction in optic neuritis. Premortem visual acuity data provided by Groebke-Lorenz[155] showed that acuity correlated inversely with amount of demyelination, but occasionally the visual acuity was surprisingly good in the presence of severe myelin loss. Although most eyes with recovered optic neuritis show abnormalities of optic nerve function using other tests, the visual acuity is often almost normal. Occasionally the acuity measures 20/20 throughout an attack of optic neuritis.

Of the 448 patients entered into the Optic Neuritis Treatment Trial,[103] 11 percent had 20/20 vision or better, 54 percent had 20/25 to 20/190 vision, 33 percent had 20/200 to light perception, and 3 percent had no light perception vision. Normal young adults usually see better than 20/20; this level of visual acuity in a patient with optic neuritis or MS may represent a drop from 20/15 or better. Those patients with worse acuity during the acute phase of optic neuritis tend to have a slightly worse visual outcome.[8,25]

The Optic Neuritis Treatment Trial showed that after an acute attack of optic neuritis, only 3 percent of patients were left with vision of 20/200 or less in the affected eye.[8,9] In no-light-perception optic neuritis, 20 percent of patients were left with vision under 20/200 in the affected eye.

Spatial Contrast Sensitivity

Traditional visual acuity tests measure the ability to detect high-contrast visual targets, usually with high spatial frequencies. Tests of spatial contrast sensitivity measure the ability to detect low-contrast targets at a variety of spatial frequencies. Many patients with resolved optic neuritis have difficulty seeing on cloudy days or when ambient illumination is low at dawn or dusk. Measurement of spatial contrast sensitivity is more likely to give a quantitative correlate of

such symptoms than are other tests. Most contrast sensitivity tests consist of sine-wave gratings of varying spatial frequency and contrast. These gratings are patterns of alternating dark and light lines of equal width that gradually blend into one another. The width of the lines is the spatial frequency: high-frequency gratings have narrow lines, and low-frequency gratings have wide lines. The test measures the lowest contrast between light and dark lines that can be detected at each spatial frequency. Patients with optic neuritis may have normal detection at high frequencies (correlating with normal visual acuity), but they may require a higher than normal contrast for detection at other frequencies.

Several methods are available for measuring contrast sensitivity. Those that use a computer and video monitor to generate sine-wave-modulated gratings are quite expensive. Arden and Gucukoglu[3] devised a series of printed sheets (Arden gratings) that can be used. Regan and Neima[116] constructed a series of letter charts at three different levels of contrast that seem to work as well as gratings. The Pelli Robson contrast sensitivity chart uses large letters of varying contrast and is widely used.

Regardless of which technique is used, testing spatial contrast sensitivity provides information about visual function that is not otherwise available and seems to be fairly sensitive in detecting optic neuropathy. Arden and Gucukoglu[3] found abnormal contrast sensitivity in 47 of 57 patients with a history of unilateral retrobulbar optic neuritis. In a subgroup of 24 patients, the contrast sensitivity was found to be abnormal in 71 percent, and VEP was abnormal in only 54 percent. Regan and colleagues[117] found that 27 of 38 patients with clinically definite or probable MS had abnormal contrast sensitivity. Zimmern and associates[163] studied eight patients with a subjective disorder of vision yet normal Snellen acuity test. All had an abnormal contrast sensitivity function in the affected eye. Fleishman and associates[46] looked at patients with recovered optic neuritis and found that abnormal contrast sensitivity correlated better with persistent subjective visual complaints than did abnormalities of visual field, color vision, or stereopsis. The

Optic Neuritis Study Group[103] found abnormal contrast sensitivity in 98.2 percent of the 448 eyes with optic neuritis. We measure contrast sensitivity in all patients that we see at the MS Clinic.

Color Vision

Patients with optic neuritis often have abnormal color vision in the affected eye. They may describe colors as "paler," "washed-out," or "darker" with the affected eye. Color vision may be tested at the bedside by having the patient compare the appearance of a red object (such as the red cap of a bottle of dilating drops) between the two eyes. Quantitative clinical tests of color vision include pseudoisochromatic plates and the Farnsworth-Munsell 100-Hue Test. This test is better for detecting color loss in optic neuropathy, but it is time-consuming and expensive. We use Ishihara pseudoisochromatic plates under fluorescent lights, and we have established our own normal values for these lighting conditions.

Mullen and Plant[97] found that color contrast detection was more impaired than luminance contrast (as in the contrast sensitivity gratings described previously) in patients with optic neuritis. Fallowfield and Krauskopf[44] used a different technique with similar results. Griffin and Wray[61] found an abnormal score on the 100-hue test in 30 of 30 eyes with previous optic neuritis. However, Burde and Gallin[19] found abnormal 100-hue test results in only three of nine patients with recovered optic neuritis, and Fleishman and associates[46] found abnormal scores in 20 of 35 eyes with previous neuritis. Engell and colleagues[43] found color vision testing to be much less sensitive than the VEP in the detection of subclinical optic neuropathy in MS, but Harrison and associates[63] and Frederiksen and associates[48] found a significant number of patients with normal VEP and abnormal color vision. The Optic Neuritis Study Group[11,103] found abnormal Ishihara plates in 88.2 percent of patients with optic neuritis and an abnormality on the Farnsworth-Munsell 100-Hue Test in 93.8 percent of these patients. Careful color vision testing will reveal abnormalities in most patients with optic neuritis, which persist even after return of visual acuity to normal.

Visual Fields

The visual field is usually abnormal in acute optic neuritis, but defects are more difficult to detect after recovery. The most typical visual field defect in the acute phase is a central scotoma (Fig. 7–1), but various types of disk-related (i.e., arcuate or altitudinal) defects are often seen. Traditionally perimetry has been done by moving a target from nonseeing to seeing parts of the visual field. After recovery from acute optic neuritis, paracentral scotomas are not unusual, but they are often difficult to detect with these kinetic techniques. Static

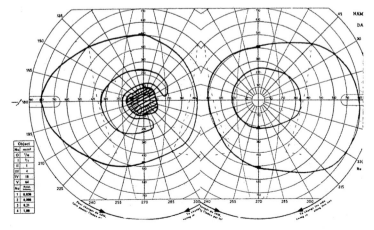

Figure 7–1. Left central scotoma. Visual field showing a left central scotoma in a patient with left optic neuritis.

perimetry is done by placing a target in the visual field and gradually increasing its intensity until the patient sees it. Automated perimeters under computer control have become generally available, and most of them use static testing techniques. Automated perimeters not only remove examiners' bias, but they also shorten examination time. At the bedside, the clinician may detect subtle central scotomas by using a red test object and confrontation techniques. A central scotoma causes relative desaturation of the target in the central visual field when compared to paracentral areas.

Burde and Gallin[19] found defects on static perimetry in eight of eight patients with recovered optic neuritis. Ellenberger and Ziegler[38] found abnormalities on perimetry (using both kinetic and static techniques) in only 56 percent of 32 eyes with previous optic neuritis. Using the tangent screen, Patterson and Heron[109] found visual field defects in 37 of 41 patients with MS (including definite, probable, and possible cases). Meienberg and colleagues[92] compared automated static perimetry with the VEP in 14 patients with MS and concluded that VEPs revealed abnormalities more often, but that perimetry can detect abnormalities in patients with normal VEPs. We have found automated perimetry to be invaluable in the detection and interpretation of visual dysfunction in MS. The Optic Neuritis Study Group[103] found abnormalities in the Humphrey Visual Field Analyzer in 97.5 percent of patients who participated in the Optic Neuritis Treatment Trial. Unlike the predominantly central defects found with manual and confrontation techniques, the Humphrey field analyzer detected more altitudinal and quadratic-type defects, with a wide variation of abnormalities found.

Relative Afferent Pupillary Defect

The relative afferent pupillary defect (RAPD, Marcus Gunn pupil, swinging flashlight test) provides objective verification of visual dysfunction (Fig. 7–2). Proper technique enhances the chances of finding an afferent pupillary defect. The patient should first be examined for anisocoria in dim light and in bright light. The alternat-

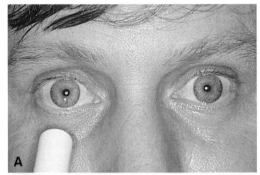
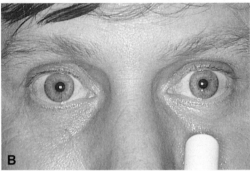

Figure 7–2. Left relative afferent pupil defect in a patient with left optic neuritis. Although both pupils react to light reasonably well, they react less well on left eye stimulation *(B)* than on right eye stimulation *(A)* when the flashlight is swung back and forth between the two eyes. **(See Color Plate I.)**

ing light test should then be done in a darkened room, with the patient looking at a target in the distance. A bright hand-held light should be used; the test does not work well when done with a penlight that has feeble batteries. The light should be shone in one eye for a few seconds, quickly moved to the other eye for the same amount of time, and then quickly back to the first eye. Care must be taken that the same spot in the visual field is stimulated in each eye. Shining a light in the temporal visual field of one eye, then in the nasal field of the other eye will create an afferent pupillary defect in the second eye. We generally hold the light centrally, just below the visual axis, and stimulate each eye for the same length of time. Holding the light longer in front of one eye will create an afferent pupillary defect in that eye due to bleaching of retinal receptors.

The normal response to the alternating light test is a small pupillary constriction followed by equivalent redilatation each time the light is moved.[28] When a patient has unilateral or asymmetrical optic nerve disease, the initial constriction will be smaller and the pupils will redilate to a larger diameter when the more diseased eye is stimulated. When the better eye is stimulated, the initial constriction is larger and the pupils redilate less.

Most patients with acute optic neuritis will have a relative afferent pupillary defect (RAPD), even when the other eye has previously been affected. RAPD can be quantified by placing neutral-density filters of increasing density over the better eye until the pupillary responses are equal.[153] Cox and associates[29] found RAPDs in 70 of 74 patients with acute optic neuritis. Two of the four patients with no RAPD had previous involvement of the other eye; the other two patients had minimal disease with good vision and mildly abnormal visual evoked potentials. These authors found that the amplitude of the pupil defect tended to decrease with recovery, but that it usually persisted unless there was clinical or subclinical involvement of the other eye. They had 11 cases in which the pupil defect resolved after clinically unilateral optic neuritis; 7 of these cases were found to have subclinical involvement in the other eye. Of patients with previous optic neuritis affecting both eyes, 66 percent had RAPDs. The patients described in this study presented with optic neuritis, and only 53 percent were known to have MS. In our MS clinic, the incidence of RAPDs is much lower (see Table 7–1) because most patients have bilateral disease, and many have not had acute optic neuritis. The Optic Neuritis Treatment Trial[9,103] had a relative afferent pupillary defect as one of the entry criteria, and therefore it was present in 100 percent of cases.

Ophthalmoscopic Appearance

Optic atrophy can be difficult to judge using the ophthalmoscope. We use three criteria for assessing atrophy: color, vascularity, and adjacent nerve fiber layer. Normal color of the temporal portion of the optic disk varies widely, with the most important determining factors being refraction of the eye, disk configuration, and background retinal

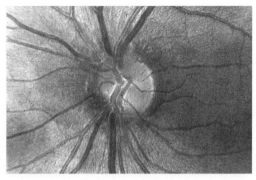

Figure 7–3. Normal hyperopic left disk. Disk is small and crowded with uniform pink color throughout. (**See Color Plate I.**)

pigmentation. Hyperopic (farsighted) patients with small, round disks with small central cups have little variation in color between temporal and nasal halves (Fig. 7–3), and relatively mild temporal pallor can be pathological in these patients. Myopic (nearsighted) patients with large or tilted disks with temporal crescents generally have normal temporal pallor (Fig. 7–4); atrophy in these patients will have to be more advanced before it can be detected by color changes alone. Comparison of disk color between the two eyes is highly sensitive in detecting unilateral optic neuropathy (Fig. 7–5).

With clear ocular media, a dilated pupil, and a good ophthalmoscope, the clinician can see tiny blood vessels on the surface of the temporal portion of the optic disk in normal subjects. Loss of these capillaries in

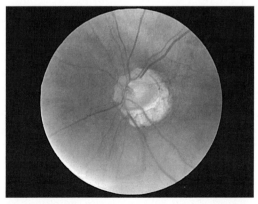

Figure 7–4. Normal myopic left disk. Normal physiological temporal pallor and peripapillary pale crescent. (**See Color Plate I.**)

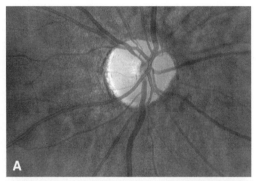
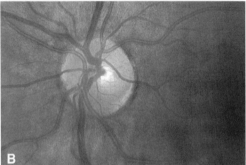

Figure 7–5. (*A*) Pathological right optic atrophy. (*B*) Normal fellow left disk for comparison. Both eyes have 20/20 vision but mild permanent nerve fiber loss has taken place on the right from previous optic neuritis. (**See Color Plate I.**)

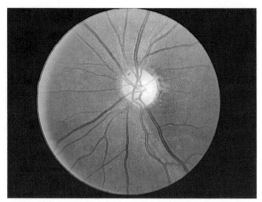

Figure 7–6. Left retinal nerve fiber layer loss. Note large area of loss of normal retinal striations temporal to the disk, which shows some temporal pallor (right side of photo). The nasal disk (left side of photo) is pinker, with normal retinal nerve fiber layer striations. (**See Color Plate II.**)

association with pallor of the disk indicates that the nerve is atrophic. Table 7–1 lists the frequency of optic atrophy in our clinic.

The detection of defects in the retinal nerve fiber layer provides objective evidence of optic neuropathy (Fig. 7–6). Such defects appear as darker slits in the arcuate nerve fiber bundles, usually best seen along the superior and inferior temporal bundles within two-disk diameters of the optic disk.[50] Nerve fiber layer defects are seen best through the dilated pupil with an ophthalmoscope that has a halogen bulb. The red-free (green) filter provides more contrast between nerve fibers and background. Feinsod and Hoyt[45] found nerve fiber layer defects in 17 of 25 patients with MS, only 4 of whom had clinical optic neuritis.

When the disk is swollen in optic neuritis, the term *papillitis* (Fig. 7–7) is often used; when it is not swollen, it is called *retrobulbar neuritis.* But the disease is the same in either case: both papillitis and retrobulbar neuritis have the same prognosis for visual recovery

and for development of MS. One exception to this rule is the patient with simultaneous bilateral papillitis, discussed previously. One small series[108] of patients with papillitis and a macular star figure (Fig. 7–8) from intraretinal deposition of protein showed that these patients had little chance of developing MS. The condition was called neuroretinitis. A disk that is normal initially may develop edema after a few days.

Previous reports[16,70,112] suggested that 17 to 23 percent of patients have papillitis; this finding is much more common in children with optic neuritis.[78,119] The Optic Neuritis Study Group[103] found 35 percent of their study patients had papillitis, 5 percent had

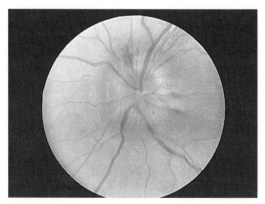

Figure 7–7. Left papillitis. Note swollen disk with blurred margins and multiple disk margin hemorrhages and a few exudates. (**See Color Plate II.**)

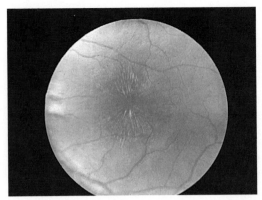

Figure 7–8. Left macular star. Note yellow radiating exudates around macula in the same eye as that in Fig. 7–7. **(See Color Plate II.)**

the afterimages may be reduced and the full spectrum of colors may not be seen. This flight of colors test can detect the optic neuropathy of multiple sclerosis.[34,82,121]

Reliable test results depend on careful control of the intensity of light used and the state of dark adaptation of the eye, and the patient must be able to report afterimages accurately. Much variability in duration and sequence of colors is seen in afterimage testing of normal patients.[18] Abnormally short afterimage times occur in a number of different conditions, including congenital color blindness; patients with macular disease may have abnormally long times.

disk or peripapillary hemorrhages, 2 percent had retinal exudates, and 3 percent had a trace of vitreous cells. Papillitis carried a lower risk for MS than does retrobulbar neuritis.

Afterimages

Subjects who close their eyes after looking at a bright light for a number of seconds usually see a colored afterimage. As time passes, the afterimage goes through a series of color changes, hence the descriptive term, "flight of colors." In patients with optic nerve disease, the total duration of

Pulfrich Phenomenon

The Pulfrich phenomenon is a subjective correlate of conduction delay in one optic nerve. A pendulum oscillating in front of a normal individual will appear to traverse an ellipse if a neutral density filter is placed over one eye (Fig. 7–9). A patient with unilateral optic neuritis may see this illusion without a filter: the disease delays conduction just as the filter does. Burde and Gallin[19] found this abnormality in five of nine patients with recovered optic neuritis. Rushton[129] found that 12 of 27 patients with definite or probable MS had an abnormal response. Slagsvold[143] found this test to be abnormal in 24 of 24 patients with unilat-

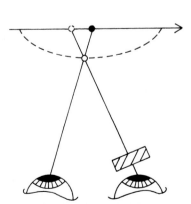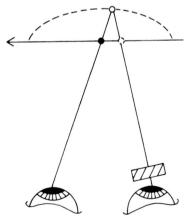

Figure 7–9. Pulfrich phenomenon, elicited by a neutral density filter over the right eye to mimic right optic neuritis. The subject views a pendulum as it swings left and right. The filter delays the visual signal from the right eye. When the signals are combined in the visual cortex, the image of the pendulum is displaced away from the subject when moving left and toward the subject when moving right.

eral optic neuritis. The last two authors used an oscilloscope to generate the illusion.

Double Flash and Flicker Detection

Double flash and flicker detection techniques have not found wide application in neuroophthalmology, although they measure a function, temporal resolution of vision, that is not measured by other visual tests, and they are easy to do, given the right equipment.

Double flash resolution is the ability to detect two brief pulses of light that are separated by a brief interval of darkness. In flicker tests, the pulses of light are continuous, with equal intervals of darkness. Critical fusion frequency is determined by increasing the number of pulses per second (hertz) until the subject can no longer see the flicker—the pulsating light appears to stay on continuously. Critical flicker frequency is determined by starting at a flicker rate above threshold (making the light look continuous) and decreasing the frequency until the flicker is just perceptible. Generally the critical flicker frequency is more reproducible. Some investigators average critical flicker and fusion frequencies together and use the terms *flicker, fusion,* and *flicker fusion* interchangeably.

Galvin and colleagues[52] measured double flash perception using a red light-emitting diode (LED) subtending 0.3-degree visual angle. They tested several areas of the central 6 degrees of the visual field of 14 patients with optic neuritis and found abnormalities in 13. These same authors[53] measured the effect of body temperature on double flash pereception in four patients with MS, only one of whom had Uhthoff's symptom affecting vision. In eyes with ophthalmoscopic evidence of optic atrophy, double flash perception deteriorated with heat and improved with cold. In another study,[51] these authors found abnormal double flash perception in 9 of 11 patients with MS with "normal fundi" and no prior history of optic neuritis. No results of VEP testing were given.

Several groups have conducted studies of flicker in patients with MS. Daley and colleagues[33] measured critical fusion frequency in 122 patients with MS using a centrally fixated red LED with a continuous red background light and with the background light flickering at 10 Hz. The results were abnormal in 48 percent of patients using the steady background and 78 percent using the flickering background. Salmi[132] found abnormal flicker frequencies in 9 of 18 patients with MS and 5 of 9 patients with optic neuritis. All of the patients with MS had abnormal flicker frequencies and abnormal VEPs, but two patients with optic neuritis had abnormal flicker frequencies and normal evoked potentials. Namerow[99] found that increasing body temperature caused a fall in flicker frequency in patients with MS. Mason and colleagues[89] compared chromatic and luminance critical flicker frequencies in patients with MS. They used red and green LEDs to generate a chromatic stimulus that consisted of alternation of red and green light and a luminance stimulus that consisted of red and green lights on and off simultaneously. They found that luminance flicker frequency was more abnormal than chromatic flicker frequency. A new test based on matching the intensity of a continuously illuminated field to the perceived intensity of a flickering field has been reported to yield abnormal findings only in patients with optic neuritis.[23]

There is little evidence in any of these studies that double flash and flicker contribute significantly to the clinical evaluation of patients with MS. None of the studies has shown abnormalities when all other aspects of the examination (including VEPs) are normal, and patients do not have complaints known to be caused by impaired temporal resolution.

Other Subjective Visual Tests

Patients with optic nerve disease, including optic neuritis, have been found to have diminished stereopsis.[49] Several tests of stereoacuity are commercially available, and most ophthalmologists have at least one. The usefulness of this test in the diagnosis of MS is limited by the fact that many normal individuals have poor stereopsis.

Patients with optic nerve disease often notice diminished brightness when using the affected eye.[131] This diminished brightness sense can be tested by having the patient look at a penlight or a white sheet of paper while the eyes are alternately covered. Care must be taken to keep the level of retinal adaptation equal in the two eyes by stimulating each eye equally.

The Amsler grid is commonly used in ophthalmology to detect scotomas within the central 10 degrees of fixation. The sensitivity of this test in optic nerve disease may be improved by decreasing the brightness of the grid using filters in front of each eye.[157]

Visual Evoked Potential

Visual evoked potential is recorded from an electrode placed on the scalp over the occipital cortex.[148] A shifting checkerboard pattern is usually used for visual stimulation, but other types of visual stimuli have been used. Optic nerve disease increases the latency and decreases the amplitude of the response. Although most investigators use similar techniques for recording and stimulation, the reported incidence of VEP abnormalities after optic neuritis has varied from 54 to 100 percent. One explanation for these disparate results is patient selection. VEP is usually abnormal in acute optic neuritis and tends to improve but remain abnormal. Those series of patients with longer follow-up are likely to have a higher frequency of normal VEPs.

Changes in latency and amplitude of the VEP are not unique to optic neuritis; similar VEP abnormalities are found in many other optic nerve diseases. However, VEP can be helpful in the differential diagnosis of some optic nerve lesions. For example, VEP latency changes are more prominent in optic neuritis than in ischemic optic neuropathy.[160] The typical VEP in recovered optic neuritis has a considerably delayed latency with a normal or nearly normal amplitude; the typical VEP in ischemic optic neuropathy has a noticeably reduced amplitude with normal latency. But there is considerable overlap in VEP abnormalities in these two diseases; some ischemic patients have delayed latencies and some neuritis patients have mainly amplitude changes.[30]

Visual evoked potential is often abnormal in MS, even in the absence of a history of acute optic neuritis. Kayed and associates[76] summarized the results of 10 studies of VEP in MS in addition to their own. Abnormal VEPs occurred in 57 to 100 percent of patients with definite MS, 33 to 100 percent of patients with probable MS, and 19 to 75 percent of patients with possible MS. Paty and colleagues[110] found an abnormal VEP in 87 percent of patients with optic neuritis and suspected MS.

Visual evoked potential is best used in conjunction with a complete eye examination. Refractive error, amblyopia, macular disease, poor cooperation (especially in factitious visual loss) and any optic neuropathy can cause an abnormal VEP. Patients who have had optic neuritis occasionally have a normal VEP and an abnormal eye examination. Hely and colleagues[65] found that 89 of 98 eyes with optic neuritis had an abnormal eye examination, but 79 of 98 had an abnormal VEP. In contrast, Brooks and Chiappa[17] found that 30 percent of 138 patients with abnormal VEPs also had no visual symptoms and a normal clinical examination.

A careful clinical examination of visual function to include best corrective visual acuity, Ishihara color vision testing, Pelli Robson contrast sensitivity testing, color and brightness comparison, visual fields, and pupil and fundus examination will almost always detect any case of clinical and subclinical optic neuritis. Ancillary electrophysiological or psychophysical testing or both may be used to confirm the clinical diagnosis.

Pattern Electroretinogram

The pattern electroretinogram (ERG) is a relatively new technique for measuring optic nerve function. The standard ERG measures the function of the outer retinal layers (the photoreceptor and bipolar cell layers) by recording the changes in corneal potential induced by a diffuse light flash. Pattern ERG uses the same contrast reversal stimulus as is used in pattern VEP testing. The amplitude of pattern ERG waves is reduced in eyes with optic nerve disease. With current techniques, pattern ERG adds little to the evaluation of patients with MS.[113] The test is neither sensitive nor specific.

Retinal Venous Sheathing and Pars Planitis

Rucker first described retinal venous sheathing in MS in 1944; he subsequently found that 10 percent of 1100 patients had this sign.[124] Bamford and associates[6] found the incidence to be 11 percent in 127 patients. In a recent study, 31 of 51 patients had sheathing.[80] Because venous sheathing is more common in the retinal periphery, indirect ophthalmoscopy or fundus biomicroscopy using the slit-lamp biomicroscope and 3-mirror contact lens is required to detect all cases. Even with the direct ophthalmoscope, sheathing of the retinal veins can be seen occasionally in the MS clinic (see Table 7–1), particularly when patients' pupils are dilated.

Pathologically, areas of venous sheathing consist of lymphocytes and plasma cells infiltrating the vein wall and the surrounding nerve fiber layer.[4,42] The cause may be an antigen shared between white matter and retina. Fluorescein angiography may show staining of vessel walls and dye leakage consistent with a breakdown of the blood-retinal barrier in areas of sheathing.[162] However, dye leakage sometimes resolves even though sheathing persists.

Retinal venous sheathing may signal a more generalized breakdown of the blood-brain barrier. Engell and associates[41] found that patients with MS with venous sheathing (periphlebitis retinae) often had abnormal technetium brain scans, suggesting a concomitant disruption of the blood-brain barrier. Arnold and associates[4] found CNS periphlebitis in all three of their cases of retinal venous sheathing in which the brain was examined.

Most authors have found no association between the development of venous sheathing and onset of an exacerbation of the disease. Bamford and colleagues[6] found no association between the presence of venous sheathing and the degree of neurologic disability. However, they did find that patients with progressive courses were more likely to have sheathing. Engell[39] found that 26 of 27 patients with retinal venous sheathing had progressive MS and that a malignant course was more common in this group. Bamford and associates[6] noted that sheathing remained unchanged for periods varying from 5 to 11 months. Rucker found that sheathing occasionally disappears completely after 1 or 2 years.[124] Engell and Hvidberg documented recurrence of sheathing in four patients.[40] Lightman and associates[85] found retinal venous sheathing in 14 of 50 patients with acute optic neuritis. Eight of the 14 patients developed MS after a mean follow-up period of 3.5 years, whereas only 5 of 32 patients without sheathing developed MS. The Optic Neuritis Study Group[103] found retinal exudates in 1.8 percent of the 448 optic neuritis treatment trial patients and vitreous cells in 3.3 percent. Because other disorders, such as sarcoidosis and syphilis, can cause retinal venous sheathing, the physician cannot rely on this sign to make the diagnosis of MS; however, it is important to realize that retinal venous sheathing does not exclude the diagnosis.

Pars planitis (chronic cyclitis, peripheral uveitis) is an ocular inflammatory disease that occurs in a small percentage of patients with MS;[6] however, most cases of pars planitis are not associated with neurological disease. The hallmark of pars planitis is an inflammatory exudate overlying the inferior pars plana and peripheral retina associated with inflammatory cells scattered throughout the vitreous. The condition is bilateral in 80 percent of cases. Cystoid macular edema occurs in 28 percent of eyes with pars planitis;[147] patients with macular edema have central scotomas and decreased visual acuity, simulating optic neuritis. The edema is often difficult to see with the ophthalmoscope; fluorescein angiography is usually needed to demonstrate the macular changes. Macular edema in this disease improves with locally injected or systemic steroids.[56] Other complications of pars planitis include cataract, glaucoma, retinal detachment, and vitreous hemorrhage. In severe cases, there is an associated anterior uveitis. In most cases, pars planitis is a chronic condition, lasting months to years.[146]

Retinal venous sheathing and pars planitis may represent different severities of the same condition. Some patients with venous sheathing have cells in the vitreous, and nearly all patients with MS and pars planitis have retinal venous sheathing. Pars planitis may be the first evidence of MS in rare instances; one of our patients developed his first neurological findings more than 20 years after having the ocular inflammatory disorder.

INFRANUCLEAR DISORDERS OF OCULAR MOTILITY

Pareses of cranial nerves III, IV, or VI occur in MS, but not often. Sixth nerve involvement is most common, and sixth nerve palsy can be the first evidence of the disease. Shrader and Schlezinger[142] reported 104 patients with isolated sixth nerve paralysis, of whom 13 had MS. In 7 cases, sixth nerve paralysis was the initial neurological event. The paralysis lasted 3 to 24 weeks (average 11 weeks) in these patients. In 419 cases reported by Rush and Younge,[128] MS was the cause in 18. Rucker[125,126] reported 924 sixth nerve palsies, of which 51 were caused by MS. Moster and colleagues[96] restricted their survey to isolated sixth nerve palsies in patients aged 15 to 50 years; 6 of 49 later developed MS. The paralysis resolved completely in five of these six patients; one patient showed no improvement. Even though MS is a possible cause, a young adult with an isolated sixth nerve palsy should be investigated for a compressive etiology.

Oculomotor paralysis is uncommon in MS. Green and associates[59] reported 130 patients with isolated oculomotor palsy; none had MS as a cause. Rucker[125,126] reported that 8 of 609 patients with third nerve palsy had MS, and Rush and Younge[128] reported MS as a cause in 8 of 290 cases; associated neurological findings were not mentioned. Two cases have been reported of oculomotor palsy as the initial evidence of MS.[36,154]

Paralysis of the fourth cranial nerve is a rare event in MS. None of the 172 cases of fourth nerve palsy in the series of Rush and Younge[128] had MS. Rucker[125,126] reported MS as an etiology in 1 of 151 cases of trochlear paralysis.

SUPRANUCLEAR DISORDERS OF OCULAR MOTILITY

Saccades and Pursuit

Abnormalities of saccadic eye movements in MS include delayed initiation time, decreased velocity, ocular dysmetria, and hypometric and hypermetric saccades.[93,102,118,149] Ocular dysmetria is an oscillation of the eyes at the end of a saccade; the eyes initially overshoot the target, followed by subsequent overshooting saccades of diminishing amplitude to either side of the target until the eyes rest on target.

Testing of smooth pursuit reveals substitution by saccades in many patients with MS.[90,102] However, Meienberg and associates[93] found that many normal subjects had similar abnormalities; they recommended that smooth-pursuit testing not be used for routine diagnosis.

Internuclear Ophthalmoplegia

Internuclear ophthalmoplegia (INO) is a common finding in MS (see Table 7–1). Müri and Meienberg[98] found INO in 34 of 100 patients without performing eye movement recordings. Using oculography, these authors found INO in 21 (44 percent) of 48 patients with definite or probable MS. This eye movement abnormality occurs when a lesion affects the medial longitudinal fasciculus (MLF), the tract containing fibers that connect the abducens nucleus in the pons with the contralateral medial rectus subdivision of the oculomotor nucleus in the mesencephalon. The pontine gaze center, located in the paramedian pontine reticular formation, mediates horizontal conjugate gaze to the ipsilateral side. Output from this area goes to the abducens nucleus, where synapses occur with abducens motor neurons that go to the ipsilateral lateral rectus muscle. Other synapses in the abducens nucleus connect the pontine gaze center with interneurons whose axons decussate and enter the contralateral MLF. Other fibers in the MLF are concerned with vertical eye movements, especially smooth pursuit, vertical vestibulo-ocular responses and vertical gaze position.[83]

A lesion in the MLF causes defective adduction of the ipsilateral eye (Fig. 7–10). This defect varies from slow adducting saccades detectable only with eye movement recording to complete absence of adduction of the eye past the vertical midline. Associated eye movement abnormalities include an irregular (ataxic) abducting nystagmus in the eye contralateral to the lesion, skew deviation and vertical nystagmus, manifested by upbeat nystagmus on gaze up or downbeat nystagmus on gaze down. If vertical nystagmus occurs in unilateral INO, it is generally apparent in up or down gaze (usually up) but not both. Bilateral INO is almost always associated with vertical nystagmus in one direction or the other, often both.[83]

In MS, INO is more often bilateral than unilateral. Other causes of INO[24,57,83,145] include stroke, trauma, the Miller Fisher variant of Guillain-Barré syndrome, CNS lupus, tumor, Wernicke's encephalopathy and encephalitis. An appearance identical to INO occurs in ocular myasthenia.

Skew Deviation

Skew deviation is a vertical divergence of the two eyes that is not explainable by a ver-

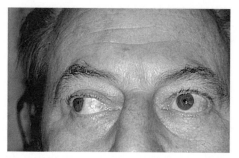

Figure 7–10. Left internuclear ophthalmoplegia. Defective adduction of left eye on right gaze with associated abducting nystagmus of right eye due to left medial longitudinal fasciculus (MLF) lesion. **(See Color Plate II.)**

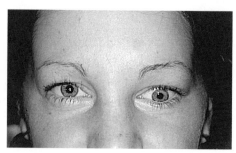

Figure 7–11. Skew deviation. A vertical misalignment of the eyes that does not fit the pattern of an isolated cyclovertical muscle palsy. **(See Color Plate II.)**

tical muscle paralysis (Fig. 7–11). The higher eye is more often ipsilateral to the lesion when there is an INO and contralateral to the lesion otherwise.[77] Skew deviation occurs more often with unilateral than with bilateral INO.[145]

Pretectal Syndrome

MS rarely causes Parinaud's ophthalmoplegia (sylvian aqueduct) syndrome. One patient with MS had limited upward gaze, pupillary light-near dissociation, convergence-retraction nystagmus, and skew deviation.[144] Another patient with upgaze paralysis and convergence-retraction nystagmus had a plaque in the dorsal midbrain that was demonstrated by MRI.[27]

Gaze Palsies

Paralysis of conjugate gaze is an uncommon finding in MS (Table 7–2). Savitsky and Rangell[137] reported paresis of lateral conjugate gaze in 10 of 264 of their cases. Three other patients had external ophthalmoplegia, and nine others had defective upward gaze. Hennerici and Fromm[66] reported a patient with complete gaze palsy.

Visual-Vestibular Interaction

Visual suppression of the vestibulo-ocular response (VOR)[140] is often abnormal in MS (see Table 7–1), particularly when pursuit is abnormal.[21] Some patients with abnormal visual-vestibular interaction complain of vi-

Table 7–2. **GAZE PALSIES AT THE UNIVERSITY OF BRITISH COLUMBIA MULTIPLE SCLEROSIS CLINIC**

Classification of Patients	No. (%) of Patients*
Total with gaze palsies	17 (4.5%)
Definite MS	13
Probable MS	2
Possible MS	2

*N = 381.
Source: UBC MS Costar[151a] Databank.

sual blurring with movement, such as difficulty reading signs in the grocery store while walking down the aisle. The only objective correlate of this visual complaint in these patients is abnormal visual suppression of the VOR.

Nystagmus

Nystagmus is the most common ocular motor finding in MS, having been reported in 28.5 percent (40 of 140) of Croll's cases,[23] 60 percent (158 of 264) of Savitsky and Rangell's cases,[137] 63 percent (57 of 91) of Wybar's cases,[161] and 45 percent of Marshall's 822 cases.[88] Many different types of nystagmus occur in MS (see Tables 7–1 and 7–3).

Table 7–3. **PRIMARY POSITION NYSTAGMUS AT THE UNIVERSITY OF BRITISH COLUMBIA MULTIPLE SCLEROSIS CLINIC**

Type of Nystagmus	No. of Patients*
Acquired pendular	13
Convergence-evoked	12
Rebound†	6
Torsional	1
Periodic alternating	1
Other‡	8
Total	41 (10.8%)

*N = 381.
†Clinical observation without magnification
‡Jerk nystagmus (vertical or horizontal).
Source: UBC MS Costar[151a] Databank.

Gaze-evoked nystagmus (see Table 7–1) is elicited by gaze right, left, up, or down. The usual pattern is nystagmus in both horizontal directions and upward, occasionally with nystagmus on downgaze. The fast phase is in the direction of gaze. This type of nystagmus is non-localizing and occurs with disease in the brain stem or cerebellum.

Rebound nystagmus[68] is caused by cerebellar disease. In this condition, gaze-evoked horizontal nystagmus occurs, but with sustained eccentric gaze the nystagmus fatigues. On return to primary position, the eyes transiently exhibit nystagmus in the opposite direction.

Acquired pendular nystagmus[5,60] sometimes occurs in MS. Aschoff and colleagues[5] found this abnormality in 25 of 644 cases of MS. This nystagmus may be monocular or binocular. It may be linear (horizontal or vertical), circular, or elliptical, and occasionally the direction of oscillation is different in the two eyes. Even though the waveform and direction in the two eyes are dissociated, the oscillations are phase-locked. Patients with this disorder often complain of oscillopsia and have difficulty reading. Unilateral abduction eye nystagmus is also seen as a feature of INO.

Convergence-evoked nystagmus is another cause of visual difficulty in MS. The waveform most frequently seen is upbeat nystagmus, but horizontal jerk and downbeat also occur. The patient reported by Sharpe and associates[141] had pendular oscillations of alternating convergence and divergence that were abolished by covering either eye. Convergence-evoked eyelid nystagmus[136] is a rhythmic jerking of the upper eyelids elicited by convergence of the eyes; it occurs almost exclusively in patients with cerebellar disease.

Saccadic Intrusions and Oscillations

Saccadic intrusions (square wave jerks, saccadic pulses, and double saccadic pulses) and saccadic oscillations (macro-square wave jerks, macrosaccadic oscillations, and ocular flutter) that occur in MS (Table 7–4) are a result of the inappropriate initiation of saccadic eye movements

Table 7–4. **SACCADIC OSCILLATIONS AT THE UNIVERSITY OF BRITISH COLUMBIA MULTIPLE SCLEROSIS CLINIC**

Type of Oscillations	No. of Patients*
All saccadic oscillations	42 (11.0%)
Square wave jerks	37
Macrosaccadic oscillations	6
Flutter	3

*N = 381.
Source: UBC MS Costar[151a] Databank.

during fixation or change in gaze position.[37] They differ from nystagmus in which ocular oscillations are generated by slow eye movement systems. These abnormalities are discussed in an excellent review article by Sharpe and Fletcher.[139]

A square wave jerk consists of a small amplitude conjugate saccade away from fixation with a saccade back to fixation after a latency delay of about 200 ms. Saccadic pulses are isolated saccades away from fixation with a slow drift back to fixation, the reverse of nystagmus. They are seen most often as abducting pulses in the eye contralateral to the MLF in INO.[67] Double saccadic pulses are isolated back-to-back saccades.[37]

The saccadic abnormalities discussed here have no specific localizing significance, although they are usually associated with disease of the cerebellum or brain stem. Many of these fixation abnormalities are difficult to distinguish without eye movement recording.[35,55,138]

EXAMINATION OF THE OCULAR MOTOR SYSTEM

Ideally, every patient being assessed for MS should have quantitative oculography using electro-oculography (EOG), infrared oculography, or scleral search coil techniques, but good eye movement recordings are generally unavailable. Fortunately, a complete and careful clinical examination of ocular motility will detect many of the abnormalities described previously. Clinical testing detects about half of the saccadic disorders detected by infrared oculography.[93] Tables 7–1 to 7–4 give the frequencies of some eye movement abnormalities detected by clinical examination in our patients.

The following discussion is meant for those who rely on clinical examination to assess eye movements. The scheme summarized in Table 7–5 is that used for neuro-ophthalmic assessment in our clinic. Additional material on the clinical examination can be found in Leigh and Zee.[83]

Fixation

To test fixation, the patient is asked to look at a distant fixation target. The eyes are observed for fixation instability caused by nystagmus, saccadic intrusions, or square wave jerks. If the eyes are misaligned from another cause, alternate fixation may mimic square wave jerks, and therefore, one eye should be covered to be sure these persist in the monocular situation. The physician can better detect subtle nystagmus and other fixation abnormalities with

Table 7–5. **A SCHEME FOR CLINICAL ASSESSMENT OF OCULAR MOTILITY**

- Observe eyes during distant fixation; supplement with observation of the fundus if necessary.
- Test convergence: Is there gaze-evoked ocular or lid nystagmus?
- Check range of motion, simultaneously checking for nystagmus.
- Check horizontal smooth pursuit.
- Assess 20° saccades, horizontal and vertical, centripetal, and across fixation.
- Test for internuclear ophthalmoplegia by looking at large-amplitude horizontal saccades.
- Elicit optokinetic nystagmus.
- Assess visual suppression of the vestibulo-ocular response.

the magnification of the ophthalmoscope while looking at the retina. It should be remembered when interpreting these abnormalities that the retina beats in the opposite direction of the anterior part of the eye. If necessary, the ocular fundus is observed in one eye while the other eye looks at the target.

Convergence

In convergence testing, a target is moved close to the eyes to the limit of convergence. The eyes are observed for convergence-evoked ocular or eyelid nystagmus.

Ductions

Ductions assess range of eye movement. Because it is sometimes difficult to know when the range of movement of the eyes is limited, the punctum of the lower lid can be used as an objective marker. Generally about 40 percent of the cornea will move past the punctum with extreme adduction. In many normal patients, abduction brings the lateral limbus of the cornea just to the lateral canthus so that no sclera is visible laterally. However, congenital or acquired (proptosis, facial palsy) widening of the palpebral fissure makes this landmark unreliable. Similar landmarks are not available for elevation or depression, and estimate of the angle through which the eye moves must be made. The average normal ranges of ductions are 54 degrees downward, 46 degrees inward, 42 degrees outward, and 34 degrees upward, with considerable individual variation.[20] Because of this variation it is much more accurate to examine the eye movements relative to one another so that the abnormal eye movement may be compared to the contralateral normal eye movement. When both eyes are symmetrically involved, this becomes more difficult to interpret. If movement of only one eye is impaired, the normal eye can be used for comparison.

If the patient experiences diplopia and testing of ductions does not provide an obvious cause, cover testing or red-glass testing will be necessary. With alternate cover testing, the patient is asked to look at a target while first one eye, then the other is covered. If the patient has a mild right sixth nerve palsy, the affected eye will not abduct normally, and the patient will have an esotropia (the eyes will be turned toward each other). As the patient's eyes are alternately occluded, the eye that has just been uncovered will move out to pick up the target. The amount of movement will be maximal when the patient looks to the right (the field of action of the paretic muscle). If the patient has limited adduction from a left INO, there will be an exotropia (the eyes will be turned away from each other) when the patient looks to the right. During alternate cover testing, the uncovered eye will move in to take up fixation.

When cover testing does not reveal the cause of diplopia, red-glass testing should be done. The success of red-glass testing depends on the patient's ability to report what is seen. The convention in ophthalmology is to place the red glass over the right eye of the patient. If the patient has a right sixth nerve palsy and is looking at a white light source with his left eye, the right eye will be looking somewhere to the left of the light source because the right eye is turned toward the nose, and the red image formed by the light in the right eye will seem to be in his temporal visual field. The patient will report two images: a white light directly ahead seen with the left eye and a red light off to the right seen with the right eye. This is called *uncrossed diplopia,* because the image seen by the left eye is to the left and the image seen by the right eye is to the right.

If the patient has a right medial rectus palsy and is looking at the target with the left eye, the red image seen by the right eye will be in its nasal visual field; the red image will be to the left and the white image seen by the left eye will be to the right. This is called *crossed diplopia.* One way to remember this is to associate the "x" of exotropia with the "cross" of crossed diplopia.

If the patient has vertical diplopia, the same principles apply. If the right eye is higher, as might be seen in a right fourth nerve palsy, red-glass testing will reveal a vertical separation of the two images. If the left eye is looking directly at the target, the right eye will be looking above the target, and the red image will be seen below the white image. The image seen by the higher eye is always below the image seen by the lower eye.

Diagnosing horizontal diplopia is relatively easy. If the patient has horizontal diplopia that is worse on looking left, either a right medial rectus palsy or a left lateral rectus palsy is present. Cover testing will show either an exodeviation or an esodeviation, and red-glass testing will show crossed or uncrossed diplopia.

Diagnosing vertical diplopia is more difficult. A variation on the three-step test will help sort out vertical diplopia:

Step 1: Determine which is the higher eye. A patient with a right hypertropia could have paresis of one of four muscles: right inferior rectus, right superior oblique, left superior rectus, or left inferior oblique. At this point, a right superior oblique palsy would be statistically most likely because the right superior oblique muscle is the only one that is supplied by a single cranial nerve.

Step 2: Determine the horizontal direction of maximal vertical deviation. A right hypertropia that is worse on left gaze is caused by either a right superior oblique palsy or a left superior rectus palsy (of the four above mentioned muscles).

Step 3: Determine the vertical direction of maximal vertical deviation. A right hypertropia that is worse on downgaze must be caused by a right superior oblique palsy (of the two above mentioned muscles).

Step 4: Determine whether vertical deviation increases with head tilt toward either shoulder. Of the two suspected muscles (from Step 2), maximum vertical deviation on right head tilt implicates the right superior oblique, because it will be stimulated by the vestibular system on right head tilt, whereas the left superior rectus will not.

Step 5: To confirm a right superior oblique palsy, ask the patient if there is subjective intorsion of the right image, which will occur in the eye with a superior oblique palsy. Thus, an acute right

superior oblique palsy will cause a right hypertropia that is worse on left gaze, downgaze, and right head tilt, and the right image will be intorted (Fig. 7–12). Standard ophthalmology texts explain this in greater detail.[20]

After the range of movement is assessed, the patient is examined for nystagmus in the various directions of gaze. If the patient has gaze-evoked nystagmus to the right or left, an assessment for rebound nystagmus should be made by having the patient maintain gaze eccentrically for approximately 20 seconds, then returning gaze to the primary position. Detection of rebound nystagmus is enhanced by observing the eyes with the magnification provided by slit-lamp biomicroscopy or ophthalmoscopy of the ocular fundus.

Pursuit

To test pursuit, the patient should observe a target moving back and forth horizontally in front of the eyes. The examiner should hold the target at least 50 centimeters from the patient and should move it slowly and evenly. Because pursuit has a maximum speed of 40 degrees per second, more rapid pursuit targets will always elicit catch-up saccades that will appear abnormal when in fact this is a normal function. Pursuit is difficult to assess clinically in the presence of nystagmus.

Saccades

Saccadic velocity and accuracy should be assessed by having the patient look back and forth between two targets held 20 degrees apart, both vertically and horizontally. Some patients with cerebellar problems have inaccurate saccades when moving the eyes back to primary position from eccentric gaze. In fact, the only oculomotor sign of cerebellar disease may be hypermetric saccades from 20 degrees up or down back to the primary position. A good way to detect the subtle adduction lag of mild INO is to observe the patient's eyes during saccades from far right to far left and back.

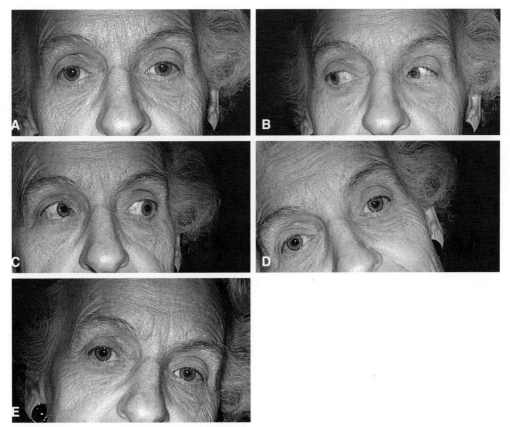

Figure 7–12. Right fourth nerve palsy. Note right hypertropia in the primary position (*A*), which decreases on right gaze (*B*), increases on left gaze (*C*) and right tilt (*D*), and decreases on left tilt (*E*). This deviation was worse in downgaze and the right image was subjectively intorted. (**See Color Plate III.**)

Optokinetic Nystagmus

Optokinetic nystagmus (OKN) is virtually never impaired in isolation; however, this response can confirm INO and asymmetrical pursuit and can help to distinguish congenital from acquired nystagmus. Either a homemade OKN cloth or an OKN drum is moved in front of the patient's eyes and the patient is asked to look (not "stare") at the stripes. If the response is not optimal, the patient is asked to count the darker lines or squares. The normal response is nystagmus with slow phase in the direction of target movement. If one eye has INO, the amplitude of induced adduction saccades in that eye will be reduced, and OKN will be less prominent than in the other eye. If there is a pursuit deficit to one side, OKN with the slow phase in that direction will be less prominent than OKN

in the opposite direction. Patients with congenital nystagmus have inverted OKN; the direction of induced nystagmus is opposite to the normal response. A patient with upbeat nystagmus will have reduced OKN downward (target movement up), because the spontaneous upbeat nystagmus tends to cancel the induced downbeat nystagmus.

Visual Suppression of the Vestibulo-Ocular Response

The patient looks at his thumbs with arms extended and turns smoothly at the waist, so that the thumbs move directly in front of the face.[21] Velocity of movement should be about 30 degrees per second. Normal individuals will exhibit no movement of the eyes with respect to the head.

An abnormal result is nystagmus with the fast phase in the direction of movement.

PUPILLARY DISORDERS

The most common pupillary abnormality in MS is RAPD, as discussed previously. Approximately 30 percent of the normal population have pupils that are noticeably different in diameter.[81] This simple (essential, physiological) anisocoria accounts for most of the unequal pupils that occur in patients with MS.

Other pupillary disorders are uncommon in MS. Bamford and colleagues[7] reported three patients with Horner's syndrome in their population of 125 to 130 patients with MS. All three had other evidence of spinal cord disease. Pharmacological testing indicated a preganglionic lesion in each case: the affected pupil dilated after instillation of hydroxyamphetamine. The Argyll Robertson pupillary syndrome is a rare occurrence in MS.[1,86] Savitsky and Rangell[137] reported that in one of their three cases, it was associated with a lesion in the periaqueductal region at the level of the colliculi. Pupillary abnormalities that occur as part of the pretectal syndrome or third nerve palsy are diagnosed by the accompanying abnormalities of ocular motility.

REFERENCES

1. Abramson JL, and Teitelbaum MH: The Argyll Robertson phenomenon in multiple sclerosis. Am J Ophthalmol 15:676–682, 1933.
2. Alvarez SL, Jacobs NA, and Murray IJ: Visual changes mediated by beer in retrobulbar neuritis: An investigative case report. Br J Ophthalmol 70:141–146, 1986.
3. Arden GB, and Gucukoglu AG: Grating test of contrast sensitivity in patients with retrobulbar neuritis. Arch Ophthalmol 96:1626–1629, 1978.
4. Arnold AC, Pepose JS, Hepler RS, and Foos RY: Retinal periphlebitis and retinitis in multiple sclerosis. 1. Pathologic characteristics. Ophthalmology 91:255–262, 1984.
5. Aschoff JC, Conrad B, and Kornhuber HH: Acquired pendular nystagmus with oscillopsia in multiple sclerosis: A sign of cerebellar nuclei disease. J Neurol Neurosurg Psychiatry 37:570–577, 1974.
6. Bamford CR, Ganley JP, Sibley WA, and Laguna JF: Uveitis, perivenous sheathing and multiple sclerosis. Neurology 28:119–124, 1978.
7. Bamford CR, Smith MS, and Sibley WA: Horner's syndrome, an unusual manifestation of multiple sclerosis. Can J Neurol Sci 7:65–66,1980.
8. Beck RW, and Cleary PA: The Optic Neuritis Study Group: One year follow-up results. Arch Ophthalmol 111:773–775, 1993.
9. Beck RW, Cleary PA, Anderson PAC Jr: A randomized, controlled trial of corticosteroids in the treatment of acute optic neuritis. N Engl J Med 326:581–588, 1992.
10. Beck RW, Cleary PA, and Trobe JD: The effect of corticosteroids for acute optic neuritis on the subsequent development of multiple sclerosis. N Eng J Med 1764–1769:1993.
11. Beck RW, Kupersmith MJ, and Cleary PA: Fellow eye abnormalities in acute unilateral optic neuritis. Ophthalmology 100:691–698, 1993.
12. Beck RW, Savino PJ, Schatz NJ, Smith CH, and Sergott RC: Plaque causing homonymous hemianopsia in multiple sclerosis identified by computed tomography. Am J Ophthalmol 94:229–234, 1982.
13. Becker FO, Michael JA, and Davis FA: Acute effects of oral phosphate on visual function in multiple sclerosis. Neurology 24:601–607, 1974.
14. Boldt HA, Haerer AF, Tourtellotte WW, Henderson JW, and DeJong RN: Retrochiasmal visual field defects from multiple sclerosis. Arch Neurol 8:565–575, 1963.
15. Bowden AN, Bowden PM, Friedmann AJ: A trial of corticotrophin gelatin injection in acute optic neuritis. J Neurol Neurosurg Psychiatry 37:869– 873, 1974.
16. Bradley WG, and Whitty CW: Acute optic neuritis: Its clinical features and their relation to prognosis for recovery of vision. J Neurol Neurosurg Psychiatry 30:531–538, 1967.
17. Brooks EB, and Chiappa KH: A comparison of clinical neuroophthalmological findings and pattern shift visual evoked potentials in multiple sclerosis. In Courjon J, Mauguiere F, Revol M (eds): Clinical Applications of Evoked Potentials in Neurology. Raven Press, New York, 1982, pp 453–457.
18. Brown JL: Afterimages. In Graham CH (ed): Vision and Visual perception. John Wiley & Sons, New York,1965, pp 479–503.
19. Burde RM, and Gallin PF: Visual parameters associated with recovered retrobulbar optic neuritis. Am J Ophthalmol 79:1034–1037, 1975.
20. Burian HM, and von Noorden GK: Binocular vision and ocular motility. CV Mosby, 1974, p 81.
21. Chambers BR, and Gresty MA: The relationship between disordered pursuit and vestibulo-ocular reflex suppression. J Neurol Neurosurg Psychiatry 46:61–66, 1983.
22. Chamlin M, and Davidoff LM: Homonymous hemianopia in multiple sclerosis. Neurology 4:429–437, 1954.
23. Christ T, Pillunat LE, and Stodtmeister R: The 'flicker test' according to Aulhorn in the diagnosis of acute optic neuritis. Ophthalmologica 192:220–227, 1986.
24. Cogan DG: Internuclear ophthalmoplegia, typical and atypical. Arch Ophthalmol 84:583–589, 1970.

25. Cohen MM, Lessell S, and Wolf PA: A prospective study of the risk of developing multiple sclerosis in uncomplicated optic neuritis. Neurology 29:208–213, 1979.

26. Compston DA, Batchelor JR, Earl CJ: Factors influencing the risk of multiple sclerosis developing in patients with optic neuritis. Brain 101:495–511, 1978.

27. Constantino A, Black SE, Carr T: Dorsal midbrain syndrome in multiple sclerosis with magnetic resonance imaging correlation. Can J Neurol Sci 13:62–65, 1986.

28. Cox TA: Pupillography of a relative afferent pupillary defect. Am J Ophthalmol 101:320–324, 1986.

29. Cox TA, Thompson HS, and Corbett JJ: Relative afferent pupillary defects in optic neuritis. Am J Ophthalmol 92:685–690, 1981.

30. Cox TA, Thompson HS, Hayreh SS, and Snyder JE: Visual evoked potential and pupillary signs. A comparison in optic nerve disease. Arch Ophthalmol 100:1603–1607, 1982.

31. Cox TA, and Woolson RF: Steroid treatment of optic neuritis. Arch Ophthalmol 99:338, 1981.

32. Croll M: The ocular manifestations of multiple sclerosis. Am J Ophthalmol 60:822–829, 1965.

33. Daley ML, Swank RL, and Ellison CM: Flicker fusion thresholds in multiple sclerosis: A functional measure of neurological damage. Arch Neurol 36:292–295, 1979.

34. Davis FA, Bergen D, Schauf C, McDonald I, and Deutsch W: Movement phosphenes in optic neuritis: A new clinical sign. Neurology 26:1100–1104, 1976.

35. Dell'Osso LF, Troost BT, and Daroff RB: Macro square wave jerks. Neurology 25:975–979, 1975.

36. Desai HB, and MacFadyen DJ: Multiple sclerosis presenting as third nerve palsy. Can J Neurol Sci 14:178–179, 1987.

37. Doslak MJ, Dell'Osso LF, and Daroff RB: Multiple double saccadic pulses occurring with other saccadic intrusions and oscillations. Neuro-ophthalmology 3:109–116, 1983.

38. Ellenberger C, and Ziegler SB: Visual evoked potentials and quantitative perimetry in multiple sclerosis. Ann Neurol 1:561–564, 1977.

39. Engell T: Neurological disease activity in multiple sclerosis patients with periphlebitis retinae. Acta Neurol Scand 73:168–172, 1986.

40. Engell T, and Hvidberg A: Recurrence of periphlebitis retinae in multiple sclerosis. Acta Ophthalmol 63:80–82, 1985.

41. Engell T, Hvidberg A, and Uhrenholdt A: Multiple sclerosis: Periphlebitis retinalis et cerebrospinalis: A correlation between periphlebitis retinalis and abnormal technetium brain scintigraphy. Acta Neurol Scand 69:293–297, 1984.

42. Engell T, Jensen OA, and Klinken L: Periphlebitis retinae in multiple sclerosis: A histopathological study of two cases. Acta Ophthalmol 63:83–88, 1985.

43. Engell T, Trojaborg W, and Raun NE: Subclinical optic neuropathy in multiple sclerosis: A neuro-ophthalmological investigation by means of visually evoked response, Farnsworth-Munsell 100 Hue Test and Ishihara Test and their diagnostic value. Acta Ophthalmol 65:735–740, 1987.

44. Fallowfield L, and Krauskopf J: Selective loss of chromatic sensitivity in demyelinating disease. Invest Ophthalmol Vis Sci 25:771–773, 1984.

45. Feinsod M, and Hoyt WF: Subclinical optic neuropathy in multiple sclerosis. J Neurol Neurosurg Psychiatry 38:1109–1114, 1975.

46. Fleishman JA, Beck RW, Linares OA: Deficits in visual function after resolution of optic neuritis. Ophthalmology 94:1029–1035, 1987.

47. Francis DA, Compston DA, Batchelor JR: A reassessment of the risk of multiple sclerosis developing in patients with optic neuritis after extended follow-up. J Neurol Neurosurg Psychiatry 50:758–765, 1987.

48. Frederiksen J, Larsson H, Olesen J: Evaluation of the visual system in multiple sclerosis. 2. Colour vision. Acta Neurol Scand 74:203–209, 1986.

49. Friedman JR, Kosmorsky GS, and Burde RM: Stereoacuity in patients with optic nerve disease. Arch Ophthalmol 103:37–38, 1985.

50. Frisen L, and Hoyt WF: Insidious atrophy of retinal nerve fibers in multiple sclerosis. Arch Ophthalmol 92:91–97, 1974.

51. Galvin RJ, Heron JR, and Regan D: Subclinical optic neuropathy in multiple sclerosis. Arch Neurol 34:666–670, 1977.

52. Galvin RJ, Regan D, and Heron JR: Impaired temporal resolution of vision after acute retrobulbar neuritis. Brain 99:255–268, 1976.

53. Galvin RJ, Regan D, and Heron JR: A possible means of monitoring the progress of demyelination in multiple sclerosis: Effect of body temperature on visual perception of double light flashes. J Neurol Neurosurg Psychiatry 39:861–865, 1976.

54. Gartner S: Optic neuropathy in multiple sclerosis. Arch Ophthalmol 50:718–726, 1953.

55. Glaser JS: Myasthenic pseudo-internuclear ophthalmoplegia. Arch Ophthalmol 75:363–366, 1966.

56. Godfrey WA, Smith RE, and Kimura SJ: Chronic cyclitis: Corticosteroid therapy. Trans Am Ophthalmol Soc 74:178–188, 1976.

57. Gonyea EF: Bilateral internuclear ophthalmoplegia. Arch Neurol 31:168–173, 1974.

58. Gould ES, Bird AC, Leaver PK: Treatment of optic neuritis by retrobulbar injection of triamcinolone. BMJ 1:1495–1497, 1977.

59. Green WR, Hackett ER, and Schlezinger NS: Neuro-ophthalmologic evaluation of oculomotor nerve paralysis. Arch Ophthalmol 72:154–167, 1964.

60. Gresty MA, Ell JJ, and Findley LJ: Acquired pendular nystagmus: Its characteristics, localising value and pathophysiology. J Neurol Neurosurg Psychiatry 45:431–439, 1982.

61. Griffin JF, and Wray SH: Acquired color vision defects in retrobulbar neuritis. Am J Ophthalmol 86:193–201, 1978.

62. Han DP, Thompson HS, and Folk JC: Differentiation between recently resolved optic neuritis and central serous retinopathy: Use of tests of visual function. Arch Ophthalmol 103:394–396, 1985.

63. Harrison AC, Becker WJ, and Stell WK: Colour vision abnormalities in multiple sclerosis. Can J Neurol Sci 14:279–285, 1987.

64. Hely MA, McManis PG, and Doran TJ: Acute optic neuritis: A prospective study of risk factors for multiple sclerosis. J Neurol Neurosurg Psychiatry 49:1125–1130, 1986.

65. Hely MA, McManis PG, and Walsh JC: Visual evoked responses and ophthalmological examination in optic neuritis: A follow-up study. J Neurol Sci 75:275–283, 1986.

66. Hennerici M, and Fromm C: Isolated complete gaze palsy: An unusual ocular movement deficit probably due to a bilateral parapontine reticular formation (PPRF) lesion. Neuro-ophthalmology 1:165–173, 1981.

67. Herishanu YO, and Sharpe JA: Saccadic intrusions in internuclear ophthalmoplegia. Ann Neurol 14:67–72, 1983.

68. Hood JD, Kayan A, and Leech J: Rebound nystagmus. Brain 96:507–515, 1973.

69. Howard CW, Osher RH, and Tomsak RL: Computed tomographic features in optic neuritis. Am J Ophthalmol 89:699–702, 1980.

70. Hutchinson WM: Acute optic neuritis and the prognosis for multiple sclerosis. J Neurol Neurosurg Psychiatry 39:283–289, 1976.

71. Ikuta F, and Zimmerman HM: Distribution of plaques in seventy autopsy cases of multiple sclerosis in the United States. Neurology 26:26–28, 1976.

72. Jacobs L, Kinkel PR, and Kinkel WR: Silent brain lesions in patients with isolated idiopathic optic neuritis: A clinical and nuclear magnetic resonance imaging study. Arch Neurol 43:452–455, 1986.

73. Jacobs L, Munschauer FE, and Samer EK: Clinical and magnetic resonance imaging in optic neuritis. Neurology 41:15–19, 1991.

74. Johns K, Lavin P, and Elliott JH: Magnetic resonance imaging of the brain in isolated optic neuritis. Arch Ophthalmol 104:1486–1488, 1986.

75. Kahana E, Leibowitz U, Fishback N, and Alter M: Slowly progressive and acute visual impairment in multiple sclerosis. Neurology 23:729–733, 1973.

76. Kayed K, Rosjo O, and Kass B: Practical application of patterned visual evoked responses in multiple sclerosis. Acta Neurol Scand 57:317–324, 1978.

77. Keane JR: Ocular skew deviation: Analysis of 100 cases. Arch Neurol 32:185–190, 1975.

78. Kennedy C, and Carroll FD: Optic neuritis in children. Transactions of the American Academy of Opthalmology and Otolaryngology 64:700–712, 1960.

79. Kinnunen E: The incidence of optic neuritis and its prognosis for multiple sclerosis. Acta Neurol Scand 68:371–377, 1980.

80. Lagoutte F, Baylac I, and Julien J: Etude systematique de la peripherie du fond d'oeil chez 51 malades porteurs d'une S.E.P. Bulletin Société Ophthalmique De France 85:239–241, 1985.

81. Lam BL, Thompson HS, and Corbett JJ: The prevalence of simple anisocoria. Am J Ophthalmol 104:69–73, 1987.

82. Larsson H, Frederiksen J, Stigsby B: Evaluation of the visual system in multiple sclerosis. 1. After-images compared to visual evoked potentials. Acta Neurol Scand 74:195–202, 1986.

83. Leigh RJ, and Zee DS: The Neurology of Eye Movements. FA Davis, Philadelphia, 1991.

84. Lessell S, and Cohen MM: Phosphenes induced by sound. Neurology 29:1524–1527, 1979.

85. Lightman S, McDonald WI, and Bird AC: Retinal venous sheathing in optic neuritis: Its significance for the pathogenesis of multiple sclerosis. Brain 110:405–414, 1987.

86. Loewenfeld IE: The Argyll Robertson pupil, 1869–1969: A critical survey of the literature. Surv Ophthalmol 14:199–299, 1969.

87. MacKarell P: Interior journey and beyond: An artist's view of optic neuritis. In Hess RF, and Plant GT (eds): Optic Neuritis. Cambridge University Press, New York, 1986, pp 283–293.

88. Marshall D: Ocular manifestations of multiple sclerosis and relationship to retrobulbar neuritis. Trans Am Ophthalmol Soc 48:487–525, 1950.

89. Mason RJ, Snelgar RS, and Foster DH: Abnormalities of chromatic and luminance critical flicker frequency in multiple sclerosis. Invest Ophthalmol Vis Sci 23:246–252, 1982.

90. Mastaglia FL, Black JL, and Collins DW: Quantitative studies of saccadic and pursuit eye movements in multiple sclerosis. Brain 102:817–834, 1979.

91. McDonald WI, and Barnes D: The ocular manifestations of multiple sclerosis. 1. Abnormalities of the afferent visual system. J Neurol Neurosurg Psychiatry 55:747–752, 1992.

92. Meienberg O, Flammer J, and Ludin HP: Subclinical visual field defects in multiple sclerosis. J Neurol 227:125–133, 1982.

93. Meienberg O, Muri R, and Rabineau PA: Clinical and oculographic examinations of saccadic eye movements in the diagnosis of multiple sclerosis. Arch Neurol 43:438–443, 1986.

94. Miller DH, Johnson G, and McDonald WI: Detection of optic nerve lesions in optic neuritis with magnetic resonance imaging. Lancet 1:1490–1491, 1986.

95. Miller DH, Newton MR, and van der Poel JC: Magnetic resonance imaging of the optic nerve in optic neuritis. Neurology 38:175–179, 1988.

96. Moster ML, Savino PJ, Sergott RC, Bosley TM, and Schatz NJ: Isolated sixth-nerve palsies in younger adults. Arch Ophthalmol 102:1328–1330, 1984.

97. Mullen KT, and Plant GT: Colour and luminance vision in human optic neuritis. Brain 109:1–13, 1986.

98. Muri RM, and Meienberg O: The clinical spectrum of internuclear ophthalmoplegia in multiple sclerosis. Arch Neurol 42:851–855, 1985.

99. Namerow NS: Temperature effect on critical flicker fusion in multiple sclerosis. Arch Neurol 25:269–275, 1971.

100. Nikoskelainen E: Prognostic indicators in optic neuritis. Ann Neurol 11:324–325, 1982.

101. Nikoskelainen E, Frey H, and Salmi A: A prognosis of optic neuritis with special reference to cere-

brospinal fluid immunoglobulins and measles virus antibodies. Ann Neurol 9:545–550, 1981.

102. Ochs AL, Hoyt WF, Stark L, and Patchman MA: Saccadic initiation time in multiple sclerosis. Ann Neurol 4:578–579, 1978.

103. Optic Neuritis Study Group: The clinical profile of optic neuritis: Optic neuritis treatment trial. Arch Ophthalmol 109:1673–1678, 1991.

104. Ormerod IA, and McDonald WI: Multiple sclerosis presenting with progressive visual failure. J Neurol Neurosurg Psychiatry 47:943–946, 1984.

105. Ormerod IE, McDonald WI, Du Boulay GH: Disseminated lesions at presentation in patients with optic neuritis. J Neurol Neurosurg Psychiatry 49:124–127, 1986.

106. Page NG, Bolger JP, and Sanders MD: Auditory evoked phosphenes in optic nerve disease. J Neurol Neurosurg Psychiatry 45:7–12, 1982.

107. Parkin PJ, Hierons R, and McDonald WI: Bilateral optic neuritis: A long-term follow-up. Brain 107:951–964, 1984.

108. Parmley VC, Schiffman JS, and Maitland CG: Does neuroretinitis rule out multiple sclerosis? Arch Neurol 44:1045–1048, 1987.

109. Patterson VH, and Heron JR: Visual field abnormalities in multiple sclerosis. J Neurol Neurosurg Psychiatry 43:205–208, 1980.

110. Paty DW, Oger JJF, and Kastrukoff LF: MRI in the diagnosis of MS: A prospective study with comparison of clinical evaluation, evoked potentials, oligoclonal banding, and CT. Neurology 38: 180–185, 1988.

111. Percy AK, Nobrega FT, and Kurland LT: Optic neuritis and multiple sclerosis. Arch Ophthalmol 87:135–139, 1972.

112. Perkin GD, and Rose FC: Optic Neuritis and Its Differential Diagnosis. Oxford University Press, New York, 1979.

113. Plant GT, Hess RF, and Thomas SJ: The pattern evoked electroretinogram in optic neuritis: A combined psychophysical and electrophysiological study. Brain 109:469–490, 1986.

114. Poser CM, Alter M, Sibley WA, and Scheinberg LC: Multiple sclerosis. In Rowland LP (ed): Merritt's Textbook of Neurology. Lea & Febiger, pp 593–611, 1984.

115. Rawson MD, and Liversedge LA: Treatment of retrobulbar neuritis with corticotrophin. Lancet 2:222, 1969.

116. Regan D, and Neima D: Low-contrast letter charts as a test of visual function. Ophthalmology 90:1192–1200, 1983.

117. Regan D, Silver R, and Murray TJ: Visual acuity and contrast sensitivity in multiple sclerosis: Hidden visual loss. Brain 100:563–579, 1977.

118. Reulen JP, Sanders EA, and Hogenhuis LA: Eye movement disorders in multiple sclerosis and optic neuritis. Brain 106:121–140, 1983.

119. Riikonen R, Donner M, and Erkkila H: Optic neuritis in children and its relationship to multiple sclerosis: A clinical study of 21 children. Dev Med Child Neurol 30:349–359, 1988.

120. Rizzo JF, and Lessell S: Risk of developing multiple sclerosis after uncomplicated optic neuritis: A long-term prospective study. Neurology 38: 185–190, 1988.

121. Rolak LA: The flight of colors test in multiple sclerosis. Arch Neurol 42:759–760, 1985.

122. Roseman R, and Ellenberger C: Slowly progressive optic neuritis. Neuro-ophthalmology 2:183–194, 1982.

123. Rosenblatt MA, Behrens MM, and Zweifach PH: Magnetic resonance imaging of optic tract involvement in multiple sclerosis. Am J Ophthalmol 104:74–79, 1987.

124. Rucker CW: Retinopathy of multiple sclerosis. Trans Am Ophthalmol Soc 45:564–570, 1947.

125. Rucker CW: Paralysis of the third, fourth and sixth cranial nerves. Am J Ophthalmol 46:787–794, 1958.

126. Rucker CW: The causes of paralysis of the third, fourth and sixth cranial nerves. Am J Ophthalmol 61:1293–1298, 1966.

127. Rudick RA, Jacobs L, and Kinkel PR: Isolated idiopathic optic neuritis: Analysis of free k-light chains in cerebrospinal fluid and correlation with nuclear magnetic resonance findings. Arch Neurol 43:456–458, 1986.

128. Rush JA, and Younge BR: Paralysis of cranial nerves 3, 4 and 5: Cause and prognosis in 1000 cases. Arch Ophthalmol 99:76–79, 1981.

129. Rushton D: Use of the Pulfrich pendulum for detecting abnormal delay in the visual pathway in multiple sclerosis. Brain 98:283–296, 1975.

130. Sacks JG, and Melen O: Bitemporal visual field defects in presumed multiple sclerosis. JAMA 234:69–72, 1975.

131. Sadun AA, and Lessell A: Brightness-sense and optic nerve disease. Arch Ophthalmol 103:39–43, 1985.

132. Salmi T: Critical flicker frequencies in MS patients with normal or abnormal pattern VEP. Acta Neurol Scand 71:354–358, 1985.

133. Sandberg-Wollheim M: Optic neuritis: Studies on the cerebrospinal fluid in relation to clinical course in 61 patients. Acta Neurol Scand 52: 167–178, 1975.

134. Sanders EA, Bollen EL, and Van der Velde EA: The course of multiple sclerosis after optic neuritis. Neuro-ophthalmology 4:249–253, 1984.

135. Sanders EA, Reulen JP, and Hogenhuis LA: Electrophysiological disorders in multiple sclerosis and optic neuritis. Can J Neurol Sci 12:308–313, 1985.

136. Sanders MD, Hoyt WF, and Daroff RB: Lid nystagmus evoked by ocular convergence: An ocular electromyographic study. J Neurol Neurosurg Psychiatry 31:368–371, 1968.

137. Savitsky N, and Rangell L: The ocular findings in multiple sclerosis. Res Publ Assoc Res Nerv Ment Dis 28:403–413, 1950.

138. Selhorst JB, Stark L, and Ochs AL: Disorders in cerebellar ocular motor control. 2. Macrosaccadic oscillation: An oculographic, control system and clinico-anatomical analysis. Brain 99: 509–522, 1976.

139. Sharpe JA, and Fletcher WA: Saccadic intrusions and oscillations. Can J Neurol Sci 11:426–433, 1984.

140. Sharpe JA, Goldberg HJ, and Lo AW: Visual-vestibular interaction in multiple sclerosis. Neurology 31:427–433, 1981.

141. Sharpe JA, Hoyt WF, and Rosenberg MA: Convergence-evoked nystagmus. Arch Neurol 32: 191– 194, 1975.

142. Shrader EC, and Schlezinger NS: Neuro-ophthalmologic evaluation of abducens nerve paralysis. Arch Ophthalmol 63:108–115, 1960.

143. Slagsvold JE: Pulfrich pendulum phenomenon in patients with a history of acute optic neuritis. Acta Ophthalmol 56:817–826, 1978.

144. Slyman JF, and Kline LB: Dorsal midbrain syndrome in multiple sclerosis. Neurology 31:196–198, 1981.

145. Smith JL, and Cogan DG: Internuclear ophthalmoplegia. Arch Ophthalmol 61:687–694, 1959.

146. Smith RE, Godfrey WA, and Kimura SJ: Chronic cyclitis. 1. Course and visual pognosis. Transactions of the American Academy of Ophthalmology and Otolaryngology 77:760–768, 1973.

147. Smith RE, Godfrey WA, and Kimura SJ: Complications of chronic cyclitis. Am J Ophthalmol 82:177–182, 1976.

148. Sokol S: Visual evoked potentials. In Aminoff MJ (ed): Electrodiagnosis in Clinical Neurology. Churchill Livingstone, New York 1986, pp 441–466.

149. Solingen LD, Baloh RW, Myers L, and Ellison G: Subclinical eye movement disorders in patients with multiple sclerosis. Neurology 27:614–619, 1977.

150. Spector RH, Glaser JS, and Schatz NJ: Demyelinative chiasmal lesions. Arch Neurol 37:757–762, 1980.

151. Stendahl-Brodin L, and Link H: Optic neuritis: Oligoclonal bands increase the risk of multiple sclerosis. Acta Neurol Scand 67:301–304, 1983.

151a. Studney D, Lublin F, Marcucci L, et al: MS COSTAR: A computerized record for use in clinical research in multiple sclerosis. J Neuro Rehab 7:145–152, 1993.

152. Tagami Y, Ohnuma T, and Isayama Y: Visual fatigue phenomenon and prescribing tinted lenses in patients with optic neuritis. Br J Ophthalmol 68:208–211, 1984.

153. Thompson HS, Corbett JJ, and Cox TA: How to measure the relative afferent pupillary defect. Surv Ophthalmol 26:39–42, 1981.

154. Uitti RJ, and Rajput AH: Multiple sclerosis presenting as isolated oculomotor nerve palsy. Can J Neurol Sci 13:270–272, 1986.

155. Ulrich J, and Groebke-Lorenz W: The optic nerve in multiple sclerosis. Neuro-ophthalmology 3:149–159, 1983.

156. Vedel-Jensen N: Optic tract neuritis in multiple sclerosis. Acta Ophthalmol 37:537–545, 1959.

157. Wall M, and Sadun AA: Threshold Amsler grid testing: Cross-polarizing lenses enhance yield. Arch Ophthalmol 104:520–523, 1986.

158. Warren KG, Catz I, and McPherson TA: CSA myelin basic protein levels in acute optic neuritis and multiple sclerosis. Can J Neurol Sci 10:235–238, 1983.

159. Wikström J, Poser S, and Ritter G: Optic neuritis as an initial symptom in multiple sclerosis. Acta Neurol Scand 61:178–185, 1980.

160. Wilson WB: Visual-evoked response differentiation of ischemic optic neuritis from the optic neuritis of multiple sclerosis. Am J Ophthalmol 86:530–535, 1978.

161. Wybar KC: The ocular manifestations of disseminated sclerosis. Proc Roy Soc Med 45:315–320, 1952.

162. Younge BR: Fluorescein angiography and retinal venous sheathing in multiple sclerosis. Can J Ophthalmol 11:31–36, 1976.

163. Zimmern RL, Campbell FW, and Wilkinson IM: Subtle disturbances of vision after optic neuritis elicited by studying contrast sensitivity. J Neurol Neurosurg Psychiatry 42:407–412, 1979.

CHAPTER 8

NEUROPATHOLOGY AND PATHOPHYSIOLOGY OF THE MULTIPLE SCLEROSIS LESION*

G. R. Wayne Moore, MD, CM, FRCPC

*This work has been supported in part by grant NS 27461 from the National Institute of Neurological Disorders and Stroke, by a grant from the Multiple Sclerosis Society of Canada, and by grants from the Mr. and Mrs. P. A. Woodward's Foundation and the British Columbia Medical Services Foundation (Vancouver Foundation).

257

Multiple sclerosis (MS) is the best known of the demyelinating diseases. Although it produces its greatest changes in the white matter, it is in fact a disorder of the myelin sheath, whether located in the white matter or gray matter. MS is also an inflammatory disorder. As of late, this feature has assumed a prominent position in the molding of our current concepts of the pathogenesis of MS lesions. The relationship of these inflammatory demyelinating lesions to the clinical presentation of a relapsing-remitting illness has amazed and frustrated students of clinicopathological correlation.

This chapter presents what is known about the gross and microscopic pathology of the MS lesion with regard to its initiation and maturation and the relationship (or often, lack thereof) to its clinical manifestations. Although many observations have been made, the appropriate interpretations of these observations are often unclear and thus subject to controversy.

A widely held view is that MS is a disorder with an immunologic pathogenesis directed against myelin and instigated by an as yet unknown etiology—viral or otherwise—in the early development of an individual. This perspective of MS is reflected in this chapter. The various theories concerning the etiology and pathogenesis of MS are considered in other chapters of this volume and in reviews of the subject.[271,376,444,499,531]

THE OLIGODENDROCYTE AND THE MYELIN SHEATH

The targets of attack in the MS lesion are the myelin sheath and the cell responsible for its production and maintenance, the oligodendrocyte. It is not entirely clear whether the primary event in MS is an attack on the myelin sheath, the oligodendrocyte, or both. However, the bulk of evidence suggests that the myelin sheath is the initial target and the oligodendrocyte dies secondarily to the loss of myelin.[389]

Excellent reviews are available on the normal morphology and chemistry of the oligodendrocyte and the myelin sheath,[297,336,375] and the reader is referred to these for details. In brief, each oligodendrocyte myelinates some 30 to 50 axons. How the oligodendrocyte accomplishes this enormous task is not entirely known. It is believed a broad flattened oligodendroglial cell process (which, in turn, is joined to the cell body by a thin, narrow process) wraps around the axon in a jelly-roll-like fashion (Fig. 8–1). A fusion of its cell membranes forms the multilamellated structure of myelin, comprised of alternating "major dense" and "intraperiod" lines. The major dense line results from a fusion of the cytoplasmic or inner aspects of the cell membrane of the same cell process; the intraperiod line results from a contact of the external aspects of cell membranes (Fig. 8–2).

The oligodendrocyte has a small rounded nucleus and relatively scant cytoplasm, which contains 20-nm microtubules. Unlike the astrocyte, the oligodendrocyte does not possess intermediate filaments. It expresses a number of markers, which can be demonstrated immunocytochemically in vitro[222] and in a specific sequence during myelination in the developing individual. In vitro studies of the developing central nervous system (CNS) in rodents[133,371] have shown that the oligodendrocyte derives from a precursor that is capable of differentiating along astrocytic or oligodendroglial lines. Before axonal ensheathment, the oligodendrocyte expresses galactocerebroside (GC)[111,287] and the enzyme 2',3'-cyclic nucleotide 3'-phosphohydrolase[400,413] (CNP, which is probably identical to Wolfgram protein W1[109]), followed by carbonic anhydrase (CA),[154] myelin basic protein (MBP),[111,400] and myelin-associated glycoprotein (MAG).[111,400,466] When myelination commences, GC, MBP, and MAG are no longer demonstrable in the cell body.[413,465,466] However, GC remains an important surface marker, and CNP and CA remain in the cytoplasm of the adult

Figure 8–1. The relationships of the oligodendrocyte to the myelin sheath, as originally schematized by M.B. Bunge, R.P. Bunge and H. Ris.[79] The oligodendroglial cell body (g) extends narrow processes (c) to several axons. These processes expand into broad flat processes which spiral around the axon (a). The elimination of cytoplasm (cy) between the plasma membranes (pm) of the oligodendroglial process results in a fusion of internal aspects of the cell membrane to form the major dense line of myelin, which is shown as a heavy black line. The juxtaposition of adjacent external aspects of the plasma membrane results in the intraperiod line. Note the external (ol) and internal oligodendroglial loops or tongues. The internal tongue is adjacent to the internal mesaxon (im), which is continuous with the extracellular space around the axon, the adaxonal space. Loops of oligodendroglial cytoplasm also occur at the termination of major dense lines in the paranodal regions of the myelin sheath next to the nodes of Ranvier (n), which is unmyelinated. The portion of the axon covered by the myelin sheath is referred to as the internode. The pm indicated at the node of Ranvier refers to the plasma membrane of the axon, the axolemma. r = ridge formed by the external oligodendroglial loop. (Reproduced from Bunge MB, Bunge RP, and Ris H: Ultrastructural study of remyelination in an experimental lesion in adult cat spinal cord. Journal of Biophysical and Biochemical Cytology 10:67–94, 1961 p 79, by copyright permission of the Rockefeller University Press.)

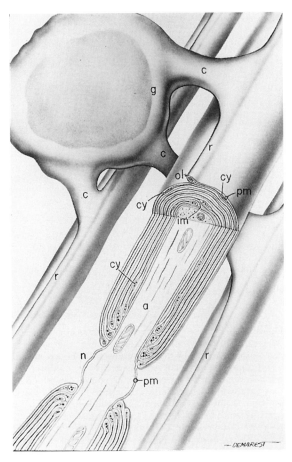

oligodendrocyte.[154,400] Proteolipid protein[111,181,287] and myelin-oligodendrocyte glycoprotein (MOG)[77,431] are markers expressed after MBP. Other oligodendrocyte markers include oligodendrocyte-myelin glycoprotein,[280] myelin/oligodendrocyte-specific protein,[116] and a protein recognized by the C1G5F2 monoclonal antibody.[55] Immature glial cells, including oligodendrocyte progenitors,[514] express a carbohydrate epitope recognized by the monoclonal antibody HNK-1, which also recognizes natural killer (NK) cells and certain T lymphocytes[2] and probably functions in cell-cell interactions.[228] However, many oligodendrocytes lose this marker during their maturation.[272,514]

The acquisition of the myelin sheath represents a major advance in the evolution of the nervous system. It allows saltatory conduction of the axonal action potential to proceed from one node of Ranvier (the portion of the axon not covered by myelin) to the next in a much more rapid fashion than in the unmyelinated axon. In the unmyelinated axon, conduction of the action potential occurs as a continuous spread of inwardly directed transmembrane current mediated by sodium channels located throughout the axolemma. On the other hand, in the myelinated fiber, the sodium channels are confined to the nodes of Ranvier, the internodal axolemma containing mainly potassium channels.[507] It is thus not difficult to envisage profound problems with action potential conduction associated with those illnesses that result in a loss of the myelin sheath. While this is true of the MS lesion, surprisingly there is often a lack of correlation between these regions of demyelination and clinical involvement, and it may well turn out that some

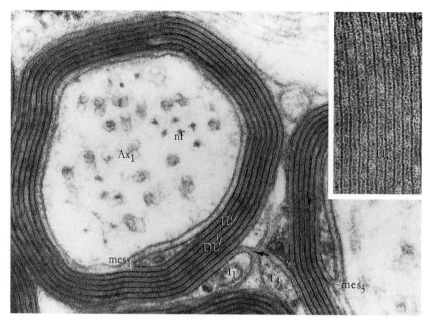

Figure 8–2. Electron micrograph (×120,000) of a myelinated CNS axon in cross-section. Note the lamellated structure of the myelin sheath, comprised of alternating major dense lines (DL) and intraperiod lines (IL). The internal mesaxon (mes$_1$) is continuous with the extracellular space between the axon and the myelin sheath (referred to as the adaxonal space), and is also continuous with the intraperiod line. The internal aspects of the plasma membrane of the external oligodendroglial loop or tongue (T$_1$) and the internal loop (just to the right of mes$_1$) are continuous with the major dense line. The external mesaxon is indicated by the arrow. Ax$_1$ = cytoplasm of axon (also termed axoplasm). nf = neurofilaments. T$_3$ and mes$_3$ = outer tongue and internal mesaxon, respectively, of adjacent myelinated fiber. The insert (×240,000) shows a higher magnification of the myelin sheath. Note the intraperiod line (IL) consists of two lines which represent the external faces of the plasma membranes which fuse to form it. (Adapted from Peters A, Palay SL, and Webster H deF. The Fine Structure of the Nervous System: The Neurons and Supporting Cells. WB Saunders, Philadelphia, 1976, p 201, with permission.)

of the clinical symptoms and signs in this disease are unrelated to demyelination per se.

THE LESIONS OF MULTIPLE SCLEROSIS

The Multiple Sclerosis Plaque

Classically, the lesions in an advanced case of MS are characterized by focal regions (or *plaques*) of light gray discoloration of the CNS. Less advanced plaques may have a pink tinge. Depending on their age, the multiple lesions demonstrate varying degrees of firmness. The more advanced lesions are quite firm and are responsible for the designation *sclerosis*.

The plaques of MS may be found wherever there is CNS myelin. The white matter contains numerous plaques of various sizes,

some of which may show a tendency to confluence. Particularly prominent and frequently present in long-standing cases are periventricular plaques (Fig. 8–3). Those plaques located between the body of the caudate nucleus and corpus callosum have been referred to as the *Wetterwinkel*, or "storm center."[377,464] However, focal areas of myelin loss may be seen in virtually any region of the hemispheres[75] and corpus callosum.[41] Lesions may also be present in the midbrain, pons, medulla oblongata, and cerebellum (Fig. 8–4).

Within the spinal cord white matter, the plaques tend to be subpial in location. The cervical spinal cord is particularly vulnerable, but plaques may be seen at all levels (Fig. 8–5).[328] Correlating with the frequent finding of visual symptoms and signs in MS, the optic nerves and chiasm are involved. In fact, when carefully examined, lesions in the visual pathways can be found in the

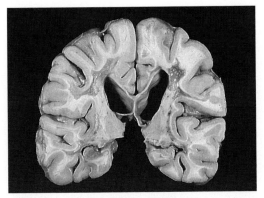

Figure 8–3. Formalin-fixed coronal slice of cerebral hemispheres from a patient with MS. Note the extensive demyelination of the periventricular regions of the lateral ventricles. Focal smaller plaques of demyelination are also evident in the parasagittal white matter. **(See Color Plate III.)**

majority of cases[483] and, in some series, in virtually every case.[252] In advanced cases, the optic nerves may show atrophy on gross examination.

Both cortical and subcortical gray matter may demonstrate MS plaques. In the mature brain, virtually all CNS axons are myelinated throughout their extent, except for the initial segment, nodes of Ranvier, and the terminal portion.[336] Thus, myelin

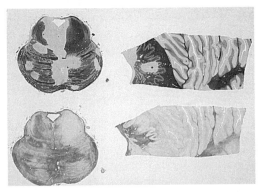

Figure 8–4. Horizontal section of rostral pons (left) and sagittal section through cerebellum and dentate nucleus (right) of a case of MS. The upper half of the figure is stained with Heidenhain stain, which stains myelin dark blue. Note the focal regions of demyelination, which do not respect anatomical boundaries in the pontine tegmentum and basis pontis. A plaque is also evident in the hilum of the dentate nucleus. The lower half shows the Holzer stain, which demonstrates gliosis in the areas of myelin loss. (Courtesy of Dr. G. Mathieson, Memorial University of Newfoundland.) **(See Color Plate IV.)**

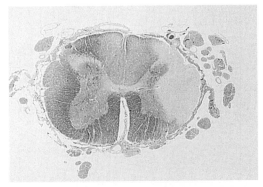

Figure 8–5. Cross-section of lumbar spinal cord stained with Luxol fast blue (LFB)-Cresyl Violet. The LFB stains myelin blue and cresyl violet stains nucleic acids (such as nuclei and neuronal Nissl substance). Note the MS plaque in the right lateral funiculus, which extends into the gray matter. The anterior horn cells are preserved in the lesion. The faint myelin pallor in the posterior columns may be due to loss of fibers from axonal involvement in a more destructive lesion or lesions caudal to this level (wallerian degeneration), or may be a shadow plaque. The same is also true of the myelin pallor of the left lateral corticospinal tract, which could be produced by axonal involvement of this tract by lesion or lesions at more rostral levels. The anatomical localization of these two latter lesions would favor wallerian degeneration and point out that, although many lesions, such as that in the right lateral funiculus, are demyelinative, axonal loss can also occur. **(See Color Plate IV.)**

pathology can be also found in fibers running within the large collections of neurons in gray matter structures.

Major Components of the Multiple Sclerosis Lesion

The major histological features of MS lesions are inflammation, demyelination, and gliosis. These features have been emphasized to varying degrees in reviews of the subject.* The inflammatory infiltrate is comprised of lymphocytes and monocytes, is multifocal, and is seen in plaques as well as in undemyelinated CNS. It is particularly prominent in the perivascular spaces (Fig. 8–6) but is also frequently seen in the leptomeninges (Fig. 8–7); in both these compartments it incites varying degrees of fibrosis.[50,341] Much work has been done to

---

*References 7, 14, 19, 20, 23, 236, 252, 338, 351, 355, 356, 373, 377, 435, 511.

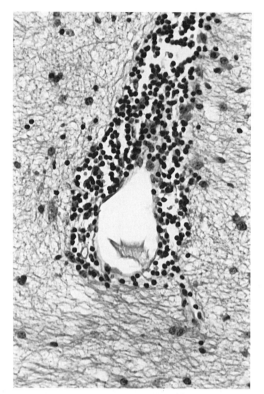

Figure 8–6. A perivascular cuff of inflammatory cells comprised of lymphocytes and monocytes within a chronic active MS plaque. Hematoxylin-eosin-Luxol fast blue. ×300.

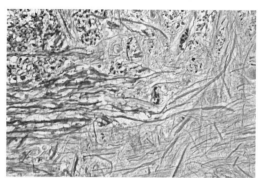

Figure 8–8. The relatively well demarcated border of a chronic silent MS plaque stained with Luxol fast blue and Bodian stains. The Luxol fast blue stains myelin sheaths blue; the Bodian stain produces dark brown axons. Note the abrupt loss of myelin sheaths, but the relative preservation of axons which have been demyelinated within the lesion (right). **(See Color Plate IV.)**

characterize the nature of these inflammatory cells (see discussion following). Within the parenchyma of the lesion, lymphocytes, monocytes, and macrophages may be seen; their relative distribution and composition depend on the duration of the lesion.

The second important feature of the MS lesion is demyelination. The clearing of myelin from chronic plaques is evident even under low-power magnification of such lesions (see Figs. 8–4 and 8–5). Axons are relatively spared (Fig. 8–8). However, axonal loss of varying degree can also be observed.

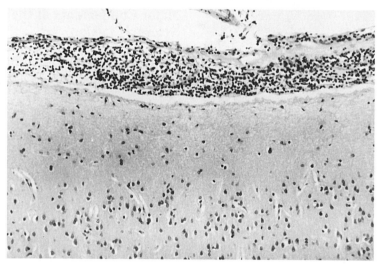

Figure 8–7. Leptomeningeal inflammatory infiltrate in MS. Lymphocytes and monocytes permeate the arachnoid and subarachnoid space. The superficial layers of the cerebral cortex are free of inflammatory cells. Hematoxylin-eosin. ×50.

While gliosis is a prominent feature of the MS lesion (see Fig. 8–4), it is best regarded as a secondary phenomena. Large reactive astrocytes abound in actively demyelinating lesions, whereas in more chronic lesions, isomorphic fibrillary gliosis is characteristic.

All these histopathological changes may play a role in the expression of clinical manifestations in MS. In the future, it may be possible to dissect, to some degree, these phenomena on a clinical and radiologic basis. Most of the remainder of this chapter discusses the initiation and progression of these inflammatory demyelinative lesions.

Immunologic Markers Studied In Multiple Sclerosis Lesions

Table 8–1 presents a brief glossary of some of the more common immunologic terms used in this discussion; others will be described as they are introduced. Over the last decade, much work has been directed toward elucidating the immunopathogenesis of MS by in situ study of MS plaques. Various immunologic markers have been studied, and functional characteristics have been ascribed to many cell markers based on in vitro studies. However, whether such markers indicate the same functions in situ when detected by immunocytochemical studies is unknown, although it is frequently assumed they are equivalent. This caveat should be borne in mind when considering the immunocytochemical findings to be described, particularly those pertaining to lymphocyte subsets.[454]

Types of Multiple Sclerosis Plaques

From the point of view of pathogenesis, it is convenient to classify MS plaques into three types:[377] (1) the acute MS plaque, (2) the chronic active MS plaque, and (3) the chronic silent MS plaque. This classification is based on the age of the plaque as assessed by histopathological changes and, to some extent, on clinical duration of the illness or exacerbation. As our knowledge of the pathogenesis of MS progresses, alterna-

tive classification systems will probably take into account immunologic markers and the degree of myelin breakdown to determine the age of the lesion and to reflect the dynamic nature of the lesion.[419]

THE ACUTE MULTIPLE SCLEROSIS PLAQUE

Acute MS presents as a monophasic episode of neurological deficit that is often quite fulminating and from which the patient frequently succumbs. In contrast to classic relapsing-remitting MS, it usually comprises one clinical episode only. The duration of the disease is generally weeks to months. Most believe it to be a variant of MS, and it is frequently termed *Marburg type* after the author who discussed this in 1906.[258] Acute MS is rare, with only occasional case reports appearing in the literature.[278] The rarity of the condition has restricted its histopathological study.

The quest for the "early" lesion of MS has proceeded since the disease has been known and, in truth, what exactly constitutes the initial change in the pathogenesis of the MS lesion is unknown. It has been assumed that the study of lesions producing a short neurological history before death will reveal the initial change. As pointed out by several authorities,[262,353,377] such early lesions are present for some time—at least weeks. Because, clinically, the neurological deficit in MS may often be established within a day, the initial event may escape notice in these lesions. Early detection of lesions by magnetic resonance imaging (MRI), together with appropriate pathological correlation, may help resolve this dilemma.

Although the lesions described as acute MS plaques are seen primarily in acute MS, similar lesions may be seen in some patients with relapsing-remitting MS with a rapidly evolving relapse. However, these latter cases also show chronic active lesions, indicating the presence of previous long-standing disease activity. The relationship between acute MS, cases of chronic MS with a rapidly evolving relapse, and classic relapsing-remitting MS is uncertain. These are probably all forms of the same disease,

Table 8–1. IMMUNOLOGIC MARKERS STUDIED IN MULTIPLE SCLEROSIS LESIONS

Marker	Description
CD4 (or OKT4)	This marker is found on lymphocytes. It indicates an inducer function.[398] It is usually a helper/inducer cell aiding in the propagation of an immune response.
4B4	This marker indicates a subset of CD4 cells with a helper/inducer function.[298] These cells aid in perpetuating the immune response.
2H4	This marker indicates a subset of CD4 cells with suppressor/inducer function.[472] These cells aid in suppressing the immune response.
CD8 (or OKT8)	This marker indicates a population of lymphocytes with two functional subsets: suppressor (dampen an ongoing immune response) or cytotoxic (directly target the offending cell perceived as immunologically foreign and lyse it).[53]
	At present, no marker differentiates these two functionally different populations of CD8 lymphocytes.[398]
	In immunocytochemical studies in MS, the function of cells bearing this marker is often surmised from their location or numbers.
OKT3 and OKT11	These markers stain all subtypes of T lymphocytes (pan-T-cell markers).
MHC class I antigen	These MHC molecules are seen on many cell types outside the CNS,[151] but inside the CNS, they are detected only on endothelial cells and probably some glial and perivascular cells.[455]
	Cytotoxic (CD8) T lymphocytes recognize antigen in the context of MHC class I antigen molecules and are thus said to be MHC class I antigen-restricted.[151]
MHC class II (or Ia) antigen	These MHC molecules are expressed by cells engaged in antigen processing and are presented to specifically sensitized CD4 helper cells[151]; thus the CD4 lymphocyte is MHC class II antigen-restricted.
	MHC class II antigen expression had been reported as minimal to nil in the normal CNS in some studies.[186,190,455,485,490]
	Using different fixation techniques, white matter microglia and, to a much lesser extent, gray matter microglia have been demonstrated to express MHC class II antigen in normal brain.[261,273] Thus, the immunocytochemical detection of MHC class II antigen in tissue depends on fixation[261] but is not influenced by postmortem intervals up to 24 hr.[455]
	The presence of infectious diseases accompanying chronic debilitation can upregulate MHC class II antigen expression.[261]
Interleukin-1 (IL-1)	A cytokine produced by activated macrophages and B cells involved in an ongoing immunologic response.[422]
	It activates T lymphocytes,[448] which then produce interleukin-2. IL-1 can also be produced by astrocytes.[139]
Interleukin-2 (IL-2)	IL-2 is a cytokine produced by activated T lymphocytes. It induces proliferation of antigen-stimulated T lymphocytes.[205,449]
	Its receptor may be localized by various monoclonal antibodies; one frequently used for this purpose is designated "anti-Tac."[492]
Prostaglandin E	A hormone produced by macrophages[182] and also reactive astrocytes.[139]
Interferons	There are three classes of interferons (Interferon-alpha [INF-α], Interferon-beta [INF-β], Interferon-gamma [INF-γ]), each of which has a different effect on modulation of the immune response.[335,488]
	Interferon-alpha and interferon-beta tend to suppress immune responses, whereas interferon-gamma enhances them.
Tumor necrosis factor (TNF)	TNF is a cytokine produced by macrophages,[15,260] which, in addition to its ability to induce necrosis in transplantable tumors, has a variety of effects on the inflammatory response, generally to enhance it.[51a]
Lymphotoxin (LT)	LT is a lytic cytokine produced by lymphocytes.[15]

CNS = central nervous system; MHC = major histocompatibility complex.

which appears to be more fulminant in some cases.

In the literature, terms referring to types of MS based on the duration of relapse or on the disease are often used loosely, and it is frequently impossible to tell their context. In this chapter, the term *acute MS lesion* is used in the context of acute MS (that is, cases with a rapid short history which is usually monophasic); however, the reader should bear in mind that similar lesions may also be seen in the chronic form of the disease during a rapidly developing attack. The term *active* will imply ongoing demyelination. It can also be used to imply the presence of inflammatory infiltrates.

Histopathology

Correlating with the rapid rate of the clinical presentation, the lesions of acute MS tend to have a more uniform appearance than those of chronic active MS. However, even in acute MS, variability in lesion age is often evident,[356,365] and some lesions may show a histological picture consistent with their appearance before the onset of the clinical presentation.[356]

The acute lesion[377] is characterized by an intense hypercellularity throughout a focal region of myelin loss (Figs. 8–9 and 8–10). The numerous cells are composed of lipid-laden macrophages, macrophages containing myelin debris, monocytes, lymphocytes, and reactive astrocytes. Reactive astrocytes are also seen around the white matter adjacent to the ill-defined margin of the lesion. There is intense perivascular cuffing by lymphocytes and monocytes (Fig. 8–11).

Shadow plaques have been described in acute MS[538] and appear to be a more frequent phenomenon in the acute form than the chronic form.[236] The shadow plaque, which appears as a region of myelin pallor instead of complete myelin loss, was originally thought to be a region of incomplete demyelination. Studies,[355,377] however, have shown that most of these lesions are actually regions of remyelination. Indeed, remyelination is a common finding in acute MS lesions.[392] These remyelinated lesions can undergo subsequent myelin breakdown, as evidenced by a focal area or areas of superimposed demyelination with histological features similar to those just described.[359]

Increased numbers of oligodendrocytes have also been described in the acute MS

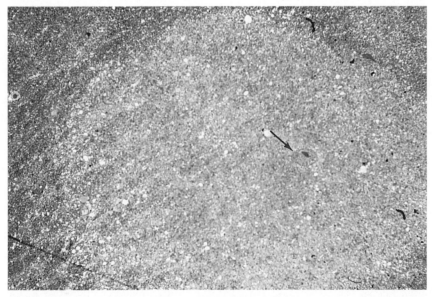

Figure 8–9. An acute MS plaque characterized by a focal region of demyelination, centered on a venule (arrow) with an inflammatory cuff. Normal white matter is seen on the far left and at the corners of the photomicrograph. This lesion was seen in a patient who also had lesions of Baló's concentric sclerosis. 1 μm epoxy section. Toluidine blue. ×30.

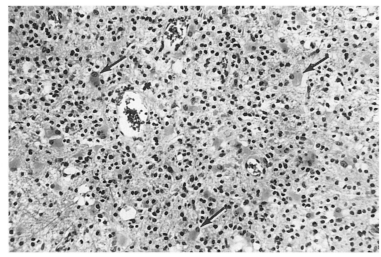

Figure 8–10. An acute MS plaque showing intense hypercellularity throughout. Reactive astrocytes with prominent cytoplasm are readily apparent (arrows). The remaining cell types are numerous lymphocytes, monocytes, macrophages, and oligodendrocytes. Hematoxylin-eosin.

plaque.[12,365] This is thought to be due to proliferation of the oligodendrocyte and seems to occur more frequently in acute than chronic MS. Evidence suggests that this proliferation may be in response to demyelination and extensive oligodendrocyte death occurring in the very early stages of the acute lesion.[355,358,365] These features (discussed further in the section on remyelination) suggest that the potential for myelin regeneration is greatest in the acute form of the disease.

Myelin stains of the acute MS lesion demonstrate the demyelination and show that many macrophages contain myelin debris. Active demyelination is evident by the immunocytochemical demonstration of macrophages with myelin debris staining positively for MBP.[356,365] The MBP positivity indicates that the macrophage has just ingested the myelin. Slightly older lesions in which active demyelination has ceased still show macrophages with myelin debris, but this is MBP negative,[356,365] indicating that the macrophage has partially degraded the myelin.

In acute MS, in addition to demyelination, there may also be a significant degree of axonal damage (see Fig. 8–11) and loss.[165,239,330a] This destructive process may also involve other tissue elements, such as astrocytes and oligodendrocytes[239] and may, in fact, progress to frank necrosis, sometimes leading to cavitation.[81,330,418,471,535] These severe changes are presumably related to the intense inflammatory infiltrate,

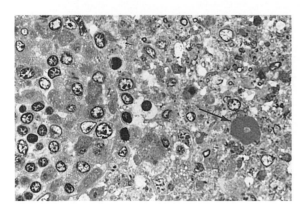

Figure 8–11. Perivascular inflammatory cuff in an acute MS plaque (high magnification of venule in Fig. 8–9). The perivascular space (left one-third of photomicrograph) is stuffed with lymphocytes and mononuclear cells, which percolate into the adjacent parenchyma. The arrow points to an axonal retraction ball, which is probably the forerunner of axonal death. 1 μm epoxy section. Toluidine blue. ×480. (From Moore GRW, Neumann PE, Suzuki K, Lijtmaer HN, Traugott U, and Raine CS: Baló's concentric sclerosis: new observations on lesion development. Annals of Neurology 17:604–611, 1985, p 607, with permission).

and the action of enzymes and cytokines and may be seen in the clinical setting of acute MS or relapsing-remitting MS with a fulminating attack associated with rapidly developing lesions. Such lesions may present as mass lesions.[330,418,535]

Immunocytochemistry

Perivascular inflammatory infiltrates are a prominent feature of MS, and demyelination is almost invariably associated with inflammation in all forms of MS. In an extensive series,[171] only 17 of 143 cases (12 percent) with demyelination showed no evidence of inflammation. Immunocytochemical studies showed that CD8 (cytotoxic/suppressor T lymphocytes, formerly referred to as OKT8), CD4 (helper/inducer T lymphocytes, formerly referred to as OKT4), and OKT11 (total T-cells marker) lymphocytes were present throughout the acute lesion, being somewhat more numerous in the center.[490] Many of the CD4 cells appear activated as evidenced by staining for interleukin-2 (IL-2) receptor.[485] The CD8 cell predominates in number over the CD4 cell.[187,485,530] The T-cell receptor usually comprises alpha and beta chains.[191] However, some T cells in the acute lesion possess the more recently recognized gamma and delta chains.[191,437,529] The latter are thought to recognize heat shock proteins.[63] Heat shock proteins are constitutively expressed in normal CNS in a variety of cell types[71a,393a] and are upregulated in various neurological diseases, including MS.[56,71a,393a]

The repertoire of the alpha-beta T-cell receptor in acute MS, as analyzed by polymerase chain reaction techniques, has been shown to be polyclonal.[530] Some of the sequences appear to have specificity for MBP.[325] However, the question of limited heterogeneity of T-cell alpha-beta receptor usage in MS in general is controversial.[171a] Analysis of T-cell receptor sequences of peripheral blood or MS tissue obtained from several laboratories appears to indicate restriction of heterogeneity within an individual patient but not between patients.[171a] A study of the gamma-delta receptor in acute MS has found evidence to indicate that some of the T-cell clones bearing this receptor have expanded, suggesting that they are recognizing a common antigen, possibly a heat shock protein.[529]

The heat shock protein 60 (hsp60) is expressed on most cell types in the acute MS lesion.[393a] This includes hypertrophic astrocytes, oligodendrocytes, and prominent astrocytes with internalized oligodendrocytes.[393a] The latter intriguing oligodendrocyte-astrocyte relationship is discussed further in the section on remyelination. It is possible that at this early stage of lesion development, hsp 60 may have a protective effect on the oligodendrocyte but may be pathogenic later on.[393a]

Lymphocytes and other inflammatory cells were not detected in the normal-appearing white matter in one study[490] but have been seen there in other studies.[128,187] This finding is in contrast to chronic MS, where lymphocytes have been demonstrated in the normal-appearing white matter in all studies where this issue has been addressed. The discrepancy in the acute MS studies may be related to the often unavoidable difficulty of differentiating early and rapidly progressive lesions in cases of relapsing-remitting MS from those of monophasic acute MS. An alternative explanation is that early in acute MS, immunologically competent cells are confined to the lesions but later populate the normal-appearing white matter. It may be that all cases of MS go through an acute stage, some of which clinically manifest as acute MS and others of which remain subclinical until the first attack of chronic relapsing-remitting MS. Further studies of the rare lesions of acute MS must be carried out before a firm understanding of their relationship to the chronic disease can be achieved.

Cells expressing MHC class II (Ia) antigen[187,485] are seen in great numbers in the acute MS lesion, particularly in the center. This marker is usually seen on macrophages that are tightly packed in the lesion (Fig. 8–12). The origin of macrophages in the MS lesion has been a matter of controversy. Both hematogenous and microglial origins have been proposed. Concepts of the origin, function, and differentiation of microglia and their relationship to CNS macrophages are continuing to evolve.[107a] From the point of view of MS research, an immunocytochemical study of the acute lesion[12] has presented evidence that the mac-

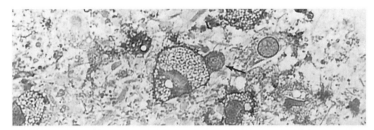

Figure 8–12. A 1 μm epoxy section of an acute MS plaque immunocytochemically stained for Ia (MHC class II). Note dark reaction product, indicating Ia-positivity on the surface of three lipid-laden macrophages (center, lower left and lower right of center). The arrow points to a lymphocyte in close proximity to an Ia-positive macrophage. This appearance may represent the morphologic basis of antigen presentation by macrophages to MHC class II-restricted T helper/inducer lymphocytes. ×750. (From Raine CS: Multiple sclerosis: Immunopathologic mechanisms in the progression and resolution of inflammatory demyelination. In Waksman BH (ed): Immunologic Mechanisms in Neurologic and Psychiatric Disease, Raven Press, New York, 1990, p 44, with permission.)

rophage initially expresses markers for hematogenous cells that are subsequently lost but does not exclude the possibility of population of the lesion by CNS microglia in the later stages of lesion formation. Another study of lesions from patients who had MS for 2 to 26 years has shown that the phagocytic cells in the lesions express markers associated with microglia.[492b] Moreover, the demonstration of MHC class II antigen on process-bearing (rodlike) microglia in the white matter surrounding the lesion suggests not only that these microglia may have an early role in antigen presentation as the lesion extends centrifugally, but also that these microglia may transform into the Ia-positive rounded macrophages that will characterize the established lesion.[61] Thus, the origin of the so-called macrophages in MS lesions is uncertain. Hematogenous monocytes may be important in the early stages of lesion development, and microglia in later stages, but more work must be done in this area before the controversy is resolved. Putting the matter of their origin aside, macrophages demonstrate various markers that are expressed at different time points in the inflammatory process.[75a,128] This finding may permit an estimation of the age of a given MS lesion.[75a,128]

Functionally, research has shown that both endothelial cells[264] and astrocytes[138] can present antigen to sensitized T lymphocytes in vitro. Because cells related to blood vessels in acute MS lesions were positive for Ia antigen, it was initially thought that these were endothelial cells.[485,491] However, studies employing confocal microscopy[61] or plastic sections,[384] which allow more precise localization of staining, have indicated that the Ia positivity in MS occurs in perivascular microglia and in macrophages. Possibly localization of other markers to endothelial cells by conventional light microscopic immunocytochemical studies of MS (see discussion following) may have to be modified after study by more precise techniques.

The degree to which astrocytes express Ia in acute MS lesions is unclear. Some studies have shown that they do express Ia antigen,[485,491] but other investigators did not confirm this finding.[61] Because oligodendrocytes do not express Ia antigen in these lesions,[244] they probably have no role in the presentation of antigen.

The costimulatory molecule B7, important in the activation of CD4 cell responses in conjunction with Class II MHC molecules, has been detected in MS lesions, including those of patients with short duration histories.[518a] This molecule is discussed in more detail in the section on the chronic active MS plaque.

Compared to its expression in normal endothelium, the endothelial expression of MHC class I antigen is slightly reduced in the center of the acute MS plaque.[485] Astrocytes express MHC class I antigen in acute lesions to a greater extent than in chronic lesions.[485]

Matrix metalloproteinases, which comprise a family of enzymes important in the remodeling of the extracellular matrix and include collagenases and gelatinases, have been demonstrated in macrophages in acute MS lesions.[256a] They have also been found to a much lesser degree on astrocytes in the lesions, as well as constitutively in endothelial cells and microglia in normal white matter.[256a] These enzymes may serve important roles in the propagation of the MS lesion and the concomitant changes in the extracellular matrix.[256a]

Polymerase chain reaction and immunocytochemical studies have detected the cytokines interleukin-1 (IL-1), interleukin-2 (IL-2), interleukin-4 (IL-4), and interleukin-12 (IL-12) messenger RNA or protein in acute or early MS lesions.[83,518a,530] Interferons (alpha, beta, and gamma) have been demonstrated immunocytochemically in acute MS lesions on endothelial cells and macrophages.[83,488] Interferon-beta, which has an immunosuppressive function, is expressed by endothelial cells in unaffected areas.[488] Tumor necrosis factor (TNF) is found on lipid-laden macrophages within the acute lesion, on astrocytes and endothelial cells at the lesion edge, and on astrocytes and microglia in the adjacent white matter.[83,438] Lymphotoxin (LT) is demonstrable on lymphocytes in perivascular cuffs at the lesion edge and on microglia near and within the edge.[438] An inhibitory cytokine, interleukin-10 (IL-10), is found on astrocytes.[83] IL-4, another immunodulatory cytokine, is seen on microglial cells, foamy macrophages, and perhaps even oligodendrocytes at the lesion edge.[83] Another cytokine noted for its ability to downregulate immune responses, transforming growth factor-β (TGF-β), is detected in the extracellular perivascular space and on some endothelial cells.[83]

Although B lymphocytes are seen in much fewer numbers than T lymphocytes in MS lesions,[187] they are present in the acute lesion and are responsible for the production of IgG, which has been demonstrated immunocytochemically in these lesions.[367] In addition to plasma cells, IgG is found on astrocytes, where it is thought to be bound nonspecifically.[367]

Adhesion molecules and their appropriate integrins are present in the acute MS lesion and adjacent parenchyma.[83] These molecules may have an important role in the initiation and propagation of an MS lesion and are discussed in detail in the section on the chronic active MS plaque.

Vitronectin, an intravascular and extracellular matrix glycoprotein, has been im-

munocytochemically demonstrated on demyelinated axons and on endothelial cells in acute MS lesions.[455a] The significance of this finding is unknown. It is unclear whether the axonal localization, which so far appears unique for MS, might have a protective or destructive effect on the axons.[455a]

Because of the numbers of inflammatory cells within the acute MS lesion, the blood-brain barrier is disrupted in these areas. The immunocytochemical demonstration of fibrinogen around vessels with inflammatory cuffs supports this notion.[12]

Summary

The acute MS lesion, correlating with the short clinical history, shows a picture of acute demyelination and intense inflammation. The intensity of the inflammatory response may be sufficient to destroy some axons in addition to myelin sheaths. Oligodendroglial proliferation and remyelination are frequently features of these lesions.

THE CHRONIC ACTIVE MULTIPLE SCLEROSIS PLAQUE

The chronic active MS plaque is seen in classic relapsing-remitting MS. The particular pathological features responsible for primary chronic progressive MS, where the clinical course is one of steady deterioration without superimposed exacerbations and remissions, has not been determined to date. However, histological studies of inflammatory infiltrates (see discussion following), immunocytochemical studies of T-cell subsets (see discussion following), and serial MRI scans[479] suggest that its pathogenesis may differ from the lesion of the relapsing-remitting form.

The chronic active plaque is characterized by histological changes showing that it has been present for some time and by an active border of demyelination advancing into the adjacent normal-appearing myelin. It should be noted that chronic plaques may show regions of active demyelination at the edge, whereas other regions of the plaque border may show no evidence of ongoing demyelination (that is, areas indistinguishable from that seen in a chronic inactive MS plaque). Thus, in contrast to the plaques of acute MS, chronic MS plaques may show considerable heterogeneity of features, both at their borders and throughout their topography, reflecting their protracted clinical course.

Histopathology

The chronic active MS plaque is a study in disease chronology. There is a gradient from the center to the border of the lesion, progressing from older to more recent disease. In the center of the lesion are numerous demyelinated axons separated by processes of fibrillary astrocytes and variable numbers of lipid-laden macrophages (Fig. 8–13). In more established lesions, the macrophages may have cleared from the central lesion parenchyma and reside in perivascular spaces, presumably en route to the venous circulation. Axonal loss may be evident[165] but not nearly as impressive as the loss of myelin. However, some cases of chronic relapsing-remitting MS can occasionally show lesions with destruction of axons and other tissue elements, to the point of cavitation.[284a]

As one proceeds more peripherally, the macrophage population becomes denser and resides within the demyelinated parenchyma. The more peripheral macrophages show less advanced stages of myelin degradation.[340] In peripheral regions of the plaque, the astrocyte possesses very prominent cytoplasm (Fig. 8–14); when this is quite pronounced, the term *gemistocytic astrocyte* is frequently used. Thus, with time, the astrocyte assumes densely fibrillar thin cytoplasmic processes and loses its "reactive" features as the region of demyelination moves more peripherally from its locale.

The border of the chronic active MS plaque is an area of considerable interest. It is relatively hypercellular in comparison to other regions of the plaque (see Fig. 8–14). However, increased cellularity at the plaque border and indeed within the lesion is less frequent in primary chronic progressive MS than secondary progressive MS, in which there are superimposed relapses and remissions.[399] At the plaque border, the active myelin breakdown occurs and the lesion advances into the surrounding myelinated parenchyma. Because acute MS plaques are so rare, a logical alternative in the examination of the early stages of the demyelinating process is the border of the chronic MS plaque, which is a much more

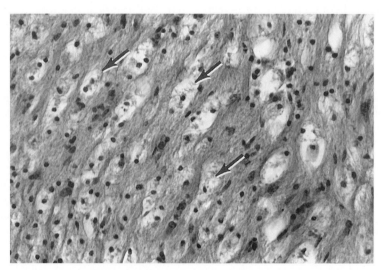

Figure 8–13. Center of chronic active MS plaque showing macrophages containing myelin debris and lipid (arrows). The numerous thin processes running diagonally in the background are predominantly those of fibrillary astrocytes. Luxol fast blue-Hematoxylin-eosin. ×440.

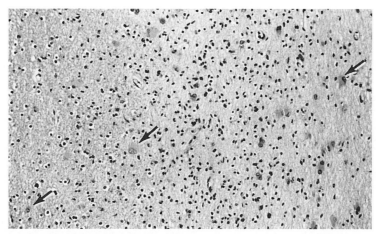

Figure 8–14. Low-power photomicrograph demonstrating the hypercellularity at the border of a chronic active MS plaque. Three zones are evident: the periphery of the lesion itself (far right); the hypercellular border, where active demyelination is taking place (middle); and the adjacent normal-appearing white matter (far left). Note that many large gemistocytic astrocytes (arrows) are seen near the border, within the border, and even within the normal-appearing white matter. Hematoxylin-eosin. ×160.

common lesion. Many studies,* particularly those using electron microscopy, have scrutinized this area. The border of the chronic active MS plaque contains many macrophages, which phagocytose and subsequently degrade myelin (Fig. 8–15).[360,363,368,373] Large reactive astrocytes are a prominent feature at the border of a chronic active MS lesion (Fig. 8–14). They have been shown to participate in the phagocytosis of myelin,[243] albeit much less than macrophages. The mechanisms of demyelination are discussed further in a later section.

Oligodendrocytes can be present in increased numbers at the edges of chronic active MS plaques (see Fig. 8–15). This increase was initially suggested by silver impregnation and enzyme histochemistry studies[208,209] and later shown in an electron microscopic study.[389] Moreover, remyelination occurs at the borders of chronic active plaques (Fig. 8–16).[363,389] This remyelinated myelin can also undergo demyelination by macrophages.[363] Unfortunately, in most instances, demyelination results in, or is accompanied by, oligodendrocyte death evident in more central (and older) regions of the plaque where oligodendrocytes are markedly reduced or absent.

In addition to remyelination with CNS myelin, remyelination by Schwann cells,

originating from nerve roots, has also been documented. This peripheral remyelination can also be seen in the presence of active demyelination.[211,214] In particular, it occurs in large spinal cord plaques, in severe lesions with partial necrosis, and in lesions where the astrocytic response (as judged by staining for glial fibrillary acidic protein) has been subdued.[211] Its occurrence in the last instance suggests that astroglial hyperplasia and hypertrophy may inhibit remyelination—at least by Schwann cells. The proliferation of Schwann cells in MS is seen in its most spectacular form as "onion bulbs" (concentric lamination of hyperplastic Schwann cells most commonly seen in hypertrophic neuropathies) in a few isolated cases.[430] Such cases appear to have concomitant hypertrophic peripheral neuropathy, except for one, where the CNS onion bulbs could not be related to coexisting peripheral nerve disease.[430]

The parenchyma adjacent to the chronic active plaque contains reactive astrocytes (see Fig. 8–14). In addition, inflammatory cells, including lymphocytes, although they may be less obvious in routine histological stains, can be readily demonstrated by immunocytochemistry in the periplaque white matter. However, particularly evident in periplaque white matter are perivascular cuffs of lymphocytes. These cuffs are thought to be extensions of lymphocytic infiltrates from the adjacent MS plaque. One

*References 4, 6, 7, 236, 252, 253, 353, 355, 360, 361, 363, 368, 373, 389, 468.

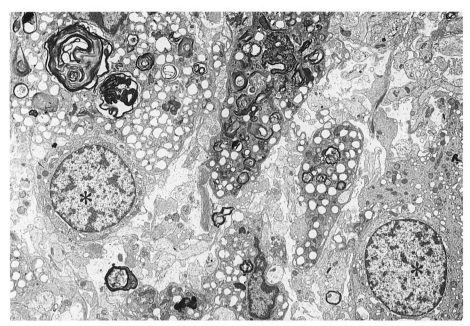

Figure 8–15. Electron micrograph of the edge of a chronic active MS plaque, showing several macrophages containing myelin debris within tertiary lysosomes. The large, clear droplets in these cells represent neutral lipid, the final degradation product. The two cells indicated with an asterisk are oligodendrocytes, which are present in increased numbers at the edge of the lesion. ×3900. (From Raine CS, Scheinberg L, and Waltz JM: Multiple Sclerosis: Oligodendrocyte survival and proliferation in an active established lesion. Laboratory Investigation 45(6):534–546, 1981, p 539, copyright by the United States and Canadian Academy of Pathology, Inc., with permission.)

frequently sees a small rim of demyelination around such cuffs. These extensions of lesions have been referred to as "Dawson's fingers," after the pathologist who described them in 1914 in a classic and magnificently illustrated monograph on the pathology of MS.[104] They provide strong suggestive evidence that the progression of the chronic MS lesion is related to the perivascular lymphocytic cuff.[5,6] An extensive study[136] has documented that MS plaques follow the course of veins. This finding appears to be true even of periventricular plaques, which have also been thought to be related to diffusion of a substance toxic to myelin from the CSF.[9,18] Furthermore, as with acute MS, there is a relationship between active demyelination and the presence of lymphocytic perivascular cuffs.[171] Whereas the composition of the inflammatory cuff outside the lesion is predominantly lymphocytic, within the plaque, it is a mixture of lymphocytes and macrophages.[6,476] This observation suggests that the lymphocyte might be the important immune cell in the early stages of chronic active plaque extension. Most lymphocytes remain in the perivascular spaces, even in the plaque,[353] although some can be demonstrated in the parenchyma by immunocytochemistry. As is true of inflammation throughout the lesion in primary chronic progressive MS, the perivascular inflammatory cuffs are less prominent than in secondary progressive disease with superimposed exacerbations and remissions.[399] Fibrin deposition within the walls of veins with lymphocytic-mononuclear cuffs occurs particularly in active lesions.[13] The vessel walls eventually undergo fibrosis, and reticulin deposition in their walls begins first in the older, more central areas of the lesion.[341]

Aside from extension of a lesion from an existing plaque, small lesions arise around lymphocytic cuffs along a vein, like a "string of beads."[252] Such lesions are not continuous and presumably represent the early stages of formation of independent plaques, which may later coalesce. Thus, in chronic

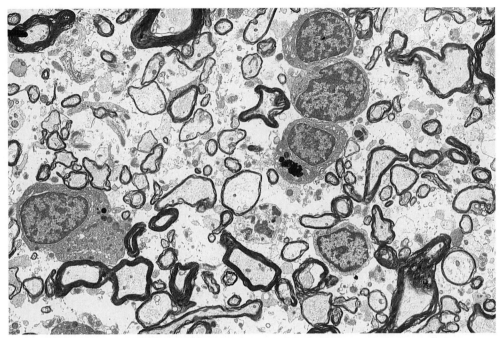

Figure 8–16. Electron micrograph of remyelination at the edge of a chronic, active MS plaque. The five nucleated cells are oligodendrocytes. Remyelination is evident as very thin myelin sheaths seen in cross-section. ×10,600. (Adapted from Raine CS, Scheinberg L, and Waltz JM: Multiple Sclerosis. Oligodendrocyte survival and proliferation in an active established lesion. Laboratory Investigation 45(6):534–546, 1981, p 543, copyright by the United States and Canadian Academy of Pathology, Inc., with permission.)

MS, plaque extension can occur by progressive demyelination at the edge, by finger-like extensions of lesions into the adjacent parenchyma, or by coalescence of two or more neighboring plaques.

Immunocytochemistry

In the early 1980s, reports emerged documenting T-cell infiltration in MS lesions.[13,70,321,489,490] Subsequent reports showed that B cells are present in only small numbers[187] but plasma cells increase with chronicity of the lesion.[239] T-cell subsets within chronic active MS lesions have been analyzed in detail.* The first detailed study[490] showed that CD4 (then termed OKT4) helper T lymphocytes were present in small numbers in the lesion center, increased in numbers more peripherally, with

larger numbers in the parenchyma of the lesion edge, and infiltrated deeply into tissue adjacent to the lesion. On the other hand, CD8 (then designated OKT8) cyto-toxic/suppressor T cells showed an increasing gradient of density from center to lesion periphery, but at the lesion edge were mainly confined to perivascular cuffs and did not penetrate far into the periplaque parenchyma.[490] Based on these findings, it was concluded that the CD4 lymphocyte was the more important cell in the pathogenesis of the chronic active lesion.[490] The centrifugal spread of the plaque border could be attributed to demyelination by macrophages, which have been activated by cytokines, particularly interferon-gamma, produced by certain helper-inducer T cells.[205] Downregulation of this immune response could be carried out by the perivascular CD8 (presumed suppressor) cells at the periphery of the lesion.

However, subsequently other workers found that the CD8 cells predominated over CD4 cells in all regions of the MS

---

*References 62, 70, 187, 189, 203, 263, 321, 457, 484, 489, 490.

plaque and in the nonplaque white matter,[62,187,189,263,525,530] and the T cells expressed MHC class I antigen.[189] Thus, they felt that the immunopathogenesis of the lesion was related to MHC class I-restricted cytotoxic T lymphocytes, which could directly target the offending myelin or oligodendrocytic antigen. One study has shown chronic active lesions with the helper-inducer population predominating at the lesion edge,[203] another study noted plaque borders where either CD4 or CD8 cells may predominate,[263] and still another has found the CD4 cell to predominate in perivascular inflammatory cuffs in the lesion edge, but CD4 and CD8 cells to be present in equal numbers in the parenchyma.[129] Possible explanations for these discrepancies include differences in the immunocytochemical techniques employed, reduced density of the CD4 marker on the cell surface, the presence of concomitant systemic infections, and differences in the definition of the activity and age of plaques between different laboratories.[539] The last point is quite important, because chronic active MS plaques can vary considerably in age within a single patient and, of course, between patients. Indeed, a group[457] previously reporting CD8 predominance has found CD4 cells to be more frequent than CD8 cells in a later study of a different series of lesions, and the discrepancies were attributed to lesions of various ages. The problem is further compounded by the inability to separate cytotoxic and suppressor cell populations expressing the CD8 marker. It may well be that the immunopathogenesis of chronic active MS lesions is related to a preponderance of CD4 cells in enlarging lesions[490] and to a predominance of suppressor cells in regressing lesions that are being immunologically downregulated.[376] The ratio of the cell types would then depend on when in the disease process the lesion was sampled.

In cases where the clinical presentation is that of chronic progressive (versus relapsing-remitting) MS, the CD8 phenotype predominates in the lesions.[242,384,484] Whether this phenotype is serving a cytotoxic or suppressor function in these lesions is unclear. However, in the lesions of tropical spastic paraparesis, which also presents with a progressive course referable to spinal cord in-

volvement, the CD8 phenotype also predominates.[294] It has been postulated that a cytotoxic mechanism may underlie the immunopathogenesis of both these progressive inflammatory disorders of white matter.[294]

The CD4 subset has been further analyzed in the chronic active lesion. It has been found that the suppressor-inducer (2H4) subset is reduced in MS when compared to the infiltrate in viral encephalitis, whereas the 4B4 (helper-inducer) subset is comparable in numbers in both conditions.[456,457] This finding suggests that there is a reduction in suppression of the ongoing immune response within the active MS plaque, allowing immune-directed demyelination to proceed relatively unchecked.

Molecules important in CD4 T-cell interactions with B cells and in activation of macrophages, namely CD40 and its ligand, have been immunocytochemically demonstrated in MS lesions, which were not further characterized as to type or age.[151b] CD40 was found on macrophages and a few B lymphocytes and its ligand was seen on CD4 T lymphocytes.[151b] The juxtaposition of cells showing positivity for CD40 with those positive for the ligand suggested ongoing interaction between the cells bearing these molecules.[151b]

One study has found that the alpha-beta T-cell receptor repertoire is not as diverse as in acute MS.[530] Recent work has shown that many of the lymphocytes in the chronic active MS plaque use gamma and delta chains in their T-cell receptors.[46b,207b,437,529] A study of chronic active lesions has shown a dominant gamma-delta T-cell receptor sequence, indicating clonal expansion in response to a specific antigen (possibly a heat shock protein),[46b] whereas another has found heterogeneity in the gamma-delta receptor repertoire.[207b]

Hsp60 is expressed in astrocytes in the center of the chronic active lesion, but is particularly strongly expressed in reactive astrocytes and oligodendrocytes at the lesion edge.[393a] The colocalization of this heat shock protein and MBP to cells at the lesion edge suggests that remyelinating oligodendrocytes are expressing this protein.[437] It has been suggested that in the chronic stages of lesion enlargement, hsp-60 expression by these cells may make them susceptible to attack by T gamma-delta cells, causing their demise.[71a,393a,437] Furthermore, the smaller heat shock protein alpha B-crystallin is also detected in astrocytes and oligodendrocytes at the edge of MS lesions, oligodendroglial expression being more prominent than astrocytic expression in earlier lesions.[493a] The latter protein is immunogenic for T cells,[439a] again raising the possibility that lesion expansion is mediated in part by non-myelin antigens expressed by oligodendrocytes or in myelin during the maturation of the lesion.[393a]

MHC class II (Ia) antigen expression in the chronic active MS lesion is well documented. It is generally agreed that macrophages or microglia in this lesion express the marker,* and demonstration of the intracellular invariant chain of the molecule (VIC-41 marker) suggests that these cells are actually synthesizing it, and not just passively absorbing it.[525] Ia-positive macrophages are in greater numbers in the center of the lesion and in somewhat fewer numbers at the margin.[485,490] Some of the Ia-positive cells may also be B lymphocytes and activated T lymphocytes. Ia-bearing macrophages[246a,485,490] and cells with long processes consistent with microglia[61,68,246a] are also seen in periplaque parenchyma. Some studies[203,485] have shown that at the edges of the chronic active plaque, astrocytes may express this marker, but to a lesser degree in more central regions of the lesion. Others, however, have not found Ia-positive astrocytes[61,68,189,492a] or could only demonstrate them in small numbers.[190,525] Thus, based on current evidence, expression of Ia antigens by astrocytes in MS lesions is an unusual event.[379]

As in acute MS, antigen presentation as judged by expression of MHC class II antigen is a feature of the chronic MS plaque, but this is by no means exclusive to MS and, in fact, can be detected in degenerative CNS diseases.[273] Although the antigen being presented in MS is unknown, there have been some recent insights into the cell type that may be important in the initial presentation of antigen in the early stages of lesion development. Experimental studies have proposed initial antigen presenta-

tion is carried out by perivascular microglia that are bone marrow derived.[195,196] This notion is supported by immunocytochemical studies of MS tissue in plastic sections[384] or using confocal microscopy,[61,492a] which better delineate microscopic anatomical relationships than the frozen sections employed previously. As noted in acute MS, these investigations showed Ia positivity of perivascular microglia and macrophages rather than the endothelium.[61,384,492a] In some experimental studies,[195,279,510] activated T lymphocytes have been shown to enter the CNS where they could come in contact with such perivascular cells. Contrary to the conventional concept of "immunologic privilege" of the CNS, a new concept is emerging that the CNS is constantly being patrolled by activated T cells (which recognize any number of CNS and non-CNS antigens) that readily breach the blood-brain barrier.[279,510] Trafficking activated T lymphocytes, which come in contact with MHC class II-positive perivascular cells presenting the putative CNS antigen, could then initiate the cascade of immunologic events, including macrophage or microglial activation, to create a new demyelinating plaque or to extend a previously existing one. Once the plaque is well established, antigen presentation presumably could be carried out by lesion macrophages expressing MHC class II antigen.

Costimulatory molecules, which together with MHC class II molecule expression, are necessary for a CD4 T-cell response, have been studied in MS lesions.[105a,518a] It has been shown that the costimulatory molecule B7 is expressed on microglia and macrophages in MS lesions.[105a] Further analysis of early and chronic MS lesions has defined this phenomenon further by demonstrating cells (probably T cells) that stain for B7-1, the costimulatory molecule associated with the induction of the Th1 CD4 cells which mediate the immune response as helper T cells secreting the pro-inflammatory cytokines IL-2, TNF-α, LT, and interferon gamma.[518a] In contrast, B7-2, involved in the induction of Th2 cells that secrete the immunomodulatory cytokines IL-4, IL-10, and TGF-β, is detected on macrophages in MS lesions as well as in infarcts, consistent with the recovery or repair function of this immune response.[518a]

---

*References 61, 68, 128, 187, 189, 190, 246a, 485, 490, 492a, 525.

MHC class I expression by endothelial cells is reduced in chronic active MS lesions as well as in the non-lesioned white matter as compared with normal control tissue.[485] However, astrocytes express MHC class I antigen within the lesion and in few numbers at the edge.[485] This expression is not as dramatic as in the central portion of the acute plaque, where they have been found in fair abundance.[485] In another study,[189] MHC class I antigen has been shown only on endothelial cells and T cells and not on astrocytes in chronic active MS.

CD1 molecules have been speculated to function similar to MHC class I and class II molecules but on antigen-presenting cells for T cells that express neither CD4 nor CD8 and are involved in immune responses to nonpeptide antigens. These CD1 molecules have been studied in chronic active MS lesions.[46a] Of this class of molecules, CD1b is found on inflammatory cells in perivascular cuffs and on hypertrophic astrocytes at the lesion border.[46a] The cell population is different from that staining for MHC class I and class II molecules.[46a] Moreover, the cytokine granulocyte-macrophage colony stimulating factor (GM-CSF), a known inducer of CD1 molecules, is also found on these hypertrophic astrocytes.[46a] Thus this sub-system of the immune response may be important in lesion propagation from antigen presentation of nonpeptide antigens (such as lipids) to CD1-restricted T cells.[46a]

Matrix metalloproteinases, as in the acute lesion, are found in macrophages, particularly at the lesion edge and to some degree in astrocytes.[256a]

With the significant numbers of inflammatory cells of various types in the chronic active lesion, not surprisingly cytokines and markers indicating lymphocytic stimulation have been demonstrated immunocytochemically in these lesions. IL-2 and its receptor have been found particularly at the plaque edge and follow a distribution similar to the CD4 infiltrate.[51,203,485,525] The number of such activated cells, however, is not large and, in fact, in some studies have been undetectable.[189] Some IL-2-positive cells appear to be reactive astrocytes, although it is possible these cells may have endocytosed the marker.[525] IL-1 has also been detected at the edge of the chronic active MS plaque.[203] Its origin could be from macrophages, activated astrocytes, or B cells in the region. Prostaglandin E is found within the lesion, at the lesion edge and within the adjacent white matter.[203] All these findings are consistent with an active ongoing immunologic response in MS.

Interferons have been demonstrated on various cell types in chronic active MS lesions.[488] In some studies, interferon-gamma was found on astrocytes in a distribution similar to that of MHC class II antigen, a finding which correlated with the capacity of this cytokine to induce Ia.[207,487,488] Interferon-alpha is found mainly on macrophages, and interferon-beta is seen on astrocytes and macrophages.[488] Endothelial cells rarely stain for interferons.[488]

Several other cytokines have been immunocytochemically analyzed—including TNF and LT. TNF staining is seen in macrophages and astrocytes within the lesion, and TNF-positive astrocytes abound at the edge.[202,438] A recent abstract has reported that different forms of LT may have different affinities for various glial cells.[81a] IL-4, IL-10, and TGF-β are also present in chronic active MS lesions on the same cell types as they are in acute MS, but less intensely.[83] Messenger RNAs for most of the above cytokines have been reported in MS lesions.[525a] In addition, messenger RNA for interleukin-6 (IL-6),[525a] which functions in the acute phase response and in B cell differentiation,[51a] and for interleukin-12 (IL-12), which plays a role in the Th1 cell differentiation,[518a] have also been detected. The demonstration of cytokines suggests they could have a role in the pathogenesis of the MS lesion.[72a]

The localization of vitronectin to endothelial cells and axons is similar to acute MS.[455a] As discussed above, the function of vitronectin in MS lesions is not known.[455a]

In an effort to understand how circulating immune competent cells can adhere to the CNS endothelial cell and thus enter the parenchyma in chronic MS, several immunocytochemical studies have demonstrated molecules with known adhesive properties. One[458] has shown fibronectin staining on the vessel wall in lesions as well as within the parenchyma of the lesion. Fibronectin receptor was demonstrated on macrophages. It was postulated that fibronectin might have a role in mononuclear adhesion to the endothelium via this receptor. Fibronectin may also aid in myelin phagocytosis by a similar mechanism.[458] The intercellular adhesion molecule-1 (ICAM-1) is upregulated on endothelial cells and can be detected on macrophages and some astrocytes in active MS plaques.[459] ICAM-1 can be demonstrated in a wide zone around the lesion as well.[486] Its leukocyte integrin, lymphocyte function-associated antigen-1 (LFA-1), is also detected.[83] In experimental allergic encephalomyelitis (EAE), an experimental analogue of MS and an autoimmune disease mediated by T cells directed against myelin components,[26,373] endothelial ICAM-1 expression precedes inflammation[460] and is downregulated during a clinical remission.[82] A similar pattern has been shown for several adhesion-related molecules in the mouse.[82] Moreover, certain cytokines upregulate expression of ICAM-1 by human cerebral endothelial cells in vitro,[522] a mechanism that may be important in the early events of lesion formation in MS. Vascular cell adhesion molecule-1 (VCAM-1) can also be detected on blood vessels and microglial cells.[83] Very late activation antigen-4 (VLA-4), the leukocyte integrin for VCAM-1, has also been found on mononuclear cells in the MS lesion.[83] The VCAM-1/VLA-4 adhesion pathway is maximal in chronic active MS lesions as compared with acute lesions.[83] This differential expression, however, is not evident with the ICAM-1/LFA-1 pathway.[83] Another study has demonstrated high endothelial venule antigen (detected by the HECA-452 monoclonal antibody[115]), an antigen usually expressed at the site of entry of lymphocytes from the circulation into peripheral lymph nodes, in the lesions, and in the periplaque parenchyma of a case of chronic progressive MS.[242,384] Experimental investigations[93,381,384] have further dissected these important early phenomena in vivo by studying the homing, attachment, and migration of lymphocytes across the endothelium in EAE. As is true of most of the immunologic markers in MS lesions, these are not necessarily specific for MS or autoimmune demyelination, and to date, no immunologic marker specific for CNS immunopathology has been documented.[379]

Summary

The chronic active MS plaque shows a gradient of pathological changes. Its central regions reflect older events, and its border shows ongoing active demyelination and attempts at remyelination. The evidence to date favors an immunopathogenesis in which CD4 lymphocytes activate macrophages to carry out the demyelination, although several studies have suggested a cytotoxic mechanism cannot be excluded. These different findings may be due to sampling of lesions at different ages. Remyelination can be seen at the border of chronic active plaques.

THE CHRONIC SILENT MULTIPLE SCLEROSIS PLAQUE

The chronic silent MS plaque is frequently referred to as "burnt out." It shows no evidence of ongoing demyelination. This, however, does not necessarily imply that it may not become active in the future.[6,359]

Histopathology

The chronic silent plaque is characterized by extensive numbers of demyelinated axons. Frequently, axonal loss is evident,[42] more conspicuously in the center than in the periphery,[377] and occasionally central cystic areas may be evident. These changes are usually interpreted as being due to excessive degrees of previous inflammation, which had resulted in destruction not only of the myelin sheath but of varying numbers of axons and other tissue elements as well. Nevertheless, the myelin loss in the chronic silent plaque is much more evident than the reduction in axons. Oligodendrocytes are absent, and demyelinated axons are seen in a sea of numerous fibrillary astrocytic processes (Fig. 8–17). Although one study[360] has shown these chronically demyelinated axons to have a smaller diameter than normal, another[443] found them to be larger. The dense gliosis may occasionally be accompanied by deposition of Rosenthal fibers,[193] which are probably a degenerative phenomenon. Small desmosomal junctions are evident between

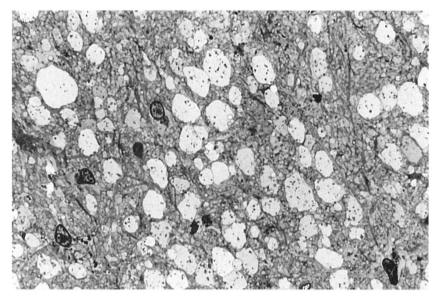

Figure 8–17. 1 μm epoxy section of a chronic, silent MS lesion. There are numerous demyelinated axons (clear circular profiles) amidst densely packed processes of fibrillary astrocytes. The nuclei are astrocytic and no oligodendrocytes are evident. Toluidine blue. ×1100. (From Raine CS: Demyelinating Diseases. In Davis RL, and Robertson DM (eds). Textbook of Neuropathology, ed 2. copyright 1991, Williams & Wilkins, Baltimore, pp 535–620, p 554, with permission.)

astrocytes and axons in long-standing plaques.[372,461] In some lesions, the extracellular space may be quite prominent.[42] Wandering through this glial scar-axonal mosaic are occasional lipid-laden macrophages, presumably making their way to the perivascular spaces to enter the systemic circulation (Fig. 8–18). Scattered lymphocytes may be evident, usually in the perivascular spaces, but the prominent inflammatory

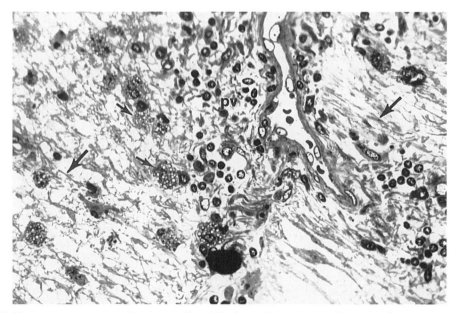

Figure 8–18. 1 μm epoxy section of a chronic silent MS plaque. Several macrophages (small arrows) are making their way to the perivascular space (pv) of a venule. Within the perivascular space there are a few lymphocytes, plasma cells and mononuclear cells. The parenchyma shows numerous processes of fibrillary astrocytes (large arrows). Toluidine blue. ×275.

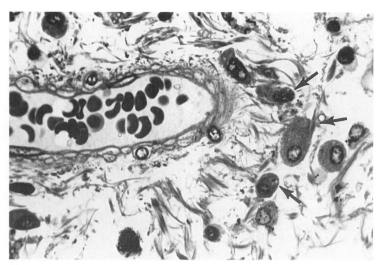

Figure 8–19. Plasma cells (arrows) in the perivascular space of a venule in a chronic silent MS plaque. 1 μm epoxy section. Toluidine blue. ×600.

cuffs that typify the active lesion are usually no longer evident (see Fig. 8–18).

An ultrastructural study[354] has shown that these perivascular spaces of the chronic silent lesion have a structure similar to that of the medullary region of lymph nodes. This is comprised of thin-walled channels, within which there are lymphocytes and macrophages, and external to which there are plasma cells. Thus, in the MS lesion, there is lymphoid tissue, which is probably autonomous. Moreover, these findings imply that the CNS has a lymphatic drainage.

In chronic silent MS plaques, the immune response appears relatively quiescent. However, plasma cells may be present in significant numbers (Fig. 8–19).[369] Deposition of IgG in the form of Russell bodies is an exceptionally unusual finding associated with plasma cells.[416] Occasionally mast cells may be seen.[104,326] The reticulin formation, which was beginning in vessels within the chronic active lesion, reaches its endpoint in the silent lesion, where a significant degree of fibrosis of vessel walls may be seen (Fig. 8–20). This finding is presumably a response to,

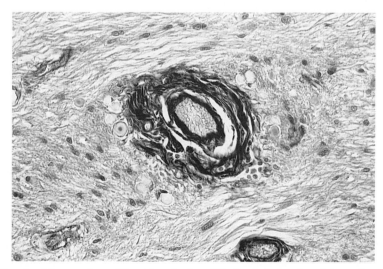

Figure 8–20. Fibrosis of the vascular wall in a chronic silent MS plaque. Intensely staining collagen is seen in the wall of a venule. Mallory trichrome. ×150.

and hence an indicator of, previous inflammatory infiltrates within these vessel walls.

The chronic silent plaque border is well demarcated, and there is an abrupt transition between myelin loss and myelinated parenchyma (see Fig. 8–8). Occasionally, oligodendrocytes can be seen at the border and, with them, evidence of remyelination[377] (Fig. 8–21). If this shelf of remyelination is substantial, a pale staining edge is evident on myelin stains and such lesions have been termed *shadow plaques* (Fig. 8–22). Sometimes an entire lesion may be remyelinated. In chronic MS lesions, remyelination by peripheral nerve myelin from Schwann cells has also been shown to survive to the chronic inactive stage.*

It has been shown that silent healed areas remyelinated by oligodendrocytes may undergo subsequent reactivation with the development of a region of demyelination within the remyelinated zone.[359] Such areas of demyelination show the same histopathology as chronic active MS plaques and may offer a histological explanation for recurring lesions at the same site, which have been documented clinically as well by MRI.[333,359] A recent abstract has suggested that this expansion of the lesion may be related to the expression of a previously unexpressed MBP peptide by oligodendrocytes in the remyelinated area.[83a] The emergence of new epitopes as targets for autoimmune demyelination during the course of the disease (referred to as "epitope spreading") has been demonstrated in chronic EAE,[93a] and may be very pertinent to the propagation of the MS lesion after the initial immune response to the original instigating antigen[393a]—whether this be reactivation of a chronic silent lesion or the progressive expansion of a chronic active plaque.

The parenchyma adjacent to the chronic inactive MS plaque can show hypertrophic astrocytes.[377] There are also a few plasma cells and lymphocytes in this region.

Large chronic inactive plaques, which are found in the periventricular region, often are associated with discontinuities in the ependyma through which tufts of fibrous astrocytic processes protrude—so-called "granular ependymitis" (Fig. 8–23). This phenom-

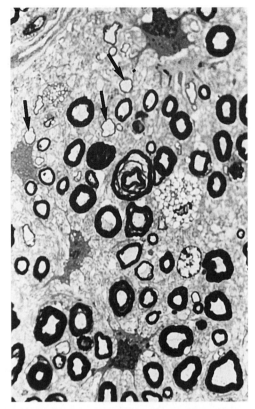

Figure 8–21. Edge of a chronic silent MS plaque showing remyelination, characterized by thin myelin sheaths (arrows). The cells with prominent processes are astrocytes. A lipid-laden macrophage is seen just to the right of center. 1 μm epoxy section. Toluidine blue. ×2400. (From Raine CS: Demyelinating Diseases. In Davis RL, and Robertson DM (eds). Textbook of Neuropathology, ed 2. copyright 1991, Williams & Wilkins, Baltimore, pp 535–620, p 558, with permission.)

enon, a marker of chronicity, is a less common feature in cases with demyelinative activity but is nonspecific for MS.[9] It is believed to be a residuum from the pre-existing inflammatory activity within the parenchyma adjacent to the ependyma.

Immunocytochemistry

Work on immunocytochemical labeling of immune markers in chronic silent MS lesions has shown that that the lesion center contains only small numbers of CD4 cells but no CD8 cells.[485,488,490,491] At the lesion edge there are more CD4 cells and a few CD8 cells, and throughout the non-lesioned white matter, both types of T lymphocytes may be detected in small num-

---

*References 131, 132, 157, 211, 214, 324.

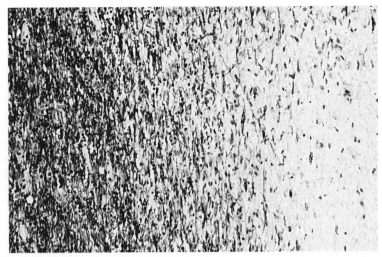

Figure 8–22. Edge of a shadow plaque. The adjacent normal-appearing white matter is on the left. The middle zone of fainter staining myelinated tissue is responsible for the "shadow" appearance. Recent studies have shown that, in most cases, this is an area of remyelination. The demyelinated region of the plaque is on the right. Hematoxylin-eosin-Luxol fast blue. ×120.

bers.[490] The early immunocytochemical studies employing routine microscopy of frozen sections have reported that the distribution of MHC class II molecules was the same as was found in chronic active lesions in these studies, but not as pronounced in degree.[485,491] Expression of the costimulatory molecule B7 is markedly reduced.[105a]

Only a few lipid-laden macrophages stain for MHC class I antigen.[485] CD1b staining is also markedly reduced, being demonstra-

ble only on occasional foot processes of astrocytes and perivascular macrophages.[46a] Macrophages with metalloproteinases are also few in number.[256a] Hsp60 staining greater than constituent levels is confined to astrocytes.[393a] VCAM-1 and ICAM-1 and their integrins are still present in the chronic silent lesion.[83]

Correlating with the marked reduction in the inflammatory infiltrate in these lesions, cytokine expression is reduced.[83,488]

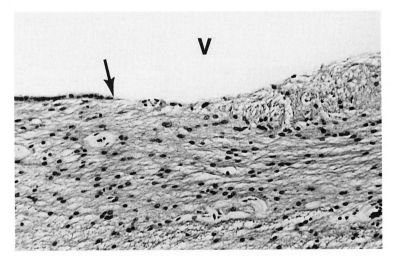

Figure 8–23. "Granular ependymitis" in a periventricular chronic silent MS plaque. The ependyma abruptly stops at the arrow, where it is replaced by a tuft of fibrillar astrocytic processes which protrude into the ventricle (V). Hematoxylin-eosin. ×140.

All of these findings point out that the immune response in the chronic silent lesion is muted.

Summary

The chronic silent plaque shows no evidence of ongoing demyelination and is primarily characterized by demyelinated axons superimposed on a background of severe fibrillary gliosis. Few immune-competent cells are present in the lesion. It can, however, become active again at any time.

IMMUNOGLOBULINS AND COMPLEMENT IN THE MULTIPLE SCLEROSIS LESION

The immunocytochemical studies noted previously have established the T cell as the predominant lymphocyte in the MS plaque. However, there is clearly evidence of B-cell activity in the lesion, even though B cells are much fewer in number. Their product, IgG, can be demonstrated in MS plaques by biochemical analysis[481] and by immuno-fluorescence techniques.[446] In addition to diffuse immunoglobulin throughout the lesion, which can be readily eluted, cells with cycloplasmic IgG have been demonstrated in active demyelinating lesions as well as in chronic inactive plaques.* Some of these cells are plasma cells; others are B cells not yet matured into plasma cells.[127,304] They are usually confined to perivascular cuffs in older lesions, may be found in the lesion parenchyma in early plaques,[127] and are occasionally seen in the adjacent normal-appearing white matter.[127,304] Plasma cells correlate with the presence of oligoclonal bands of IgG in the cerebrospinal fluid (CSF).[130] These IgG-synthesizing cells usually demonstrate light chains more frequently than heavy chains and kappa chains more frequently than lambda.[127] Astrocytes have also been shown to stain for IgG.[87,113,367,526] Probably this finding represents binding of IgG to Fc receptors on the

*References 87, 113, 126, 127, 253, 304, 478, 494, 526.

astrocyte surface. Although IgG is the predominant immunoglobulin class in MS plaques, some IgA- and, to a much lesser extent, IgM-containing cells may be seen.[126,127,304]

The relevant antigen or antigens against which the immunoglobulin is directed is unknown. Anti-MBP or anti-proteolipid protein IgG[501a] and anti-MBP producing B cells[151a] have been reported in MS tissue, but the relationship to disease etiology is unclear. It was thought that the demyelinating activity of MS sera observed in CNS tissue cultures[64,69] might be due to immunoglobulin, but this appears not to be the case.[168] This lack of specificity is also true of the demyelination induced by normal human serum.[445] Although IgG may not account for lysis of myelin in tissue culture, it still may play an important role in the removal of myelin by macrophages in the active MS lesion (see discussion following).

Complement in the form of C1q,[526] C3,[13] C3d,[148] C5–9,[527] C9[89,148] and the terminal component neoantigen[89] has been localized immunocytochemically in blood vessel walls in MS lesions. C1q has also been found in macrophages and microglia, and C5–9 in microglia.[527] SP40,40 (a complement inhibitor), has been localized to reactive astrocytes,[527] but these astrocytes do not stain for complement, suggesting that SP40,40 function is not related to protection from complement effects in these cells.[527] The co-localization of C1q with IgG[526] and C3d and C9 with IgM and IgG[148] suggests immune complex deposition occurs in the MS lesion.

Human oligodendrocytes have been shown to be resistant to complement-induced lysis in vitro, due to the presence of the complement regulatory protein CD59 on their surface.[537a] CD59 has been detected in white matter in normal adult CNS and in MS, but at relatively low levels compared to myelinating areas in the developing CNS.[537a] On the other hand, a recent abstract reported on oligodendrocytes with deposits of the terminal complement complex in MS lesions in which glial cells, including oligodendrocytes, and endothelial cells did not express CD59.[15a] Whether complement-mediated lysis of oligodendrocytes is an important mechanism in the pathogenesis of the MS lesion is unresolved at the present time.

THE VASCULATURE AND BLOOD-BRAIN BARRIER IN THE MULTIPLE SCLEROSIS LESION

Positive technetium brain scans, transient enhancing lesions seen with large-dose contrast computed tomography (CT) scans, and transient gadolinium enhancement of MRI lesions in patients with MS are indicative of breakdown of the blood-brain barrier.[16,124,227,241,282,432] Morphologic evidence of leakage of the blood-brain barrier may be found in the demonstration of fibrinogen,[148,526] fibrin,[13] albumin,[89] and transferrin[127] around and within blood vessel walls in the MS lesion. (Such high-molecular-weight substances are normally excluded from CNS perivascular regions.) Using trypan blue as a high-molecular-weight dye for the perfusion of postmortem MS brain, leakage of the dye has been demonstrated around veins within MS plaques.[71] In addition, the demonstration of uptake of native or oxidized low-density lipoproteins by macrophages is indicative of transgression of the damaged blood-brain barrier by low-density lipoproteins, normally confined to the plasma.[317a] Some studies,[446,478,482] however, have been unable to show evidence of blood-brain barrier disturbance in these lesions. These differences are probably related to the fact that the breakdown of the blood-brain barrier is not massive, as evidenced by minimal, if any, elevation of the CSF albumin concentration and the transient nature of this phenomenon, as shown by MRI studies.

The ultrastructural basis for the blood-brain barrier is tight junctions between adjacent endothelial cells that effectively separate the perivascular and intravascular spaces, preventing the passive diffusion of high-molecular-weight substances.[108,336] Blood-brain barrier function is also related to the fact that cerebral endothelial cells have many fewer vesicles than endothelial cells in other organs.[108,336]

An in vitro model of the human blood-brain barrier has been developed,[108a] and it has been shown that these monolayers of cultured human cerebral microvascular endothelial cells respond to various cytokines.[207,207a,522] Interferon gamma induces the expression of MHC class II molecules on these cells[207] and this effect is abolished by co-incubation with interferon beta.[207a] As discussed in Chapter 12, interferon beta has been shown to have a beneficial effect on the course of relapsing-remitting MS.[333a,478a] The results of these in vitro studies suggest that this effect may be due to an interferon beta–mediated dampening of interferon gamma–induced MHC class II molecule expression.[207a]

An electron microscopic study[74] of a single actively demyelinating MS lesion showed that the tight junctions were intact. However, the count of vesicles in endothelial cells was markedly increased, suggesting that there may be enhanced transendothelial transport.[74] Similar findings have also been observed in lesions of chronic EAE with breakdown of the blood-brain barrier demonstrated by transendothelial vesicular transport of gadolinium.[188] The fenestrations seen in the endothelium of guinea pigs with chronic EAE[453] have not been described in MS to date.

The secretion of enzymes, cytokines, and toxic free radicals (see discussion following) by the inflammatory infiltrates within and around the walls of vessels could result in weakening of the vessel wall,[13] and this process may be the basis of blood-brain barrier breakdown. The relationship between inflammation and the blood-brain barrier is the subject of intensive experimental investigation.[237] In MS, a correlation can be found between the presence of perivascular inflammatory infiltrates in the retina and positivity of the technetium brain scan, suggesting that inflammation and blood-brain barrier disruption are related.[124] Moreover, a postmortem study of reactivated MS lesions, which enhanced with gadolinium on the MRI scan, revealed extensive inflammatory infiltrates in the region of enhancement.[219] Most likely, the lymphocyte-mononuclear infiltrate in the vessel wall is responsible for the blood-brain barrier leakage. It is possible that this early breakdown may be initiated by cytokines or other mediators from these cells just before or at the time of their penetration of the endothelium. Certain cytokines can induce changes in retinal and cerebral endothelial cells that could increase their permeability.[73,121] In MS, primary disruption in the barrier unrelated to inflammation is a less likely scenario, but we cannot completely dismiss this possibility.

Although blood-brain barrier breakdown is usually thought to be associated with active MS lesions, there is immunocytochemical evidence of a blood-brain barrier disturbance in some chronic silent plaques.[87a,232] This finding is believed to be due to persistent damage to the barrier induced by inflammatory infiltrates that had previously resolved.[232] As in active lesions, the endothelial cells show increased numbers of pinocytotic vesicles.[87a] It has been speculated that the reduction of mitochondria in these endothelial cells may be a primary phenomenon in blood-brain barrier breakdown.[87a]

Rarely does damage to the vessel wall result in frank hemorrhage into the MS plaque. Small, fresh petechial hemorrhages have been described.[13,255] Moreover, stainable iron has been documented in MS lesions, to both a mild[500] and a moderate degree.[8,92] In the latter instance, this is evident particularly near the plaque edge. These findings are consistent with the previous occurrence of minor hemorrhages in these lesions. To date, few cases in the literature have reported frank CNS hemorrhage in the setting of MS. In two of these,[3] it was believed to be unrelated to MS, and in others,[62,215] there was hemorrhage into an MS plaque.

In summary, varying degrees of damage to blood vessels occur in MS, ranging from transient opening of the blood-brain barrier to rare frank hemorrhage. These vascular phenomena are probably all related to the presence of the vascular inflammatory infiltrate.

MECHANISMS OF DEMYELINATION IN MULTIPLE SCLEROSIS

A variety of approaches have contributed to our present understanding of the process of demyelination in MS. These approaches have included biochemical, histochemical, and ultrastructural studies.

Biochemical and Histochemical Studies of Demyelinated Plaques

As discussed previously, the more central regions of the chronic active plaque represent older stages of the disease process. Thus, it is not surprising that histochemical and biochemical studies have shown decreased or absent components of myelin in these areas. For instance, MBP is lost in these lesions* as is MAG.[149,212,316,366] Low-molecular-weight proteins in plaques are thought to be proteolytic breakdown products of MBP,[315,316] and MBP-degradation products have been demonstrated by immunocytochemistry.[246a] Degradation of proteolipid has also been found.[94,315,415]

Lipid components of myelin are also reduced in the chronic active plaque. This fact is true of phospholipids in general,[95,532] total cholesterol,[11,532] cerebrosides,[11,152,532] ethanolamine plasmalogen,[532] and $C_{20:1}$ fatty acid.[152] A reduction in the cerebroside-sulfatide ratio occurs in these lesions,[119] and this finding may be related to gliosis or to demyelinated axons.[319] Some investigators[200] have found an elevation of lactic dehydrogenase activity, which they have attributed to an increased number of astrocytes, whereas others have attributed the finding of reduced levels of this enzyme to oligodendroglial depletion.[143] However, decreased levels of the enzymes CNP (a marker of oligodendrocytes and myelin[229]) and cytoplasmic glycerol phosphate dehydrogenase also reflect the myelin and oligodendroglial loss.[198,245,404,415] The same is probably true of reduced acid lipase activity.[200,201] The reason for reduction in cytosolic phospholipase A_2 activity, but not its total content, in plaques and in grossly normal appearing white matter is unclear.[206a] The esterified cholesterol invariably found in MS plaques[95,339,532] is the biochemical correlate of the contents of numerous lipid-laden macrophages, which can be demonstrated by stains such as Sudan black

---

*References 10, 149, 175, 178, 212, 316, 366, 416, 516.

(stain), oil red O (stain), and variations of the Marchi technique.

Biochemical and histochemical studies have demonstrated a variety of enzymes in chronic plaques. The presence of acid proteinase or cathepsin A* and acid phosphatase[22,200,416] has been well documented. The lysosomal form of phospholipase A_2[206a] and the neutral proteinase cathepsin B[54a] are also increased in MS plaques. Some investigators[67,513] believe that, most likely, their origin is the numerous macrophages throughout these lesions. Because of a lack of correlation between plaque activity (as judged by hypercellularity) and hydrolase activity, others[22,200,274] have suggested that these hydrolytic enzymes are of astrocytic origin. Both schools of thought are probably correct. Indeed, astrocytes and macrophages were found to contain acid phosphatase activity in a study that used a combination of histochemical and routine histological staining techniques.[22]

Other enzymes with elevated activity in MS plaques have included carboxylic acid esterase,[416] β-glucuronidase,[98,274,416] β-galactosidase,[274] a thiol-dependent proteinase (probably carboxypeptidase B),[201] plasmalogenase,[29] arylsulfatase,[99] and n-acetyl-β-D-glucosaminidase.[274] The last enzyme correlated well with gliosis,[274] as did glucuronidase.[416]

Biochemical and Histochemical Studies of Macroscopically Normal-Appearing White Matter

Biochemical and histochemical studies have focused on the macroscopically normal-appearing white matter in MS, to determine if there is an inherent chemical abnormality in MS myelin. Acid hydrolases, including acid proteinase,[34,99,118,403,404,408] acid phosphatase,[22,403] β-glucuronidase,[98,99,274,403] and n-acetyl-β-D-glucosaminidase,[274] have been shown to have increased activity in the grossly normal-appearing white matter. This finding is also true of cathepsin B,[54a] β-galactosidase,[274] arylsulfatase,[99] plasmalogenase,[29] phospholipase A_1[313] and the lysosomal form of phospholipase A_2.[206a]

*References 67, 98, 118, 200, 274, 403, 415, 416.

One study, however, has found that acid hydrolases are normal,[200] and still another has noted lysosomal fragility, with an increased tendency to rupture in MS,[24] suggesting that the unaffected myelin may be more susceptible to the pathogenetic process of MS.

Biochemical analyses of normal-appearing white matter in MS have revealed decreased total phospholipid,[95,153,408] cerebroside,[11,403,408] sulfatide,[25] phosphatidyl serine,[313] and phosphatidyl inositol.[313] Moreover, gangliosides G_{M4} (a myelin-oligodendrocyte ganglioside), G_{M1}, G_{D1b}, and G_{Q1b} are reduced.[536] CNP has also been found to be reduced.[162] Much excitement was generated with the demonstration of the reduction of fatty acids, particularly lineolic acid, in lesions,[152] in normal-appearing white matter[36,153] and serum.[37,49,447] This observation was followed by a clinical trial wherein sunflower seed oil was administered to patients with MS to correct the alleged deficiency of lineolic acid[281] and reinforced the idea that there was an intrinsic metabolic defect in MS myelin. The finding of inclusions thought to be lipid in cells in MS white matter was also consistent with this.[47]

Cholesterol esters have been detected in normal-appearing white matter.[95,512,536] Other studies have shown reduced levels of MBP[315] and Wolfgram proteolipid[315] in normal-appearing white matter and in isolated myelin.[402]

Contrary to these studies, other workers found that normal-appearing white matter in MS has normal levels of total phospholipids,[532] total cholesterol,[532] cerebroside,[99] sulfatide,[99] ethanolamine phospholipids,[99] esterified cholesterol,[532] and acid hydrolases.[200] Most analyses of the chemical composition of isolated myelin have demonstrated normal levels[98,469,521] of most constituents tested.

The most likely explanation for these discrepancies is the inadvertent inclusion of microscopic areas of demyelination (or other pathology) in the samples used for the studies showing abnormalities.[319,469] Indeed, such areas are frequent in the grossly normal-appearing white matter[252] and have been found in histochemical and biochemical studies, which included light microscopic[24,274] and electron microscopic examination.[34,403,408] Such areas show diffuse gliosis, vascular fibrosis, perivascular cuffing by inflammatory cells, perivascular deposition of lipofuscin, and sometimes demyelination.[21] Astrocytes or inflammatory cells in these areas are probably the explanation for increased DNA content in normal-appearing white matter.[201]

Under the electron microscope, a frequent finding has been increased numbers of lysosomes, particularly in astrocytes,[34,403,408] but macrophages and other cell types may also show this feature. Even microscopically normal white matter may show high levels of n-acetyl-β-D-glucosominidase, probably related to activation of astrocytic lysosomes.[274] Lysosomes are thought to account for many of the increases in enzymes seen in the macroscopically normal-appearing white matter, and these enzymes, in turn, are thought to be responsible for generating the myelin breakdown products. Thus, the myelin breakdown in MS does not differ from simple myelin degradation seen with demyelinating conditions in general.[434] This process is a multifocal one, and it is generally accepted that this is not the result of a generalized metabolic derangement of myelin.[262]

However, physiochemical data[523] have shown that MBP from MS myelin cannot promote organization of phospholipid bilayers into lamellar structures as efficiently as normal MBP can. A study[300] of MBP charge isomeres suggests that MS myelin is structurally equivalent to that of an individual at 6 years of age or less. Such physiochemical studies have challenged the idea that myelin is developmentally mature prior to the demyelinating event in MS. The significance of elevated levels of certain metals, such as calcium, manganese, and zinc,[91] and radioactivity thought to be emanating from trace elements[306] in the white matter of patients with MS is unclear at this time.

Histochemical Studies of Active Plaque Margins

As mentioned previously, the edges of chronic active MS plaques have been examined repeatedly to determine the early stages of demyelination as it extends into the adjacent parenchyma. Enzyme histochemi-

cal studies have also looked at these active plaque edges. Oxidative enzyme activity at the plaque edge has been attributed to oligodendroglial hyperplasia.[142,143,208,209] The plaque border also shows increased acid phosphatase activity,[142,176] and proteolysis at the plaque border has been well documented.[175,176] Initially, the acid proteinase activity was attributed to oligodendrocytes at the plaque edge.[176] However, another study[67] has shown this enzyme in macrophages, and this cell probably is the major source of the enzyme at the plaque border.

It has been shown that nitric oxide synthase activity is detected in astrocytes in the borders of chronic active lesions, and one hypothesis is that the resulting toxic free radicals may be important in the pathogenesis of demyelination in MS by mediating oligodendrocyte death.[60,71b,278a] Nitric oxide synthase is also found in astrocytes[60] and endothelial cells[71b] throughout the lesion in the case of more actively demyelinating[60] and acute[71b] lesions. The nitric oxide synthesase activity co-localizes to cells with IL-1 and TNF positivity[71b] correlating with the ability of these cytokines to induce this enzyme.[303a] In situ polymerase chain reaction has also demonstrated its messenger RNA in macrophage cytoplasm at the lesion edge and within the lesion.[35a]

Histochemical and immunocytochemical studies have shown a loss of MBP in the white matter surrounding MS plaques.[11,178,516] Acid proteinase activity can be demonstrated in this region,[200] and this enzyme can degrade MBP.[117] Moreover, the finding of MBP fragments in the CSF of patients with MS[515] is also consistent with enzymatic digestion of MBP. One proposal held that degradation of MBP by acid proteinase was an early event in the demyelination process. The loss of basic protein could then be followed by changes in the phospholipid myelin membrane with loss of lipids and demyelination.[11]

In addition to acid proteinases, macrophages also produce neutral proteinases. This group of enzymes, particularly plasminogen activator, has also been implicated in demyelination.[80] Plasminogen activator can cause the release of plasmin, which is also known to degrade MBP.[80] Fibrinolytic activity referable to this enzyme has been demonstrated in MS tissue.[199] Further evidence that proteinases are important in demyelination is found in the observation that proteinase inhibitors suppress the development of EAE.[72]

Demyelination by macrophages is nonspecific with respect to the target, because any tissue containing the substrates for their enzymes will be digested, and in fact, proteolytic enzymatic digestion can lead to tissue necrosis,[497] a possible explanation for necrotic lesions and axonal loss in MS. The concept of nonspecific demyelination[519] has been termed "bystander demyelination." Although enzymatic digestion by macrophages is a nonspecific phenomenon, their activation in the lesion may have an immunologically specific basis, if stimulated by cytokines produced by helper-inducer T cells sensitized to an antigen in myelin.

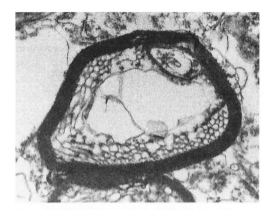

Figure 8–24. Electron micrograph of "vesicular demyelination." Note the circular vesicle-like profiles in the myelin sheath. The changes within the axon are post-mortem artifacts. (From Dr. J.W. Prineas, Veterans Administration Medical Center, East Orange, New Jersey; and University of Medicine and Dentistry of New Jersey–New Jersey Medical School, Newark, New Jersey.)

Ultrastructural Studies

The concept of enzymatic digestion of myelin in MS finds support in the fact that "myelin buds," similar to those described at the edge of active MS lesions[252,434] have been produced experimentally by proteolysis of myelin by trypsin.[177] Ultrastructurally, these abnormalities have been termed "skeins of myelin"[252] or "vesicular demyelination"[100,223,224](Fig. 8–24), and have been mentioned or illustrated in a few other cases,[28,105] all of which had a rather rapid clinical course. Some electron microscopists contend that this vesicular myelin change is a postmortem artifact and point out that it has not been observed in optimally fixed MS tissue.[363] It has, however, been observed in instantaneously fixed animal tissue, where it was usually associated with macrophages; enzymatic digestion was a speculated mechanism.[100] Other ultrastructural changes early in the demyelinating process in MS include an increase in the width of spacing between myelin lamellae,[20,161,355] fragmentation, and formation of electron-dense debris[20,252,468] while the myelin still encompasses the axon. These observations, together with the finding of unbound extracellular myelin fragments[243] in active MS lesions, are also suggestive evidence of lysis of myelin mediated by enzymes or possibly cytokines. How much extracellular enzymatic digestion of myelin

by macrophages or other cells that contain lysosomes (for example, astrocytes) contributes to the overall picture is unclear, but it has become increasingly apparent from electron microscopic studies that the macrophage is also actively involved in removing myelin fragments (see discussion following).

Indeed, the ultrastructural study of acute plaques, early lesions, and the borders of established chronic active plaques has resulted in major contributions to our understanding of the pathogenesis of MS. Early electron microscopic studies of MS were performed in the 1960s.[135,334] Many of the ultrastructural studies that followed were concerned with the search for the ever-elusive virus thought to be responsible for MS. In 1972, paramyxovirus-like particles were reported in demyelinating lesions of a case of MS.[352] Subsequent workers* described similar or other inclusions in MS tissues, and this finding generated a fair amount of excitement and controversy at the time. Many of these inclusions turned out to be normal structures, nonspecific structures, or artifacts, and the ultrastructural demonstration of virus was never established.

---

*References 27, 40, 103, 112, 134, 197, 224, 225, 234, 246, 283, 284, 308, 309, 310, 332, 382, 386, 387, 403, 407, 474, 475, 477, 502, 508.

"Polelike bodies," which are probably in macrophages, have also been described.[410] Their linear structure is unusual, and they appear to originate from the endophasic reticulum. Their significance is unknown.

In the early ultrastructural studies, the appearance of the paramyxovirus-like particles was quite convincing, but these subsequently were found in several other conditions.[387] This list has since expanded to include many inflammatory and noninflammatory disorders.[353] The abnormal material may be altered nucleoprotein related to treatment with corticosteroids or cytotoxic agents.[78,353] Thus, despite numerous studies, a virus has not been convincingly demonstrated by the electron microscope. This fact, of course, does not preclude incorporation of a portion of the viral genome into that of the patient with MS, nor does it rule out the possibility of a previous viral infection that has long been cleared by the immune system but that has resulted in an ongoing immune response to an epitope of viral antigen which cross-reacts with a component of human CNS myelin.[144] Aside from ultrastructural studies attempting to demonstrate virus in MS tissue, numerous other technologies have been employed to investigate the possible role of viruses in MS; the virology of the disease is discussed in detail in Chapter 10.

Although in the long-run electron microscopy did not demonstrate virus, it has made important contributions to our understanding of the mechanisms of myelin loss in MS. For some time, considerable controversy has focused on whether the myelin sheath or the cell which maintains it, the oligodendrocyte, is the primary target in MS. However, a seminal electron microscopic study by Raine and colleagues[389] demonstrated surviving and increased numbers of oligodendrocytes at the edge and within a chronic active lesion. Oligodendrocyte survival has also been reported in chronic relapsing EAE.[293] These findings are consistent with the myelin sheath being the target, and with subsequent oligodendrocyte death being secondary to myelin damage and loss. Some studies[76,330a] have reported oligodendrocyte survival in early lesions of some patients with MS but also pointed out that in others, there is oligodendroglial loss and suggested the pathogenesis of the disease may differ from patient to patient. Some published electron micrographs showing degenerating oligodendrocytes in close contact with macrophages or lymphocytes[355] suggest that direct attack on oligodendrocytes may occur. Moreover, some immunocytochemical analyses and radioimmunoassay of MAG have shown loss of this protein extends beyond the loss of MBP in the plaque,[212,217] which is consistent with an early loss of MAG in the pathogenesis of the lesion. Because MAG is located in the periaxonal and paranodal regions of the adult oligodendrocytic process, these data have been cited as evidence of early oligodendroglial death. This finding is further supported by the ultrastructural demonstration of degenerating distal oligodendrocytic processes before myelin loss both in MS[161,410,411] and in experimental demyelination produced by cuprizone, a substance toxic to oligodendrocytes.[249] On the other hand, other studies have shown equivalent areas of MBP and MAG involvement[366] and some lesions where MAG loss is excessive and others where it is not.[149] In addition, it is apparent that during demyelination a given myelin internode shows nonuniform partial myelin loss (suggesting an attack directed against the myelin sheath itself) rather than a complete loss of the entire internode (which would be anticipated if antecedent oligodendroglial death had occurred).[355] Ultrastructural studies of cells engaged in removal of myelin also favor a direct attack on the myelin sheath.

Early electron microscopic studies did not show cells involved in active myelin removal,[161,334,406,468] but showed features indicative of myelin breakdown and in some cases remyelination.[334, 468] Thus, as we have seen, because hydrolytic enzymes were readily demonstrated histochemically and biochemically in MS lesions and ultrastructural studies had shown astrocytes with large numbers of lysosomes in periplaque or normal-appearing white matter, it was thought that enzymatic digestion of myelin was important in demyelination and that the astrocyte might be the important cell in this function.[34,403,408] Some investigators[175] suggested that the proteolytic activity might be attributed to oligodendrocytes proliferating at the lesion edge. However, it soon

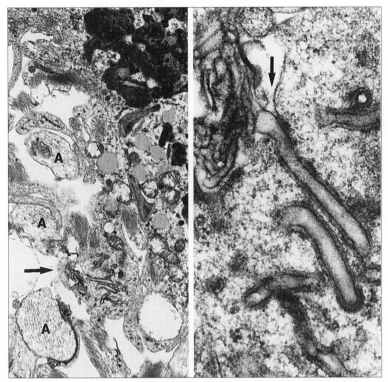

Figure 8–25. Electron micrograph of a macrophage in a chronic active MS plaque (left half of figure) near three axons (A), two of which have been demyelinated. The axon in the lower left is partially demyelinated and is in close proximity to wormlike configurations on the macrophage surface (arrow). This phenomenon has been termed "micropinocytosis vermiformis." On the right, this is shown at higher magnification. These structures represent infolding of the cell membrane of the macrophage. The membranous contents of these invaginations are continuous with extracellular membranous debris (arrow), the appearance of which is consistent with degenerating myelin. The ruffled appearance of the internal aspect of these structures is thought to represent clathrin. Left × 10,500; Right × 67,500. (From Prineas JW, and Connell F: The fine structure of chronically active multiple sclerosis plaques. Neurology 28(2):68–75, 1978, p 74, with permission.)

became clear that myelin breakdown occurred in association with contact of the myelin sheath by macrophages.[367,368]

The destruction of myelin by macrophages has been well demonstrated by immunocytochemistry, where macrophages were shown to phagocytose MBP-positive and MAG-positive fragments of myelin.[366] Further electron microscopic studies[363,389] have confirmed phagocytosis of myelin by macrophages. Moreover, in acute and early MS lesions, macrophages have been shown to penetrate into the myelin sheath.[236,367] The initial events in the attack on myelin are uncertain. Thus, it is possible the macrophage first directly attaches itself to the myelin sheath and then extirpates a fragment of myelin. Alternatively, enzyme- or cytokine-mediated lysis of myelin may be necessary to produce a free floating or partially damaged fragment of myelin, which is then engulfed by the macrophage. As discussed previously, ultrastructural evidence suggests that at least the second scenario may occur. In any event, careful examination of the surfaces of macrophages engaged in myelin removal reveals highly specialized membrane structures where the cell membrane attaches itself to the myelin fragment being phagocytosed. These structures and the associated myelin fragments which are bound at the extracellular face of the intraperiod line, have wormlike appearances. These have been termed *micropinocytosis vermiformis* (Fig. 8–25) and were described in MS by Prineas and Connell.[36] This method of phagocytosis is a variant of receptor-mediated phagocytosis, which employs clathrin-coated pits. The structures of micropinocytosis vermiformis are regarded as elongated clathrin-coated pits. Clathrin-coated pits have been demonstrated in EAE[125] but are not specific for autoimmune demyelination (Fig. 8–26).[374] Each comprises an invagination of the cell membrane, within which resides the material phagocytosed (in this case, myelin) separated from the cell membrane by a finely granular electron-dense substance (Fig. 8–26). This substance is thought to be the ligand that binds the material to receptors clustered in the clathrin-coated pit membrane at the time of formation of the ligand-receptor complex.[517] Clathrin is a latticelike network of electron-dense material on the cytoplasmic aspect of the cell membrane of the coated pit. It has

an intimate relationship with the filamentous cytoskeleton of the macrophage. Once bound to the clathrin-coated pit, material may be readily phagocytosed. Thus, the existence of clathrin-coated pits on phagocytic cells in MS implies that there is a receptor for myelin on these cells, and that there must be a ligand that binds the myelin to its receptor. The identification of this ligand-receptor complex may be of importance in understanding the mechanism of myelin removal in MS.

It has been postulated that IgG serves as the ligand responsible for receptor-mediated phagocytosis of myelin in MS.[362] Indeed, macrophages engaged in demyelina-

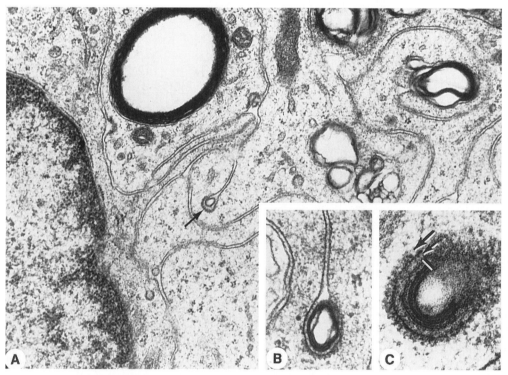

Figure 8–26. (*A*) Electron micrograph of an actively demyelinating lesion in a guinea pig with acute allergic encephalomyelitis. The arrow points to a clathrin-coated pit within a crypt formed by highly complex infoldings of the macrophage surface. The circular membranous material within the coated pit is myelin. ×23,000. (*B*) Higher magnification of a clathrin-coated pit with myelin. The coated pit is at the termination of a crypt formed by two opposing macrophage cell membranes. ×47,500. (*C*) A clathrin-coated pit showing the components of this structure. The black and white bar straddles the myelin lamellae within the coated pit. The major dense and intraperiod lines are still visible in this myelin "droplet," which is about to be phagocytosed. The small arrow points to the electron-dense material between the myelin and the macrophage membrane. This material represents the ligand responsible for binding the tissue being phagocytosed to receptors, which cluster at the underlying macrophage membrane. The large arrow indicates the lattice-like appearance of the clathrin on the internal aspect of the cell membrane. ×118,500. (Adapted from Moore GRW, and Raine CS: Immunogold localization and analysis of IgG during immune-mediated demyelination. Laboratory Investigation 59(5):641–648, 1988, p 642, copyright by the United States and Canadian Academy of Pathology, Inc., with permission.)

tion show capping of surface IgG, and it has been suggested that this is a result of clustering of IgG-Fc-receptor complexes into clathrin-coated pits on the macrophage surface.[362] In this manner, IgG would be bound nonspecifically by the Fc portion to the membrane Fc receptor, which receptor is known to exist on macrophages in MS lesions.[320,492c] The binding of the Fab portion of the IgG molecule to the myelin fragment would be specific via the antigen-binding site that would recognize the putative antigen of myelin. Evidence indicates that antibodies directed against myelin lipids may be responsible for demyelination in EAE,[292,391] in CNS cultures[383] and in the optic nerve in vivo.[440] IgG, however, could also bind nonspecifically to MBP in the myelin sheath.[350] As discussed previously, IgG is readily demonstrable in MS lesions, and its oligoclonality is consistent with its being directed against a specific antigen. An immu-

noelectron microscopic study[291] of acute EAE has shown IgG within clathrin-coated pits of macrophages engaged in demyelination. However, this was not a frequent finding, and it was suggested that the macrophage might also use a mechanism of progressive engulfing of IgG-coated myelin by means of Fc receptors in a zipperlike manner.[291] One possibility is that the receptor-mediated phagocytosis of myelin might be the morphologic equivalent of antigen processing by macrophages expressing MHC class II antigen in the MS lesion.[388] To date, no ultrastructural immunocytochemical studies in MS have been carried out to delineate the nature of the ligand binding myelin to the macrophage surface.

The astrocyte has also been shown to engage in receptor-mediated phagocytosis of myelin,[243] but this function appears mainly delegated to the macrophage. Given the preponderance of data favoring a CD4

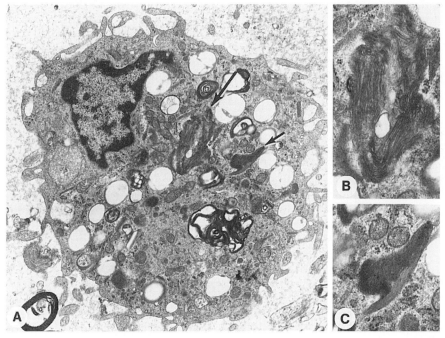

Figure 8–27. (*A*) Electron micrograph of a macrophage in an acute MS lesion. Note the myelin debris in various stages of degradation. The final product is neutral lipid, which is seen in the figure as clear vacuoles from which the lipid has been removed during processing for electron microscopy. Two of the lysosomes containing myelin debris are shown at a higher magnification in B (large arrow) and C (small arrow). ×7,200. (*B*) Note that the myelin within the tertiary lysosome has been altered and consists of thick, electron-dense lines flanked by lines of lesser density. ×20,000. (*C*) This lysosome shows myelin which has undergone even further degradation. Periodicity is hardly evident, and in the lower portion it is comprised of a granular material with reduced electron density. ×20,000.

helper-inducer T lymphocyte predominating in the chronic active plaque,[203,378,457,490] it would seem likely that macrophages are stimulated at the site by lymphokines released by activated lymphocytes. (However, some[322] have argued that because the macrophages demonstrate Fc receptor, but not complement C3b or C3d receptors, they are not T cell-activated.) It is indeed an intriguing thought that the Fc receptor may be the means by which the macrophage removes myelin. The evidence is circumstantial, and more confirmatory evidence awaits further studies.

Once internalized, the myelin undergoes degradation within the lysosomes of the macrophage (Fig. 8–27).[235] The myelin fragments separate into individual layers consisting of a central electron-dense line and lines of lesser density.[235] Further changes consist of transformation into broad bands and finely granular lines, which have been described as laminar[235] or tubular.[31] Some ultrastructural evidence suggests that initial myelin digestion takes place in macrophages in the lesion parenchyma, whereas the process is completed in macrophages in the Virchow-Robin spaces about blood vessels.[355,369] Esterification of cholesterol is a major process occurring in macrophages in MS lesions—a phenomenon well established by chemical studies discussed previously. In addition to myelin degradation, another source of esterified cholesterol is native and oxidized low density lipoproteins phagocytosed by the macrophage.[317a] Eventually, macrophages are stuffed with neutral lipid. These lipid filled macrophages have been variously termed *compound granular corpuscles*, *foamy macrophages*, *lipid-laden macrophages*, and *gitterzellen*. As we have seen, macrophages abound in the central portion of chronic active plaques (see Fig. 8–13) and are present in small numbers in well-established chronic inactive plaques (see Fig. 8–18). In the latter case, most have presumably exited to the systemic circulation.

REMYELINATION IN MULTIPLE SCLEROSIS

Evidence for CNS remyelination was reported in early ultrastructural studies in MS.[334,468] Remyelination by Schwann cells also occurs in MS, and the reader is referred to the section on the chronic active plaque for a discussion of this phenomenon. Remyelination is characterized by disproportionally thin myelin sheaths forming short internodes (see Figs. 8–16 and 8–28).[79,180,248,361,363] Other features that may be seen in remyelination include premature termination of major dense lines into oligodendroglial cytoplasmic loops on the external or internal aspects of the myelin sheath at various points along the internode (Fig. 8–29),[28,373] uncompacted oligodendroglial cytoplasm around the axon (Fig. 8–30),[373,468] and myelination of cell bodies, usually of oligodendrocytes (Fig. 8–31).[28,468] Gradual tapering of the myelin sheath as it approaches the nodes of Ranvier has also been interpreted as evidence of remyelination, but this may also be related to partial demyelination. However, the oligodendroglial cytoplasmic loops associated with premature tapering of the myelin sheath have been shown to form junctional complexes between one another.[361] Periodic densities, similar to transverse bars at the normal paranode, have also been seen between these oligodendroglial loops and nearby demyelinated axons.[361] These features suggest that tapering myelin sheaths comprise remyelinated myelin, whereby the oligodendrocyte attempts to form new paranodal structures.

As noted previously, remyelination is seen at the edge of chronic active MS plaques[361,389] but may be quite prolific and widespread in acute lesions[236,355] and lesions of subacute duration.[330a,363] However, it is now recognized that these remyelinated internodes also undergo demyelination (Fig. 8–32).[359,363] Remyelination that survives the demyelinating process would account for the "shadow plaques," which may be seen in chronic silent lesions. Thus, the rim of pale-staining myelin at the edge of some of these shadow plaques (see Fig. 8–22) represents remyelination in a previous chronic active plaque, whereas more diffusely remyelinated lesions may represent previously active lesions in which the demyelination process was aborted, allowing the remyelination to persist throughout the lesion.[358,376] The reasons for remyelination

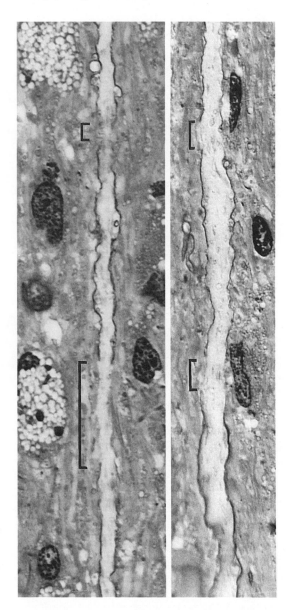

Figure 8–28. Remyelination is seen as short internodes of thin myelin separated by areas of bare axon (bars) which may represent regenerating nodes of Ranvier. ×1460. (From Prineas JW, Kwon EE, Cho E-S, and Sharer LR. Continual breakdown and regeneration of myelin in progressive multiple sclerosis plaques. Annals of the New York Academy of Sciences, 436:11–32, 1984, p 15, with permission.)

persisting in some lesions but not in others are unknown.[357]

Remyelination is thought to be carried out by surviving[330a] or proliferating[357] oligodendrocytes within the MS lesion. A recent abstract reporting on markers associated with the apoptosis (programmed cell death) suggested that oligodendrocyte survival in MS may be related to their expression of Bcl-2,[61a] an inhibitor of apoptosis.[531a] As discussed previously, oligodendroglia have been reported in increased numbers in acute plaques,[236,365] lesions of subacute duration,[363] and chronic active MS lesions.[389]

Other workers have found that oligodendrocytes are not present in increased numbers, but in significant, although somewhat reduced, numbers in the early stages of the plaque.[330a] Nevertheless, most investigators would agree that significant or complete oligodendrocyte loss is a feature of more advanced disease.

When increased numbers of oligodendrocytes have been noted, it is thought that their increased presence is due to their proliferation, and immunocytochemical studies of cell proliferation support[299] or do not support[393a] this conclusion. Oligodendrocytes

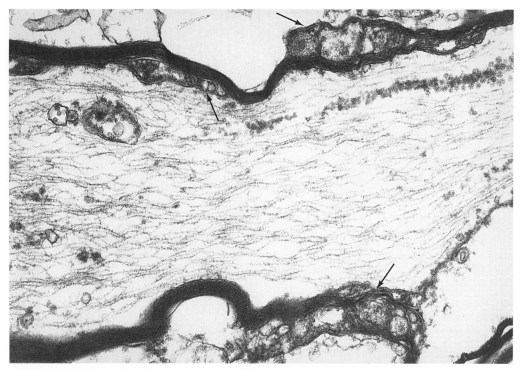

Figure 8–29. Electron micrograph showing a longitudinally sectioned, remyelinated axon in a band of myelin from a lesion of Baló's concentric sclerosis. Note the thin myelin sheath and the loops of oligodendroglial cytoplasm (arrows) formed at premature terminations of myelin lamellae. ×12,300. (From Moore GRW, Neumann PE, Suzuki K, Lijtmaer HN, Traugott U, and Raine CS. Balo's concentric sclerosis: new observations on lesion development. Annals of Neurology, 17:604–611, 1985, p 608, with permission.)

may have undergone cell division before the time of sampling in the study where they were negative for a cell proliferation marker.[393a] It has been postulated that oligodendroglial proliferation occurs in oligodendrocytes that have survived.[236,389] It has also been suggested that newly generated oligodendrocytes are responsible for the proliferation and that this is in response to massive oligodendrocyte death[355] (which, as discussed previously, could result from the myelin loss or a primary attack on the oligodendrocyte itself). Studies of lesions of varying duration[355,358,365] have suggested that acute lesions can be considered to evolve through several phases in the early development of the MS plaque—namely, demyelination with massive oligodendrocyte death, followed by proliferation of immature oligodendrocytes, which, in turn, then execute the remyelination. It has been shown that during the phase of oligodendroglial hyperplasia in acute lesions, oligodendrocytes may be found within the cell bodies of astrocytes.[364] This finding was interpreted as astrocytic phagocytosis of the oligodendrocyte and a possible mechanism responsible for the failure of extensive remyelination evident in older, more established lesions.[364] However, work in other laboratories would indicate that this finding may simply be protective sequestration of the oligodendrocyte by the astrocyte,[528] possibly mediated by hsp60,[393a] or, alternatively, by emperipolesis (active penetration of one cell by another).[156] The phenomenon is not specific for MS, and has also been reported in a biopsy of an acute demyelinating disease of uncertain nature in a 15-year-old boy[159] and has been described in a variety of other disease processes that appear to have inflammation as a common feature.[528] It has also been described in chronic, as well as acute, MS plaques, although it is more frequent in the latter.[528] Thus, its relationship to the early events

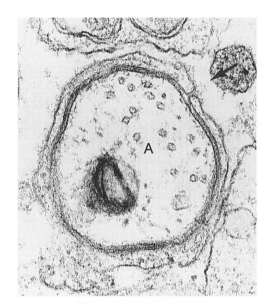

Figure 8–30. Electron micrograph of a chronic MS plaque showing an oligodendrocyte process encompassing an axon (*A*) during very early remyelination. The arrow points toward the future mesaxon. ×67,000. (From Suzuki K, Andrews JM, Waltz JM, and Terry RD: Ultrastructural studies of multiple sclerosis. Laboratory Investigation 20(5):444–454, 1969, p 452, copyright by the United States and Canadian Academy of Pathology, Inc., with permission.)

in MS lesion formation has been questioned.[528]

In many ways, the immature oligodendrocyte in the acute MS lesion resembles the oligodendrocyte seen during development of the CNS. Immunocytochemical studies have shown that such cells stain very intensely for HNK-1, CNP,[365] and MAG[244] before axonal ensheathment and remyelination. However, in contrast to the developing oligodendrocyte, cytoplasmic MBP is not evident. The latter may simply relate to technical difficulties or may be due to differences in these two cells[365]; MBP and MAG are seen in oligodendroglial cytoplasm during experimental remyelination.[250] As remyelination commences in MS, cytoplasmic HNK-1 and CNP are reduced.[365] The upregulation of HNK-1 in oligodendrocytes before ensheathment in these lesions provides further evidence that this molecule may be important in cell adhesion.

It is unknown whether the increased numbers of oligodendrocytes in MS derive from differentiated oligodendrocytes that

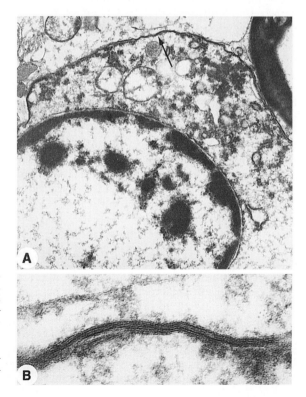

Figure 8–31. (*A*) Electron micrograph of an oligodendrocyte within a band of remyelination in a lesion of Baló's concentric sclerosis. The cell is encompassed by a few lamellae of myelin (arrow). ×13,000. (*B*) Higher magnification of the aberrant myelin. ×57,000. (From Moore GRW, Neumann PE, Suzuki K, Lijtmaer HN, Traugott U, and Raine CS: Balo's concentric sclerosis: new observations on lesion development. Annals of Neurology 17:604–611, 1985, p 609, with permission.)

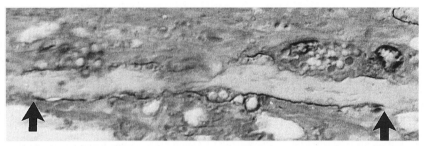

Figure 8–32. The myelin sheath of the internode between the arrows is both thin and short. It thus fulfills the criteria for a remyelinated internode. A macrophage containing myelin and lipid debris is seen contacting the myelin sheath (center right). Toluidine blue. ×1450. (From Prineas JW, Kwon EE, Cho E-S, and Sharer LR: Continual breakdown and regeneration of myelin in progressive multiple sclerosis plaques. Annals of the New York Academy of Sciences 436:11–32, 1984, p 21, with permission.)

acquire the immature characteristics described previously or whether they arise from oligodendroglial precursors that evolve into these immature oligodendrocytes. It is also not evident at what stage of differentiation cell division could occur in the MS lesion. An early study of experimental remyelination[79] demonstrated cells with the ultrastructural features of oligodendrocytes and others resembling astrocytes in remyelinating lesions. It has since been shown that cultured glial cell precursors can differentiate into oligodendrocytes or astrocytes depending on the composition of their growth media.[133,371] In remyelinated chronic EAE lesions, oligodendrocytes in unusual perivascular locations near astrocytes suggest that they may have originated from a common progenitor cell.[385] Experimental models of demyelination and remyelination show dividing oligodendrocytes in remyelinating lesions, but again, their origin is not entirely clear.[58,247,248] If they originate from the parenchyma around the demyelinated lesion, they must have migrational abilities to reach the site of remyelination,[248] and some experimental evidence suggests that this might be the case.[32,169] Thus, while we assume that the increased numbers of oligodendrocytes in the MS lesion are related to proliferation, migration may be an additional or alternative explanation.

The molecular stimulus that may be responsible for oligodendroglial hyperplasia is unknown. One possibility is a cytokine produced by inflammatory cells within the MS lesion. For example, some workers[52] have shown that IL-2 can stimulate proliferation of oligodendrocytes, but others[420,534] have found an inhibitory or no effect. Another possibility is that the oligodendrocyte is responding to myelin breakdown products. Extracts from neonatal and adult rat brain are mitogenic for oligodendrocytes in vitro.[421] The exact component responsible for this has not yet been determined. To date, axons have been shown to induce oligodendroglial proliferation,[524] but myelin-enriched fractions[86] and MBP[289] do not. A further group of mitogens to be considered are growth factors.[110,370] These include platelet-derived growth factor,[166,318] fibroblast growth factor,[110] and insulin-like growth factor,[303] which have been reported to cause proliferation of oligodendroglial precursors.

A remarkable degree of oligodendroglial hyperplasia and remyelination, accompanied by clinical improvement, has been demonstrated in the strain 13 guinea pig model of chronic relapsing EAE after treatment with a MBP-GC mixture made up in incomplete Freund's adjuvant.[390] Evidence suggests that IgG raised against spinal cord components plays a role in the induction of similar findings in the murine Theiler's virus model.[409] Immune suppression also allows remyelination to occur.[409a] Clearly, further research into the nature of the factor or factors responsible for oligodendroglial hyperplasia and remyelination would have significant implications for future therapeutic approaches to MS.

CLINICOPATHOLOGICAL CORRELATIONS IN MULTIPLE SCLEROSIS

The Accuracy of the Clinical Diagnosis

An extensive study in Denmark[122] has determined that the diagnosis of MS was confirmed by postmortem examination in 94 percent of cases diagnosed as clinically definite MS, and in 66 percent of cases diagnosed as clinically probable MS. Misdiagnoses encompass a wide variety of conditions that can simulate the acute, relapsing-remitting, and chronic progressive forms of MS, including spinocerebellar degenerations, olivopontocerebellar degeneration, encephalititides, subacute combined degeneration, syringomyelia and syringobulbia, vascular malformations, tumors, cerebral infarction, cerebral hemorrhage, lymphogranulomatosis, Alzheimer's disease,[122] neuroenteric cysts,[495] and collagen vascular disorders.[442] In this era of neuroimaging with CT and MRI, many of these conditions will be more readily diagnosable.

However, several cases are on record where the CT scan* or MRI[129,218,220,312,537] appearance of an active demyelinating lesion with edema simulated that of a cerebral tumor. Moreover, because of the presence of numerous astrocytes, biopsies of such lesions may initially suggest a diagnosis of an astrocytic tumor.[206] The reverse, a clinical diagnosis of MS in patients with diffuse astrocytomas, has also been reported.[417] In a small number of cases, the coexistence of MS and gliomas has been documented.[97,256b,494a]

The Relationship between Lesion Location and Clinical Manifestations

Generally one may find a lesion or lesions in the CNS to explain a specific symptom or sign in a given case of MS. The involvement of the medial longitudinal fasiculus in internuclear ophthalmoplegia, a lesion in the trigeminal root entry zone or nucleus in trigeminal neuralgia,[216,240] interruption of the lateral corticospinal tract in spastic paresis, demyelination of the posterior column in proprioceptive sensory loss, lesions within the dentatothalamic pathways and red nucleus responsible for intention myoclonus,[184,401] and the perivenous inflammatory infiltrate producing retinal venous sheathing[33,441] are but a few examples. The last example poses a problem for those of us who consider MS to be an immunologic disease directed against myelin, because there is usually no myelin in the human retina.[444] Moreover, the retinal perivascular inflammatory cuffs are not necessarily continuous with those in the optic nerve and may occur independently of optic neuritis.[33]

It has been long recognized that the peripheral nervous system (PNS) is occasionally involved in MS.[221,342] Rare cases have signs and symptoms of demyelinating polyneuritis superimposed on the CNS features.[140,238] In some instances, the clinical presentation is entirely referrable to the PNS, and the CNS lesions are subclinical.[54,277] The coexistence of these two conditions has been documented pathologically.[54,238] Other MS cases have been associated with a peripheral neuropathy attributable to cachexia.[185] A demyelinating neuropathy can be demonstrated in some cases of less debilitating MS, where the peripheral demyelination appears to be subclinical and unrelated to nutritional status.[344] Concomitant hypertrophic neuropathy has also been described,[430] implying that there are repetitive episodes of demyelination and attempts at remyelination in the PNS of such cases. The occurrence of demyelination in the PNS and CNS of the same patient raises the possibility that this may not be simply a coincidence and that these phenomena may share a common etiology and pathogenesis. A spectrum of demyelinating diseases may be present in the nervous system with pure CNS involvement and pure PNS involvement at either extreme and unusual combinations in between.[277,347]

---

*References 1, 206, 220, 259, 311, 312, 330, 405, 418, 493, 496, 501, 535, 537.

Where wallerian degeneration has been found in peripheral nerves in MS, it has been thought to be secondary to involvement of more proximal portions of the fibers in spinal cord plaques.[262] Its occurrence indicates axonal destruction within these lesions.

What is surprising in the clinicopathological correlation of the CNS lesions of MS is that the number of lesions demonstrated postmortem frequently greatly exceeds the number predicted clinically.[307] Moreover, the literature provides examples of benign MS where the patient had remote neurological symptoms but no or minimal symptoms just before death,[137,158,256,498] and of asymptomatic MS where there were no previous neurological symptoms,* but MS lesions were evident postmortem. Many of these cases have predominantly periventricular demyelinative plaques and spare more clinically evident areas, such as the long descending tracts.[123] Thus, the subclinical nature of many of these cases may be simply due to the fact that they reside in a clinically silent area. However, as discussed later, clinical, pathological, and electrophysiological evidence suggests that even demyelination of areas critical for normal CNS function may not necessarily result in lasting clinical manifestations.

The Relationship between Pathology, Physiology, and Clinical Manifestations

Each of the histological features of the MS plaque may contribute to the clinical expression of the lesion. The precise mechanisms, however, are unknown; this is particularly true of some remissions characterized by a complete and rapid reversal of profound neurological deficits. Extrapolation from clinical and pathological observations and from clinical and experimental physiological studies allows for some insight into the complex interactions of these processes. The actively demyelinating lesion is a highly dynamic process, and the clinical manifestation of a given lesion is

related not only to its location but to the interaction of many electrophysiological, immunologic, and morphologic factors operating at that time.

For a detailed discussion of the physiology of MS, the reader is referred to the excellent reviews by Waxman[503–505] and by McDonald and colleagues.[173,265,268,269] In this section, the concepts advanced by these and other investigators are correlated with the pathology of the MS plaque. Many of these concepts have been based on experimental studies.

As previously discussed, the major histological features of the actively demyelinating MS lesion are demyelination, inflammation, and gliosis. Each of these is discussed in relation to the neurophysiology and clinical manifestations of MS.

THE ROLE OF DEMYELINATION AND REMYELINATION

The most obvious morphologic feature of the MS lesion is loss of myelin sheaths, and it would seem that this should account for most or all of the clinical manifestations of MS. This, however, is not the case. From the physiologist's point of view, demyelination produces many perturbations of conduction of the axon potential, including slow conduction, temporal dispersion of the compound action potential (due to varying degrees of slowing in different fibers), complete block of conduction, and a relative block of conduction (where only high-frequency trains are not conducted).[270,503,505] Of these, complete conduction block is usually associated with clinical manifestations,[173,265,394,503,505] particularly those of the motor and sensory systems. Even paranodal demyelination is sufficient to produce conduction block.[233]

Some neural systems, where timing is important in processing information, may fail owing to the slowing of conduction.[265,503] Others, such as vibration sense, depend more on transmission of high-frequency trains[173] and disruption of the the latter may explain, in part, the loss of vibration sense early in MS.[173] Thus, whether an MS lesion will manifest itself clinically depends on the function and electrophysiological modus operandi of the system in which it resides, and whether it has induced

*References 35, 123, 150, 160, 256, 296, 343.

complete or partial conduction block or merely slowing of conduction.

Clinical manifestations of MS can fluctuate both in degree and quality over a matter of hours. This variability is thought to be related to the exquisite sensitivity of the demyelinated axon to exogenous metabolic and physical factors. In addition to the well-known temperature effect (Uhthoff's phenomenon), changes in the metabolic milieu produced by hyperventilation, oral intake of phosphate, or intravenous bicarbonate have been shown to affect the clinical expression of an MS lesion.[48,101]

Aside from the negative symptoms of MS, many patients also experience paroxysmal positive symptoms, both sensory and motor. These positive symptoms are thought to have their basis in the generation of ectopic and reflected impulses in demyelinated axons or in cross-talk *(ephaptic transmission)* between adjacent demyelinated axons.[395,396,503] Lhermitte's symptom is thought to be due to the increased mechano-sensitivity of demyelinated cervical cord axons, which are deformed during neck flexion.[452,503] A similar effect on the optic nerve is believed to be responsible for phosphenes induced by eye movement in cases with optic neuritis.[102,268]

Not surprisingly, such symptoms and signs could result from demyelinated plaques. What is surprising, as mentioned previously, is that many plaques appear to be asymptomatic. Although many of these may be located in clinically silent areas,[498] some show demyelination in pathways critical for normal neurological function.[35,158] Other evidence that conduction of action potentials occurs in many of these demyelinated lesions comes from studies of visual evoked potentials, which have shown that slowing of the potential (indicating demyelination is present) does not necessarily have a clinical effect.[173,174,505] Moreover, pathologically verified extensively demyelinated optic nerves can have some preserved visual function.[520] Although restoration of conduction in MS lesions is the most likely explanation for these findings, alternative proposals have included utilization of preserved redundant pathways, resolution of edema within the lesion, synapse sprouting, presence of normally unmyelinated axons in the CNS, and adaptive synaptic changes.[268,505]

That continuous conduction of the axon potential can occur along demyelinated axons has been shown experimentally in the PNS, and this finding can occur as early as 4 to 6 days after the demyelinating event.[66] The demonstration of continuous conduction implies that there must be a redistribution or reinsertion of sodium channels (which were formerly only located at the nodes of Ranvier[507]) to the demyelinated internodal axolemma.[504] Morphologic evidence for this is the demonstration of sodium channels throughout regions of demyelinated axolemma in experimental models of peripheral nerve demyelination. This observation has been shown both with the ferric ion-ferrocyanide technique[141] and by monoclonal antibodies to the sodium channel.[276] This finding has also been demonstrated in experimentally demyelinated CNS axons.[57] In this instance, it was noted that sodium channels were detected in axolemma ensheathed by uncompacted processes of oligodendrocytes or Schwann cells but not in segments of axons that were not associated with glia.[57] It is unknown whether these sodium channels located in former internodal axolemma are redistributed from the nodes of Ranvier or whether they are newly synthesized channels inserted into the membrane,[504] but experimental evidence tends to favor the latter possibility.[57] Using tritiated saxitoxin as a ligand for sodium channels, sodium channels have been shown to be in high concentration in MS plaques at the light microscopic level.[285,286] Because normal white matter does not show saxitoxin binding by this technique,[302] the finding is certainly consistent with redistribution of the sodium channel, but whether this redistribution is continuous along the demyelinated axolemma must await electron microscopic studies using similar technologies.

In addition to continuous propagation of the action potential, discontinuous (i.e., saltatory) conduction has also been demonstrated in experimentally demyelinated fibers in the PNS,[451] and these studies have been extrapolated to the CNS. The focal regions of inwardly directed current, termed *phi nodes,* are seen as early as 4 days, have a short internodal distance, and are thought to be due to collections of sodium channels in new nodes of Ranvier. These *phi nodes* show nodal properties in electron microscopy and freeze-fracture studies of the CNS.[59,412] Interestingly, these are seen before formation of the remyelinated myelin sheath.[451] When the myelin sheath is regenerated, dense collections of sodium channels remain at the new nodes of Ranvier.[509]

Because recovery from neurological deficits in MS can occur very quickly—within 48 hours in some cases of optic neuritis—it is probable that remyelination does not play a role in such a rapid remission.[266] Such rapid recovery may be related to clearing of edema[266] or reduction of inflammatory cells within the lesion (see discussion following). However, as pointed out previously, remyelination is frequent in acute and early plaques.[236,355,363,392] In EAE remyelination may begin as early as 6 days after plaque formation, and by two weeks, many axons have thin myelin sheaths.[236] Axons with thin myelin sheaths as well as those with remyelinated myelin sheaths with short internodes can conduct action potentials.[226,450]

The role of remyelination in restoration of function during a clinical remission in MS is unclear at this time, but it probably has a much more important role than we had previously considered. Even the small rim of remyelination confined to the border of the chronic active MS plaque or shadow plaque may have clinical significance. In this regard, it is important to point out that even though continuous conduction may occur along demyelinated axons, in some instances, the action potential cannot enter the demyelinated segment from the normally myelinated axon.[504] However, using computer simulation, it has been shown that the insertion of two short internodes in the transition zone between demyelination and the normally myelinated axon allows for the entry of the action potential into the demyelinated area.[506] Propagation of the action potential by continuous conduction then could proceed through the demyelinated lesion. In this manner, the few short internodes of remyelinated myelin seen at the borders of chronic MS plaques may serve an impor-

tant function in allowing conduction to occur in these chronic lesions.

Therefore, the physiology of the MS lesion and its clinical expression can be regarded as the dynamic interplay of the effects of demyelination on conduction, the subsequent redistribution of axolemmal membrane ionic channels, and the regeneration of the myelin sheath.

THE ROLE OF INFLAMMATION

The inflammatory infiltrate in MS lesions can be considerable, particularly in acute and chronic active plaques with active demyelination. The role of this lymphocytic-mononuclear infiltrate in the production of symptoms and signs in MS has received more attention than previously. It is highly probable that inflammation is responsible for an effect on the neurophysiology of the axon—demyelinated or otherwise. We know that products of the immune response can produce electrophysiological dysfunction, but to what extent and by what means this may come about in the MS lesion is unclear.

The MRI scanner has proved to be sensitive for the detection of MS lesions[227,333] and has shown that lesions can appear and disappear or fade in a random fashion in a given patient and frequently are subclinical.[518] The relationship between MRI images and the pathology of MS lesion is discussed in detail in Chapter 9. However, we shall briefly consider these short-lived lesions here. While static chronic demyelinated lesions may be detected by the MRI scanner,[317,467] the pathological basis for these evanescent lesions is unknown.

In EAE, it has been shown experimentally that MRI can detect changes in the blood-brain barrier even before clinical signs.[188,323] Breakdown of the blood-brain barrier, as noted previously, occurs in the MS lesion. Its radiologic correlates are lesions that enhance on delayed high-dose contrast CT scans[16,432] and gadolinium-enhanced MRI scans.[282] Possibly the transient MRI lesions represent extracellular water due to the disturbance of the blood-brain barrier.[317] Inflammatory infiltrates, as discussed previously, are probably in themselves responsible for the blood-brain barrier disturbance in MS. The disappearance or fading of the lesion could thus be attributed to clearing of the inflammation.[333] Their temporal profile of rapid increase over 4 weeks followed by a gradual decline over the next 4 to 8 weeks[518] would be consistent with the influx and clearing of inflammation and subsequent restoration of blood-brain barrier function.

On the other hand, in view of the recent knowledge concerning the degree and rapidity of remyelination occurring in some lesions,[236,355,363,392] the transience of these lesions could be related to their remyelination. In view of the frequent numbers of these MRI lesions, if the latter were the case, we should expect to see shadow plaques much more frequently than we do. The elucidation of the pathology of these transient MRI lesions remains a challenge but is of considerable importance because they probably provide the key to the determination of the initial event in the pathogenesis of the chronic MS lesion. Inflammation and associated blood-brain barrier disturbance would certainly be a primary possibility.

Evidence from experimental studies shows that inflammation alone may produce clinical signs. Guinea pigs with acute EAE, induced by relatively low doses of MBP, can show significant neurological deficits, but extensive examination of their CNS reveals perivascular inflammatory infiltrates and no parenchymal demyelination.[292,295,391] Thus, in this instance, inflammation alone is sufficient to cause clinical neurological dysfunction.

The concept that inflammatory infiltrates or their products might be responsible for some of the clinical phenomenology of MS received considerable impetus in the 1960s. It was shown that serum from patients with MS, as well as from animals with EAE, can produce alterations in evoked bioelectric responses in CNS tissue cultures.[65] These effects appeared to be on synapses and were complement dependent. Similar results have been found using isolated frog spinal cord[85] and have been shown to be due to the IgG fraction of serum.[423] Others[254] have suggested that while the effect is antisynaptic, the presence of myelin in the culture experiments was also necessary to produce an effect. It

has subsequently been shown that the bioelectric blocking effect can also be produced by normal human serum and is not MS specific.[433] This nonspecificity still does not detract from the inevitable conclusion that serum factors, probably IgG, can directly disturb normal neurophysiology. Therefore, the IgG in MS lesions could play a role in the clinical expression of this disorder.

Edema may also contribute to symptomatology.[267,268] It is possible that alterations in the ionic concentrations in the excessive extracellular water may disturb nerve conduction.[268] Edema might induce ischemia to nerve fibers by vascular compression, particularly in the optic nerve, which has little room for expansion in the optic canal and at its point of entry into the sclera.[267,268]

Interest has focused on the role of cytokines in the clinical manifestations of MS. As noted previously, immunocytochemical evidence indicates the presence of various cytokines in MS lesions, which is not surprising in view of the extensive inflammatory infiltrates. Neurophysiological effects have been demonstrated for TNF, interferon-gamma, and IL-1; intraocular inoculation of these cytokines produces slowing of the visual evoked response in rabbits.[73] This study demonstrated changes in the vasculature and suggested that the physiological disturbances were due to increased permeability of the blood-brain barrier, which would allow the entry of neuroelectrical blocking factors (such as those discussed previously).[73] It has been shown that cytokines from T lymphocytes of patients with MS damage myelin in CNS cultures.[436,439] In the case of TNF,[439] the ultrastructural appearance was reminiscent of internodal change induced by an agent known to effect ionic channels.[288] Electroencephalographic studies have demonstrated that IL-1 can enhance slow-wave activity during sleep[480]—a further example of a neurophysiological effect of a cytokine. Because products of the humoral immune response and cytokines are capable of producing electrophysiological abnormalities, it would seem reasonable to conclude that such effects probably occur in the MS lesion.

In addition to these electrophysiological disturbances, the inflammatory infiltrate is possibly responsible for other abnormalities in the lesion. For example, axonal loss in MS may well be related to the toxic effects of enzymes, cytokines and toxic free radicals produced by the lymphocyte and macrophage population in the plaque. Such products of the inflammatory infiltrate, cytotoxic T lymphocytes, or both might result in focal destruction of the axon and subsequent wallerian degeneration. Axonal loss is a reasonable explanation for some of the permanent neurological deficits in MS[269] (see discussion following).

THE ROLE OF GLIOSIS

Astrocytes are the cells responsible for the "scarring" of MS lesions. However, they appear to have many more functions than simply providing the scaffolding for old lesions in the CNS. In contrast to the passive role assigned to them in the past, a flourishing body of literature has demonstrated that astrocytes have ionic channels,[44,45,46] have receptors for various neurotransmitters,[204] and take up, release, and possibly synthesize some neurotransmitters.[44,194] They show calcium waves in response to certain neurotransmitters.[44,194] Induction of early response genes in astrocytes can also be mediated by neurotransmitters.[30] Astrocytes are thought to take up potassium ions that have accumulated in the extracellular space as a result of action potential activity in the axolemma.[44,46,114,167,172,192] They are also important in regulating the volume and pH of the extracellular space.[470] Many of these phenomena appear to be mediated by a syncytium of astrocytes connected by gap junctions.[106] All these findings are consistent with the emerging notion that in the CNS, there are numerous functional interactions between neurons and astrocytes and vice versa.[44,194] In the case of MS, this concept is reinforced by the presence of desmosome-like membrane specializations between adjacent astrocytes and between astrocytes and demyelinated axons.[372,461]

How astrocytes participating in gliosis in diseases of the CNS contribute to the physiology of these disorders is an area of research still in its infancy. However, such research may provide some exciting insights into some aspects of MS pathophysiology.

VARIANTS OF MULTIPLE SCLEROSIS

A number of variants of MS have historically been given special status, either because of the peculiar location of their lesions or because of their unusual morphologic appearances. These include Baló's concentric sclerosis, neuromyelitis optica (Devic's syndrome), cases of MS with extensive confluent demyelination in the cerebral hemispheres, and rare cases with demyelination confined to the subpial regions.

Baló's Concentric Sclerosis

In 1906, Marburg first described peculiar concentric rings of demyelination alternating with rings of myelin.[230,258] This phenomenon was subsequently noted by Barré and colleagues in 1926.[43,230] These lesions were eventually named after Baló, who described them in a case report in 1927[38] and 1928.[39] Since then, a number of case reports have been published on the subject, and these reports have been reviewed by Courville[90] and Kuroiwa.[230]

The classic lesion of Baló's concentric sclerosis consists of rings (or actually globes when three-dimensional space is considered) of myelin separated by rings of demyelination (Fig. 8–33). The lesion is usually centered on a blood vessel, and there is an age gradient of demyelinating rings from older to more recent from the center to the periphery. Other lesions can have a lamellar appearance or can take on the pattern of a rose or carnation.[90] The lesions of concentric sclerosis have been described in the cerebral hemispheres,[90] cerebellum,[90] pons,[163,414] medulla oblongata,[290] spinal cord,[14,213,290] and optic chiasm.[213,290]

A variety of explanations has been advanced for the patterns of the lesions in Baló's concentric sclerosis.[90,230] A study of a case employing electron microscopy

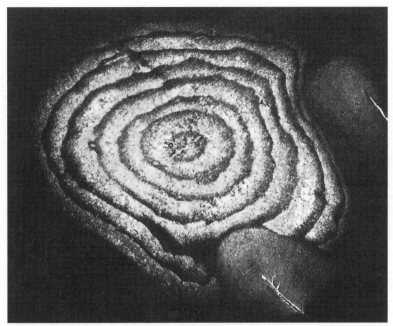

Figure 8–33. The classic appearance of a lesion of Baló's concentric sclerosis, as illustrated by Baló in his 1928 publication of "encephalitis periaxialis concentrica". Note that concentric bands of demyelination alternate with bands of myelin. Lesions can also assume a lamellar appearance or take on more complex, ornate patterns. (From Baló J: Encephalitis periaxialis concentrica. Archives of Neurology and Psychiatry. 19:242–264, 1928, p 247. Copyright 1928, American Medical Association, with permission.)

showed rings of myelin largely comprised of remyelinated axons (Figs. 8–29, 8–31, and 8–34).[290] Examination of the interface of the zone of remyelinated myelin with the ring of demyelination revealed removal of myelin by macrophages, astrogliosis, lymphocytes, and large numbers of oligodendrocytes, in a pattern similar to that seen at the edge of a chronic active MS plaque.

Observations in other cases have led to the conclusion that the bands of myelin represent early stages of demyelination rather than remyelination.[533] These seemingly divergent views may not necessarily be mutually exclusive, because, as we have seen before, discrepancies in the interpretation of MS pathology may be related to studying lesions of varying age.

The reason for the alternating pattern of rings remains an enigma. In view of the increased number of perivascular CD8 cells at the border of the chronic active MS lesion,[490] it might be hypothesized that immune suppression allows remyelination or incomplete demyelination to occur at borders of the plaque, while the next wave of demyelination breaks through the region of immune suppression to the adjacent white matter. The latter then becomes the next ring of demyelination, the border of which subsequently becomes populated with suppressor cells and the cycle repeats itself again. To date, however, there have been no immunocytochemical studies of T-cell subsets in these lesions. The mechanisms of demyelination seen in the band of demyelination are thought to be no different from those described in MS.[170,290]

In some cases, lesions similar to those seen in acute MS coexist but are separate from the larger concentric lesions.[290,426] There are also acute lesions with Baló-like rings at their periphery.[179] Based on these observations, it has been suggested that cases of Baló's concentric sclerosis may represent an intermediary or transitional form between acute MS and the classic remitting-relapsing form.[290] If this is so, in the case of most patients where Baló's lesions are discovered, death supervenes at that stage,[90] whereas in those that survive, the demyelinating process eventually consumes

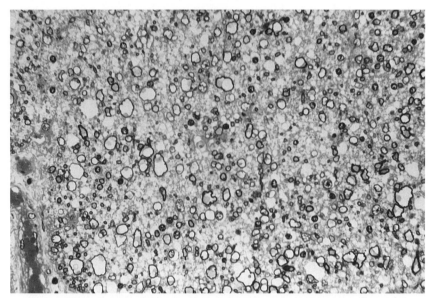

Figure 8–34. A band of myelin in a Baló's concentric sclerosis lesion shows that numerous axons have thin myelin sheaths. This finding, taken together with the ultrastructural findings illustrated in Figures 8–29 and 8–31, is indicative of remyelination. 1 μm epoxy section. Toluidine blue. ×300. (From Moore GRW, Neumann PE, Suzuki K, Lijtmaer HN, Traugott U, and Raine CS: Balo's concentric sclerosis: new observations on lesion development. Annals of Neurology 17:604–611, 1985, p 608, with permission.)

the rings of remyelination or partial demyelination, and the classic chronic active MS plaque is established.

Baló's concentric sclerosis is usually seen in patients with an acute monophasic neurological illness—that is, the clinical profile of acute MS. The patients are usually young and frequently initially exhibit a disorder of high cortical function or signs of increased intracranial pressure.[90,230] Focal neurological signs may supervene later.[230] The CSF may be hemorrhagic, and indeed the lesions themselves, in some instances, may show hemorrhage.[230] The lesions are seen on CT scan,[84,146,290] but their concentric pattern is not evident. Usually the diagnosis of Baló's concentric sclerosis is made postmortem, but it has been diagnosed by biopsy antemortem.[146,155] The concentric pattern has been detected by MRI scan antemortem[155,462] and by MRI scan of formalin-fixed tissue postmortem.[305]

The notion that these lesions are a variant of MS is reinforced by their inflammatory and demyelinative nature and the fact that they frequently coexist with MS

plaques (reviewed by Itoyama et al.[213]). They may also be seen in association with large hemispheric plaques.[345,473]

An entity referred to as *concentric lacunar leukoencephalopathy* closely resembles Baló's concentric sclerosis[96,164] but differs in having extensive loss of axons in addition to the demyelination. The bands comprise zones of cavitation with intervening bands of gliosis, within which there is little or no surviving myelin. The relationship between these two conditions is unclear. The extensive cavitation and myelin and axonal loss seen in concentric lacunar leukoencephalopathy might be the result of massive inflammation early in the course of the illness. The coexisting demyelinating lesions in one case[96] suggest that this is a demyelinating disorder akin to MS. Another case[164] with a progressive history in the absence of illustrated inflammatory lymphocytic infiltrates, however, is more difficult to classify. The progressive course may be related to progressive axonal loss resulting from the nonspecific enzymatic effects of the extensive macrophage population in this condition.

Neuromyelitis Optica

The occurrence of bilateral visual impairment and spinal cord signs separated by, at the most, several weeks is referred to as *neuromyelitis optica,* or *Devic's syndrome.* The association of optic nerve and spinal cord signs and symptoms was first discussed by Allbutt in 1870.[17,88,231] The bulk of his article concerned cases of spinal trauma, but he does refer to one case of "acute myelitis" where an "eye disorder" supervened. In 1894, Gault,[88,147,231] with the encouragement of his teacher Devic,[107] reviewed the published cases. Since then, the subject has been reviewed by Peters[337] in German and by Cloys and Netsky[88] and Kuroiwa[231] in English.

The history of neuromyelitis optica is one of a disorder in search of a nosological position. Controversy has centered on whether it comprises a variant of MS,[231] whether it is an entity distinct from MS,[183,463] or whether it consists of several disorders, one of which is MS.[19,88,96,329] Many cases showing plaques in addition to the optic and spinal lesions are variants of MS. Other cases show features of perivenous (postvaccinal or postinfectious) encephalomyelitis[19] and possibly other categories of disease,[88,329] including concentric lacunar leukoencephalopathy.[96] Still others show spinal cord necrosis associated with optic nerve demyelination without any other lesions in the CNS.[257] Thus, it is prudent to consider neuromyelitis optica as a clinical syndrome that is the clinical expression of several disease entities, one of which is MS. However, it has been suggested that the use of this diagnosis be restricted to those cases with evidence of spinal cord necrosis and optic nerve demyelination without any lesions elsewhere in the CNS, thus excluding MS and other disseminated CNS diseases from this designation.[257]

The pathology, then, depends on the underlying disease. The lesions may be inflammatory and demyelinative in those associated with MS, but frequently, even in the MS variant, they show extensive necrosis and even cavitation. The latter manifests as an acute often fulminating clinical presentation of an ascending myelopathy. Why such destructive lesions should involve the spinal cord and optic nerves and should be seen in a variety of conditions is uncertain. However, it has been suggested that the edema associated with the lesion within the close confines of the pia in the case of the spinal cord and the optic canal in the case of the optic nerve might be responsible for ischemia leading to necrosis in these regions.[327] The edema then would be the common denominator in a variety of conditions, which, although they may affect multiple regions of the CNS, manifest themselves clinically as neuromyelitis optica because of the critically compromised situation at these two locations.

Variants with Extensive Hemispheric Demyelination

Leukodystrophies, which are inherited metabolic disorders of white matter, characteristically produce widespread demyelination. They are, of course, unrelated to MS, although some forms may simulate chronic progressive MS clinically.[120,430a] However, MS, particularly in the young, can produce extensive loss of myelin within the cerebral hemispheres. Great confusion has pervaded this field of study mainly as a result of semantics and the realization that both inherited and acquired diseases of the myelin sheath can produce extensive confluent demyelination. The problem has been well delineated by Poser and the reader is referred to his most recent review[346] for a detailed unraveling of the literature that has evolved into our current concept of these unusual cases.

The controversy centers on what constitutes *Schilder's disease.* This term in the past was used to designate those cases involving extensive bilateral confluent hemispheric demyelination. This observation was indeed what Schilder described in 1912, for which he used the term "encephalitis periaxialis diffusa."[427] However, he described two further cases in 1913[428] and 1924,[429] which retrospectively turned out to be quite different from the entity described in his initial paper,[346] being probably a leukodystrophy[349] and subacute sclerosing panencephalitis,[251] respectively. Further confusion over terminology resulted from the use of the term *diffuse sclerosis* for a variety of conditions, including cases similar to Schilder's initial description of 1912.[346]

Much of this nosological turmoil was resolved when it was shown that the vast majority of cases previously termed "Schilder's disease" were, in fact, adrenoleukodystrophy, a sex-linked disorder affecting the adrenal cortex and white matter.[424,425] This condition would account for most of the males with Schilder's disease, and possibly some females as well, because adrenoleukodystrophy has more recently been described in girls.[331] It has also been pointed out that the lymphocytic inflammatory infiltrate, which can be quite pronounced in these cases, is seen in the almost completely demyelinated areas but not at the peripheral rim of active demyelination.[424] This description implies that the immune response is secondary and responding to a breakdown product of the myelin. In this regard, the pathology differs from MS where the lymphocyte abounds at (and probably precedes) the advancing edge of demyelination.

Nevertheless, there remain a few cases of Schilder's disease which do not fit the pathological criteria for adrenoleukodystrophy. These are, in all likelihood, a variant of MS and have been referred to as "myelinoclastic diffuse sclerosis" by Poser.[346] According to Poser, such cases show extensive confluent regions of demyelination in the hemispheric white matter and may spare the subcortical U-fibers but, in contrast to the leukodystrophies, may involve them as well as extending into the adjacent cerebral cortex. The lesion is predominantly demyelinating, but axons may be destroyed and frank tissue necrosis and eventual cavitation may be evident.[346] Perivascular inflammation is a prominent component but may not be present in cases that are no longer active.[346] Gliosis, which may manifest itself in the form of giant multinucleated astrocytes, is a prominent feature.[346] In some instances, the smaller plaques of MS are seen in addition to the large hemispheric lesions; these cases are frequently referred to as *transitional sclerosis*.

The diagnosis of this rare variant of MS is a diagnosis of exclusion; a leukodystrophy must be excluded. Adrenoleukodystrophy has been shown to be a disorder of long-chain fatty acid metabolism,[301] and biochemical assays for long-chain fatty acids performed on plasma or cultured skin fibroblasts confirm the diagnosis. Using the criterion of exclusion of adrenoleukodystrophy by biochemical means, only a few reported cases[275,348] to date qualify as MS with diffuse confluent hemispheric involvement. No doubt, more clarification will be forthcoming in the future.

Disseminated Subpial Demyelination

In the literature, two cases[145,314] have been reported in which foci of demyelination are confined to the subpial region, without involvement of subependymal regions. Both were characterized by loss of myelin with preservation of axons. In one, inflammation was minimal to absent,[314] and in the other, it was a prominent feature.[145] One showed extensive involvement of the cerebral cortex and brain stem,[145] whereas the other involved the brain stem and some subcortical structures.[314] Both demonstrated changes in mental status and various focal neurological signs. The exact classification of these cases is uncertain, but because they show inflammatory (at least in one case) and demyelinating lesions of varying ages separated in space, they may well turn out to be variants of MS with disseminated subpial demyelination. Examination of further cases is necessary to clarify their status in the group of demyelinating diseases of the CNS.

AN OVERVIEW

Current concepts of the immunopathogenesis of the MS lesion have been reviewed and schematized by Raine.[374,379,380] Many of these concepts are reiterated here, and the reader is referred to Raine's reviews for details of how the immune system orchestrates these events in the MS plaque.

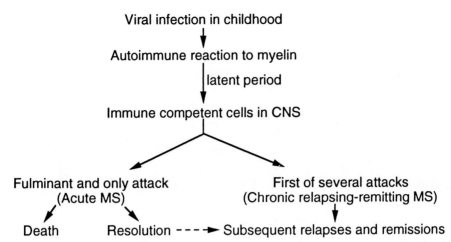

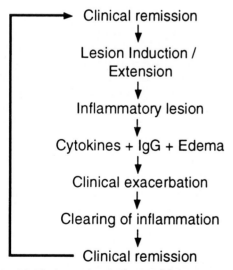

Figure 8–35. A postulated schema for early events in the pathogenesis of MS. (The dashed arrow refers to the occasional case of acute MS which goes on to a relapsing-remitting course and suggests the possibility that classic relapsing-remitting cases of MS may go through a clinically silent "acute" phase.) CNS = central nervous system.

What follows is an attempt to integrate and summarize the morphologic and physiological data presented in this chapter into a schema. It is hoped that this schema may provide a useful framework to modify as newer or more certain data emerge. The approach is summarized in Figures 8–35 through 8–37.

If we believe that MS is an autoimmune disease, then a number of mechanisms

Figure 8–36. A postulated schema of the sequence of events in a purely inflammatory (non-demyelinating) lesion in chronic relapsing-remitting MS.

could be considered important in the instigation of autoimmunity to myelin.[531] One school of thought holds that MS is the result of cross-reactivity between a virus (or other exogenous antigen) and a myelin component and that this cross reaction occurs during a viral illness in childhood in a genetically susceptible individual.[374] This is the model considered here, but the sequence of events at the onset of the clinical disease would be equally applicable to any instigating factors of autoimmunity.

As shown in Figure 8–35, a long latent period after the childhood infection could precede the first attack of MS.[374,380] In some patients, this first attack is a fulminant monophasic insult, which represents acute MS, from which they succumb, completely recover, or survive with a permanent neurological deficit. In exceptional circumstances, patients with fulminant acute MS who recover may later demonstrate the relapsing-remitting form of the disease.

In most patients, however, the first attack is not fulminating, and there are probably patients whose first episode of the disease is subclinical but whose lesions could theoretically be detected by MRI. Both these groups of patients then experience further episodes of the chronic relapsing-remitting form of MS.

Induction of a new lesion or extension of a pre-existing chronic MS lesion could occur

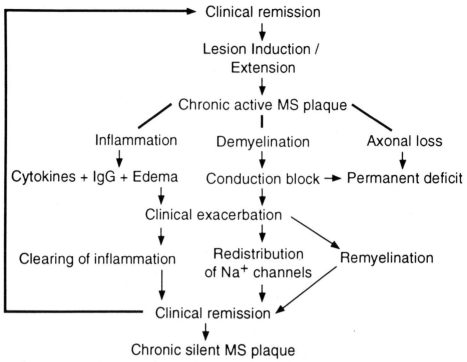

Figure 8–37. A postulated schema of the sequence of events in a chronic MS plaque with inflammation and demyelination.

with microglial or macrophage expression of MHC class II molecules, which can be upregulated by various factors such as interferon gamma[488] during an intercurrent viral illness, allowing presentation of the putative antigen to trafficking or residential antigen-specific helper-inducer T lymphocytes. In the case of induction of a new lesion, current concepts[195,196,279,510] would predict that this antigen-presenting event occurs at the level of the perivascular microglial cell. The induction and extension of the lesion probably also involves the interaction of multiple other molecules in addition to MHC class II and the T-cell receptor, such as integrins and adhesion molecules,[105a,518a] other putative antigen-presenting molecules,[46a] costimulatory molecules,[105a,518a] and other molecules involved in the interaction of T cells with other cell types.[151b] Proinflammatory and immunomodulatory cytokines[72a,83] are another group of molecules with important roles in this process.

In some of the lesions of chronic MS, as illustrated in Figure 8–36, only inflammation may be evident and the process does not proceed to demyelination. The clinical symptoms or the appearance of lesions on MRI scan would be thus due to edema[267,268] from blood-brain barrier breakdown and the secretion of cytokines[73,436,439,480] and IgG[65,423] by the inflammatory infiltrate. Possibly instigated initially by the emergence of a suppressor T lymphocyte population in the lesion[376] or the secretion of immunomodulatory cytokines[83] by Th2 cells,[380,518a] the clearance of the inflammatory infiltrate and the associated edema would reverse the radiologic appearance, and the clinical symptoms and the lesion would then have undergone a remission.

In other lesions, as illustrated in Figure 8–37, helper-inducer T lymphocytes stimulate sufficient macrophages to bring about demyelination. The demyelination is carried out by macrophages[363,389] by the nonspecific actions of enzymes[11,519] or cytokines[439] and by utilization of ligand-receptor complexes to engulf the myelin.[360,362] Oligodendrocyte destruction by toxic nitrogen free radicals produced by astrocytes and possibly macrophages may also play a role in demyelination.[60,71b,278a] We also cannot exclude the possibility of a cytolytic effect on oligodendrocytes or the myelin sheath mediated by cytotoxic T lymphocytes as a mechanism. If the enzymatic or cytolytic activity is excessive, axonal destruction may result, and if in a clinically important region, such axonal loss would be expected to be responsible for a permanent neurological deficit.[269] However, most of the deficit during a relapse would probably be due to conduction block or other disturbances of action potential conduction as a consequence of demyelination.[173,265,503,505] With redistribution of sodium channels through the demyelinated regions of axolemma, conduction could return, conduction block be overcome, and reversal of the clinical deficit would ensue.[503] Remyelination could also restore function.[503,504] These effects on the axon, together with resolution of the inflammatory infiltrate, would result in the clinical remission attributed to this lesion. Permanent conduction block, failure of remyelination, and in some instances, axonal loss could account for the permanent deficits retained after some exacerbations and the deficits of chronic progressive MS.

After remission, the patient is stable until a preexisting lesion is reactivated or a new lesion induced, and the cycle begins again.[374,380] The clinical symptoms and radiologic lesions depend on the location of the focus of activation.

Throughout this process, gliosis is occurring.[374] Eventually the inflammation and active demyelination becomes quiescent, and the result is a chronic silent plaque in which there is extensive gliosis and demyelinated axons. Whether such a plaque will manifest permanent chronic clinical signs would depend on the factors responsible for restoration of function discussed above.

Our current knowledge of the pathology of the MS lesion is consistent with the notion that this disease has an immune pathogenesis. The disability the patient manifests is due to complex interactions between the immune response, the physiology of normal and demyelinated axons, and the processes of repair and scarring in the CNS.

REFERENCES

1. Abbott RJ, Howe JG, Currie S, and Holland I: Multiple sclerosis plaque mimicking tumour on computed tomography. BMJ 285:1616–1617, 1982.
2. Abo T, and Balch CM: A differentiation antigen of human NK and K cells identified by a monoclonal antibody (HNK-1). J Immunol 127:1024–1029, 1981.
3. Abroms IF, Yessayan L, Shillito J, and Barlow CF: Spontaneous intracerebral haemorrhage in patients suspected of multiple sclerosis. J Neurol Neurosurg Psychiatry 34:157–162, 1971.
4. Adams CWM: The onset and progression of the lesion in multiple sclerosis. J Neurol Sci 25:165–182, 1975.
5. Adams CWM: The progression of the lesion in multiple sclerosis (abstract). Neurology 26(6 pt 2):33–34, 1976.
6. Adams CWM: Pathology of multiple sclerosis: Progression of the lesion. Br Med Bull 33:15–20, 1977.
7. Adams CWM: The general pathology of multiple sclerosis: Morphological and chemical aspects of the lesions. In Hallpike JF, Adams CWM, and Tourtellotte WW (eds): Multiple Sclerosis: Pathology, Diagnosis and Management. Williams & Wilkins, Baltimore, 1983, pp 203–240.
8. Adams CWM: Perivascular iron deposition and other vascular damage in multiple sclerosis. J Neurol Neurosurg Psychiatry 51:260–265, 1988.
9. Adams CWM, Abdulla YH, Torres EM, and Poston RN: Periventricular lesions in multiple sclerosis: Their perivenous origin and relationship to granular ependymitis. Neuropathol Appl Neurobiol 13:141-152, 1987.
10. Adams CWM, Bayliss OB, Hallpike JF, and Turner DR: Histochemistry of myelin. XII. Anionic staining of myelin basic proteins for histology, electrophoresis and electron microscopy. J Neurochem 18:389–394, 1971.
11. Adams CWM, Hallpike JF, and Bayliss OB: Histochemistry of myelin. XIII. Digestion of basic protein outside acute plaques of multiple sclerosis. J Neurochem 18:1479–1483, 1971.
12. Adams CWM, Poston RN, and Buk SJ: Pathology, histochemistry and immunocytochemistry of lesions in acute multiple sclerosis. J Neurol Sci 92:291-306, 1989.
13. Adams CWM, Poston RN, Buk SJ, Sidhu YS, and Vipond H: Inflammatory vasculitis in multiple sclerosis. J Neurol Sci 69:269–283, 1985.
14. Adams RD, and Kubik CS: The morbid anatomy of the demyelinative diseases. Am J Med 12:510–546, 1952.
15. Aggarwall BB, and Eessalu TE: Human tumor necrosis factor and lymphotoxin: Their structural and functional similarities. In Bonavida B, and Collier RJ (eds): Membrane-Mediated Cytotoxicity. Alan R Liss, New York, 1987, pp 297–307.
15a. Ahdab-Barmada M, and Rozin L: Deficiency of complement regulatory proteins in multiple

sclerosis lesions (abstract). J. Neuropathol Exp Neurol 55:641, 1996.

16. Aita JF, Bennett DR, Anderson RE, and Ziter F: Cranial CT appearance of acute multiple sclerosis. Neurology 28:251–255, 1978.

17. Allbutt TC: On the ophthalmoscopic signs of spinal disease. Lancet 1:76–78, 1870.

18. Allen IV: The pathology of multiple sclerosis—fact, fiction and hypothesis. Neuropathol Appl Neurobiol 7:169–182, 1981.

19. Allen IV: Demyelinating diseases. In Adams JH, Corsellis JAN, and Duchen LW (eds): Greenfield's Neuropathology, ed 4. John Wiley & Sons, New York, 1984, pp 338–384.

20. Allen IV: Pathology of multiple sclerosis. In Matthews WB (ed): McAlpine's Multiple Sclerosis, ed 2. Churchill Livingstone, Edinburgh, 1991, pp 341–378.

21. Allen IV, Glover G, and Anderson R: Abnormalities in the macroscopically normal white matter in cases of mild or spinal multiple sclerosis (MS). Acta Neuropathol [Suppl] (Berlin) 7:176–178, 1981.

22. Allen IV, Glover G, McKeown SR, and McCormick D: The cellular origin of lysosomal enzymes in the plaque in multiple sclerosis. II. A histochemical study with combined demonstration of myelin and acid phosphatase. Neuropathol Appl Neurobiol 5:197–210, 1979.

23. Allen IV, and Kirk J: Demyelinating diseases. In Adams JH, and Duchen LW (eds): Greenfield's Neuropathology, ed 5. Oxford University Press, New York, 1992, pp 447–520.

24. Allen IV, and McKeown SR: A histological, histochemical and biochemical study of the macroscopically normal white matter in multiple sclerosis. J Neurol Sci 41:81–91, 1979.

25. Alling C, Vanier M-T, and Svennerholm L: Lipid alterations in apparently normal white matter in multiple sclerosis. Brain Res 35:325–336, 1971.

26. Alvord EC Jr, Kies MW, and Suckling AJ: Experimental Allergic Encephalomyelitis, A Useful Model for Multiple Sclerosis. Alan R Liss, New York, 1984.

27. Andrews JM, and Andrews RL: The significance of dense core particles in subacute demyelinating disease in an adult. Lab Invest 28:236–243, 1973.

28. Andrews JM, and Cancilla PA: Subacute demyelinating disease in an adult (diffuse-disseminated sclerosis): Electron microscopic findings. Bulletin of the Los Angeles Neurological Societies 38:49–59, 1973.

29. Ansell GB, and Spanner S: Plasmalogenase activity in normal and demyelinating tissue of the central nervous system. Biochem J 108:207–209, 1968.

30. Arenander A, and deVellis J: Early response gene induction in astrocytes as a mechanism for encoding and integrating neuronal signals. In Yu ACH, Hertz L, Norenberg MD, Syková E, and Waxman SG (eds): Neuronal-Astrocytic Interactions: Implications for Normal and Pathological CNS Function. Progress in Brain Research, Vol 94. Elsevier, Amsterdam, 1992, pp 177–188.

31. Argyrakis A: Glial cell alterations in multiple sclerosis. In Bauer HJ, Posner S, and Ritter G (eds): Progress in Multiple Sclerosis Research. Springer-Verlag, Berlin, 1980, pp 355–359.

32. Armstrong RC, Harvath L, and Dubois-Dalcq ME: Type 1 astrocytes and oligodendrocyte-type 2 astrocyte glial progenitors migrate toward distinct molecules. J Neurosci Res 27:400–407, 1990.

33. Arnold AC, Pepose JS, Hepler RS, and Foos RY: Retinal periphlebitis and retinitis in multiple sclerosis. 1. Pathologic characteristics. Ophthalmology 91:255–262, 1984.

34. Arstila AU, Riekkinen P, Rinne UK, and Laitinen L: Studies on the pathogenesis of multiple sclerosis: Participation of lysosomes on demyelination in the central nervous system white matter outside plaques. Eur Neurol 9:1–20, 1973.

35. Auer RN, Gallagher JC, and Butt JC: Solitary asymptomatic plaque of demyelination in the medulla oblongata. Clin Neuropathol 7:225–227, 1988.

35a. Bagasra O, Michaels FH, Zheung YM, et al: Activation of the inducible form of nitric oxide synthase in the brains of patients with multiple sclerosis. Proc Natl Acad Sci USA 92:12041–12045, 1995.

36. Baker RWR, Thompson RHS, and Zilkha KJ: Fatty-acid composition of brain lecithins in multiple sclerosis. Lancet 1:26–27, 1963.

37. Baker RWR, Thompson RHS, and Zilkha KJ: Serum fatty acids in multiple sclerosis. J Neurol Neurosurg Psychiatry 27:408–414, 1964.

38. Baló J: A leukoenkephalitis periaxialis concentrica (tricaról). Magyar orvosi Archivum, 1927.

39. Baló J: Encephalitis periaxialis concentrica. Archives of Neurology and Psychiatry 19:242–264, 1928.

40. Barbosa LH, and Hamilton R: Studies with multiple-sclerosis brain. Lancet 1:1415–1417, 1973.

41. Barnard RO, and Triggs M: Corpus callosum in multiple sclerosis. J Neurol Neurosurg Psychiatry 37:1259–1264, 1974.

42. Barnes D, Munro PMG, Youl BD, Prineas JW, and McDonald WI: The longstanding MS lesion: A quantitative MRI and electron microscopic study. Brain 114:1271–1280, 1991.

43. Barré, Morin, Draganesco, and Reyes: Encéphalite périaxiale diffuse (type Schilder): Syndrome tétraplégique avec stase papillaire. Rev Neurol (Paris) II:541–557, 1926.

44. Barres BA: New roles for glia. J Neurosci 11:3685–3694, 1991.

45. Barres BA, Chun LLY, and Corey DP: Ion channels in vertebrate glia. Annu Rev Neurosci 13:441–474, 1990.

46. Barres BA, Koroshetz WJ, Chun LLY, and Corey DP: Ion channel expression by white matter glia: The type-1 astrocyte. Neuron 5:527–544, 1990.

46a. Battistini L, Fischer FR, Raine CS, and Brosnan CF: CD1b is expressed in multiple sclerosis lesions. J Neuroimmunol 67:145–151, 1996.

46b. Battistini L, Selmaj K, Kowal C, et al: Multiple sclerosis: limited diversity of the Vδ2-Jδ3 T-cell receptor in chronic active lesions. Ann Neurol 37:198–203, 1995.

47. Bayliss OB, and Adams CWM: Cellular lipid inclusions in the white matter in multiple sclerosis. Nature 233:264–265, 1971.

48. Becker FO, Michael JA, and Davis FA: Acute effects of oral phosphate on visual function in multiple sclerosis. Neurology 24:601–607, 1974.

49. Belin J, Pettet N, Smith AD, Thompson RHS, and Zilkha KJ: Linoleate metabolism in multiple sclerosis. J Neurol Neurosurg Psychiatry 34:25–29, 1971.

50. Bell RA, Robertson DM, Rosen DA, and Kerr AW: Optochiasmatic arachnoiditis in multiple sclerosis. Arch Ophthalmol 93:191–193, 1975.

51. Bellamy AS, Calder VL, Feldmann M, and Davison AN: The distribution of interleukin-2 receptor bearing lymphocytes in multiple sclerosis: evidence for a key role of activated lymphocytes. Clin Exp Immunol 61:248–256, 1985.

51a. Benveniste EN: Inflammatory cytokines within the central nervous system: Sources, function, and mechanism of action. Am J Physiol 263 (Cell Physiol 32): C1–C16, 1992.

52. Benveniste EN, and Merrill JE: Stimulation of oligodendroglial proliferation and maturation by interleukin-2. Nature 321:610–613, 1986.

53. Berke G: Functions and mechanisms of action of cytolytic lymphocytes. In Paul WE (ed): Fundamental Immunology, ed 3. Raven Press, New York, 1993, pp 965-1014.

54. Best PV: Acute polyradiculoneuritis associated with demyelinated plaques in the central nervous system: report of a case. Acta Neuropathol (Berl) 67:230–234, 1985.

54a. Bever CT, and Garver DW: Increased cathepsin B activity in multiple sclerosis brain. J Neurol Sci 131:71–73, 1995.

55. Birling M-C, Nussbaum F, and Nussbaum J-L: A new oliogodendrocyte specific plasma membrane surface protein identified by a monoclonal antibody produced in vitro. J Neurosci Res 38:538–550, 1994.

56. Birnbaum G, Clark HB, and Psihos D: Expression of heat shock proteins in the brains of patients with multiple sclerosis and other neurological diseases (abstract). Ann Neurol 30:305, 1991.

57. Black JA, Felts P, Smith KJ, Kocsis JD, and Waxman SG: Distribution of sodium channels in chronically demyelinated spinal cord axons: immuno-ultrastructural localization and electrophysiological observations. Brain Res 544:59–70, 1991.

58. Blakemore WF: Myelination, demyelination and remyelination in the CNS. In Smith WT, and Cavanagh JB (eds): Recent Advances in Neuropathology, no. 2. Churchill-Livingstone, Edinburgh, 1982, pp 53–81.

59. Blakemore WF, and Smith KJ: Node-like axonal specialisations along demyelinated central nerve fibers: Ultrastructural observations. Acta Neuropathol (Berl) 60:291–296, 1983.

60. Bö L, Dawson TM, Wesselingh S, Mörk S, Choi S, Kong PA, Hanley D, and Trapp BD: Induction of nitric oxide synthase in demyelinating regions of multiple sclerosis brains. Ann Neurol 36:778–786, 1994.

61. Bö L, Mörk S, Kong PA, Nyland H, Pardo CA, and Trapp BD: Detection of MHC class II-antigens on macrophages and microglia, but not on astrocytes and endothelia in active multiple sclerosis lesions. J Neuroimmunol 51:135–146, 1994.

61a. Bonetti B, and Raine CS: Bcl-2 and Fas system molecule expression in multiple sclerosis lesions (abstract). J Neuropathol Exp Neurol 55:641, 1996.

62. Booss J, Esiri MM, Tourtellotte WW, and Mason DY: Immunohistological analysis of T lymphocyte subsets in the central nervous system in chronic progressive multiple sclerosis. J Neurol Sci 62:219–232, 1983.

63. Born W, Happ MP, Dallas A, et al: Recognition of heat shock proteins and cell function. Immunol Today 11:40–43, 1990.

64. Bornstein MB: The immunopathology of demyelinative disorders examined in organotypic cultures of mammalian central nerve tissues. In Zimmerman HM (ed): Progress in Neuropathology, Vol II. Grune & Stratton, New York, 1973, pp 69–90.

65. Bornstein MB, and Crain SM: Functional studies of cultured brain tissues as related to "demyelinative disorders." Science 148:1242–1244, 1965.

66. Bostock H, and Sears TA: The internodal axon membrane: Electrical excitability and continuous conduction in segmental demyelination. J Physiol (Lond) 280:273–301, 1978.

67. Bowen DM, and Davison AN: Macrophages and cathepsin A activity in multiple sclerosis brain. J Neurol Sci 21:227–231, 1974.

68. Boyle EA, and McGeer PL: Cellular immune response in multiple sclerosis plaques. Am J Pathol 137:575–584, 1990.

69. Bradbury K, Aparicio SR, Sumner DW, et al: Comparison of in vitro demyelination and cytotoxicity of humoral factors in multiple sclerosis and other neurological diseases. J Neurol Sci 70:167–181, 1985.

70. Brinkman CJJ, terLaak HJ, Hommes OR, Poppema S, and Delmotte P: T-lymphocyte subpopulations in multiple-sclerosis lesions. (Letter to the Editor). N Engl J Med 307:1644–1645, 1982.

71. Broman T: Blood-brain barrier damage in multiple sclerosis: Supravital test-observations. Acta Neurol Scand Suppl 10:21–24, 1964.

71a. Brosnan CF, Battistini L, Gao Y-L, Raine CS, and Aquino DA: Heat shock proteins and multiple sclerosis: A review. J Neuropathol Exp Neurol 55:389–402, 1996.

71b. Brosnan CF, Battistini L, Raine CS, Dickson DW, Casadevall A, and Lee SC: Reactive nitrogen intermediates in human neuropathology: An overview. Dev Neurosci 16:152–161, 1994.

72. Brosnan CF, Cammer W, Norton WT, and Bloom BR: Proteinase inhibitors suppress the development of experimental allergic encephalomyelitis. Nature 285:235–237, 1980.

72a. Brosnan CF, Cannella B, Battistini L, and Raine CS: Cytokine localization in multiple sclerosis lesions: Correlation with adhesion molecule expression and reactive nitrogen species. Neurology 45 (suppl 6):S16–S21, 1995.

73. Brosnan CF, Litwak MS, Schroeder CE, Selmaj K, Raine CS, and Arezzo JC: Preliminary studies of cytokine-induced functional effects on the visual pathways in the rabbit. J Neuroimmunol 25: 227–239, 1989.

74. Brown WJ: The capillaries in acute and subacute multiple sclerosis plaques: A morphometric analysis. Neurology 28(2):84–92, 1978.

75. Brownell B, and Hughes JT: The distribution of plaques in the cerebrum in multiple sclerosis. J Neurol Neurosurg Psychiatry 25:315–320, 1962.

75a. Brück W, Porada P, Poser S, et al: Monocyte/macrophage differentiation in early multiple sclerosis lesions. Ann Neurol 38:788–796, 1995.

76. Brück W, Schmied M, Suchanek G, et al: Oligodendrocytes in the early course of multiple sclerosis. Ann Neurol 35:65–73, 1994.

77. Brunner C, Lassmann H, Waehneldt TV, Matthieu J-M, and Linington C: Differential ultrastructural localization of myelin basic protein, myelin/oligodendroglial glycoprotein, and 2'-3' cyclic nucleotide 3'-phosphodiesterase in the CNS of adult rats. J Neurochem 52:296–304, 1989.

78. Buja LM, Ferrans VJ, and Rabson AS: Unusual nuclear inclusions (letter). Lancet 1:402–403, 1974.

79. Bunge MB, Bunge RP, and Ris H: Ultrastructural study of remyelination in an experimental lesion in adult cat spinal cord. Journal of Biophysical and Biochemical Cytology 10:67–94, 1961.

80. Cammer W, Bloom BR, Norton WT, and Gordon S: Degradation of basic protein in myelin by neutral proteinases secreted by stimulated macrophages: A possible mechanism of inflammatory demyelination. Proc Natl Acad Sci USA 75:1554–1558, 1978.

81. Cancilla PA, Andrews JM, and Rose AS: Subacute demyelinating disease in an adult (diffuse-disseminated sclerosis): Clinical course, response to therapy, and neuropathological findings. Neurology 21:825–832, 1971.

81a. Cannella B, Browning J, and Raine CS: Differences in cellular affinity between lymphotoxin α (LTα) and LTβ in the CNS of multiple sclerosis (MS) and non-MS subjects (abstract). J Neuropathol Exp Neurol 55:641, 1996.

82. Cannella B, Cross AH, and Raine CS: Adhesion-related molecules in the central nervous system: Upregulation correlates with inflammatory cell influx during relapsing experimental autoimmune encephalomyelitis. Lab Invest 65:23–31, 1991.

83. Cannella B, and Raine CS: The adhesion molecule and cytokine profile of multiple sclerosis lesions. Ann Neurol 37:424–435, 1995.

83a. Capello E, Voskuhl R, McFarland HF, and Raine CS: Differential expression of a novel candidate autoantigen, X2MBP, in multiple sclerosis (MS) lesions (abstract). J Neuropathol Exp Neurol 55:640, 1996.

84. Castaigne P, Escourolle R, Chain F, et al: Sclérose concentrique de Baló. Rev Neurol (Paris) 140: 479–487, 1984.

85. Cerf JA, and Carels G: Multiple sclerosis: Serum factor producing reversible alterations in bioelectric responses. Science 152:1066–1068,1966.

86. Chen S-J, and DeVries GH: Mitogenic effect of axolemma-enriched fraction on cultured oligodendrocytes. J Neurochem 52:325–327, 1989.

87. Chou SM: Pathogenesis of MS from a neuropathologist's vista. In Kuroiwa Y, and Kurland LT (eds): Multiple Sclerosis: East and West. Kyushu University Press, Fukuoka, Japan, 1982, pp 317–337.

87a. Claudio L, Raine CS, and Brosnan CF: Evidence of persistent blood-brain barrier abnormalities in chronic-progressive multiple sclerosis. Acta Neuropathol (Berl) 90:228–238, 1995.

88. Cloys DE, and Netsky MG: Neuromyelitis optica. In Vinken PJ, and Bruyn GW (eds): Handbook of Clinical Neurology, Vol 9, Multiple Sclerosis and Other Demyelinating Diseases. North-Holland, Amsterdam, 1970, pp 426–436.

89. Compston DAS, Morgan BP, Campbell AK, et al: Immunocytochemical localization of the terminal complement complex in multiple sclerosis. Neuropathol Appl Neurobiol 15:307–316, 1989.

90. Courville CB: Concentric sclerosis. In Vinken PJ, and Bruyn GW (eds): Handbook of Clinical Neurology, Vol 9, Multiple sclerosis and Other Demyelinating Diseases. North-Holland, Amsterdam, 1970, pp 437–451.

91. Craelius W, Jacobs RM, and Jones AOL: Mineral composition of brains of normal and multiple sclerosis victims. Proc Soc Exp Biol Med 165: 327–329, 1980.

92. Craelius W, Migdal MW, Luessenhop CP, Sugar A, and Mihalakis I: Iron deposits surrounding multiple sclerosis plaques. Arch Pathol Lab Med 106:397–399, 1982.

93. Cross AH, Cannella B, Brosnan CF, and Raine CS: Homing to central nervous system vasculature by antigen-specific lymphocytes. I. Localization of ^{14}C-labelled cells during acute, chronic, and relapsing experimental allergic encephalomyelitis. Lab Invest 63:162–170, 1990.

93a. Cross AH, Touhy VK, and Raine CS: Development of reactivity to new myelin antigens during chronic relapsing autoimmune demyelination. Cell Immunol 146:261–269, 1993.

94. Csejtey C, Hallpike JF, Adams CWM, and Bayliss OB: Degraded proteolipid in multiple sclerosis plaques—histochemical electrophoretic observations. Histochem J 7:599–604, 1975.

95. Cumings JN: Lipid chemistry of the brain in demyelinating diseases. Brain 78:554–563, 1955.

96. Currie S, Roberts AH, and Urich H: The nosological position of concentric lacunar leukoencephalopathy. J Neurol Neurosurg Psychiatry 33:131–137, 1970.

97. Currie S, and Urich H: Concurrence of multiple sclerosis and glioma. J Neurol Neurosurg Psychiatry 37:598–605, 1974.

98. Cuzner ML, Barnard RO, MacGregor BJL, Borshell NJ, and Davison AN: Myelin composition in acute and chronic multiple sclerosis in relation to cerebral lysosomal activity. J Neurol Sci 29: 324–334, 1976.

99. Cuzner ML, and Davison AN: Changes in cerebral lysosomal enzyme activity and lipids in multiple sclerosis. J Neurol Sci 19:29–36, 1973.

100. Dal Canto MC, Wiśniewski HM, Johnson AB, Brostoff SW, and Raine CS: Vesicular disruption of myelin in autoimmune demyelination. J Neurol Sci 24:313–319, 1975.

101. Davis FA, Becker FO, Michael JA, and Sorensen E: Effect of intravenous sodium bicarbonate, disodium edetate (Na$_2$ EDTA), and hyperventilation on visual and oculomotor signs in multiple sclerosis. J Neurol Neurosurg Psychiatry 33:723–732, 1970.

102. Davis FA, Bergen D, Schauf C, McDonald I, and Deutsch W: Movement phosphenes in optic neuritis: A new clinical sign. Neurology 26:1100–1104, 1976.

103. Davis RL: Intranuclear structures in acute multiple sclerosis (abstract). J Neuropathol Exp Neurol 32:178, 1972.

104. Dawson JW: The histology of disseminated sclerosis. Transactions of the Royal Society of Edinburgh 50:517-740, 1916.

105. de Preux J, and Mair WGP: Ultrastructure of the optic nerve in Schilder's disease, Devic's disease and disseminated sclerosis. Acta Neuropathol (Berl) 30:225–242, 1974.

105a. De Simone R, Giampaolo A, Giometto B, et al: The costimulatory molecule B7 is expressed on human microglia in culture and in multiple sclerosis acute lesions. J Neuropathol Exp Neurol 54:175–187, 1995.

106. Dermietzel R, Hertzberg EL, Kessler JA, and Spray DC: Gap junctions between cultured astrocytes: immunocytochemical, molecular, and electrophysiological analysis. J Neurosci 11:1421–1432, 1991.

107. Devic E: Myélite subaiguë compliquée de névrite optique (abstract). Le Bulletin Médical 8:1033–1034, 1894.

107a. Dickson DW, Mattiace LA, Kure K, Hutchins K, Lyman WD, and Brosnan CF: Biology of disease: Microglia in human disease, with an emphasis on acquired immunodeficiency syndrome. Lab Invest 64:135–156, 1991.

108. Dorovini-Zis K, Anders JJ, and Brightman MW: Cerebral endothelium, blood-brain-barrier and the astrocyte membrane. In Cunha-Vaz JG (ed): The Blood-Retinal Barriers. Plenum, New York, 1980, pp 65–79.

108a. Dorovini-Zis K, Prameya R, and Bowman PD: Culture and characterization of microvascular endothelial cells derived from human brain. Lab Invest 64:425–436, 1991.

109. Drummond RJ, and Dean G: Comparison of 2'-3' cyclic nucleotide 3' phosphodiesterase and the major component of Wolfgram protein W1. J Neurochem 35:1155–1165, 1980.

110. Dubois-Dalcq M, and Armstrong R: The cellular and molecular events of central nervous system remyelination. Bioessays 12:569–576, 1990.

111. Dubois-Dalcq M, Behar T, Hudson L, and Lazzarini RA: Emergence of three myelin proteins in oligodendrocytes cultured without neurons. J Cell Biol 102:384–392, 1986.

112. Dubois-Dalcq M, Schumacher G, and Sever JL: Acute multiple sclerosis: Electron-microscopic evidence for and against a viral agent in the plaques. Lancet 2:1408–1411, 1973.

113. Dubois-Dalcq M, Schumacher G, and Worthington EK: Immunoperoxidase studies on multiple sclerosis brain (abstract). Neurology 25:496, 1975.

114. Duffy PE: Astrocytes: Normal, Reactive, and Neoplastic. Raven Press, New York, 1983.

115. Duijvestijn AM, Horst E, Pals ST, et al: High endothelial differentiation in human lymphoid and inflammatory tissues defined by monclonal antibody HECA-452. Am J Pathol 130:147–155, 1988.

116. Dyer CA, Hickey WF, and Geissert EE Jr: Myelin/oligodendrocyte-specific protein: a novel surface membrane protein that associates with microtubules. J Neurosci Res 28:607–613,1991.

117. Einstein ER, and Csejtey J: Degradation of encephalitogen by purified brain acid proteinase. FEBS Lett 3:191–195, 1968.

118. Einstein ER, Csejtey J, Dalal KB, Adams CWM, Bayliss OB, and Hallpike JF: Proteolytic activity and basic protein loss in and around multiple sclerosis plaques: Combined biochemical and histochemical observations. J Neurochem 19:653–662, 1972.

119. Einstein ER, Dalal KB, and Csejtey J: Increased protease activity and changes in basic proteins and lipids in multiple sclerosis plaques. J Neurol Sci 11:109–121, 1970.

120. Eldridge R, Anayiotos CP, Schlesinger S, et al: Hereditary adult-onset leukodystrophy simulating chronic progressive multiple sclerosis. N Engl J Med 311:948–953, 1984.

121. Ellison MD, Krieg RJ, and Povlishock JT: Differential central nervous system responses following single and multiple recombinant interleukin-2 infusions. J Neuroimmunol 28:249–260, 1990.

122. Engell T: A clinico-pathoanatomical study of multiple sclerosis diagnosis. Acta Neurol Scand 78: 39–44, 1988.

123. Engell T: A clinical patho-anatomical study of clincally silent multiple sclerosis. Acta Neurol Scand 79:428–430, 1989.

124. Engell T, Hvidberg A, and Uhrenholdt A: Multiple sclerosis: periphlebitis retinalis et cerebrospinalis: A correlation between periphlebitis retinalis and abnormal technetium brain scintigraphy. Acta Neurol Scand 69:293–297, 1984.

125. Epstein LG, Prineas JW, and Raine CS: Attachment of myelin to coated pits on macrophages in experimental allergic encephalomyelitis. J Neurol Sci 61:341–348, 1983.

126. Esiri MM: Immunoglobulin-containing cells in multiple-sclerosis plaques. Lancet 2:478–480, 1977.

127. Esiri MM: Multiple sclerosis: A quantitative and qualitative study of immunoglobulin-containing cells in the central nervous system. Neuropathol Appl Neurobiol 6:9-21, 1980.

128. Esiri MM, and Reading MC: Macrophage populations associated with multiple sclerosis plaques. Neuropathol Appl Neurobiol 13:451–465, 1987.

129. Estes ML, Rudick RA, Barnett GH, and Ransohoff RM: Stereotactic biopsy of an active multiple sclerosis lesion: Immunocytochemical analysis and neuropathologic correlation with
magnetic resonance imaging. Arch Neurol 47:
1299–1303, 1990.

130. Farrell MA, Kaufmann JCE, Gilbert JJ, Noseworthy JH, Armstrong HA, and Ebers GC: Oligoclonal bands in multiple sclerosis: Clinical-
pathologic correlation. Neurology 35:212–218,
1985.

131. Feigin I, and Ogata J: Schwann cells and peripheral myelin within human central nervous tissues: The mesenchymal character of Schwann
cells. J Neuropathol Exp Neurol 30:603–612,
1971.

132. Feigin I, and Popoff N: Regeneration of myelin
in multiple sclerosis: The role of mesenchymal
cells in such regeneration and in myelin formation in the peripheral nervous system. Neurology 16: 364–372, 1966.

133. ffrench-Constant C, and Raff MC: Proliferating
bipotential glial progenitor cells in adult rat optic nerve. Nature 319:499–502, 1986.

134. Field EJ, Cowshall S, Narang HK, and Bell TM:
Viruses in multiple sclerosis? Lancet 2:280–281,
1972.

135. Field EJ, and Raine CS: Examination of multiple
sclerosis biopsy specimens (abstract). In Third
European Regional Conference on Electron Microscopy. Publishing House of the Czechoslovak
Academy of Sciences, Prague, 1964, p 289.

136. Fog T: The topography of plaques in multiple
sclerosis, with special reference to cerebral
plaques. Acta Neurol Scand Suppl 15:1–161,
1965.

137. Fog T, Hyllested K, and Andersen SR: A case of
benign multiple sclerosis, with autopsy. Acta
Neurol Scand Suppl 51:369–370, 1972.

138. Fontana A, Fierz W, and Wekerle H: Astrocytes
present myelin basic protein to encephalitogenic T-cell lines. Nature 307:273–276, 1984.

139. Fontana A, Kristensen F, Dubs R, Gemsa D, and
Weber E: Production of prostaglandin E and an
interleukin-1 like factor by cultured astrocytes and
C$_6$ glioma cells. J Immunol 129:2413–2419,1982.

140. Forrester C, and Lascelles RG: Association between polyneuritis and multiple sclerosis. J Neurol Neurosurg Psychiatry 42:864–866, 1979.

141. Foster RE, Whalen CC, and Waxman SG: Reor-
ganization of the axon membrane in demyelinated peripheral nerve fibers: Morphological
evidence. Science 210:661–663, 1980.

142. Friede RL: Enzyme histochemical studies in
multiple sclerosis. Arch Neurol 5:433–443,1961.

143. Friede RL, and Knoller M: Quantitative enzyme
profiles of plaques of multiple sclerosis. Experi-
entia 20:130–132, 1964.

144. Fujinami RS: Virus-induced autoimmunity
through molecular mimicry. Ann NY Acad Sci
540:210–217, 1988.

145. Galaburda AM, Waxman SG, Kemper TL, and
Jones HR: Progressive multifocal neurologic
deficit with disseminated subpial demyelination. J Neuropathol Exp Neurol 35:481–494,
1976.

146. Garbern J, Spence AM, and Alvord EC Jr: Balo's
concentric demyelination diagnosed premortem.
Neurology 36:1610–1614, 1986.

147. Gault F: De la neuromyélite optique aiguë. Thesis, Lyon 1894.

148. Gay D, and Esiri M: Blood-brain barrier damage
in acute multiple sclerosis plaques: An immuno-
cytological study. Brain 114:557–572, 1991.

149. Gendelman HE, Pezeshkpour GH, Pressman NJ,
et al: A quantitation of myelin-associated glycoprotein and myelin basic protein loss in different demyelinating diseases. Ann Neurol 18:324–
328, 1985.

150. Georgi W: Multiple Sklerose. Pathologisch-
anatomische Befunde multipler Sklerose bei
klinisch nicht diagnostizierten Krankheiten.
Schweiz Med Wochenschr 91:605–607, 1961.

151. Germain RN: Antigen processing and presentation. In Paul WE (ed): Fundamental Immunology, ed 3. Raven Press, New York, 1993, pp629–
676.

151a. Gerritse K, Deen C, Fasbender M, Ravid R,
Boersma W and Claassen E: The involvement of
specific anti myelin basic protein antibody-
forming cells in multiple sclerosis. J Neuroimmunol 49:153–159, 1994.

151b. Gerritse K, Laman JD, Noell RJ, et al: CD40-
CD40 ligand interactions in experimental aller-
gic encephalomyelitis and multiple sclerosis.
Proc Natl Acad Sci USA 93:2499–2504, 1996.

152. Gerstl B, Eng LF, Tavaststjerna M, Smith JK, and
Kruse SL: Lipids and proteins in multiple sclerosis white matter. J Neurochem 17:677–689,
1970.

153. Gerstl B, Kahnke MJ, Smith JK, Tavaststjerna MG,
and Hayman RB: Brain lipids in multiple sclerosis and other diseases. Brain 84:310–319,1961.

154. Ghandour MS, Vincendon G, Gombos G, et al:
Carbonic andydrase and oligodendroglia in developing rat cerebellum: A biochemical and im-
munohistologic study. Dev Biol 77:73–83, 1980.

155. Gharagozloo AM, Poe LB, and Collins GH: Antemortem diagnosis of Baló concentric sclerosis:
correlative MR imaging and pathologic features. Radiology 191:817–819, 1994.

156. Ghatak NR: Occurance of oligodendrocytes
within astrocytes in demyelinating lesions. J
Neuropathol Exp Neurol 51:40–46, 1992.

157. Ghatak NR, Hirano A, Doron Y, and Zimmerman HM: Remyelination in multiple sclerosis
with peripheral type myelin. Arch Neurol
29:262–267, 1973.

158. Ghatak NR, Hirano A, Lijtmaer H, and Zimmerman HM: Asymptomatic demyelinated plaque.
Arch Neurol 30:484–486, 1974.

159. Ghatak NR, Leshner T, Price AC, and Felton WL
III: Remyelination in the human central nervous system. J Neuropathol Exp Neurol 48:507–
518, 1989.

160. Gilbert JJ, and Sadler M: Unsuspected multiple
sclerosis. Arch Neurol 40:533–536, 1983.

161. Gonatas NK: Ultrastructural observation in a case
of multiple sclerosis (abstract). J Neuropathol
Exp Neurol 29:149, 1970.

162. Göpfert E, Pytlik S, and Debuch H: 2',3'-cyclic
nucleotide 3'-phosphohydrolase and lipids of

myelin from multiple sclerosis and normal brains. J Neurochem 34:732–739, 1980.

163. Gray F, Léger JM, Duyckaerts C, and Bor Y: Sclérose concentrique de Bal: Lésions uniquement pontines. Rev Neurol (Paris) 141:43–45,1985.

164. Grcevic N: Concentric lacunar leukoencephalopathy. Arch Neurol 2:266–273, 1960.

165. Greenfield JG, and King LS: Observations on the histopathology of the cerebral lesions in disseminated sclerosis. Brain 59:445–458, 1936.

166. Grinspan JB, Stern JL, Pustilnik SM, and Pleasure D: Cerebral white matter contains PDGF-responsive precursors to O2A cells. J Neurosci 10: 1866–1873, 1990.

167. Grossman RG, and Seregin A: Glial-neural interaction demonstrated by the injection of Na$^+$ and Li$^+$ into cortical glia. Science 195:196–198, 1977.

168. Grundke-Iqbal I, and Bornstein MB: Multiple sclerosis: Serum gamma globulin and demyelination in organ culture. Neurology 30:749–754, 1980.

169. Gumpel M, Gout O, Lubetzki C, Gansmuller A, and Baumann N: Myelination and remyelination in the central nervous system by transplanted oligodendrocytes using the shiverer model: Discussion on the remyelinating cell population in adult mammals. Dev Neurosci 11:132–139, 1989.

170. Guo Yu-pu, and Gao Shu-fang: Concentric sclerosis: Report of a case with light and electron microscopic examination. Chin Med J (Engl) 95:884–890, 1982.

171. Guseo A, and Jellinger K: The significance of perivascular infiltrations in multiple sclerosis. J Neurol 211:51–60, 1975.

171a. Hafler DA, Saadeh MG, Kuchroo VK, Milford E, and Steinman L: TCR usage in human and experimental demyelinating disease. Immunol Today 17:152–159, 1996.

172. Haljamäe H, and Hamberger A: Potassium accumulation by bulk prepared neuronal and glial cells. J Neurochem 18:1903–1912, 1971.

173. Halliday AM, and McDonald WI: Pathophysiology of demyelinating disease. Br Med Bull 33: 21–27, 1977.

174. Halliday AM, McDonald WI, and Mushin J: Visual evoked response in diagnosis of multiple sclerosis. BMJ 4:661–664, 1973.

175. Hallpike JF, and Adams CWM: Proteolysis and myelin breakdown: a review of recent histochemical and biochemical studies. Histochem J 1:559–578, 1969.

176. Hallpike JF, Adams CWM, and Bayliss OB: Histochemistry of myelin. VIII. Proteolytic activity around multiple sclerosis plaques. Histochem J 2:199–208, 1970.

177. Hallpike JF, Adams CWM, and Bayliss OB: Histochemistry of myelin. X. Proteolysis of normal myelin and release of lipid by extracts of degenerating nerve. Histochem J 2:315–321, 1970.

178. Hallpike JF, Adams CWM, and Bayliss OB: Histochemistry of myelin. XI. Loss of basic protein in early myelin breakdown and multiple sclerosis plaques. Histochem J 2:323–328, 1970.

179. Harper CG (ed): Diagnostic dilemma: Acute central nervous system disorder mimicking stroke. Med J Aust 1:136–138, 1981.

180. Harrison BM: Remyelination in the central nervous system. In Hallpike JF, Adams CWM, and Tourtellotte WW (eds): Multiple sclerosis: Pathology, Diagnosis and Management. Williams and Wilkins, Baltimore, 1983, pp461–478.

181. Hartman BK, Agrawal HC, Agrawal D, and Kalmbach S: Development and maturation of central nervous system myelin: comparison of immunohistochemical localization of proteolipid protein and basic protein in myelin and oligodendrocytes. Proc Natl Acad Sci USA 79:4217–4220, 1982.

182. Hartung H-P, Hadding U, Bitter-Suermann D, and Gemsa D: Release of prostaglandin E and thromboxane from macrophages by stimulation with factor H. Clin Exp Immunol 56:453–458, 1984.

183. Hassin GB: Neuroptic myelitis versus multiple sclerosis: A pathologic study. Archives of Neurology and Psychiatry 37:1083–1099, 1937.

184. Hassler R, Bronisch F, Mundiger F, and Riechert T: Intention myoclonus of multiple sclerosis, its patho-anatomical basis and its stereotactic elief. Neurochirurgia (Stuttg) 18:90–106, 1975.

185. Hasson J, Terry RD, and Zimmerman HM: Peripheral neuropathy in multiple sclerosis. Neurology 8:503–510, 1958.

186. Hauser SL, Bhan AK, Gilles FH, Hoban CJ, Reinherz EL, Schlossman SF, and Weiner HL: Immunohistochemical staining of human brain with monoclonal antibodies that identify lymphocytes, monocytes and the Ia antigen. J Neuroimmunol 5:197–205, 1983.

187. Hauser SL, Bhan AK, Gilles F, Kemp M, Kerr C, and Weiner HL: Immunohistochemical analysis of the cellular infiltrate in multiple sclerosis lesions. Ann Neurol 19:578–587, 1986.

188. Hawkins CP, Munro PMG, Mackenzie F, Kesselring J, Tofts PS, duBoulay EPGH, Landon DN, and McDonald WI: Duration and selectivity of blood-brain barrier breakdown in chronic relapsing experimental allergic encephalomyelitis studied by gadolinium-DTPA and protein markers. Brain 113:365–378, 1990.

189. Hayashi T, Morimoto C, Burks JS, Kerr C, and Hauser SL: Dual-label immunocytochemistry of the active multiple sclerosis lesion: Major histocompatibility complex and activation antigens. Ann Neurol 24:523–531, 1988.

190 Hayes GM, Woodroofe MN, and Cuzner ML: Microglia are the major cell type expressing MHC Class II in human white matter. J Neurol Sci 80:25–37, 1987.

191. Hedrick SM, and Eidelman FJ: T lymphocyte antigen receptors. In Paul WE (ed): Fundamental Immunology, ed 3. Raven Press, New York, 1993, pp 383–420.

192. Henn FA, Haljamäe A, and Hamberger A: Glial cell function: Active control of extracellular K$^+$ concentration. Brain Res 43:437–443, 1972.

193. Herndon RM, Rubinstein LJ, Freeman JM, and Mathieson G: Light and electron microscopic observations on Rosenthal fibers in Alexander's disease and in multiple sclerosis. J Neuropathol Exp Neurol 29:524–551, 1970.

194. Hertz L: Neuronal-astrocytic interactions in brain development, brain function and brain disease. In Timiras PS, Privat A, Giacobini E, Lauder J, and Vernadakis A (eds): Plasticity and Regeneration of the Nervous System: Advances in Experimental Medicine and Biology, Vol 296. Plenum, New York, 1991, pp 143–159.

195. Hickey WF: T-Lymphocyte entry and antigen recognition in the central nervous system. In Ader R, Felten DA, and Cohen N (eds): Psychoneuroimmunology, ed 2. Academic Press, San Diego, 1991, pp 149–175.

196. Hickey WF, and Kimura H: Perivascular microglial cells of the CNS are bone marrow-derived and present antigen in vivo. Science 239: 290–292, 1988.

197. Hill TJ: Letter to the Editors. J Neurol Sci 20: 471–472, 1973.

198. Hirsch HE, Blanco CE, and Parks ME: Glycerol phosphate dehydrogenase: Reduced activity in multiple sclerosis plaques confirms localization in oligodendrocytes. J Neurochem 34:760–762, 1980.

199. Hirsch HE, Blanco CE, and Parks ME: Fibrinolytic activity of plaques and white matter in multiple sclerosis. J Neuropathol Exp Neurol 40:271–280, 1981.

200. Hirsch HE, Duquette P, and Parks ME: The quantitative histochemistry of multiple sclerosis plaques: Acid proteinase and other acid hydrolases. J Neurochem 26:505–512, 1976.

201. Hirsch HE, and Parks ME: A thiol proteinase highly elevated in and around the plaques of multiple sclerosis. Some biochemical parameters of plaque activity and progression. J Neurochem 32:505–513, 1979.

202. Hofman FM, Hinton DR, Johnson K, and Merrill JE: Tumor necrosis factor identified in multiple sclerosis brain. J Exp Med 170:607–612, 1989.

203. Hofman FM, von Hanwehr RI, Dinarello CA, Mizel SB, Hinton D, and Merrill JE: Immunoregulatory molecules and IL2 receptors identified in multiple sclerosis brain. J Immunol 136:3239– 3245, 1986.

204. Hösli E, and Hösli L: Receptors for neurotransmitters on astrocytes in the mammalian central nervous system. Prog Neurobiol 40:477–506, 1993.

205. Howard MC, Miyajima A, and Coffman R: T-cell-derived cytokines and their receptors. In Paul WE (ed): Fundamental Immunology, ed 3. Raven Press, New York, 1993, pp 763–800.

206. Hunter SB, Ballinger WE Jr, and Rubin JJ: Multiple sclerosis mimicking primary brain tumor. Arch Pathol Lab Med 111:464–468, 1987.

206a. Huterer SJ, Tourtellotte WW, and Wherrett JR: Alterations in the activity of phospholipases A_2 in post-mortem white matter from patients with multiple sclerosis. Neurochem Res 20:1335–1343, 1995.

207. Huynh HK, and Dorovini-Zis K: Effects of interferon-γ on primary cultures of human brain microvessel endothelial cells. Am J Pathol 142: 1265–1278, 1993.

207a. Huynh HK, Oger J, and Dorovini-Zis K: Interferon-β down regulates interferon-γ-induced class II MHC molecule expression and morphological changes in primary cultures of human brain microvessel endothelial cells. J Neuroimmunol 60:63–73, 1995.

207b. Hvas J, Oksenberg JR, Fernando J, Steinman L, and Bernard CCA: γδ T cell receptor repertoire in brain lesions of patients with multiple sclerosis. J Neuroimmunol 46:225–234, 1993.

208. Ibrahim MZM, and Adams CWM: The relationship between enzyme activity and neuroglia in plaques of multiple sclerosis. J Neurol Neurosurg Psychiatry 26:101–110, 1963.

209. Ibrahim MZM, and Adams CWM: The relationship between enzyme activity and neuroglia in early plaques of multiple sclerosis. Journal of Pathology and Bacteriology 90:239–243, 1965.

210. Ikuta F, and Zimmerman HM: Distribution of plaques in seventy autopsy cases of multiple sclerosis in the United States (abstract). Neurology 26:(6 pt 2) 26–28, 1976.

211. Itoyama Y, Ohnishi A, Tateishi J, Kuroiwa Y, and Webster H deF: Spinal cord multiple sclerosis lesions in Japanese patients: Schwann cell remyelination occurs in areas that lack glial fibrillary acidic protein (GFAP). Acta Neuropathol (Berl) 65:217–223, 1985.

212. Itoyama Y, Sternberger NH, Webster H deF, Quarles RH, Cohen SR, and Richardson EP Jr: Immunocytochemical observations on the distribution of myelin-associated glycoprotein and myelin basic protein in multiple sclerosis lesions. Ann Neurol 7:167–177, 1980.

213. Itoyama Y, Tateishi J, and Kuroiwa Y: Atypical multiple sclerosis with concentric or lamellar demyelinated lesions: two Japanese patients studied post mortem. Ann Neurol 17:481–487, 1985.

214. Itoyama Y, Webster H deF, Richardson EP Jr, and Trapp BD: Schwann cell remyelination of demyelinated axons in spinal cord multiple sclerosis lesions. Ann Neurol 14:339–346, 1983.

215. Jankovic J, Derman H, and Armstrong D: Haemorrhagic complications of multiple sclerosis. J Neurol Neurosurg Psychiatry 43:76–81, 1980.

216. Jensen TS, Rasmussen P, and Reske-Nielsen E: Association of trigeminal neuralgia with multiple sclerosis: Clinical and pathological features. Acta Neurol Scand 65:182–189, 1982.

217. Johnson D, Sato S, Quarles RH, Inuzuka T, Brady RO, and Tourtellotte WW: Quantitation of the myelin-associated glycoprotein in human nervous tissue from controls and multiple sclerosis patients. J Neurochem 46:1086–1093, 1986.

218. Kalyan-Raman UP, Garwacki DJ, and Elwood PW: Demyelinating disease of corpus callosum presenting as glioma on magnetic resonance scan: A case documented with pathological findings. Neurosurgery 21:247–250, 1987.

219. Katz D, Taubenberger JK, Cannella B, McFarlin DE, Raine CS, and McFarland HF: Correlation between magnetic resonance imaging and lesion development in chronic, active multiple sclerosis. Ann Neurol 34:661–669, 1993.

220. Kepes JJ: Large focal tumor-like demyelinating lesions of the brain: Intermediate entity between multiple sclerosis and acute disseminated encephalomyelitis? A study of 31 patients. Ann Neurol 33:18–27, 1993.

221. Keuter EJW: Polyneuritis and multiple sclerosis. Psychiatria, Neurologia, Neurochirurgia 70:271–279, 1967.

222. Kim SU: Human oligodendrocytes in culture: Biology and immunology. In Kim SU (ed): Myelination and Demyelination: Implications for Multiple Sclerosis. Plenum, New York, 1989,pp 1–15.

223. Kirk J: The fine structure of the CNS in multiple sclerosis. II. Vesicular demyelination in an acute case. Neuropathol Appl Neurobiol 5:289–294, 1979.

224. Kirk J: Pseudoviral hollow-cored vesicles in multiple sclerosis brain. Acta Neuropathol (Berl) 48:63–66, 1979.

225. Kirk J, and Hutchinson WM: The fine structure of the CNS in multiple sclerosis: I. Interpretation of cytoplasmic papovavirus-like and paramyxovirus-like inclusions. Neuropathol Appl Neurobiol 4:343–356, 1978.

226. Koles ZJ, and Rasminsky M: A computer simulation of conduction in demyelinated nerve fibers. J Physiol (Lond) 227:351–364, 1972.

227. Koopmans RA, Li DKB, Oger JJF, Mayo J, and Paty DW: The lesion of multiple sclerosis: Imaging of acute and chronic stages. Neurology 39:959–963, 1989.

228. Kruse J, Mailhammer R, Wernecke H, et al: Neural cell adhesion molecules and myelin-associated glycoprotein share a common carbohydrate moiety recognized by monoclonal antibodies L2 and HNK-1. Nature 311:153–155, 1984.

229. Kurihara T, and Tsukada Y: The regional and subcellular distribution of 2',3'-cyclic nucleotide 3'- phosphohydrolase in the central nervous system. J Neurochem 14:1167–1174, 1967.

230. Kuroiwa Y: Concentric sclerosis. In Koetsier JC (ed): Demyelinating Diseases. Handbook of Clinical Neurology, Vol 3 (47). Elsevier, Amsterdam, 1985, pp 409–417.

231. Kuroiwa Y: Neuromyelitis optica (Devic's disease, Devic's syndrome). In Koetsier JC (ed): Demyelinating Diseases. Handbook of Clinical Neurology, Vol 3 (47). Elsevier, Amsterdam, 1985, pp 397–408.

232. Kwon EE, and Prineas JW: Blood-brain barrier abnormalities in longstanding multiple sclerosis lesions: An immunohistochemical study. J Neuropathol Exp Neurol 53:625–636, 1994.

233. Lafontaine S, Rasminsky M, Saida T, and Sumner AJ: Conduction block in rat myelinated fibres following acute exposure to anti-galactocerebroside serum. J Physiol (Lond) 323:287–306, 1982.

234. Lampert F, and Lampert P: Multiple sclerosis. Morphologic evidence of intranuclear paramyxovirus or altered chromatin fibers (editorial)? Arch Neurol 32:425–427, 1975.

235. Lampert PW: Fine structure of the demyelinating process. In Hallpike JF, Adams CWM, and

236. Tourtellotte WW (eds): Multiple Sclerosis: Pathology, Diagnosis and Management. Williams and Wilkins, Baltimore, 1983, pp29–46.

236. Lassman H: Comparative Neuropathology of Chronic Experimental Allergic Encephalomyelitis and Multiple Sclerosis. Springer-Verlag, Berlin, 1983.

237. Lassman H (ed): Symposium: Inflammation and the blood-brain barrier. Brain Pathol 1:88-123, 1991.

238. Lassman H, Budka H, and Schnaberth G: Inflammatory demyelinating polyradiculitis in a patient with multiple sclerosis. Arch Neurol 38:99–102, 1981.

239. Lassman H, Suchanek G, and Ozawa K: Histopathology and the blood-cerebrospinal fluid barrier in multiple sclerosis. Ann Neurol 36:S42-S46, 1994.

240. Lazar ML, and Kirkpatrick JB: Trigeminal neuralgia and multiple sclerosis: Demonstration of the plaque in an operative case. Neurosurgery 5:711– 717, 1979.

241. Lebow S, Anderson DC, Mastri A, and Larson D: Acute multiple sclerosis with contrast-enhancing plaques. Arch Neurol 35:435–439, 1978.

242. Lee SC, Cross AH, and Raine CS: High endothelial venule antigen expression in multiple sclerosis lesions (abstract). J Neuropathol Exp Neurol 49:288, 1990.

243. Lee SC, Moore GRW, Golenwsky G, and Raine CS: Multiple sclerosis: A role for astroglia in active demyelination suggested by Class II MHC expression and ultrastructural study. J Neuropathol Exp Neurol 49:122–136, 1990.

244. Lee SC, and Raine CS: Multiple sclerosis: Oligodendrocytes in active lesions do not express major histocompatibility complex molecules. J Neuroimmunol 25:261–266, 1989.

245. Leveille PJ, McGinnis JF, Maxwell DS, and de Vellis J: Immunocytochemical localization of glycerol-3-phosphate dehydrogenase in rat oligodendrocytes. Brain Res 196:287–305, 1980.

246. Lhermitte F, Escourolle R, Cathala F, Hauw J-J, and Marteau R: Étude neuropathologique d'un cas de sclérose en plaques: Discussion de la nature virale de particules observées en microscopie électronique sur une biopsie cérébrale et sur cultures cellulaires. Rev Neurol (Paris) 129: 3–19, 1973.

246a. Li H, Newcombe J, Groome NP, and Cuzner ML: Characterization and distribution of phagocytic macrophages in multiple sclerosis plaques. Neuropathol Appl Neurobiol 19:214–223, 1993.

247. Ludwin SK: An autoradiographic study of cellular proliferation in remyelination of the central nervous system. Am J Pathol 95:683–696, 1979.

248. Ludwin SK: Remyelination in the central nervous system and the peripheral nervous system. In Waxman SG (ed): Functional Recovery in Neurological Disease. Advances in Neurology, Vol 47. Raven Press, New York, 1988, pp 215–254.

249. Ludwin SK, and Johnson ES: Evidence for a "dying-back" gliopathy in demyelinating disease. Ann Neurol 9:301–305, 1981.

250. Ludwin SK, and Sternberger NH: An immuno-histochemical study of myelin proteins during remyelination in the central nervous system. Acta Neuropathol (Berl) 63:240–248, 1984.

251. Lumsden CE: Fundamental problems in the pathology of multiple sclerosis and allied demyelinating diseases. BMJ 1:1035–1043, 1951.

252. Lumsden CE: The neuropathology of multiple sclerosis. In Vinken PJ, and Bruyn GW (eds): Multiple Sclerosis and Other Demyelinating Diseases. Handbook of Clinical Neurology, Vol 9. North-Holland, Amsterdam, 1970, pp 217–309.

253. Lumsden CE: The immunogenesis of the multiple sclerosis plaque. Brain Res 28:365–390, 1971.

254. Lumsden CE, Howard L, Aparicio SR, and Bradbury M: Anti-synaptic antibody in allergic encephalomyelitis. II. The synapse-blocking effects in tissue culture of demyelinating sera from experimental allergic encephalomyelitis. Brain Res 93:283–299, 1975.

255. Macchi G: The pathology of the blood vessels in multiple sclerosis. J Neuropathol Exp Neurol 13:378–384, 1954.

256. Mackay RP, and Hirano A: Forms of benign multiple sclerosis: Report of two "clinically silent" cases discovered at autopsy. Arch Neurol 17:588–600, 1967.

256a. Maeda A and Sobel RA: Matrix metalloproteinases in the normal human central nervous system, microglial nodules, and multiple sclerosis lesions. J Neuropathol Exp Neurol 55:300–309, 1996.

256b. Malmgren RM, Detels R, and Verity MA: Co-occurrence of multiple sclerosis and glioma–Case report and neuropathologic and epidemiologic review. Clin Neuropathol 3:1–9, 1984.

257. Mandler RN, Davis LE, Jeffery DR, and Kornfeld M: Devic's neuromyelitis optica: a clinicopathological study of 8 patients. Ann Neurol 34:162–168, 1993.

258. Marburg O: Die sogenannte "akute multiple sklerose" (Encephalomyelitis periaxialis scleroticans). Jahrbücher Für Psychiatrie und Neurologie 27:213–312, 1906.

259. Mastrostefano R, Occhipinti E, Bigotti G, and Pompili A: Multiple sclerosis plaque simulating cerebral tumor: Case report and review of the literature. Neurosurgery 21:244–246, 1987.

260. Matthews N: Production of anti-tumor cytotoxin by human monocytes. Immunology 44:135–142, 1981.

261. Mattiace LA, Davies P, and Dickson DW: Detection of HLA-DR on microglia in the human brain is a function of both clinical and technical factors. Am J Pathol 136:1101–1114, 1990.

262. McAlpine D, Lumsden CE, and Acheson ED: Multiple sclerosis—A Reappraisal. ed 2. Churchill Livingstone, Edinburgh, 1972.

263. McCallum K, Esiri MM, Tourtellotte WW, and Booss J: T cell subsets in multiple sclerosis: Gradients at plaque borders and differences in non-plaque regions. Brain 110:1297–1308, 1987.

264. McCarron RM, Spatz M, Kempski O, Hogan RN, Muehl L, and McFarlin DE: Interaction between myelin basic protein-sensitized T lymphocytes and murine cerebral vascular endothelial cells. J Immunol 137:3428-3435, 1986.

265. McDonald WI: Pathophysiology in multiple sclerosis. Brain 97:179–196, 1974.

266. McDonald WI: Remyelination in relation to clinical lesions of the central nervous system. Br Med Bull 30:186–189, 1974.

267. McDonald WI: The symptomatology of tumors of the anterior visual pathways. Can J Neurol Sci 9: 381–390, 1982.

268. McDonald WI: The pathophysiology of multiple sclerosis. In McDonald WI, and Silberberg DH (eds): Multiple Sclerosis. Butterworths, London, 1986, pp 112–133.

269. McDonald WI: The pathological and clinical dynamics of multiple sclerosis. J Neuropathol Exp Neurol 53:338–343, 1994.

270. McDonald WI, and Sears TA: The effects of experimental demyelination on conduction in the central nervous system. Brain 93:583–598, 1970.

271. McFarlin DE, and McFarland HF: Multiple sclerosis. N Engl J Med 307:1183–1188, 1246–1251,1982.

272. McGarry RC, Riopelle RJ, Frail DE, Edwards AM, Braun PE, and Roder JC: The characterization and cellular distribution of a family of antigens related to myelin associated glycoprotein in the developing nervous system. J Neuroimmunol 10: 101–114, 1985.

273. McGeer PL, Itagaki S, Tago H, and McGeer EG: Reactive microglia in patients with senile dementia of the Alzheimer type are positive for the histocompatibility glycoprotein HLA-DR. Neurosci Lett 79:195–200, 1987.

274. McKeown SR, and Allen IV: The cellular origin of lysosomal enzymes in the plaque in multiple sclerosis: A combined histological and biochemical study. Neuropathol Appl Neurobiol 4:471–482, 1978.

275. Mehler MF, and Rabinowich L: Inflammatory myelinoclastic diffuse sclerosis. Ann Neurol 23:413–415, 1988.

276. Meiri H, Pri-Chen S, and Korczyn AD: Sodium channel localization in rat sciatic nerve following lead-induced demyelination. Brain Res 359:326–331, 1985.

277. Mendell JR, Kolkin S, Kissel JT, Weiss KL, Chakeres DW, and Rammohan K: Evidence for central nervous system demyelination in chronic inflammatory demyelinating polyradiculoneuropathy. Neurology 37:1291–1294, 1987.

278. Mendez MF, and Pogacar S: Malignant monophosic multiple sclerosis or "Marburg's disease." Neurology 38:1153–1155, 1988.

278a. Merrill JE, Ignarro LJ, Sherman MP, Melinek J, and Lane TE: Microglial cell cytotoxicity of oligodendrocytes is mediated through nitric oxide. J Immunol 151:2132–2141, 1993.

279. Meyermann R, Korr J, and Wekerle H: Specific target retrieval by encephalitogenic T line cells (abstract). Clin Neuropathol 5:101, 1986.

280. Mikol DD, Gulcher JR, and Stefansson K: The oligodendrocyte-myelin glycoprotein belongs to a distinct family of proteins and contains the HNK-1 carbohydrate. J Cell Biol 110:471–479, 1990.

281. Millar JHD, Zilkha KJ, Langman MJS, et al: Double-blind trial of linoleate supplementation of the diet in multiple sclerosis. BMJ 1:765–768, 1973.

282. Miller DH, Rudge P, Johnson G, et al: Serial gadolinium enhanced magnetic resonance imaging in multiple sclerosis. Brain 111:927–939, 1988.

283. Mirra SS, Miles ML, and Takei J: Paramyxovirus-like particles in three variants of multiple sclerosis (abstract). J Neuropathol Exp Neurol 34:88, 1974.

284. Mirra SS, and Takei Y: Ultrastructural identification of virus in human central nervous system disease. In Zimmerman HM (ed): Progress in Neuropathology, Vol III. Grune & Stratton, New York, 1976, pp 69–88.

284a. Miura H, Mukoyama M, and Kamei N: Multiple sclerosis with bilateral continuous cystic lesions along lateral ventricles and caudate-callosal angles (Wetterwinkel). Clin Neuropathol 12:191–195, 1993.

285. Moll C, Mourre C, Lazdunski M, and Ulrich J: Increase of sodium channels in demyelinated lesions of multiple sclerosis. Brain Res 556:311–316, 1991.

286. Moll C, and Ulrich J: Ion channels in MS-plaques. Schweiz Arch Neurol Psychiatr 140:27–29, 1988.

287. Monge M, Kadiiski D, Jacque CM, and Zalc B: Oligodendroglial expression and deposition of four major myelin constituents in the myelin sheath during development: An in vivo study. Dev Neurosci 8:222–235, 1986.

288. Moore GRW, Boegman RJ, Robertson DM, and Raine CS: Acute stages of batrachotoxin-induced neuropathy: a morphologic study of a sodium-channel toxin. J Neurocytol 15:573–583, 1986.

289. Moore GRW, Kim SU, Chang E, and Kim M: Myelin basic protein does not have a mitogenic effect on adult oligodendrocytes. Acta Neuropathol (Berl) 89:431–437, 1995.

290. Moore GRW, Neumann PE, Suzuki K, Lijtmaer HN, Traugott U, and Raine CS: Balo's concentric sclerosis: new observations on lesion development. Ann Neurol 17:604–611, 1985.

291. Moore GRW, and Raine CS: Immunogold localization and analysis of IgG during immune-mediated demyelination. Lab Invest 59:641–648,1988.

292. Moore GRW, Traugott U, Farooq M, Norton WT, and Raine RS: Experimental autoimmune encephalomyelitis: Augmentation of demyelination by different myelin lipids. Lab Invest 51:416–424, 1984.

293. Moore GRW, Traugott U, and Raine CS: Survival of oligodendrocytes in chronic relapsing experimental autoimmune encephalomyelitis. J Neurol Sci 65:137–145, 1984.

294. Moore GRW, Traugott U, Scheinberg LC, and Raine CS: Tropical spastic paraparesis: A model of virus-induced, cytotoxic T-cell-mediated demyelination? Ann Neurol 26:523–530, 1989.

295. Moore GRW, Traugott U, Stone SH, and Raine CS: Dose-dependency of MBP-induced demyelination in the guinea pig. J Neurol Sci 70:197–205, 1985.

296. Morariu M, and Klutzow WF: Subclinical multiple sclerosis. J Neurol 213:71–76, 1976.

297. Morell P, Quarles RH, and Norton WT: Myelin formation, structure and biochemistry. In Siegel GJ, Agranoff BW, Albers RW, and Molinoff PB (eds): Basic Neurochemistry: Molecular, Cellular and Medical Aspects, ed 5. Raven Press, New York, 1994, pp 117–143.

298. Morimoto C, Letvin NL, Boyd AW, Hagan M, Brown HM, Kornacki MM, and Schlossman SF: The isolation and characterization of the human helper inducer T cell subset. J Immunol 134:3762–3769, 1985.

299. Morris CS, Esiri MM, Spinkle TJ, and Gregson N: Oligodendrocyte reactions and cell proliferation markers in human demyelinating diseases. Neuropathol Appl Neurobiol 20:272–281, 1994.

300. Moscarello M, Wood DD, Ackerley C, and Boulias C: Myelin in multiple sclerosis is developmentally immature. J Clin Invest 94:146–154,1994.

301. Moser HM, Moser AE, Singh I, and O'Neill BP: Adrenoleukodystrophy: survey of 303 cases: biochemistry, diagnosis and therapy. Ann Neurol 16:628–641, 1984.

302. Mourre C, Moll C, Lombet A, and Lazdunski M: Distribution of voltage-dependent Na$^+$ channels identified by high affinity receptors for tetrodotoxin and saxitoxin in rat and human brains: Quantitative autoradiographic analysis. Brain Res 448:128–139, 1988.

303. Mozell RL, and McMorris FA: Insulin-like growth factor-I stimulates regeneration of oligodendrocytes in vitro. Ann NY Acad Sci 540:430–432, 1988.

303a. Murphy S, Simmons ML, Agullo L, et al: Synthesis of nitric oxide in CNS glial cells. Trends Neurosci 16:323–328, 1993.

304. Mussini J-M, Hauw J-J, and Escourolle R: Immunofluorescence studies of intra cytoplasmic immunoglobulin binding lymphoid cells (CILC) in the central nervous system: Report of 32 cases including 19 multiple sclerosis. Acta Neuropathol (Berl) 40:227–232, 1977.

305. Nagara H, Inoue T, Koga T, Kitaguchi T, Tateishi J, and Goto I: Formalin fixed brains are useful for magnetic resonance imaging (MRI) study. J Neurol Sci 81:67–77, 1987.

306. Najbauer J, Pálffy G, and Kuntár L: Positive autoradiographic findings in brains of four MS patients. Acta Neurol Scand 79:476–481, 1989.

307. Namerow NS, and Thompson LR: Plaques, symptoms and the remitting course of multiple sclerosis. Neurology 19:765–774, 1969.

308. Narang HK: Comparative morphology of measles virus and paramyxovirus-like tubules in multiple sclerosis using ruthenium red stain. Neuropathol Appl Neurobiol 7:411–420, 1981.

309. Narang HK, and Field EJ: An electron-microscopic study of multiple sclerosis biopsy material: Some unusual inclusions. J Neurol Sci 18: 287–300, 1973.

310. Narang HK, and Field EJ: Paramyxovirus like tubules in multiple sclerosis biopsy material. Acta Neuropathol (Berl) 25:281–290, 1973.

311. Nelson MJ, Miller SL, McLain LW Jr, and Gold LHA: Multiple sclerosis: Large plaque causing

mass effect and ring sign. J Comput Assist Tomogr 5:892–894, 1981.

312. Nesbit GM, Forbes GS, Scheithauer BW, Okazaki H, and Rodriguez M: Multiple sclerosis: Histopathologic and MR and/or CT correlation in 37 cases at biopsy and three cases at autopsy. Radiology 180:467–474, 1991.

313. Neu I, and Woelk H: Investigations of the lipid metabolism of the white matter in multiple sclerosis: changes in glycero-phosphatides and lipid-splitting enzymes. Neurochem Res 7:727-735, 1982.

314. Neumann PE, Mehler MF, Horoupian DS, and Merriam AE: Atypical psychosis with disseminated subpial demyelination. Arch Neurol 45: 634–636, 1988.

315. Newcombe J, Cuzner ML, Röyttä M, and Frey H: White matter proteins in multiple sclerosis. J Neurochem 34:700–708, 1980.

316. Newcombe J, Glynn P, and Cuzner ML: The immunological identification of brain proteins on cellulose nitrate in human demyelinating disease. J Neurochem 38:267–274, 1982.

317. Newcombe J, Hawkins CP, Henderson CL, et al: Histopathology of multiple sclerosis lesions detected by magnetic resonance imaging in unfixed post mortem central nervous system tissue. Brain 114:1013–1023, 1991.

317a. Newcombe J, Li H, and Cuzner ML: Low density lipoprotein uptake by macrophages in multiple sclerosis plaques: implications for pathogenesis. Neuropathol Appl Neurobiol 20: 152–162, 1994.

318. Noble M, Murray K, Stroobant P, Waterfield MD, and Riddle P: Platelet-derived growth factor promotes division and motility and inhibits premature differentiation of the oligodendrocyte/type-2 astrocyte progenitor cell. Nature 333:560–562, 1988.

319. Norton WT, and Cammer W: Chemical pathology of diseases involving myelin. In Morell P (ed): Myelin, ed 2. Plenum, New York, 1984, pp 369–403.

320. Nyland H, Matre R, and Mørk S: Fc receptors on microglial lipophages in multiple sclerosis (letter). N Engl J Med 302:120–121, 1980.

321. Nyland H, Matre R, Mørk S, Bjerk J-R., and Næss A: T-lymphocyte populations in multiple-sclerosis lesions (Letter to the Editor). N Engl J Med 307:1643–1644, 1982.

322. Nyland H, Mörk S, and Matre R: In-situ characterization of mononuclear cell infiltrates in lesions of multiple sclerosis. Neuropathol Appl Neurobiol 8:403–411, 1982.

323. O'Brien JT, Noseworthy JH, Gilbert JJ, and Karlik SJ: NMR changes in experimental allergic encephalomyelitis: NMR changes precede clinical and pathological events. Magn Reson Med 5: 109–117, 1987.

324. Ogata J, and Feigin I: Schwann cells and regenerated peripheral myelin in multiple sclerosis: An ultrastructural study. Neurology 25:713–716,1975.

325. Oksenberg JR, Panzara MA, Begovich AB, et al: Selection for T-cell receptor Vβ-Dβ-Jβ gene rearrangements with specificity for a myelin basic protein peptide in brain lesions of multiple sclerosis. Nature 362:68–70, 1993.

326. Olsson Y: Mast cells in plaques of multiple sclerosis. Acta Neurol Scand 50:611–618, 1974.

327. Oppenheimer DR: Demyelinating diseases. In Blackwood W, and Corsellis JAN (eds): Greenfield's Neuropathology, ed 3. Edward Arnold, London, 1976, pp 470–499.

328. Oppenheimer DR: The cervical cord in multiple sclerosis. Neuropathol Appl Neurobiol 4:151–162, 1978.

329. Ortiz de Zárate JC, Tamaroff L, Sica REP, and Rodriguez JA: Neuromyelitis optica versus subacute necrotic myelitis: Part II. Anatomical study of two cases. J Neurol Neurosurg Psychiatry 31:641–645, 1968.

330. Otsuka S-I, Nakatsu S, Matsumoto S, et al: Multiple sclerosis simulating brain tumor on computed tomography. J Comput Assist Tomogr 13: 674–678, 1989.

330a. Ozawa K, Suchanek G, Breitschopf H, et al: Patterns of oligodendroglia pathology in multiple sclerosis. Brain 117:1311–1322, 1994.

331. Palmucci L, Anzil AP, and Schiffer D: A case of adrenoleukodystrophy in a girl: Genetic considerations. J Neurol Sci 53:233–240, 1982.

332. Pathak S, and Webb HE: Paramyxovirus-like inclusions in brain of patient with severe multiple sclerosis. Lancet 2:311, 1976.

333. Paty DW: Magnetic resonance imaging in the assessment of disease activity in multiple sclerosis. Can J Neurol Sci 15:266–272, 1988.

333a. Paty DW, Li DKB, the UBC MS/MRI Study Group, and the IFNB Multiple Sclerosis Study Group: Interferon beta-1b is effective in relapsing-remitting multiple sclerosis. II. MRI analysis results of a multicenter, randomized, double-blind, placebo-controlled trial. Neurology 43: 662–667, 1993.

334. Périer O, and Grégoire A: Electron microscopic features of multiple sclerosis lesions. Brain 88: 937–952, 1965.

335. Pestka S, and Baron S: Definition and classification of the interferons. In Pestka S (ed): Interferons: Part A. Methods in Enzymology, Vol 78. Academic Press, New York, 1981, pp 3–14.

336. Peters A, Palay SL, and Webster H deF: The Fine Structure of the Nervous System: Neurons and Their Supporting Cells, ed 3. Oxford University Press, New York, 1991.

337. Peters G: Neuromyelitis optica. In Lubarsch O, Henke F, and Rössle R (eds): Handbuch der speziellen pathologischen Anatomie und Histologie, XIII. IIA. Erkrankungen des zentralen Nervensystems II. Springer-Verlag, Berlin, 1958, pp 630–644.

338. Peters G: Multiple sclerosis. In Minckler J (ed): Pathology of the Nervous System. McGraw-Hill, New York, 1968, pp 821–843.

339. Petrescu A: Histochemistry of lipids in multiple sclerosis. Wien Z Nervenheilk/Suppl II:38–52, 1969.

340. Petrescu A: Progressive oil-spot-like lesion in multiple sclerosis. Acta Neuropathol [Suppl] (Berl) 7:182–184, 1981.

341. Petrescu A, and Marcovici G: Correlation between demyelination stages and vascular reticulin proliferation in multiple sclerosis. Revue Roumaine de Neurologie 8:61–67, 1971.

342. Pette H: Klinische und anatomische Studien: über die Pathogenese der multiplen Sclerose. Deutsche Zeitschrift für Nervenheilkunde 105: 76-132, 1928.

343. Phadke JG, and Best PV: Atypical and clinically silent multiple sclerosis: A report of 12 cases discovered unexpectedly at necropsy. J Neurol Neurosurg Psychiatry 46:414–420, 1983.

344. Pollock M, Calder C, and Allpress S: Peripheral nerve abnormality in multiple sclerosis. Ann Neurol 2:41–48, 1977.

345. Poser CM: Diffuse-disseminated sclerosis in the adult. J Neuropathol Exp Neurol 16:61–78, 1957.

346. Poser CM: Myelinoclastic diffuse sclerosis. In Koetsier JC (ed): Demyelinating Diseases. Handbook of Clinical Neurology, Vol 3 (47). Elsevier, Amsterdam, 1985, pp 419–428.

347. Poser CM: The peripheral nervous system in multiple sclerosis: A review and pathogenetic hypothesis. J Neurol Sci 79:83–90, 1987.

348. Poser CM, Goutières F, Carpentier M-A, and Aicardi J: Schilder's myelinoclastic diffuse sclerosis. Pediatrics 77:107–112, 1986.

349. Poser CM, and van Bogaert L: Natural history and evolution of the concept of Schilder's diffuse sclerosis. Acta psychiatrica et neurologia scandinavica 31:285-331, 1956.

350. Poston RN: Basic proteins bind immunoglobulin G: A mechanism for demyelinating disease? Lancet 1:1268–1271, 1984.

351. Powell HC, and Lampert PW: Pathology of multiple sclerosis. Neurol Clin 1:631–644, 1983.

352. Prineas J: Paramyxovirus-like particles associated with acute demyelination in chronic relapsing multiple sclerosis. Science 178:760–763, 1972.

353. Prineas J: Pathology of the early lesion in multiple sclerosis. Hum Pathol 6:531–554, 1975.

354. Prineas JW: Multiple sclerosis: Presence of lymphatic capillaries and lymphoid tissue in the brain and spinal cord. Science 203:1123–1125, 1979.

355. Prineas JW: The neuropathology of multiple sclerosis. In Koetsier JC (ed): Demyelinating Diseases: Handbook of Clinical Neurology, Vol 3 (47). Elsevier, Amsterdam, 1985, pp 213–257.

356. Prineas JW: Pathology of multiple sclerosis. In Cook SD (ed): Handbook of Multiple Sclerosis. Marcel Dekker, New York, 1990, pp 187–218.

357. Prineas JW: Multiple sclerosis: Pathology of the early lesion. In Herndon RM, Seil FJ (eds): Multiple Sclerosis: Current Status of Research and Treatment. Demos, New York, 1994, pp 113–130.

358. Prineas JW, Barnard RO, Kwon EE, Sharer LR, and Cho E-S.: Multiple sclerosis: Remyelination of nascent lesions. Ann Neurol 33:137–151, 1993.

359. Prineas JW, Barnard RO, Revesz T, Kwon EE, Sharer L, and Cho E-S: Multiple sclerosis: Pathology of recurrent lesions. Brain 116:681–693, 1993.

360. Prineas JW, and Connell F: The fine structure of chronically active multiple sclerosis plaques. Neurology 28(2):68–75, 1978.

361. Prineas JW, and Connell F: Remyelination in multiple sclerosis. Ann Neurol 5:22–31, 1979.

362. Prineas JW, and Graham JS: Multiple sclerosis: capping of surface immunoglobulin G on macrophages engaged in myelin breakdown. Ann Neurol 10:149–158, 1981.

363. Prineas JW, Kwon EE, Cho E-S, and Sharer LR: Continual breakdown and regeneration of myelin in progressive multiple sclerosis plaques. Ann NY Acad Sci 436:11–32, 1984.

364. Prineas JW, Kwon EE, Goldenberg PZ, Cho E-S, and Sharer LR: Interaction of astrocytes and newly formed oligodendrocytes in resolving multiple sclerosis lesions. Lab Invest 63:624–636, 1990.

365. Prineas JW, Kwon EE, Goldenberg PZ, Ilyas AA, Quarles RH, Benjamins JA, and Sprinkle TJ: Multiple sclerosis: Oligodendrocyte proliferation and differentiation in fresh lesions. Lab Invest 61:489–503, 1989.

366. Prineas JW, Kwon EE, Sternberger NH, and Lennon VA: The distribution of myelin-associated glycoprotein and myelin basic protein in actively demyelinating multiple sclerosis lesions. J Neuroimmunol 6:251–264, 1984.

367. Prineas JW, and Raine CS: Electron microscopy and immunoperoxidase studies of early multiple sclerosis lesions (abstract). Neurology 26(6 pt 2):29–32, 1976.

368. Prineas JW, and Raine CS: Mechanism of myelin breakdown in multiple sclerosis (abstract). J Neuropathol Exp Neurol 38:336, 1979.

369. Prineas JW, and Wright RG: Macrophages, lymphocytes and plasma cells in the perivascular compartment in chronic multiple sclerosis. Lab Invest 38:409–421, 1978.

370. Raff MC: Glial cell diversification in the rat optic nerve. Science 243:1450–1455, 1989.

371. Raff MC, Miller RH, and Noble M: A glial progenitor cell that develops in vitro into an astrocyte or an oligodendrocyte depending on culture medium. Nature 303:390–396, 1983.

372. Raine CS: Membrane specialisations between demyelinated axons and astroglia in chronic EAE lesions and multiple sclerosis plaques. Nature 275:326–327, 1978.

373. Raine CS: Multiple sclerosis and chronic relapsing EAE: Comparative ultrastructural neuropathology. In Hallpike JF, Adams CWM, and Tourtellotte WW (eds): Multiple Sclerosis: Pathology, Diagnosis and Management. Williams & Wilkins, Baltimore, 1983, pp 413460.

374. Raine CS: Biology of disease: Analysis of autoimmune demyelination: Its impact upon multiple sclerosis. Lab Invest 50:608–635, 1984.

375. Raine CS: Morphology of myelin and myelination. In Morell P (ed): Myelin, ed 2. Plenum, New York, 1984, pp 1–50.

376. Raine CS: Multiple sclerosis: Immunopathologic mechanisms in the progression and reso-

lution of inflammatory demyelination. In Waksman BH (ed): Immunologic Mechanisms in Neurologic and Psychiatric Disease. Raven Press, New York, 1990, pp 37–54.

377. Raine CS: Demyelinating diseases. In Davis RL, and Robertson DM (eds): Textbook of Neuropathology, ed 2. Williams & Wilkins, Baltimore, 1991, pp 535–620.

378. Raine CS: Multiple sclerosis: A pivotal role for the T cell in lesion development. Neuropathol Appl Neurobiol 17:265–274, 1991.

379. Raine CS: The Dale E. McFarlin memorial lecture: the immunology of the multiple sclerosis lesion. Ann Neurol 36:S61-S72, 1994.

380. Raine CS: Multiple sclerosis: Immune system molecule expression in the central nervous system. J Neuropathol Exp Neurol 53:328–337, 1994.

381. Raine CS, Cannella B, Duijvestijn AM, and Cross AH: Homing to central nervous system by antigen-specific lymphocytes. II. Lymphocyte/endothelial cell adhesion during the initial stages of autoimmune demyelination. Lab Invest 63:476–489, 1990.

382. Raine CS, and Field EJ: Nuclear structures in nerve cells in multiple sclerosis. Brain Res 10: 266–268, 1968.

383. Raine CS, Johnson AB, Marcus DM, Suzuki A, and Bornstein MB: Demyelination in vitro: Absorption studies demonstrate that galactocerebroside is a major target. J Neurol Sci 52:117–131, 1981.

384. Raine CS, Lee SC, Scheinberg LC, Duijvestijn AM, and Cross AH: Adhesion molecules on endothelial cells in the central nervous system: An emerging area in the neuroimmunology of multiple sclerosis. Clin Immunol Immunopathol 57:173–187, 1990.

385. Raine CS, Moore GRW, Hintzen R, and Traugott U: Induction of oligodendrocyte proliferation and remyelination after chronic demyelination: Relevance to multiple sclerosis. Lab Invest 59:467–476, 1988.

386. Raine CS, Powers JM, and Suzuki K: Acute multiple sclerosis: Confirmation of "paramyxovirus-like" intranuclear inclusions. Arch Neurol 30: 39–46, 1974.

387. Raine CS, Schaumburg HH, Snyder DH, and Suzuki K: Intranuclear "paramyxovirus-like" material in multiple sclerosis, adreno-leukodystrophy and Kuf's disease. J Neurol Sci 25:29–41, 1975.

388. Raine CS, and Scheinberg LC: On the immunopathology of plaque development and repair in multiple sclerosis. J Neuroimmunol 20: 189–201, 1988.

389. Raine CS, Scheinberg L, and Waltz JM: Multiple sclerosis: Oligodendrocyte survival and proliferation in an active established lesion. Lab Invest 45:534–546, 1981.

390. Raine CS, and Traugott U: Chronic relapsing experimental autoimmune encephalomyelitis: Ultrastructure of the central nervous system of animals treated with combinations of myelin components. Lab Invest 48:275–284, 1983.

391. Raine CS, Traugott U, Farooq M, Bornstein MB, and Norton WT: Augmentation of immune-mediated demyelination by lipid haptens. Lab Invest 45:174–182, 1981.

392. Raine CS, and Wu E: Multiple sclerosis: remyelination in acute lesions. J Neuropathol Exp Neurol 52:199–204, 1993.

393. Raine CS, Wu E, and Brosnan CF: Heat shock protein 65 (hsp 65) expression in multiple sclerosis (MS) lesions (abstract). J Neuropath Exp Neurol 52:311, 1993.

393a. Raine CS, Wu E, Ivanyi J, Katz D, and Brosnan CF: Multiple sclerosis: A protective or a pathogenic role for heat shock protein 60 in the central nervous system? Lab Invest 75:109–123, 1996.

394. Rasminsky M: The effects of temperature on conduction in demyelinated single nerve fibers. Arch Neurol 28:287–292, 1973.

395. Rasminsky M: Physiology of conduction in demyelinated axons. In Waxman SG (ed): Physiology and Pathobiology of Axons. Raven Press, New York, 1978, pp 361–376.

396. Rasminsky M: Hyperexcitability of pathologically myelinated axons and positive symptoms in multiple sclerosis. In Waxman SG, and Ritchie JM (eds): Demyelinating Disease: Basic and Clinical Electrophysiology. Advances in Neurology, Vol 31. Raven Press, New York, 1981, pp 289–297.

397. Rasminsky M, and Sears TA: Functional consequences of demyelination. J Neurol 236:436–437, 1989.

398. Reinherz EL, and Schlossman SF: The differentiation and function of human T lymphocytes. Cell 19:821–827, 1980.

399. Revesz T, Kidd D, Thompson AJ, Barnard RO, and McDonald WI: A comparison of the pathology of primary and secondary progressive multiple sclerosis. Brain 117:759–765, 1994.

400. Reynolds R, and Wilkin GP: Development of macroglial cells in rat cerebellum. II. An *in situ* immunohistochemical study of oligodendroglial lineage from precursor to mature myelinating cell. Development 102:409–425,1988.

401. Riechert T, Hassler R, Mundiger F, Bronisch F, and Schmidt K: Pathologic-anatomical findings and cerebral localization in stereotactic treatment of extrapyramidal motor disturbances in multiple sclerosis. Confinia Neurologica 37:24–40, 1975.

402. Riekkinen PJ, Palo J, Arstila AU, et al: Protein composition of multiple sclerosis myelin. Arch Neurol 24:545–549, 1971.

403. Riekkinen PJ, Rinne UK, and Arstila AU: Neurochemical and morphological studies on demyelination in multiple sclerosis with special reference to etiological aspects. Zeitschrift für Neurologie 203:91–104, 1972.

404. Riekkinen PJ, Rinne UK, Arstila AU, Kurihara T, and Pelliniemi TT: Studies on the pathogenesis of multiple sclerosis. 2',3'-cyclic nucleotide 3-phosphohydrolase as marker of demyelination and correlation of findings with lysosomal changes. J Neurol Sci 15:113–120, 1972.

405. Rieth KG, DiChiro G, Cromwell LD, et al: Primary demyelinating disease simulating glioma of the corpus callosum: Report of three cases. J Neurosurg 55:620–624, 1981.

406. Rinne UK, Arstila A, and Riekkinen P: Ultrastructural studies of multiple sclerosis brain biopsies. Acta Neurol Scand Suppl 43:237, 1970.

407. Rinne UK, Arstila AU, and Riekkinen PJ: Electron microscopic study on nuclear changes in multiple sclerosis brain biopsies. Acta Neurol Scand 48:529–537, 1972.

408. Rinne UK, Riekkinen PJ, and Arstila AU: Biochemical and electron microscopic alterations in the white matter outside demyelinated plaques in multiple sclerosis. In Leibowitz U (ed): Progress in Multiple Sclerosis. Academic Press, New York, 1972, pp 76–98.

409. Rodriguez M, and Lennon VA: Immunoglobulins promote remyelination in the central nervous system. Ann Neurol 27:12–17, 1990.

409a. Rodriguez M, and Lindsley M: Immunosuppression promotes central nervous system remyelination in chronic virus-induced demyelinating disease. Neurology 42:348–357, 1992.

410. Rodriguez M, and Scheithauer B: Ultrastructure of multiple sclerosis. Ultrastruct Pathol 18:3–13, 1994.

411. Rodriguez M, Scheithauer BW, Forbes G, and Kelly PJ: Oligodendrocyte injury is an early event in lesions of multiple sclerosis. Mayo Clinic Proc 68:627–636, 1993.

412. Rosenbluth J, and Blakemore WF: Structural specializations in cat of chronically demyelinated spinal cord axons as seen in freeze-fracture replicas. Neurosci Lett 48:171–177, 1984.

413. Roussel G, and Nussbaum JL: Comparative localization of Wolfgram W1 and myelin basic proteins in the rat brain during ontogenesis. Histochem J 13:1029–1047, 1981.

414. Roussel J: Sclérose en plaques à évolution subaiguë avec sclérose concentrique pontobulbaire et lésions médullaires atypiques. Acta Neurologica et Psychiatrica Belgica 59:781–787, 1959.

415. Röyttä M, Frey H, Riekkinen P, and Rinne UK: Pathogenesis of multiple sclerosis: Neurochemical and morphological studies on MS biopsies and autopsies. Eur Neurol 14:209–218, 1976.

416. Röyttä M, Frey H, Riekkinen P, and Rinne UK: Topographic analysis of MS and control brains. Adv Exp Med Biol 100:569–583, 1978.

417. Röyttä M, and Latvala M: Diagnostic problems in multiple sclerosis: Two cases with clinical diagnosis of MS showing only a diffusely growing malignant astrocytoma. Eur Neurol 25:197–207, 1986.

418. Sagar HJ, Warlow CP, Sheldon PWE, and Esiri MM: Multiple sclerosis with clinical and radiological features of cerebral tumour. J Neurol Neurosurg Psychiatry 45:802–808, 1982.

419. Sanders V, Conrad AJ, and Tourtellotte WW: On classification of post-mortem multiple sclerosis plaques for neuroscientists. J Neuroimmunol 46:207–216, 1993.

420. Saneto RP, Altman A, Knobler RL, Johnson HM, and deVellis J: Interleukin 2 mediates the inhibition of oligodendrocyte progenitor cell proliferation in vitro. Proc Natl Acad Sci USA 83: 9221–9225, 1986.

421. Saneto RP, and deVellis J: Effect of mitogens in various organs and cell culture conditioned media on rat oligodendrocytes. Dev Neurosci 7:340–350, 1985.

422. Scala G, Kuang YD, Hall RE, Muchmore AV, and Oppenheim JJ: Accessory cell function of human B cells. 1. Production of both interleukin 1-like activity and interleukin 1 inhibitory factor by an EBV-transformed human B cell line. J Exp Med 159:1637–1652, 1984.

423. Schauf CL, and Davis FA: Circulating toxic factors in multiple sclerosis: A perspective. In Waxman SG, and Ritchie JM (eds): Demyelinating Disease: Basic and Clinical Electrophysiology. Raven Press, New York, 1981, pp 267–280.

424. Schaumburg HH, Powers JM, Raine CS, Suzuki K, and Richardson EP Jr: Adrenoleukodystrophy: A clinical and pathological study of 17 cases. Arch Neurol 32:577–591, 1975.

425. Schaumburg HH, Richardson EP, Johnson PC, Cohen RB, Powers JM, and Raine CS: Schilder's disease: Sex-linked recessive transmission with specific adrenal changes. Arch Neurol 27:458–460, 1972.

426. Scheinker IM: Histogenesis of the early lesions of multiple sclerosis. II. Acute multiple sclerosis. Archives of Neurology and Psychiatry 50:171–182, 1943.

427. Schilder P: Zur Kenntnis der sogenannten diffusen Sklerose (Über Encephalitis periaxialis diffusa). Zeitschrift für die gesamte Neurologie und Psychiatrie 10:1–60, 1912.

428. Schilder P: Zur Frage der Encephalitis periaxialis diffusa (sogenannte diffuse Sklerose). Zeitschrift für die gesamte Neurologie und Psychiatrie 15: 359-376, 1913.

429. Schilder P: Die Encephalitis periaxialis diffusa. Archiv für Psychiatrie und Nervenkrankhelten 71:327–356, 1924.

430. Schoene WC, Carpenter S, Behan PO, and Geschwind N: "Onion bulb" formations in the central and peripheral nervous system in association with multiple sclerosis and hypertrophic polyneuropathy. Brain 100:755–773, 1977.

430a. Schwankhaus JD, Katz DA, Eldridge R, Schlesinger S, and McFarland H: Clinical and pathological features of an autosomal dominant, adult-onset leukodystrophy simulating chronic progressive multiple sclerosis. Arch Neurol 51: 757–766, 1994.

431. Scolding NJ, Frith S, Linington C, Morgan BP, Campbell AK, and Compston DAS: Myelin-oligodendrocyte glycoprotein (MOG) is a surface marker of oligodendrocyte maturation. J Neuroimmunol 22:169–176, 1989.

432. Sears ES, McCammon A, Bigelow R, and Hayman LA: Maximizing the harvest of contrast enhancing lesions in multiple sclerosis. Neurology 32: 815–820, 1982.

433. Seil FJ: Tissue culture studies of neuroelectric blocking factors. In Waxman SG, and Ritchie JM (eds): Demyelinating Disease: Basic and Clini-

cal Electrophysiology. Raven Press, New York, 1981, pp 281–288.

434. Seitelberger F: Histochemistry of demyelinating diseases proper including allergic encephalomyelitis and Pelizaeus-Merzbacher's disease. In Cumings JN (ed): Modern Scientific Aspects of Neurology. Edward Arnold, London, 1960, pp 146–187.

435. Seitelberger F: The pathology of multiple sclerosis. Ann Clin Res 5:337–344, 1973.

436. Selmaj K, Bradbury K, and Chapman J: Multiple sclerosis: effects of activated T-lymphocyte-derived products on organ cultures of nervous tissue. J Neuroimmunol 18:255–268, 1988.

437. Selmaj K, Brosnan CF, and Raine CS: Colocalization of lymphocytes bearing γδ T-cell receptor and heat shock protein hsp 65+ oligodendrocytes in multiple sclerosis. Proc Natl Acad Sci USA 88: 6452–6456, 1991.

438. Selmaj K, Raine CS, Cannella B, and Brosnan CF: Identification of lymphotoxin and tumor necrosis factor in multiple sclerosis lesions. J Clin Invest 87:949–954, 1991.

439. Selmaj KW, and Raine CS: Tumor necrosis factor mediates myelin and oligodendrocyte damage in vitro. Ann Neurol 23:339–346, 1988.

440. Sergott RC, Brown MJ, Silberberg DH, and Lisak RP: Antigalactocerebroside serum demyelinates optic nerve in vivo. J Neurol Sci 64: 297–303, 1984.

441. Shaw PJ, Smith NM, Ince PG, and Bates D: Chronic periphlebitis retinae in multiple sclerosis: A histopathological study. J Neurol Sci 77: 147–152, 1987.

442. Shepherd DI, Downie AW, and Best PV: Systemic lupus erythematosus and multiple sclerosis. Transactions of the American Neurological Association 99:173–176, 1974.

443. Shintaku M, Hirano A, and Llena JF: Increased diameter of demyelinated axons in chronic multiple sclerosis of the spinal cord. Neuropathol Appl Neurobiol 14:505–510, 1988.

444. Silberberg DH: Pathogenesis of demyelination. In McDonald WI, and Silberberg DH (eds): Multiple Sclerosis. Butterworths, London, 1986, pp 99–111.

445. Silberberg DH, Manning MC, and Schreiber AD: Tissue culture demyelination by normal human serum. Ann Neurol 15:575–580, 1984.

446. Simpson JF, Tourtellotte WW, Kokmen E, Parker JA, and Itabashi HH: Fluorescent protein tracing in multiple sclerosis brain tissue. Arch Neurol 20:373–377, 1969.

447. Smith AD, and Thompson RHS: Lipids and multiple sclerosis. In Field EJ (ed): Multiple Sclerosis, a Critical Conspectus. University Park Press, Baltimore, 1977, pp 225–244.

448. Smith KA, Lachman LB, Oppenheim JJ, and Favata MF: The functional relationship of the interleukins. J Exp Med 151:1551–1556, 1980.

449. Smith KA, and Ruscetti FW: T cell growth factor and the culture of cloned functional T cells. Adv Immunol 31:137–175, 1981.

450. Smith KJ, Blakemore WF, and McDonald WI: The restoration of conduction by central remyelination. Brain 104:383–404, 1981.

451. Smith KJ, Bostock H, and Hall SM: Saltatory conduction precedes remyelination in axons demyelinated with lysophosphatidyl choline. J Neurol Sci 54:13–31, 1982.

452. Smith KJ, and McDonald WI: Spontaneous and mechanically evoked activity due to central demyelinating lesion. Nature 286:154–155, 1980.

453. Snyder DH, Hirano A, and Raine CS: Fenestrated CNS blood vessels in chronic experimental allergic encephalomyelitis. Brain Res 100: 645–649, 1975.

454. Sobel RA: T-lymphocyte subsets in the multiple sclerosis lesion. Res Immunol 140:208–211, 1989.

455. Sobel RA, and Ames MB: Major histocompatibility complex molecule expression in the human central nervous system: Immunohistochemical analysis of 40 patients. J Neuropath Exp Neurol 47:19–28, 1988.

455a. Sobel RA, Chen M, Maeda A, and Hinojoza JR: Vitronectin and integrin vitronectin receptor localization in multiple sclerosis lesions. J Neuropathol Exp Neurol 54:202–213, 1995.

456. Sobel RA, Collins AB, Colvin RB, and Bhan AK: The *in situ* cellular immune response in acute herpes simplex encephalitis. Am J Pathol 125: 332–338, 1986.

457. Sobel RA, Hafler DA, Castro EE, Morimoto C, and Weiner HL: The 2H4 (CD45R) antigen is selectively decreased in multiple sclerosis lesions. J Immunol 140:2210–2214, 1988.

458. Sobel RA, and Mitchell ME: Fibronectin in multiple sclerosis lesions. Am J Pathol 135:161–168, 1989.

459. Sobel RA, Mitchell ME, and Fondren G: Intercellular adhesion molecule-1 (ICAM-1) in cellular immune reactions in the human central nervous system. Am J Pathol 136:1309–1316, 1990.

460. Sobel RA, Mitchell M, and Rothlein R: Intercellular adhesion molecule-1 (ICAM-1) in central nervous system (CNS) immunopathology (abstract). FASEB J 3:A1320, 1989.

461. Soffer D, and Raine CS: Morphologic analysis of axo-glial membrane specializations in the demyelinated central nervous system. Brain Res 186:301–313, 1980.

462. Spiegel M, Krüger H, Hofmann E, and Kappos L: MRI study of Baló's concentric sclerosis before and after immunosuppressive therapy. J Neurol 236:487–488, 1989.

463. Stansbury FC: Neuromyelitis optica (Devic's disease): Presentation of five cases, with pathologic study, and review of literature. Arch Ophthalmol 42:292–335; 465–501, 1949.

464. Steiner G (ed): Krankheitserreger und Gewebsbefund bei Multiple Sklerose. Springer-Verlag, Berlin, 1931.

465. Sternberger NH, Itoyama Y, Kies MW, and Webster H deF: Immunocytochemical method to identify basic protein in myelin-forming oligodendrocytes of newborn rat CNS. J Neurocytol 7:251–263, 1978.

466. Sternberger NH, Quarles RH, Itoyama Y, and Webster H deF: Myelin-associated glycoprotein demonstrated immunocytochemically in myelin

and myelin-forming cells of developing rat. Proc Natl Acad Sci USA 76:1510–1514, 1979.

467. Stewart WA, Hall LD, Berry K, and Paty DW: Correlation between NMR scan and brain slice data in multiple sclerosis. Lancet 2:412, 1984.

468. Suzuki K, Andrews JM, Waltz JM, and Terry RD: Ultrastructural studies of multiple sclerosis. Lab Invest 20:444–454, 1969.

469. Suzuki K, Kamoshita S, Eto Y, Tourtellotte WW, and Gonatas JO: Myelin in multiple sclerosis: Composition of myelin from normal-appearing white matter. Arch Neurol 28:293–297, 1973.

470. Syková E, Svoboda J, Šimonová Z, and Jendelová P: Role of astrocytes in ionic and volume homeostasis in spinal cord during development and injury. In Yu ACH, Hertz L, Norenberg MD, Syková E, and Waxman SG (eds): Neuronal-Astrocytic Interactions: Implications for Normal and Pathological CNS Function. Progress in Brain Research, Vol 94. Elsevier, Amsterdam, 1992, pp 47–56.

471. Tabira T, and Tateishi J: Neuropathological features of MS in Japan. In Kuroiwa Y, and Kurland LT (eds): Multiple Sclerosis East and West. Kyushu University Press, Fukuoka, Japan, 1982, pp 273–295.

472. Takeuchi T, Schlossman SF, and Morimoto C: The 2H4 molecule but not the T3-receptor complex is involved in suppressor inducer signals in the AMLR system. Cell Immunol 107: 107–114, 1987.

473. Tanaka J, Garcia JH, Khurana R, Kamijyo Y, and Viloria JE: Unusual demyelinating disease: A form of diffuse-disseminated sclerosis. Neurology 25:588–593, 1975.

474. Tanaka R, Iwasaki Y, and Koprowski H: Unusual intranuclear filaments in multiple-sclerosis brain. Lancet 1:1236–1237, 1974.

475. Tanaka R, Iwasaki Y, and Koprowski H: Paramyxovirus-like structures in brains of multiple sclerosis patients. Arch Neurol 32:80–83, 1975.

476. Tanaka R, Iwasaki Y, and Koprowski H: Ultrastructural studies of perivascular cuffing cells in multiple sclerosis brain. Am J Pathol 81:467–478, 1975.

477. Tanaka R, Iwasaki Y, and Koprowski H: Intracisternal virus-like particles in brain of a multiple sclerosis patient. J Neurol Sci 28:121–126, 1976.

478. Tavolato BF: Immunoglobulin G distribution in multiple sclerosis brain: An immunofluorescence study. J Neurol Sci 24:1–11, 1975.

478a. The INFB Multiple Sclerosis Study Group: Interferon beta-1b is effective in relapsing-remitting multiple sclerosis. I. Clinical results of a multicenter, randomized, double-blind, placebo-controlled trial. Neurology 43:655–661, 1993.

479. Thompson AJ, Kermode AG, Wicks D, et al: Major differences in the dynamics of primary and secondary progressive multiple sclerosis. Ann Neurol 29:53–62, 1991.

480. Tobler I, Borbely AA, Schwyzer M, and Fontana A: Interleukin-1 derived from astrocytes enhances slow wave activity in sleep EEG of the rat. Eur J Pharmacol 104:191–192, 1984.

481. Tourtellotte WW, Itabashi HH, and Parker JA: Multifocal areas of synthesis of immunoglobu-lin-G in multiple sclerosis brain tissue and the sink action of the cerebrospinal fluid. Transactions of the American Neurological Association 92:288– 290, 1967.

482. Tourtellotte WW, and Parker JA: Some spaces and barriers in postmortem multiple sclerosis. Prog Brain Res 29:493-525, 1967.

483. Toussaint D, Périer O, Verstappen A, and Bervoets S: Clinicopathological study of the visual pathways, eyes, and cerebral hemispheres in 32 cases of disseminated sclerosis. Journal of Clinical Neuro-Ophthalmology 3:211–220,1983.

484. Traugott U: Characterization and distribution of lymphocyte subpopulations in multiple sclerosis plaques versus autoimmune demyelinating lesions. Springer Seminars in Immunopathology 8:71–95, 1985.

485. Traugott U: Multiple sclerosis: relevance of class I and class II MHC-expressing cells to lesion development. J Neuroimmunol 16:283–302, 1987.

486. Traugott U, Frohman E, and Scheinberg LC: Role of adhesion molecules in the immunopathogenesis of multiple sclerosis lesions (abstract). Neurology 39(suppl 1):171, 1989.

487. Traugott U, and Lebon P: Interferon-γ and Ia antigen are present on astrocytes in active chronic multiple sclerosis lesions. J Neurol Sci 84:257– 264, 1988.

488. Traugott U, and Lebon P: Multiple sclerosis: Involvement of interferons in lesion pathogenesis. Ann Neurol 24:243–251, 1988.

489. Traugott U, Reinherz EL, and Raine CS: Multiple sclerosis: Distribution of T cell subsets within chronic active lesions. Science 219:308–310, 1983.

490. Traugott U, Reinherz EL, and Raine CS: Multiple sclerosis: Distribution of T cells, T cell subsets and Ia-positive macrophages in lesions of different ages. J Neuroimmunol 4:201–221, 1983.

491. Traugott U, Scheinberg LC, and Raine CS: On the presence of Ia-positive endothelial cells and astrocytes in multiple sclerosis lesions and its relevance to antigen presentation. J Neuroimmunol 8:1–14, 1985.

492. Tsudo M, Uchiyama T, and Uchino H: Expression of Tac antigen in activated normal human B cells. J Exp Med 160:612–617, 1984.

492a. Ulvestad E, Williams K, Bø L, Trapp B, Antel J, and Mørk S: HLA class II molecules (HLA-DR, -DP, -DQ) on cells in the human CNS studied *in situ* and *in vitro*. Immunology 82:535–541, 1994.

492b. Ulvestad E, Williams K, Mørk S, Antel J, and Hyland H: Phenotypic differences between human monocytes/macrophages and microglial cells studied *in situ* and *in vitro*. J Neuropathol Exp Neurol 53:492–501, 1994.

492c. Ulvestad E, Williams K, Vedeler C, et al: Reactive microglia in multiple sclerosis lesions have an increased expression of receptors for the Fc part of IgG. J Neurol Sci 121:125–131, 1994.

493. van der Velden M, Bots GTAM, and Endtz LJ: Cranial CT in multiple sclerosis showing a mass effect. Surg Neurol 12:307–310, 1979.

493a. van Noort JM, van Sechel AC, Bajramovic JJ, El Ouagmiri M, Polman CH, Lassmann H, and Ravid R: The small heat-shock protein αβ crystallin as candidate autoantigen in multiple sclerosis. Nature 375:798–801, 1995.

494. Vandvik B, and Reske-Nielsen E: Immunochemical and immunohistochemical studies of brain tissue in subacute sclerosing panencephalitis and multiple sclerosis. Acta Neurol Scand Suppl 51:413–416, 1972.

494a. Vieregge P, Nahser HC, Gerhard L, Reinhardt V, and Nau HE: Multiple sclerosis and cerebral tumor. Clin Neuropathol 3:10–21, 1984.

495. Vinters HV, and Gilbert JJ: Neurenteric cysts of the spinal cord mimicking multiple sclerosis. Can J Neurol Sci 8:159–161, 1981.

496. Vliegenthart WE, Sanders EACM, Bruyn GW, and Vielvoye GJ: An unusual CT-scan appearance in multiple sclerosis. J Neurol Sci 71:129–134, 1985.

497. Vogel FS: Demyelinization induced in living rabbits by means of a lipolytic enzyme preparation. J Exp Med 93:297–304, 1951.

498. Vuia O: The benign form of multiple sclerosis: Anatomo-clinical aspects. Acta Neurol Scand 55:289–298, 1977.

499. Waksman BH: Pathogenetic mechanisms in multiple sclerosis: A summary. Ann NY Acad Sci 436:125–129, 1984.

500. Walton JC, and Kaufmann JCE: Iron deposits and multiple sclerosis. Arch Pathol Lab Med 108:755–756, 1984.

501. Wang A-M, Morris JH, Hickey WF, Hammerschlag SB, O'Reilly GV, and Rumbaugh CL: Unusual CT patterns of multiple sclerosis. AJNR 4:47–50, 1983.

501a. Warren KG, Catz I, Johnson E, and Mielke B: Anti-myelin basic protein and anti-proteolipid protein specific forms of multiple sclerosis. Ann Neurol 35:280–289, 1994.

502. Watanabe I, and Okazaki H: Virus-like structure in multiple sclerosis. Lancet 2:569–570, 1973.

503. Waxman SG: Clinicopathological correlations in multiple sclerosis and related diseases. In Waxman SG, Ritchie JM (eds): Demyelinating Disease: Basic and Clinical Electrophysiology. Advances in Neurology, Vol 31. Raven Press, New York, 1981, pp 169–182.

504. Waxman SG: Biophysical mechanisms of impulse conduction in demyelinated axons. In Waxman SG (ed): Functional Recovery in Neurological Disease. Advances in Neurology, Vol 47. Raven Press, New York, 1988, pp 185–213.

505. Waxman SG: Clinical course and electrophysiology of multiple sclerosis. In Waxman SG (ed). Functional Recovery in Neurological Disease: Advances in Neurology, Vol 47. Raven Press, New York, 1988, pp 157–184.

506. Waxman SG, and Brill MH: Conduction through demyelinated plaques in multiple sclerosis: computer simulations of facilitation by short internodes. J Neurol Neurosurg Psychiatry 41:408–416, 1978.

507. Waxman SG, and Ritchie JM: Organization of ion channels in the myelinated nerve fiber. Science 228:1502–1507, 1985.

508. Webb HE, Pathak S, Oaten S, and Barnard RO: Paramyxovirus-like particles in three severe cases of multiple sclerosis. In Behan PO, and Rose FC (eds): Progress in Neurological Research: with Particular Reference to Motor Neurone Disease. Pitman, London, 1979, pp 79–97.

509. Weiner LP, Waxman SG, Stohlman SA, and Kwan A: Remyelination following viral-induced demyelination: Ferric ion-ferrocyanide staining of nodes of Ranvier within the CNS. Ann Neurol 8:580–583, 1980.

510. Wekerle H, Linington C, Lassman H, and Meyermann R: Cellular immune reactivity within the CNS. Trends Neurosci 9:271–277, 1986.

511. Weller RO: Pathology of multiple sclerosis. In Matthews WB, Acheson ED, Batchelor JR, and Weller RO (eds): McAlpine's Multiple Sclerosis. Churchill Livingstone, Edinburgh, 1985, pp 301–343.

512. Wender M, Filipek-Wender H, and Stanislawska B: Cholesteryl esters in apparently normal white matter in multiple sclerosis. Eur Neurol 10:340–348, 1973.

513. Wender M, and Kozik M: Contribution to the histoenzymatic changes in multiple sclerosis. Acta Neuropathol (Berl) 13:143–148, 1969.

514. Wernecke H, Lindner J, and Schachner M: Cell type specificity and developmental expression of the L2/HNK-1 epitopes in mouse cerebellum. J Neuroimmunol 9:115–130, 1985.

515. Whitaker JN: Myelin encephalitogenic protein fragments in cerebrospinal fluid of persons with multiple sclerosis. Neurology 27:911–920, 1977.

516. Whitaker JN: The distribution of myelin basic protein in central nervous system lesions of multiple sclerosis and acute experimental allergic encephalomyelitis. Ann Neurol 3:291–298, 1978.

517. Willingham MC, and Pastan I: Endocytosis and exocytosis: Current concepts of vesicle traffic in animal cells. Int Rev Cytol 92:51–92, 1984.

518. Willoughby EW, Grochowski E, Li DKB, Oger J, Kastrukoff LF, and Paty DW: Serial magnetic resonance scanning in multiple sclerosis: A second prospective study in relapsing patients. Ann Neurol 25:43–49, 1989.

518a. Windhagen A, Newcombe J, Dangond F, et al: Expression of costimulatory molecules B7-1 (CD80), B7-2 (CD86), and interleukin 12 cytokine in multiple sclerosis lesions. J Exp Med 182:1985–1996, 1995.

519. Wisniewski HM, and Bloom BR: Primary demyelination as a nonspecific consequence of a cell-mediated immune reaction. J Exp Med 141:346–359, 1975.

520. Wisniewski HM, Oppenheimer D, and McDonald WI: Relation between myelination and function in MS and EAE (abstract). J Neuropathol Exp Neurol 35:327, 1976.

521. Wolfgram F, and Tourtellotte WW: Amino acid composition of myelin in multiple sclerosis. Neurology 22:1044–1046, 1972.

522. Wong D, and Dorovini-Zis K: Upregulation of intercellular adhesion molecule-1 (ICAM-1) expression in primary cultures of human brain mi-

crovessel endothelial cells by cytokines and lipopolysaccharide. J Neuroimmunol 39:11–22, 1992.

523. Wood DD, and Moscarello MA: Is the myelin membrane abnormal in multiple sclerosis? J Membr Biol 79:195–201, 1984.

524. Wood PM, and Bunge RP: Evidence that axons are mitogenic for oligodendrocytes isolated from adult animals. Nature 320:756–758, 1986.

525. Woodroofe MN, Bellamy AS, Feldmann M, Davison AN, and Cuzner ML: Immunocytochemical characterization of the immune reaction in the central nervous system in multiple sclerosis: Possible role for micoglia in lesion growth. J Neurol Sci 74:135–152, 1986.

525a. Woodroofe MN, and Cuzner ML: Cytokine mRNA expression in inflammatory multiple sclerosis lesions: detection by non-radioactive in situ hybridization. Cytokine 5:583–588, 1993.

526. Woyciechowska JL, and Brzosko WJ: Immunofluorescence study of brain plaques from two patients with multiple sclerosis. Neurology 27:620–622, 1977.

527. Wu E, Brosnan CF, and Raine CS: SP-40,40 immunoreactivity in inflammatory CNS lesions displaying astrocyte/oligodendrocyte interactions. J Neuropathol Exp Neurol 52:129–134, 1993.

528. Wu E, and Raine CS: Multiple sclerosis: Interactions between oligodendrocytes and hypertrophic astrocytes and their occurrence in other, non-demyelinating conditions. Lab Invest 67:88–99, 1992.

529. Wucherpfennig KW, Newcombe J, Hong L, Keddy C, Cuzner ML, and Hafler DA: γδ T-cell receptor repertoire in acute multiple sclerosis lesions. Proc Natl Acad Sci USA 89:4588–4592, 1992.

530. Wucherpfennig KW, Newcombe J, Li H, Keddy C, Cuzner ML, and Hafler DA: T cell receptor V_α-V_β repertoire and cytokine gene expression in active multiple sclerosis lesions. J Exp Med 175:993–1002, 1992.

531. Wucherpfennig KW, Weiner HL, and Hafler DA: T-cell recognition of myelin basic protein. Immunol Today 12:277–282, 1991.

531a. Wyllie AH: The genetic regulation of apoptosis. Current Opinion in Genetics and Development 5:97–104, 1995.

532. Yanagihara T, and Cumings JN: Alterations of phospholipids, particularly plasmalogens, in the demyelination of multiple sclerosis as compared with that of cerebral oedema. Brain 92:59–70, 1969.

533. Yao D-L, Webster H deF, Hudson LD, et al: Concentric sclerosis (Baló): morphometric and in situ hybridization study of lesions in six patients. Ann Neurol 35:18–30, 1994.

534. Yong VW, Kim SU, Kim MW, and Shin DH: Growth factors from human glial cells in culture. Glia 1:113–123, 1988.

535. Youl BD, Kermode AG, Thompson AJ, et al: Destructive lesions in demyelinating disease. J Neurol Neurosurg Psychiatry 54:288–292, 1991.

536. Yu RK, Ueno K, Glaser GH, and Tourtellotte WW: Lipid and protein alterations of spinal cord and cord myelin of multiple sclerosis. J Neurochem 39:464–477, 1982.

537. Zagzag D, Miller DC, Kleinman GM, Abati A, Donnenfeld H, and Budzilovich GN: Demyelinating disease versus tumor in surgical neuropathology: Clues to a correct pathological diagnosis. Am J Surg Pathol 17:537–545, 1993.

537a. Zajicek J, Wing M, Skepper J, and Compston A: Human oligodendrocytes are not sensitive to complement: A study of CD59 expression in the human central nervous system. Lab Invest 73:128–138, 1995.

538. Zimmerman HM, and Netsky MG: The pathology of multiple sclerosis. Res Publ Assoc Res Nerv Ment Dis 28:271–312, 1950.

539. Zweiman B, and Lisak RP: Lymphocyte phenotypes in the multiple sclerosis lesions— what do they mean (editorial)? Ann Neurol 19:588–589, 1986.

CHAPTER 9

MAGNETIC RESONANCE IMAGING CHANGES AS LIVING PATHOLOGY IN MULTIPLE SCLEROSIS

Donald W. Paty, MD
G. R. Wayne Moore, MD, CM

Magnetic resonance imaging (MRI) provides a powerful new approach to objectively quantitate and characterize the pathology of MS in the living state.[43,78,105,107,131,133] Proton magnetic resonance images, to a considerable extent, reflect the water content of tissue. Differences in water content between cerebral white and gray matter contribute greatly to the exquisite anatomical definition of magnetic resonance images of the brain. The images also reflect alterations in local populations of cells and their aggregate biochemically defined constituents, particularly their lipid content and composition. The pathological features of acute and chronic MS lesions most likely account for the remarkable sensitivity for and variability of appearance of MRI lesions in this disease. Almost three decades ago, Tourtelotte and Parker[176] showed that lipid content of demyelinated plaques was reduced by three-quarters and that the lipid loss was replaced by water so that the fat-free dry weight was unchanged. Gangliosides (an axonal marker) were also reduced in plaques, which suggested axonal loss. More recently, Wilson and colleagues [188] showed that MS plaques contained only 30 percent of the lipid contained in normal white matter. Magnetic resonance spectroscopy (MRS) provides a tool that can identify specific chemicals within regions of interest in the brain, allowing identification of pathological changes as they occur. Lipids associated with the breakdown of myelin, unlike the lipids of normal myelin, which do not produce an MRS signal, should yield detectable MRS signals at short echo times. The pathological changes in MS that cause the prolonged T_1 and T_2 relaxation times obtained from MS lesions are unknown. T_1 is the spin-lattice magnetization decay time. It is determined by the rate at which protons in the body exchange thermal energy. T_1 is said to be sensitive to gliosis. T_2 is the spin-spin relaxation time and is influenced not only by the number of resonating protons present but also by the behavior of the surrounding molecular structure. T_2 abnormalities appear to arise when water protons are increased or have modified resonances owing to outside molecular influences.

Evolving data from comparative pathological, biochemical, and MRI studies of acute and chronic experimental allergic encephomyelitis (EAE) in animals[147,158] and postmortem studies of MS in humans[95,145,146] will likely define the relative contribution of these changes to the MR image of the MS plaque in the near future. In addition, MRS and relaxation techniques have the potential of identifying some of the chemical changes that occur in the evolving MS lesion, permitting an accurate in vivo assessment of MS pathology. Several reviews[105,141,142] have highlighted the contribution of MRI to the understanding of MS pathology.

CLINICAL–MRI CORRELATION (see chapter 12 for details)

T_2-weighted MRI images exquisitely define MS lesions above the level of the mid-cervical cord, and diagnostically abnormal scans can be anticipated in approximately 90 percent of patients with clinically definite MS.[148] Findings on individual MRI scans do not correlate well with clinical status at the time of imaging, as measured by disability status scales,[136] or with the prior clinical course (that is, relapsing-remitting, relapsing progressive, or occult).[99] However, benign[170] and primary chronic progressive disease have somewhat characteristic appearances. Thompson[169] suggested that the pathological process in those forms of MS is different from that seen in the typical relapsing-remitting MS (RRMS) or relapsing progressive MS (RPMS) (secondary progressive MS, SPMS). Koopmans and colleagues[82] were the first to suggest a pattern difference between these two clinical forms, with benign patients (those with RRMS) having spotted single lesions scattered throughout the white matter, and

the patients with chronic progressive MS (CPMS) having confluent periventricular lesions. Gonzalez and colleagues[46] confirmed this finding.

Serial unenhanced imaging over time often shows the accumulation of asymptomatic new lesions and lesion enlargement.[130] Serial studies[66,83,113,187] have shown that the rate of development of asymptomatic new lesions is considerably greater than the rate of clinical activity in patients with both RRMS and RPMS. In contrast to the pattern seen in relapsing patients, the patients with primary CPMS have a low rate of accumulation of new MRI lesions, and these are small and mostly nonenhancing.[171] Because MRI evidence for disease activity is demonstrated much more frequently than clinical evidence in patients with both RRMS and RPMS, it has been proposed that serial and quantitative MRI examinations will aid considerably in the ability to monitor disease activity in MS clinical trials.[109a,111] MRI activity may predict the clinical outcome.

A number of studies have shown significant correlation between MRI measurements and clinical or immunologic measurements or both. *Tofts and Kermode[174] have developed a quantitative measure of gadolinium enhancement to apply to MRI analysis of the extent of MS pathology. Serial MRI examinations would thus provide objective supportive data for clinically documented stabilization or reduction in activity. New lesions likely reflect changes in pathology, which may occur independent of changes in clinical neurologic status.[155] For example, optic nerve pathology can occur without changes in visual acuity.[44] Spinal imaging[108] does not help in the clinical correlation except with cord atrophy. Sensitive neurophysiological tests can reveal correlation with lesions thought otherwise to be silent.[98]

Some of the lack of correlation between MRI and clinical measures may be due to the insensitivity of clinical measures.[98] In a disease such as MS, whose basic pathophysiology includes an autoimmune attack on central nervous system (CNS) myelin, an effective immunomodulatory therapy would be expected to reduce the rate of accum-

---

*References 21, 22, 25, 27, 37, 57, 80, 101, 181, 183.

ulation of new lesions with time. Such an effect has recently been reported.[135] In addition, the correlations between MRI measures, treatment effect, and clinical impairment measures were highly statistically significant.[64] In several studies, the MRI activity rate predicted the clinical outcome.[133a,176a] Spinal cord and cerebral atrophy also correlate with clinical measures.[101a,101b]

In addition, the main reason we use MRI in the diagnosis of MS is the fact that MRI reveals many asymptomatic pre-existing lesions. That concept can support the diagnostic requirement for lesions disseminated in space. It just does not make sense that, at the same time, one can demand a robust correlation between MRI and clinical findings.

PATHOLOGY–MRI CORRELATION

The appearance of MRI lesions seen on coronal MRI slices in patients with MS is reminiscent of the classic appearance of periventricular demyelination seen at autopsy (Fig. 9–1). In fact, parasagittal T_2-weighted views show the corpus callosum and periventricular lesions, with Dawson's fingers (perivenular lesions that radiate out from MS plaques) very well (Fig. 9–2). The appearance on the parasagittal T_2-weighted image is so characteristic that it may be the most diagnostically specific MRI feature of MS (see Chapter 4 for details).

In postmortem pathological–MRI correlation studies, immediate postmortem imaging with the brain in situ and subsequent imaging of formalin-fixed tissue can provide accurate diagnostic information.[160] Figures 9–3 and 9–4 illustrate one pathological correlation in a brain that was formalin-fixed. The reader should note the elegant precision with which the scan reveals even the smallest brain stem lesions. Immediate postmortem cadaver MRI scans with subsequent pathological examination have provided support for the concept that MRI can measure the extent of demyelination. Pathological correlation studies have shown that even small (3 mm) demyelinating lesions can be easily seen on MRI and that areas of partial demyelination (or possibly remyelination) can also easily be seen.[161] MRI can also identify small islands of preserved myelin within large areas of demyelination.

In her studies of postmortem examinations, Stewart[156,160,161] compared the qualitative T_1 and T_2 data on postmortem and fixed brains with the histopathologic features in seven cases. Only lesions that

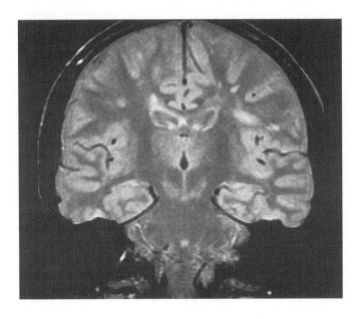

Figure 9–1. This coronal proton density (PD) scan shows how the MS lesions in life look like the periventricular demyelination seen at autopsy. The MS lesions are the bright spots. There are several periventricular ones and one brain stem one. (Figs. 9–1 through 9–11 courtesy of Dr. David Li, Department of Diagnostic Radiology, University of British Columbia.)

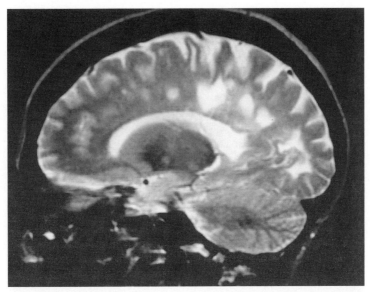

Figure 9–2. This parasagittal T_2-weighted scan shows the periventricular lesions that look like Dawson's fingers seen pathologically.

extended completely through the MRI slice were selected for comparison. T_1 and T_2 measurements were then taken from the geographic center of the selected lesions to ensure the homogeneity of tissue from which the measurements were taken. Neuropathologists who were totally unaware of the MRI quantitative data then graded the degree of histological change in demyelination, inflammation, and gliosis on a scale of

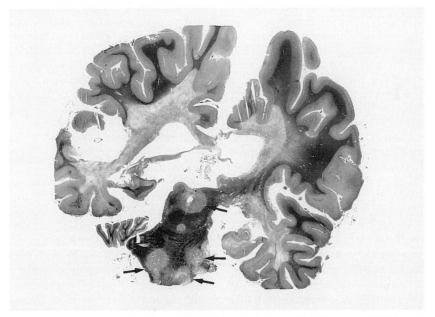

Figure 9–3. This pathological coronal section of the brain stained for myelin shows several distinct demyelinated lesions in the brain stem (*arrows*). Please ignore the hemisphere abnormalities and artifact. The diffuse periventricular demyelination is very complex and hard to interpret. (Photo courtesy of Dr. Wayne Moore, Department of Pathology, Vancouver Hospital and Health Sciences Center.)

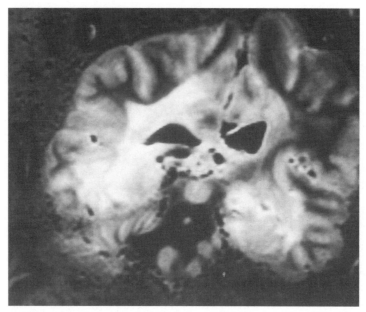

Figure 9–4. This postmortem-fixed brain MRI coronal slice is of the same area as the pathological section seen in Figure 9–3. It shows each of the brain stem lesions seen on the myelin stained section almost exactly. As in Figure 9–3, please ignore the complex hemispheric abnormalities. (Photo courtesy of Dr. Robert Nugent, Department of Diagnostic Radiology, Vancouver Hospital and Health Sciences Center.)

1 to 4. The pathological score was then compared with MRI information obtained from the same lesion. The results showed that in completely demyelinated lesions, the more heavily gliotic ones had the longest T_1 values, confirming the finding that T_1 was sensitive to gliosis.[9,156]

Generally, digitized and matched photographs of the fixed brain slices showed the areas of involvement to be larger on the actual pathological slice than was detected by the postmortem MRI scans. One-centimeter pathological slices were cut so that the plane of the surface of the pathological slice photographed corresponded to the center of the appropriate MRI slice, to minimize errors due to volume averaging. The correlation between the MRI slice and the extent of pathology was very good. The correlation coefficients for well positioned slices were mostly high (R = 0.80 – 0.94). In one case, in the top slice of the pathological specimen, many small lesions appeared near or in the cortex that were completely missed by MRI. The total error in measurement of the extent of lesions varied between 13 percent and 30 percent, slice by slice, when a set of matched digitized pho-

tographs of the fixed tissue were compared with the postmortem MRI scans. The pathological correlation varied, with some slices showing greater and some lesser extent of pathology than did the corresponding MRI slice. The errors seen were thought to be due to lack of resolution or errors in positioning, in addition to volume averaging. In future studies the errors introduced by volume averaging can be minimized by using thin-slice and volumetric techniques.

Ormerod and associates[126] also performed pathological correlation studies on six formalin-fixed MS brains. These investigators reported a good correspondence between the areas of abnormality on the magnetic resonance images and the histopathological findings. Like Stewart, they concluded that the abnormalities seen on the MRI scan originated from chronic plaques of MS. Presumably, the lipid lost by demyelination is replaced by water, and during the process of demyelination, myelin lipid is converted to neutral fat, which is eventually removed by macrophages.[141] Therefore, there is a window in time in which MRS can detect the neutral fat signal and other abnormal signals as markers for myelin breakdown. Although pathological correlation studies have been performed involving established lesions, unfortunately no such studies exist that allow valid conclusions to be drawn concerning new lesions. However, there are case reports of autopsy after CT or MRI in vivo in which an enhancing lesion on imaging was seen on pathological examination to be intensely inflammatory.[33,77] In an extensive analysis of an acute MS lesion identified on MRI scan, Estes and associates[33] reported that the area of demyelination corresponded well with the MRI appearance of the lesion.

In correlating the pathology of MS lesions with magnetic resonance findings, Barnes and colleagues[11] found that the chronic lesions were pathologically heterogeneous. "Open" lesions with an expanded extracellular space comprised the majority of chronic lesions (87 percent). Evidence of blood-brain barrier (BBB) disruption was present in only 17 percent of lesions. Their findings supported the concept that axonal loss increases with the age of the lesions.

Newcombe and co-workers[122] performed MRI scans on 17 unfixed MS brains and six control brains. Chronic plaques were well correlated with the MRI scan appearance. However, in some instances, MRI underestimated the extent of the pathology in these unfixed brains, especially in the posterior fossa. When the MRI was diffusely abnormal, the MRI changes were many times more extensive than the corresponding histological findings. The authors concluded that the extensive MRI changes were due to increased water content in white matter areas that did not have distinct histological plaque formation. Spectroscopic imaging[189] and relaxation analysis[16] studies have also suggested that much of the normal-appearing MS white matter on standard MRI is actually abnormal. It is unknown if this abnormality is due to water alone, as suggested by Newcombe and colleagues, or due to molecular and cellular abnormalities in the myelin.

Nesbit and colleagues[121] evaluated 32 MRI and 30 computed tomography (CT) scans in patients with MS who had had ei-

ther cerebral biopsies or autopsies soon after their scans. Lesions that had enhanced on the scan tended to be "histologically active," confirming the impression that BBB disruption is an important element in active MS lesions.

Hook and associates[61] reported three cases of colon cancer treated with 5-fluorouracil and levamisole in which MS-like lesions (biopsy confirmed) were seen on the MRI scan. The MRI findings resolved after withdrawal of the chemotherapy. This observation suggests that toxic agents can produce lesions on the MRI scan that look like the inflammatory demyelination of MS. Although probably no connection exists between this phenomenon and MS, understanding the mechanism of such lesions may be helpful in understanding MS.

Grafton and co-workers[48] examined the correlations between pathology and MRI on the fixed brains of seven elderly patients, three of whom were hypertensive. Some periventricular lesions seen on MRI scans, particularly the larger ones, were demyelinated and gliotic on histological examination. However, similar pathological changes were seen in brain areas in which no MRI abnormalities were seen and vice versa. The authors found no clear-cut correlations between MRI findings and the pathology of the deep white matter lesions. Another study[151a] showed axonal loss in the MRI lesions of Alzheimer's disease and normal aging.

Sappey-Marinier[151] performed MRS and relaxation studies on fresh frozen MS autopsy material. She found the relaxation times (T_1 and T_2) to be prolonged in MS lesions and in normal-appearing white matter (T_2). The reported changes paralleled the increase in water content in those areas. She also found that neutral lipids in the brain could be accurately measured by MRS techniques.

Barnes and associates[11] compared the ultrastructure in an autopsied case of MS and the MRI changes in 16 volunteers living with MS. They found heterogeneity in both samples, which they thought was due to the variable degree of axonal loss. They interpreted the findings as suggestive of progressive axonal loss with time and related chronic clinical progression to axonal loss. Larsson and his colleagues[93] also found more MRI heterogeneity in "older plaques" than in newer ones, suggesting that MRI characteristics could reflect specific pathological changes.

Orita and colleagues[125] used coronal MRI studies to document wallerian degeneration in stroke patients. The pyramidal tract degeneration secondary to hemispheric stroke can clearly be seen.

Peterson and co-workers[139] reported on four patients who received radiation therapy to intracranial masses that turned out to be MS mass lesions. All four patients with MS had unexpectedly poor clinical outcomes. Fisher[40] reported on a 40-year-old man who had radiation therapy for a reported CNS lymphoma who at autopsy had MS lesions adjacent to areas of radiation necrosis. The speculation was that active MS lesions may sensitize the brain to radiation necrosis.

ASSESSING THE BURDEN OF DISEASE BY MRI FOR CLINICAL STUDIES

A number of studies have compared the extent of disease, or burden of disease (BOD), on the cerebral MRI scan[83,135] with the degree of severity of MS as determined by clinical measurements. The initial expectation was that the extent of MRI abnormality would be strongly correlated with clinical impairment. Although one recent study[177] found an r value of 0.66 between an MRI score and the Extended Disability Status Scale (EDSS) score (p = 0.0001) using a standardized MRI protocol, other data show lower levels of correlation. At the University of British Columbia (UBC), we completed three separate studies comparing the BOD, as measured by MRI, with the clinical severity, as measured by the EDSS. The highest r value that we found was 0.5(D.W. Paty, 1988) (maximum possible r value = 1). The r values from our other studies ranged between 0.22 and 0.02. Most of the correlations reported are statistically significant, but they are not clinically relevant. The lack of strong correlation between clinically determined severity and

the extent of MRI lesions in individual cases should not be surprising, because parallel observations have long been noted in clinicopathological correlation studies. The lack of sensitivity of clinical measures has been the cornerstone for the use of diagnostic investigations such as evoked potentials and imaging.[98] Clinical severity, as measured by EDSS,[91] to a great extent is determined by the location of lesions, particularly those in the spinal cord. Because most MRI clinical correlation studies have not imaged the spinal cord, we should not expect a close correlation with the EDSS. For example, Koopmans and his associates[82] did a careful clinical–MRI correlation study contrasting 32 patients with benign MS and 32 patients with RPMS matched for age, sex, and duration of disease. The duration of disease was greater than 10 years in all patients. The patients with benign MS (mean EDSS = 1.55) showed from 0 to 4,661 mm^2 total area of MS lesions (mean = 1,162). The patients with RPMS (mean EDSS = 6.03) varied from 140 to 11,910 mm^2 total area (mean = 2,912mm^2). In six of the pairs (20 percent), the benign patient of the pair showed a heavier load of disease by MRI than did the patient with RPMS. The correlation between the location of MRI lesions in the brain stem and cerebellum and clinical symptoms was approximately 50 percent in both. For example, only 50 percent of the patients with benign MS who had brain stem lesions on MRI scan had a history of brain stem symptoms, and only approximately 50 percent of the patients with RPMS who had a history of brain stem symptoms had brain stem lesions on MRI scan. Levine and colleagues[98] showed that this correlation could be improved by sensitive neurophysiological testing. Koopmans and colleagues[85] showed that changes in MRI BOD not only increased over time but also correlated significantly with clinical worsening in a clinical trial with cyclosporine.

In a quantitative MRI study of 67 patients with CPMS, Baumhefner and his colleagues[14] found a modest correlation between lesion burden on MRI scan and the intra–blood-brain barrier IgG synthesis rate. In a controlled MRI study of eight patients who had both MS and diagnosed psychiatric disease, Honer[60] found that the psychiatric patients had a greater degree of involvement of the temporal lobe than did matched nonpsychiatric patients.

A study of spinal cord imaging[108,172] did not find a close correlation between the number and extent of spinal cord lesions and spinal disability. The authors found an average of 4.1 spinal lesions (2.2 cervical, 1.9 thoracic) per patient, using multiarray coils and fast spin-echo (SE) techniques. Of their patients, 94 percent (31 of 33) had spinal lesions, whereas none were seen in 12 healthy, age-matched controls.[22] Spinal cord and cortical atrophy have been found to correlate with clinical measurements.[101, 101a,101b] Contrary to MRI studies of the brain and spinal cord, the clinical correlation with optic nerve imaging in optic neuritis has been good.[112]

In addition to location, the severity and complexity of the histological features of the pathological process must also be considered. The clinical expression of a lesion is due not only to its location but also to a combination of additional factors operating at morphologic and physiological levels (see Chapter 8).

A computer-assisted method for measuring the extent of the abnormal areas seen on the MRI scan has been developed at UBC to follow the evolution of the pathological process over time.[127,135] Using this method, an experienced, skilled radiologic technician can trace and measure the same MRI lesions in a reasonable period of time with a reproducibility error of approximately 6 percent. The radiologist indicates the number, size, and distribution of lesions for each subject. The lesions are identified as follows:

1. Small, solitary, round or oval lesions with a maximum diameter less than 10 mm
2. Large, solitary, round or oval lesions with a diameter greater than 10 mm
3. Confluent lesions, which are relatively large and are probably formed by the merging of two or more rounded, smaller lesions to produce an irregularly shaped ("lumpy-bumpy") or thick (greater than 5 mm) linear area of abnormality on the magnetic resonance image. The periventricular confluent changes are likely permanent.[13]

The technician doing the analysis then traces the lesions using the radiologist's markings as a guide. Figures 9–5 and 9–6 illustrate the MRI quantitation process.

Subsequent MRI examinations of the same patients require careful repositioning.

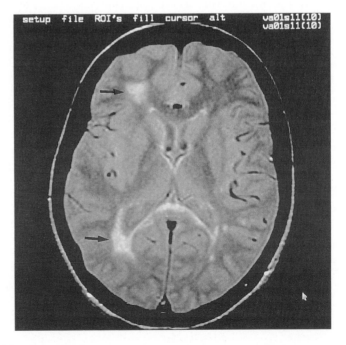

Figure 9–5. This is a proton-density axial slice as displayed on the computer screen showing several periventricular lesions (*arrows*).

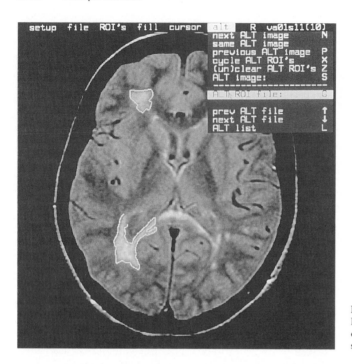

setup file ROI's fill cursor alt   R va01sl1(10)
next ALT image   N
same ALT image
previous ALT image   P
cycle ALT ROI's   X
(un)clear ALT ROI's   Z
ALT image: S
─────────────────────────────
ALT ROI file: C
prev ALT file   ↑
next ALT file   ↓
ALT list   L

Figure 9–6. This is the same slice as in Figure 9–5, showing two of the lesions outlined by the computer-assisted measurement system described in the text.

For accurate repositioning, both internal and external landmarks should be used. The process of repositioning the patient usually takes approximately 20 minutes additional time at each study. To make subsequent positioning easier, the patient should be positioned as comfortably as possible for the first examination.

To provide a more objective approach to clinical trials, the MRI quantitation method was reapplied in several studies. In one prospective evaluation of 63 patients with CPMS during a placebo-controlled therapeutic trial of interferon alpha,[76,86,89] all had MRI examinations at entry, at 6 months, and at 2 years. The MRI quantitation technique was used to analyze the MRI changes that occurred over that time. The changes in the "burden of MS" ranged from −70 to +221 percent over 2 years. The mean change in extent of MS was +21 percent over 2 years. Unfortunately, no significant difference was found between the treated and placebo groups of patients in either clinical or MRI measurements.

Patients with the smallest total lesion load had the greatest variability in MRI measurements. Therefore, a separate analysis was done of patients with large disease burden and those with minimal disease burden at baseline. The elimination of the patients with a small BOD did not change the outcome of the study. This experience clearly showed an average increase in MRI-detected lesion burden of approximately 20 percent over the 2 years of this clinical trial (approximately a 10 percent increase per year).

The quantitative MRI method[134] has also been used in a clinical trial with cyclosporine.[87,117] No therapeutic effect was shown on MRI analysis; however, the mean percent increase in MRI-detected BOD over 2 years was approximately 50 percent. In addition, the change in MRI correlated significantly with the change in clinical impairment (EDSS).[85] The MRI quantitative measure in a therapeutic trial with interferon beta[135] showed an increase in BOD of approximately 20 percent over 2 years in the placebo group, contrasted to a −4 percent change in BOD for the high-dose treatment group.

Pannizzo and associates[129] reported on an automated imaging processing method for the calculation of disease burden in 10 patients with CPMS. They looked at the effect of coil response, tip angles, patient positioning, and interslice gap thickness on the analysis of repeated images. They found an operator-independent error of 6 percent and an agreement between operators of 97 percent. Wicks and colleagues[185] reported on a segmentation method for measuring BOD with reasonable reproducibility, in addition to a promise of time savings. Others[49,67,69,70,71] have also been working on volume estimation techniques which, if reproducible and efficient, should eventually improve monitoring methods. Several automatic lesion load methods were evaluated in a meeting in Montreal in November 1995 (Workshop on evaluation of MS lesion load, Montreal Neurological Institute, Montreal, Canada, November 6–7, 1995). Even though the methods have improved over the last few years, the authors have concluded that the eye is much better than the computer in identifying and measuring lesions. Stone and colleagues[165] also evaluated one automatic method, and their findings were encouraging in that automatic methods could accurately measure disease extent. For the immediate future, however, the authors recommend the use of manual quantification techniques, because automated methods still require further refinements to ensure the accuracy of their measurements.

Filippi and co-workers[38] found that imaging thin slices (3 mm) produced a 20 percent increase in volume estimation. Goodkin and colleagues[47] and Yetkin[192] studied lesion changes on MRI scans and sounded a note of caution because of the strong chance of a positioning artifact being called biologically significant activity.

In looking at the implication of MRI lesion load, Filippi and colleagues[36] found that the lesion load at onset predicted clinical and MRI behavior at 5-year follow-up. They also identified some trends that might help to distinguish benign MS from SPMS.[34] Finally, this group[35] compared several methods of evaluating extent of involvement and found that a semiautomatic thresholding technique produced better intraobserver and interobserver agreement than a manual tracing technique or an arbitrary scoring system. However, at this time, automatic lesion detection is not reliable enough to be used as an outcome measure[67,109a,167,185] until validated against the manual system. Any automated system must

be able to detect the expected increase in BOD over time as well as any treatment effect.[135] One study has actually found a decrease in BOD in placebo patients over time,[67a] a finding which is counterintuitive.

SERIAL MRI STUDIES REVEAL THE EVOLUTION OF PATHOLOGY

Barkhof has written a useful monograph on gadolinium enhancement in MS.[5] The dynamic nature of the MS process has been dramatically shown by a number of systematic serial studies (Table 9–1). Some have been done by morphologic unenhanced methods alone and others with the addition of gadolinium enhancement. The first three systematic serial unenhanced MRI studies were performed at UBC. Twenty-four patients were repeatedly examined over 6 months. In the first study,[66] 7 patients had monthly scans. In the second[187] and third studies,[83] 17 had biweekly scans. A total of 213 MRI follow-up examinations were performed. The first study involved seven patients with RRMS who had moderate disability; the second, nine patients with RRMS who had mild impairment; and the third, eight patients with RPMS without evidence of relapses who had moderate disability.

Activity was graded as one of the following categories: (1) new lesions (Fig. 9–7), (2) reappearing lesions (reactivated), and (3) old lesions enlarging (also reactivated) (Fig. 9–8). If a lesion was continuously active (enlarging) over more than one scan, it was counted only once as an activity event. An enlarging lesion identified by consensus was usually a change of 70 percent in area for small (less than 1 cm) lesions. A change as small as 10 percent for the larger (greater than 1 cm) lesions could be perfectly obvious. In this chapter, the term *active* refers to new or enlarging lesions on the MRI scan. It may well have the same connotation as when *active* is used in the histopathological description of many lesions (see Chapter 8). However, whether this "activity" (enlargement) represents an extension of demyelination, inflammation, or both, or other morphological character-

Table 9–1. **SERIAL MAGNETIC RESONANCE IMAGING**

Year	Senior Author	No. of Patients	Duration of Study	Scanning Interval	Patient Category	Type of Activity*	Comments
1984	Johnson[†68]	3	22 mo	1 wk–22 mo	Mixed MS	M—[‡]	Four studies were performed per patient at varying times. New lesions appeared; some lesions became smaller, others enlarged.
1984	Li[†99]	3	12 mo	6–12 mo	Mixed MS	M	Two studies were performed per patient. Most lesions were asymptomatic. New lesion went away; others appeared or enlarged.
1987	Ormerod[†126]	35	12 mo	6–12 mo	Suspected MS	M—follow-up for diagnosis	Diagnostically important new lesions appeared on repeat scans in 20%.
		17	19 wks	8–19 wks	CDMS	M	Seven of 17 (41%) showed new lesions on follow-up scans.
1988	Grossman[†51]	13	16–24 mo	16–24 mo	CDMS	Gd	Two studies were performed per patient. Eight of 13 had enhancement; some lost enhancement, some developed enhancement.
1988	Isaac[66]	7	6 mo	4 wk	RRMS (mod)	M	Five clinical relapses and 18 active MRI lesions were seen. All MRI active lesions were clinically silent.
1988	Oger[124]	7	6 mo	4 wk	RRMS (mod)	Same patients as Isaac (1988)[66]	Immune function changes seemed to follow new lesions' appearance.
1988	Kappos[72]	74	6 mo	6 mo	Mixed MS	M	Part of a clinical trial, nine patients had new lesions.
1988	Palo[128]	57	2 yr	Intermittent	Mixed MS	M	New lesions were present on 20% of follow-up scans.
1988	Miller[113]	9	6 mo	3–5 wk	RRMS	Gd	All 12 new lesions enhanced.
1989	Willoughby[187]	9	6 mo	2 wk	RRMS (mild)	M	Two clinical relapses, and 12 new MRI lesions were seen. All new MRI lesions were asymptomatic.

Continued on following page

Table 9–1.—*continued*

Year	Senior Author	No. of Patients	Duration of Study	Scanning Interval	Patient Category	Type of Activity*	Comments
1989	Koopmans[83]	8	6 mo	2 wk	RPMS	M	No clinical relapses were seen. 86 active lesions were seen on MRI. All active MRI lesions were silent neurologically (see text).
1989	Uhlenbrock[179]	20	up to 40 mo	3 mo	RRMS	M	Ten percent of old lesions enlarged and asymptomatic new lesions appeared.
1990	Kermode[79]	7	3 mo	7 d–3 mo	RRMS	Gd and M	Enhancement can precede visualization of standard MRI lesion.
1990	Kermode[79]	24	3 mo	2 wk	RRMS	Gd and M	Enhancement can precede visualization of standard MRI lesion.
1990	Bastianello[12]	4	4 mo	Monthly	CDMS	Gd and M	All new lesions enhanced and some stable lesions enhanced.
1991	Harris[56]	6	8–11 mo	Monthly	RRMS—Early	Gd	One hundred thirteen new enhancing lesions were seen, most scans had at least one.
1991	Thompson[169]	12	6 mo	2 wk × 3 mo 4 wk × 3 mo	Primary CPMS	Gd and M	The 20 new and active lesions seen were small and unenhancing, seen at a low rate.
		12	6 mo	Same	RPMS	Gd and M	One hundred nine new and active lesions were large and mostly enhancing, seen at a high rate.
1991	Truyen[178]	36	22 mo	Variable	RRMS	M	Fifty-six percent of stable patients had activity; relapsing patients had more changes than did stable patients ($P = <0.001$).
1991	Thompson[171]	10	6 mo	2 wk or 4 wk	RRMS < 10 yr Benign MS	Gd and M	Early RRMS had more activity than benign disease. Clinical and MRI activity correlated.

Continued on following page

Table 9–1.—*continued*

Year	Senior Author	No. of Patients	Duration of Study	Scanning Interval	Patient Category	Type of Activity*	Comments
1992	Wiebe[186]	29	13 wk	6 wk	Mixed MS	Gd and M spinal imaging done	Enhancement increased the spinal cord activity by 5% and spinal activity increased the overall activity by 20%. Clinical and MRI activity correlated.
1992	Capra[20]	10	3 mo	2 wk	RRMS	Gd	Ninety-three enhancing lesions were found in 8 patients.
1992	Barkhof[6a]	7	4–12 mo	4 wk	RRMS	Gd and M	Morphological changes were seen in 92% of the enhancing lesions.
1993	Smith[154]	9	24–37 mo	Monthly	RRMS	Gd	The study was an extension of the Harris study. MRI activity occurred much more frequently than clinical activity. MRI and clinical activity correlated.
1993	Paty[135]	52	24 mo	6 wk	RRMS	M	MRI activity was very sensitive for detecting the treatment effect in a clinical trial.
1993	Miller[110]	25	4 mo	Monthly	RRMS or RPMS	Gd and M	MRI identified 106 active lesions; 64% were seen only by enhancement.
1994	Tas[168]	13	12 mo	Monthly	RRMS	Gd and M	All patients had active scans, with 3.8 active lesions per patient per month. MRI activity preceded clinical activity in 75% of patients.
1994	Dousset[30]	32	1 yr	Variable	Mixed MS	Mixed	MTI could detect: 1. Resolution of inflammation 2. Progressive severity, demyelination, and/or axonal loss.

Continued on following page

Table 9-1.—*continued*

Year	Senior Author	No. of Patients	Duration of Study	Scanning Interval	Patient Category	Type of Activity*	Comments
1994	van Walderveen[181]	2	9 mo	Variable	RRMS	T_2M	Activity went down in 3rd trimester of pregnancy.
1994	Khoury[80]	18	12 mo	Variable	Mixed MS	M + Gd	MRI and clinical activity correlated.
1995	van Walderveen[182]	49	24 mo	24 mo	Mixed MS	M,T_1 + Gd	MRI and clinical changes correlated. T_1 hypointensity correlated best.
1995	Weiner[183]	45	1 yr	2 wk	Mixed MS	Several T_2 and Gd	A positive correlation was found with immune function relapses, and cognitive function.
1995	Stone[165]	7	2–3 yr	Monthly	RRMS	M and Gd	Increase in abnormal white matter over time.
1996	Thorpe[173]	10	1 yr	Monthly	RRMS	Enhancing (brain and cord)	Spinal cord lesions were much more likely to correlate with clinical findings but most active lesions were in the brain.
1996	Losseff[101]	21	5-yr follow-up	Monthly	RRMS & SPMS	Enhancing lesions	Disability on 5-yr follow-up correlated with activity on MRI.
1996	Losseff[101a]	29	18 mo	6 mo	13 RRMS 16 SPMS	Cerebral atrophy	Progressive cerebral atrophy was seen that correlated with clinical worsening.

*Active MRI lesions indicates new, enlarging, or reappearing lesions, gadolinium not used.
†Early studies were not systematic.
‡M (morphological) means that the lesions were evaluated by changes seen on the proton density and T_2 weighted images; gadolinium was not used (see text).
BOD = burden of disease; CDMS = clinically definite MS; CPMS = chronic progressive MS; Gd = gadolinium enhancement; M = morphological; mod = moderate disability;
MTI = magnetic transfer imaging; RPMS = relapsing progressive MS (secondary progressive); RRMS = relapsing–remitting MS; SPMS = secondary progressive MS.

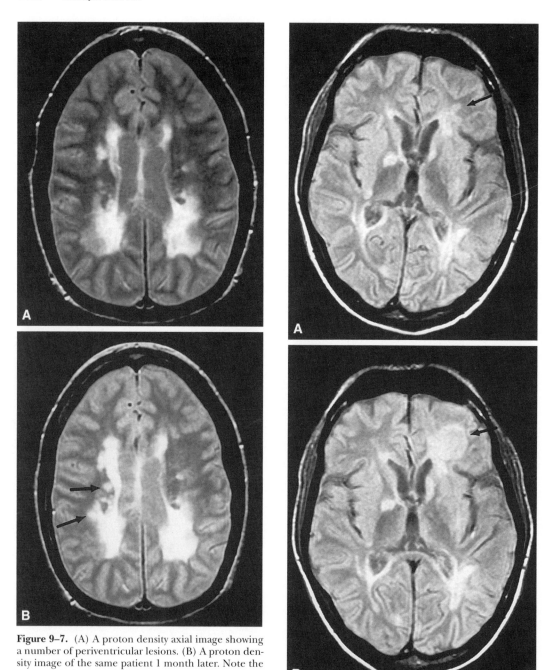

Figure 9–7. (A) A proton density axial image showing a number of periventricular lesions. (B) A proton density image of the same patient 1 month later. Note the two new lesions marked by the arrows. Figure 9–9B shows these same lesions to be enhancing.

Figure 9–8. (A) A proton density axial scan with a number of lesions. Note the small lesion marked by the arrow. (B) A follow-up scan 1 month later shows a large lesion (*arrow*) that has developed from the previously seen small one.

istics in a given lesion, is unknown, because our understanding of histological correlates of MRI signal abnormalities is incomplete. *Activity* on the MRI scan can also refer to enhancement of a lesion with gadolinium, regardless of whether it is increasing in size or not (see following). In this instance, breakdown of BBB detected by gadolinium enhancement would be a sign of disease activity.

The results of these studies showed that 79 (37 percent) of the 213 follow-up MRI examinations were positive for morphological evidence of disease activity, with 127 active lesions being identified. This activity rate is almost identical to the activity rate in the placebo limb of the reported therapeutic trial of interferon beta-1b.[135]

The average clinical relapse rate in the 24 patients was 0.6 relapses per patient per year. The average rate of active MRI lesions (evidence for total activity) was 10.6 active lesions per patient per year. There were 2 new lesions per patient per year in the minimally disabled RRMS study group, in contrast to 6.25 new lesions per patient per year in the RPMS study group. The very high rate of total activity in the RPMS group (21.5 active lesions per patient per year) is probably related to the fact that there were so many pre-existing lesions in those patients. Pre-existing lesions tended to increase in size more frequently than did new lesions. There were 2.6 active scans per patient per year in the RRMS group in contrast to 12.5 active scans per patient per year in the RPMS group. An active scan is defined as a scan with any lesion activity. The reader must remember, however, that these studies were done on patients selected for clinical activity, so the data cannot be taken as representative of all patients with MS. Figures 9–8 to 9–14 show examples of the activity that was seen in some of our serially examined patients. Another study[51] showed that enhancement on follow-up scans was likely to occur around the time of relapse.

Brannin and associates[16] did four MRI examinations with calculation of T_1 and T_2 relaxation times both before and after clinical relapses. They found that the T_1 and T_2 relaxation times in normal-appearing white matter (inversion recovery) were actually abnormal. Moreover, no consistent changes

were reported with clinical relapse or steroid therapy.

The Queen Square MS-MRI group and others[110,113,169,170,173] have done similar systematic MRI studies using gadolinium enhancement in addition to standard MRI. Gadolinium-DTPA (Gd-DTPA) is a paramagnetic contrast material that provides enhancement on certain magnetic resonance images by shortening the spin relaxation time of hydrogen. Large molecules such as gadolinium EDTA (gadolinium EDTA) are usually excluded from the brain by the BBB, so that gadolinium enhancement can be used as a marker for a disrupted BBB barrier. Barkhof and colleagues[7] looked at the effect of gadolinium on long TR SE (TE 60) images and found that the contrast (in lesions that enhanced on T_1) increased significantly, but that change did not influence their ability to detect the MS lesions on those images. They concluded that gadolinium could be given before T_2 SE sequences without influencing the detection of lesions on the T_2 weighted scan. However, they did not measure the area of the lesions to see if they were affected.

Figure 9–9 gives an example of two enhancing lesions. Kermode and associates[79] performed 15 gadolinium-enhanced MRI studies in eight patients, seven of which were follow-up scans. They found 102 enhancing lesions. Serial follow-up showed three instances in which enhancement was seen before the typical lesion was seen on the standard T_2-weighted magnetic resonance image. The same authors[79] subsequently did a systematic MRI follow-up, using both standard and gadolinium-enhanced scans once every 2 weeks for 6 months on 24 relapsing patients. Of the new lesions seen on T_2-weighted scans, 95 percent enhanced. In the latter study, there were four instances in which gadolinium enhancement appeared before the standard MRI lesion was seen. Bastianello and associates[12] also used gadolinium enhancement in four patients imaged monthly for 4 months. They found enhancement to occur in new, changing lesions and sometimes in morphologically unchanging lesions. In contrast, the serial gadolinium studies in patients with primary CPMS studied by Thompson and colleagues[171] showed that

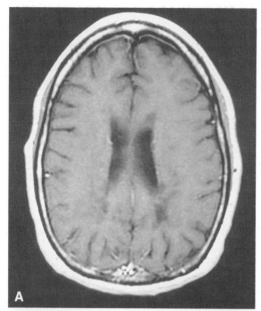

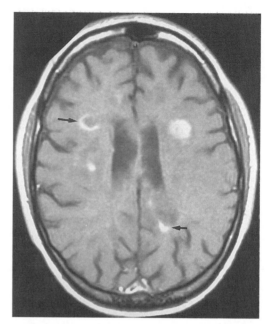

Figure 9–10. Several examples of enhanced lesions. Note how some of the low-intensity lesions on the T_1 scan have ring enhancement (*arrows*).

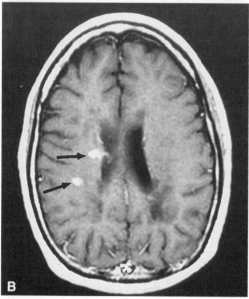

Figure 9–9. (A) A gadolinium-enhanced axial T_1 scan on the same patient on the same date as Figure 9–7A, showing no enhancing lesions. There are, however, several low-intensity (dark), nonenhancing chronic lesions. (B) This follow-up scan 1 month later shows enhancement in the two new lesions that were seen in Figure 9–7B.

enhancement was rare in this group of patients.

Figures 9–10 and 9–11 show some additional examples of gadolinium-enhanced lesions. Each type of lesion seen on the T_2-weighted scan (new, stable, enlarging) can enhance as evidence for activity. Filippi and colleagues[39] found that triple-dose gadolinium resulted in identification of 66 percent more enhancing lesions. The number of patients with enhancement increased by 28 percent, and the area and intensity of the enhancement also increased. The impact of double- and triple-dose gadolinium serial studies of disease activity is yet to be evaluated.

Thompson and his colleagues[169–171] also showed that the MRI pattern in serial studies varies according to the clinical course (Table 9–2). Patients with primary CPMS had low rates of MRI activity, with rare enhancement. Patients with early RRMS had more activity than did a long-duration benign group. Enhancement was also more frequently seen in the early patients with RRMS than in patients with longer-duration benign MS.[81] Patients with SPMS or RPMS had an MRI activity rate of 18.2 active lesions per patient per year (see Table 9–2).

Revesz and colleagues[143] looked at the pathological process in CPMS versus relapsing MS. They found less inflammation in patients with CPMS but no major differences in the distribution of lesions.

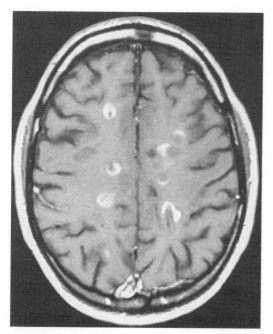

Figure 9–11. Several additional examples of enhanced lesions.

Wiebe and associates[186] performed serial (every 13 weeks) MRI examinations of both head and cord with and without gadolinium enhancement in 29 patients in various categories of clinical activity. They found that imaging the spinal cord added 20 percent to the activity detected and that only 10 percent of the activity was detected by gadolinium alone. Two-thirds of all MRI activity was detected in the head. MRI activity and clinical activity correlated.

Harris and colleagues[56] and Smith and colleagues[153] followed up 10 patients with RRMS monthly for over a year with serial gadolinium-enhanced and unenhanced MR scans. They found the duration of enhancement to be short in most instances (less than 1 month). The MRI-detected activity was more frequent than clinical activity. The MRI activity tended to come in bursts that roughly correlated with periods of clinical activity. Stone and co-workers[164] reported on 61 patients imaged monthly from 3 to 52 months (mean, 14 months) with gadolinium-enhanced scans. Eighty percent showed enhancement at some time (mostly in actively relapsing patients); 31 percent had enhancement on every scan, the mean number of enhancing lesions being 2.53 per patient per month (30.4 enhancing lesions per year). This study conclusively proves that MS disease activity is much more frequent than clinical symptoms would suggest. Stone and co-workers[166] also looked at enhancing lesions in 68 patients imaged by three monthly scans.

Table 9–2. CLINICAL COURSE AND MAGNETIC RESONANCE IMAGING ACTIVITY

		ACTIVITY RATE BY PATIENT CATEGORY*				
Date	**Senior Author**	**Benign MS**	**Early RRMS**	**Late RRMS**	**RPMS**	**I° PMS**
1988	Isaac[66]	—	—	High	—	—
1989	Willoughby[187]	—	Low	—	—	—
1989	Koopmans[83]	—	—	—	High	—
1991	Thompson[169]	—	—	—	High	Low, enhancement rare
1992	Thompson†[170]	Low	Medium	—	—	—
1994	Paty, Li and Zhao (unpublished data)	Low	Low	High	Highest	—
1994	Kidd[81]	Low	—	—	—	—

*Activity rates of low, medium, and high represent relative judgments because different techniques were used in many studies.

†Clinical and MRI activity correlated (*P*<.01).

I° PMS = primary progressive MS; RPMS = relapsing progressive MS (or secondary progressive MS = SPMS); RRMS = relapsing and remitting MS.

They found that enhancement was associated with younger age at onset of disease and more severe neurological impairment.

Tas and colleagues[168] looked at 13 patients with RRMS over an average of 12 months and found prerelapse MRI activity in 75 percent of patients. Khoury and his associates[80] also found a correlation between fluctuations in MRI and clinical activity. Thorpe and associates[173] imaged both the brain and spinal cord monthly in 10 patients with RRMS. They found that spinal cord and brain enhancement occurred together in bursts and that spinal lesions were much more likely to be associated with clinical symptoms than were brain lesions. The same group has shown that both brain and spinal cord atrophy as measured on MRI correlate with clinical disability.[101a,101b] Atrophy is probably a measure of axonal loss as well as chronic demyelination.[184] Finally, Zhao and colleagues[194] found that new lesions of the corticospinal tract were much more likely to have clinical correlation than were new lesions elsewhere in the brain.

Koopmans and his associates[83a] studied 21 patients with high-volume delayed CT (HVDCT) scans. A total of 90 CT-enhancing lesions were seen, of which 49 were followed up by unenhanced MRI. Active lesions were seen in one-half of the MRI scans. In half of the active scans, there was also evidence for some lesions enlarging while others were getting smaller. HVDCT follow-up showed that five of the initial enhancing lesions continued to enhance after 2 to 7 months. They were probably re-enhancing rather than persistently enhancing. Three enhancing lesions became smaller and then disappeared on MRI follow-up. While these changes were occurring, 13 new enhancing lesions developed on CT. About one-half of the newly seen CT-enhancing lesions had been previously seen on MRI. Of the lesions that were CT-enhancing at the start, 16 percent merged with neighboring lesions to appear confluent during follow-up. The average time from initial enhancement to confluence was 16 months. New lesions are usually rounded (spherical) or oval, whereas confluent lesions are irregularly shaped with a lumpy-bumpy appearance. Miller[113] has seen similar follow-up changes in his serial gadolinium-enhanced studies.

The evolution of new lesions is interesting to follow. New lesions tend to reach their maximum size within 4 weeks of first detection. The enhancing phase of new lesions lasts 2 to 4 weeks.[113] Typical new lesions then decline in size over the subsequent 6 to 8 weeks, either to resolve as a small area of abnormality or, in some studies, to actually disappear. Disappearing lesions have been seen in the UBC studies where 1-cm slices were imaged with an MRI machine of low field strength (0.15 T). Apparently, most new lesions seen on higher-strength machines (0.5 to 1.5 T) get smaller but do not disappear. In Wiebe and colleagues' study[186] using a 1.5-T machine, not one of approximately 1200 lesions disappeared. The difference betweeen the two studies is probably because higher-field-strength magnets give better resolution on thin slices than do low-field-strength magnets. As noted previously, 39 percent of the time some lesions enlarged while other lesions became smaller. Miller and his colleagues[110] analyzed both morphologic and enhancing changes. They found that gadolinium markedly increases the activity rate because enhancement is seen frequently in morphologically stable lesions. The evolution of lesions over time is discussed later in this chapter.

Koopmans and associates' study[83] showed that 56 percent of enhancing lesions were located in the deep (nonperiventricular) cerebral white matter, 23 percent were periventricular, and 21 percent were at the gray-white matter junction. The distribution of enhancing lesions was similar to the distribution of the new MRI lesions in the serial MRI studies, where most new lesions were also in the deep cerebral white matter, away from the ventricles. Therefore, the anatomical distribution of new lesions on MRI differed from that of the chronic demyelinating lesions usually seen at autopsy. At autopsy, the heaviest plaque burden in chronic cases is usually found in the periventricular regions. This difference in distribution between acute lesions and chronic demyelinating lesions raises questions about the ultimate fate of the new and dynamic lesions that are seen on MRI and CT.

As discussed in Chapter 8, the pathology of these interesting transient lesions is unknown at present. Serial gadolinium-enhanced studies show that 80 to 90 percent of the new lesions show breakdown of the BBB, probably the result of interaction between the cerebral vasculature and lymphocytes and monocytes. The resolution of transient lesions could be due to remyelination, but we believe that the resolution of acute lesions is most often due to reduction in inflammation. One report[77] showed an enhancing lesion that was intensely inflammatory on biopsy. Nesbit and colleagues[121] found that "histologically active" lesions at autopsy or at biopsy had been enhancing when scanned during life. These studies all support the idea that resolution or reduction of MRI lesions is due to reduced inflammation rather than remyelination.

Zhao and colleagues[193] looked at the morphologic characteristics of 150 active lesions (new, recurrent, and enlarging) on serial MRI and compared them with stable lesions. New and recurrent lesions were smaller, more likely round or oval, and did not tend to be located periventricularly. Enlarging and stable lesions were larger and more irregular in shape, had more well-defined contours, and tended to be periventricular. Occasionally diffuse acute lesions are seen that have a very subtle appearance on T_2 and an increased signal on the unenhanced T_1 (D. Li, personal communication, 1996). Since the T_1 changes resolved on follow-up, Dr. Li thinks the increased T_1 is due to neutral fat present as a consequence of early demyelination.[95]

Ebers and his associates[32] showed that the enhancement of CT lesions disappeared shortly after steroid therapy. Barkhof and colleagues[6] looked at the effect of intravenous high-dose steroid (pulse) therapy on MRI enhancement and found a correlation between clinical improvement, reduced MRI enhancement, and CSF myelin basic protein levels. These studies suggest that steroids have a biologic as well as a physiological effect.

The serial MRI method, without enhancement, has been used to monitor for treatment effects in a cohort of 52 patients at UBC in a multicenter trial of interferon beta.[135] The serial scans (every 6 weeks) revealed that the treatment markedly reduced the disease activity rate. The treatment effect was seen as a trend as early as 6 weeks (as percent active scans), and the cumulative activity rates showed statistically significant treatment effect at 1 year (Paty, unpublished data, 1993). This study has shown that MRI monitoring is not only more objective than clinical methods but is also more sensitive to treatment effects. Guidelines have been published for the use of MRI techniques in the evaluation of clinical trials.[109a,111] The correlation between MR measures and clinical measures is covered in detail in Chapter 12.

Figures 9–7 and 9–8 illustrate some of the changes that can be seen on serial MRI studies. In summary, the lessons learned from the serial MRI experience in MS are as follows:

1. **Asymptomatic new lesions are frequent in patients with both RRMS and RPMS.** The correlation between clinical events and new MRI events in individual patients is poor, but there does seem to be a significant correlation between MRI activity, MRI patterns, and the clinical state of patients. The rate of MRI activity is probably greater in patients with RPMS than in patients with RRMS. In part, the explanation for the high rate of activity in RPMS is that many more lesions are present at baseline, and most of the activity seen is reactivation of pre-existing lesions.

2. **Clear MRI evidence exists for significant and persistent asymptomatic disease activity in many clinically stable patients.** It appears that recognition of the phasic clinical expression of MS is only scratching the surface as an indicator of disease activity. The underlying disease activity is significantly greater and more persistent than that predicted by clinical symptoms. This finding agrees with the well-documented pathological observation that lesions seen postmortem are often more in number and extent than expected clinically.[117a] MS disease activity is a more continuously active phenom-

enon than was previously acknowledged, and clinical activity, in general, is just the "tip of the iceberg." It is also reminiscent of the findings of Bodian[15] regarding the pathological process involved in poliomyelitis; he always found the pathological changes to be more extensive than would be expected from the clinical examination. Of course, there are occasional patients with MS who have a single, small but intense, strategically located lesion in the spinal cord that causes paraplegia at a time when there are no lesions in the brain.[43,172] Also, corticospinal tract lesions are more likely to be associated with appropriate clinical symptoms.[194]

3. **New lesions seen on MRI almost always enhance, indicating BBB breakdown. They are probably the primary MS lesions.** Most new lesions disappear or fade over several weeks. However, no firm evidence exists regarding the pathological process occurring in these new lesions. Because BBB disruption seems to be associated with the inflammation process, most of the dynamically changing lesions seen on serial MRI studies are probably inflammatory ones.

   Alternatively, it is possible that resolution of these lesions is due to remyelination. In the future, it is hoped that correlative studies examining the pathological process using a combination of MRI, MRS, T_2 relaxation analysis, and other techniques might be able to distinguish these histopathological features at an *in-vivo* imaging level.

4. **Both the new and the enlarging MRI lesions may follow independent patterns of evolution.** Some lesions can be seen decreasing in size while others are enlarging. This phenomenon suggests that once a new lesion has developed, local factors play an important role in its subsequent evolution.

   For a disease that likely entails some systemic immune activation, it may seem surprising that lesions in the brain may behave independently of each other. Possibly the pattern of new,

enlarging, and enhancing lesions reflects the fact that the threshold for fresh activity is influenced positively and negatively by the age of the lesion. A number of factors obviously are involved in the production of a new lesion, such as T cells, B cells, avidity of cells, activated macrophages, and lymphokines such as interferon gamma, in addition to BBB disruption (endothelial cell function).

If these activities are all subthreshold, there would be no new lesion. However, if by chance the aggregate of several factors exceeds the local threshold (a stochastic process), then a new lesion or a reactivated lesion would develop. Interestingly, in pulmonary tuberculosis, where systemic cell-mediated immunity must play a major role in the evolution of pulmonary granulomas, it has been shown that individual lesions in the same lung enlarge or regress as though their behavior were completely independent of each other. Pathological observations in MS support this idea by showing that there are lymphocytes and plasma cells in small numbers distributed throughout the meninges and the normal-appearing white matter.

5. **The anatomical distribution of both the enhancing CT lesions and the dynamic MRI lesions is interesting.** Most HVDCT enhancing lesions are not periventricular or adjacent to a periventricular lesion. The same anatomical distribution has also been true of the actively changing lesions that have been seen on serial MRI follow-up. In contrast, pathological studies have shown that old established chronic lesions are most likely to be periventricular in location. These chronic lesions are also seen on MRI. The nature of the pathological process within stable periventricular lesions must be chronic demyelination. Long-term follow-up studies of new lesions will be necessary to know the fate of most of the nonperiventricular new and enhancing lesions. Do they all go

on to chronic demyelination? Although some may do so, many probably do not.

6. **Some patients with primary CPMS seem to have a remarkably different serial MRI pattern from that of patients with other forms of the disease.** These patients have low levels of MRI activity. New MRI lesions are usually small and, for the most part, nonenhancing. They also seem to have a difference in pathological process, at least from the point of view of degree of inflammation. This difference from the relapsing-remitting pattern may be a matter of degree, with a concomitantly lower-intensity inflammatory response, breakdown of the BBB, or both. Whether the stable lesions are different in terms of myelin pathology and axonal loss is not clear at this time.

7. **Patients with a benign course of RRMS tend to have a pattern of independent lesions scattered throughout the white matter, even when they have the same BOD as do matched patients with SPMS.** Patients with CPMS, in contrast, tend to have confluent periventricular lesions with fewer peripheral, isolated ones. At this moment, experience with MRI evaluation of the pattern of disease has been limited. However, very interesting questions have been raised considering the evolution of the pathological process in the various clinical categories.

8. **MRI monitoring is more objective and more sensitive to treatment effects than is clinical monitoring.**[65] Not surprisingly, the clinical manifestations do not fully reflect the MRI changes. The pathology of MS occurs throughout the CNS, whereas the tracts that involve specific neurological functions are limited in area. In fact, this phenomenon is why MRI and evoked potentials are such useful diagnostic examinations. The principle is that evoked potentials and MRI can reveal asymptomatic lesions in a high proportion of cases that are monosymptomatic, yet suggestive of MS.

MRI evaluation is actually revealing the pathology, in contrast to clinical evaluation, which is reflecting a minority of the pathological lesions.

MAGNETIC RESONANCE SPECTROSCOPIC (MRS) STUDIES

The number of MRS studies of MS has increased tremendously in the last few years. MRS techniques that permit inferences about chemical change in tissue have found abnormalities in spectroscopically detected chemical components of MS lesions. (Figs. 9–12 and 9–13). Arnold and his colleagues[3] found that the N-acetylaspartate (NAA) peak is decreased in chronic MS lesions. Because NAA is only found in neurones, they reasoned that this chemical change was a reflection of the changes associated with the loss of axons. Findings confirming axonal involvement have also been found in cerebral infarction and in Binswanger's disease.[23] Most investigators believe that MRS will aid in distinguishing among various pathologies. Richards[143a] reviewed the subject of MRS in MS, and Table 9–3 cites a number of MRS and relaxation studies done in humans over the past several years. Spectroscopic imaging may add even more to our knowledge of the pathological process involved in MS.[90,189]

The detection of neutral fat in evolving MS lesions could also help to elucidate the sequence of events. Richards and his colleagues[147] performed in vivo proton spectroscopy studies in EAE and detected lipid changes or changes attributed to myelin breakdown products. Simon and Fonte[152] showed a lipid signal associated with demyelination in animals with acute EAE. Narayana[118–120] and Wolinsky and colleagues[190,191] found fat signals in proton spectra of some MRI lesions in patients with MS. They reported evidence for the presence of cholesterol, fatty acids, or both in 5 of 21 acute MS lesions and 6 of 11 enhancing lesions. The lipid changes seen in the acute MS lesions disappeared after 2 weeks. Koopmans and his colleagues[87] con-

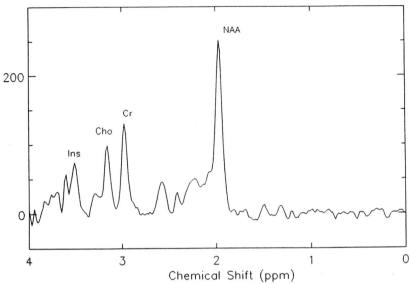

Figure 9–12. A spin-echo (SE) 20 millisecond (ms) magnetic resonance spectroscopy (MRS) spectrum from white matter in a volunteer who does not have MS. (Figs. 9–12 and 9–13 courtesy of Dr. Rob Koopmans and Dr. Peter Allen, University of Alberta.)

firmed these findings. It is unclear why the signal attributed to myelin breakdown products disappears so quickly, because the presence of lipid-laden macrophages in chronic MS lesions has been well documented pathologically to persist for months (see Chapter 8). Matthews and associates[104] performed proton MRS studies on several patients with MS. As noted previously, they found the NAA resonance intensities to be reduced in chronic irreversible MS lesions. However, in "active" lesions they found either no abnormality, an increase in tissue lactate, or an in-

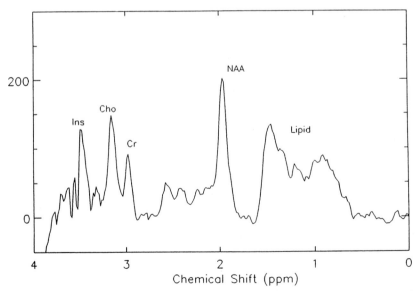

Figure 9–13. An SE 20-ms MRS spectrum from an MS lesion showing three changes from normal: (1) The *N*-acetylaspartate (NAA) peak is down; (2) new broad peaks have appeared in the lipid range; (3) the inositol (INS) peak is greater than normal (see text for explanation).

Table 9–3. MAGNETIC RESONANCE SPECTROSCOPY, RELAXATION, AND OTHER STUDIES IN HUMANS

Year	Senior Author	Technique	Pathological State (Actual or Inferred)	Type of MR Activity or Changes Found or Proposed
1989	Larsson[95]	T$_2$ relaxation times	Acute lesions	Biexponential T$_2$ changes evolve in acute lesions.
1989	Arnold[4]	²H MRS	Axonal loss	NAA levels decreased in MS patients.
1989	Narayana[119]	²H MRS	Active demyelination (lipid)	Lipid peak seen in several patients.
1989	Mooyaart[115]	³¹P MRS	PDE (phospholipids)	PDE decreased in progressive patients.
1990	Sappey-Marinier[151]	T$_2$ relaxation times	Autopsy specimens	Relaxation times were prolonged with increased water in MS lesions.
1990	Wolinsky[191]	²H MRS	Active demyelination	Lipid peak seen in 6 patients.
1991	Koopmans[88]	²H MRS	Axonal loss, demyelination	NAA levels decreased and lipid peaks were seen.
1991	Cadoux-Hudson[18a]	³¹P MRS	Active demyelination	³¹P MRS can detect changes in energy metabolism in acute MS lesions.
1991	Arnold[2]	²H MRS	Axonal loss	NAA levels decreased with time.
1991	MacKay[103]	T$_2$ relaxation times	Normal myelin	A short T$_2$ component was found on multiexponential decay analysis.
1991	Armspach[1]	T$_2$ relaxation times	Normal-appearing white matter	T$_2$ relaxation times were abnormal.
1991	Matthews[104]	²H MRS	Axonal loss	NAA peak decreased over time.
1991		²H MRS	Active demyelination	Lactate peak seen.
1991	Larsson[94]	²H MRS	Active demyelination	Lipid peak seen in evolving plaques (2–3 mo).
1991	Van Hecke[180]	²H MRS	Axonal loss	NAA peak decreased over time.
1991	Miller[111]	²H MRS	Axonal loss	NAA peak decreased.
		²H MRS	Axonal loss, active demyelination	Decreased NAA, lactate peak were seen.

Continued on following page

351

Table 9–3.—*continued*

Year	Senior Author	Technique	Pathological State (Actual or Inferred)	Type of MR Activity or Changes Found or Proposed
1991	Larsson[92]	Diffusion	Demyelination	Findings suggest increased extracellular water space, therefore, decreased myelin.
1992	Arnold[3]	^{2}H MRS	Axonal loss	NAA peak (serial observations) decreased over time.
1992	Bruhn[18]	^{2}H MRS	Children with MS	NAA and creatines low in plaques.
1992	Arnold[3]	^{2}H MRS	Active demyelination	Choline levels increased.
1992	Dousset[31]	MTI	Demyelination	Lesions were easily detected by MTI, better than standard SE.
1992	Grossman[53]	^{2}H MRS	Axonal loss and active demyelination	Decreased NAA was found in 17/21 lesions. Enhancing lesions also showed myelin breakdown products.
1993	Koopmans[84]	^{2}H MRS	Gliosis, active demyelination, and axonal loss	Decreased NAA, increased inositol, and detection of fat peaks in MS lesions.
1993	Davie[24]	^{2}H MRS	Demyelination, axonal loss	Progressive loss of NAA and detection of lipid resonances were found in 7/8 acute MS lesions.
1994	Davie[26]	^{2}H MRS	Active demyelination, axonal damage	Serial MRS showed the NAA loss to recover in some lesions. The lipid resonances appeared after 1 mo and lasted 4–8 mo (average of 5 mo).
1994	Husted[64]	^{31}P MRS ^{2}H MRS	Reduced myelin lipids	NAA levels were decreased in lesions, and in normal-appearing white matter.
1994	Husted[63]	^{31}P MRS	Reduced myelin lipids	Phospholipid broad MRS component reduced in MS.
1994	Wolinsky[189]	^{2}H MRS	Metabolic activity	"Inositol storms" seen, temporary increases in normal appearing white matter.
1995	Peters[138]	^{2}H MRS	Axonal loss	NAA reduced in MS lesions and correlated with disability.
1995	Peters[138]	^{2}H MRS	MS normal-appearing white matter	NAA levels were decreased in MS group as compared with those of volunteers.
1995	De Stefano[27]	^{2}H MRS	MS lesions	1. The NAA decrease in MS can be reversible. 2. NAA changes correlated with neurological impairment ($r = 0.73$) ($P = <.0001$).
1995	Davie[25]	^{2}H MRS	Axonal loss in cerebellar ataxia (11 patients)	Ataxia correlated with decreased NAA in the cerebellum.
1995	Loevner[100]	MTI	Normal-appearing white matter	MTI detected abnormalities missed by conventional T_2-weighted imaging.

^{2}H = proton; MR = magnetic resonance; MTI = magnetization transfer imaging; NAA = *N*-acetylaspartate; ^{31}P = phosphorus; PDE = phosphodiesterase.

creased choline-to-creatine ratio with or without a decrease in NAA level. They also found that the NAA decrease could be reversible.[28] The same group has also found that myoinositol increased reversibly in acute lesions, and that the NAA changes correlated both with brain lesion volumes and clinical disability. In one case, a single lesion evolved from an increased choline-to-creatine ratio to a decreased NAA-to-creatine ratio. They proposed that the changes seen reflected the evolution from active demyelination to a stage of axonal loss. They did not find any evidence for neutral lipid in any of their lesions. Their inability to see lipid was probably due to the lack of ability to do short-echo-time MRS (TE20MS) on their machine. They have now confirmed that, as would be expected, NAA loss occurs in MRS studies of patients with amyotrophic lateral sclerosis.[140]

Van Hecke and colleagues[180] performed proton MRS studies on 18 patients with MS and 17 control subjects. They found the normal-appearing white matter in the MS group to be normal, and they also found decreased NAA-to-choline ratios in MS lesions. Subsequent studies[26,190] showed that the NAA drop can be transient, so that the loss of NAA in the brain seen on MRS study is not necessarily a marker for axonal loss. In this regard, Genain and co-workers[45] found NAA intensities on MRS to be a sensitive marker for experimental inflammatory lesions. DeStefano and associates[27] also found decreased NAA, choline, and creatine levels and increased inositol levels in 11 patients, including a lower-than-normal NAA in normal-appearing MS white matter. Husted and colleagues[63] found biochemical alterations in MS lesions by both ^{31}P and ^{2}H MRS. Davie and colleagues[24,25,26] not only found that the NAA decrease in MS could be reversible but also that NAA decrease in the cerebellum correlated with severe ataxia.

Lenkinski and colleagues[97] performed proton MRS studies on 15 patients with MS and found extra peaks in all. They found the extra peaks at 2.1 to 2.6 ppm in lesions that also showed gadolinium enhancement. They speculated that the extra peaks (which could be γ-aminobutyric acid, gluta-

mate, or other amino acids) could reflect myelin breakdown products.[53]

Studies by Dr. Peter Allen of the University of Alberta,[87,195] in collaboration with UBC, have shown that in some new or otherwise active MRI lesions, a proton MRS fat signal can be seen at very short (TE-20) echo times. Others have now confirmed this observation.[26] The fact that no fat changes were seen in other new lesions suggests that the pathological process in MS lesions is heterogeneous. These findings are consistent with the hypothesis that many of the new lesions are inflammatory ones and do not involve demyelination. However, we have seen some new lesions on serial MRI studies in which the NAA peak was low early in the evolution of the lesion. In some of those instances, the standard T_2-visible lesion then went away. This finding suggests that in some instances, the decrease in NAA level was not due to axonal loss or that axonal destruction may be a result of toxic effects of products of the intense inflammatory infiltration. Follow-up studies are underway to explore this hypothesis. Brenner and colleagues[17] have looked at the NAA peak in acute EAE in the guinea pig, in which there is very little demyelination, and found reduced NAA levels. Minderhoud and colleagues[114] used phosphorus MRS at 1.5 T to show increased creatine phosphate levels in MS lesions. They believed that this increase was correlated to the severity of the neurological handicap, being greatest in the patients with chronic disease.

Menon and associates[109] used MRS to study NAA levels in patients with acquired immunodeficiency disease. They found decreased NAA levels in both visible lesion areas and in normal-appearing white matter, supporting the concept that MRS studies can show axonal loss or dysfunction in areas of brain that are otherwise normal on imaging. In addition, some spectroscopic studies have shown an elevation in myo-inositol in both MS lesions[84] and normal-appearing white matter.[189] Wolinsky and his colleagues[189] showed what they call "inositol storms" in normal-appearing MS white matter, suggesting a transient metabolic change that may be another measure of disease activity. Because inositol has been shown to be elevated during active astrocyte proliferation,[84] it may play a part in active gliosis.

EXPERIMENTAL MRI, MRS, AND T_1 AND T_2 RELAXATION STUDIES (HUMAN AND ANIMAL)

Many investigators believe that relapsing EAE is a valid model for MS.[149] Therefore, MRI studies using this model should help us in understanding the pathological–MRI correlation in MS. Tofts and colleagues[175] surveyed the literature until 1991 and indicated a number of other modalities that could be used to follow pathological changes in brain tissue. They cover many of the technical factors that underlie these changes. Husted and colleagues[64] found changes in normal-appearing MS white matter, suggesting decreased neuronal density that was more widespread than previously suspected.

Table 9–4 cites a number of experimental MRI studies that we have surveyed, and a more detailed description of a selected group of these studies follows. Barnes and associates[10] used MRI to look at a triethyl tin model of cytotoxic cerebral edema in cats. They showed that T_2 relaxation time increased approximately twice as much as did T_1, and that the T_2 signal was biexponential. They concluded that the slowly relaxing component of T_2 reflected edema and that the rapidly relaxing component reflected intracellular water. They also examined vasogenic edema by a cortical freezing technique and found multiexponential decay characteristics for the T_2 signal. However, they contended that the T_1 changes were more informative for gliosis than were T_2. The same group[9] studied experimental gliosis after cortical freezing in cats. In contrast to the changes seen in cytotoxic edema, the T_1 signal changed in gliosis without much change in T_2.

Stewart and her colleagues[158,162] looked at multiexponential T_2 data from guinea pigs with EAE. She found a short T_2 component at approximately 10 ms that decreased as the tissue was more demyelinated on histological examination. Fresh and fixed tissue showed much the same findings. She and Mackay[103,162] proposed that this short T_2 component reflects the water trapped in the lamellae of normal myelin.

Ford and associates[41] examined lyso-phosphatidylcholine-induced demyelinating lesions and found that lesions evolved over 7 days and had a high-signal rim. The rim pathology consisted of lipid debris and lipid-laden macrophages. The lesion intensity fell over the next 2 weeks while remyelination developed.

Hawkins and his colleagues[58] performed elegant electron micrographic studies of gadolinium passing through the BBB in their guinea pig model of EAE. They showed most convincingly that, in their model, the gadolinium passes through the BBB by active vesicular transport rather than by diffusion past tight junctions. They were also able to block the vesicular transport by using a metabolic poison, showing that the process of vesicular transport is energy dependent. These and earlier investigators have also shown that enhanced vesicular traffic can be seen in the endothelium of blood vessels located within acute MS plaques. Richards and colleagues[144,145,146] performed a series of MRI and MRS studies of primates with EAE. They found lipid changes that could be postulated as due to the accumulation of neutral lipid during active demyelination. Therefore the MS and EAE MRS studies both point to a lipid signal indicating active demyelination (see pathology chapter).

One reason for using new techniques for detecting changes in myelin in magnetic resonance studies is to look at in-vivo evolving lesions. Several patients have been examined by using a multiexponential 32-echo T_2 sequence.[103] A minor component to the T_2 signal from white matter seen at short echo times is similar to that described by Stewart in EAE. It is seen in normal-appearing white matter but not in either gray matter or in most MS lesions. Possibly this minor, but consistent, component to the T_2 signal could be a marker for normal myelin. MacKay[103] proposed that this signal component represents the water trapped in the lamellae of normal myelin. If this finding and the fat detection by spectroscopy findings are consistent, then the goal of

Table 9–4. EXPERIMENTAL MRI STUDIES

Year	Senior Author	Pathological State Postulated or Seen	Material	Type of MR Activity Found or Proposed
1984	Karlik[74]	Inflammation	GP EAE	T_1 and T_2 prolonged in EAE lesions.
1985	Stewart[157]	Inflammation	Primate EAE	EAE lesions were seen on MRI scan.
1985	Noseworthy[123]	Inflammation	GP EAE	T_1 and T_2 were prolonged in EAE lesions.
1986	Karlik[75]	Inflammation	GP EAE	T_1 correlated with inflammation. T_2 correlated with demyelination.
1986	Barnes[10]	Cytotoxic cerebral edema	Cat—TET lesion	T_2 increased twice as much as T_1 in edema.
1987	Grossman[54]	Inflammation	GP EAE	T_2 MRI lesions had definite inflammatory pathology.
1987	Richards[147]	Demyelination	Primate EAE	MRS lipid signal increased.
1988	Barnes[9]	Vasogenic cerebral edema	Cat—cortical freezing	T_1 and T_2 both increased in EAE lesions.
1988	Barnes[9]	Gliosis	Cat—cortical freezing	T_1 changes more specific for gliosis than T_2.
1988	Simon[152]	Demyelination	GP EAE	^{2}H MRS can detect lipids in active demyelination.
1988	Stewart[159]	Normal myelin	Normal GP	A short T_2 component was found on multiexponential decay analysis.
1988	Peersman[137]	Inflammation	GP EAE	T_2 changes were seen.
1990	Ford[41]	Demyelination (LPC)	Rat	T_2 sensitive to both edema and demyelination. T_1 more sensitive to edema and lipid accumulation.
1991	Stewart[158]	Inflammation	Primate EAE lesions	Lesions come and go spontaneously.

Continued on following page

Table 9–4.—continued

Year	Senior Author	Pathological State Postulated or Seen	Material	Type of MR Activity Found or Proposed
1990	Hawkins[58]	Blood-brain barrier disruption	GP EAE	Gd crosses blood-brain barrier by active vesicular transport.
1990	Ford[41]	Demyelination	Rat EAE	T_1 and T_2 prolongation with high-signal rim.
1991	Richards[146]	Active lesions	Primate EAE	Shifts in creatine, choline peaks help to define pathology.
1991	Stewart[163]	Demyelination	GP EAE	T_2 signal analysis indicated active demyelination.
1992	Dousset[31]	Demyelination	GP EAE	Magnetization transfer imaging more sensitive than SE imaging.
1992	Richards[144]	Demyelination (no axonal loss)	Primate EAE	NAA levels decreased.
1993	Koopmans[84]	Gliosis	Human lesions	Inositol levels increased as a possible marker.
1993	Stewart[162]	Demyelination	GP EAE	T_2 relaxation time studies of lesions can detect demyelination.
1994	Wolinsky[189]	Metabolic activity	Human NAWM	"Inositol storms" occur in NAWM.
1994	Genain[45]	Acute inflammation	Primate NAWM	NAWM was abnormal on ^2H MRS studies with reduced NAA.
1994	Husted[62,64]	MS lesions	Human NAWM	NAWM was abnormal on ^{31}P MRS studies.
1995	Richards[145]	Acute and chronic lesions	Primate EAE	Diffusion imaging helped to distinguish between acute inflammatory and chronic lesions.
1996	Morissey[116]	Inflammation and edema	Rat EAE	High-field MRI may distinguish between inflammation and vasogenic edema.

EAE = experimental allergic encephalomyelitis; Gd = gadolinium; GP = guinea pig; LPC = lysophosphatidylcholine; MR = magnetic resonance; NAA = N-acetyl aspartate; NAWM = normal-appearing white matter; SE = spin echo; TET = triethyl tin.

using MR techniques to document the evolution of demyelination in MS lesions may soon be attainable. Figures 9–14 and 9–15 illustrate the myelin images from MacKay's studies. The method involves detecting the loss of myelin by loss of the myelin component on T_2 relaxation and subsequently detecting the appearance of myelin breakdown products by MRS.

Magnetization transfer imaging (MTI) may also be used to look at similar biochemical changes. MTI is a way of specifying water content in its relation to macromolecules.[52] One saturates the energy level of bound protons in immobile water. Exchange of this energy with free water thus changes the intensity of signals on a subsequent MR image. Patients with MS had a low magnetization transfer (MT) rate in both lesions (26 percent) and normal-appearing white matter (37 percent). The MT rate in normal-appearing white matter was lowest (33 percent) in patients with CPMS.

Magnetization transfer imaging may be measuring, in a more gross way, the same water components as does T_2 relaxation analysis (see previous discussion).[103] It appears that MTI[31,50] changes evolve later than do T_2 changes and may reflect demyelination, axonal loss, or both. The changes seen on T_1 images may also reflect demyelination, although experimental studies suggest that T_1 is sensitive to gliosis as well. MTI and T_1 certainly reveal the more severely involved lesions, because these measures both correlate better with clinical impairment than does the extent of T_2 abnormalities.[30,182]

Dousset and colleagues,[30] using MTI, reported that demyelinated and axonal loss lesions had a low MT rating. They also found several different patterns suggesting stability; remyelination; or progressive axonal demyelination, axonal loss, or both. They felt MTI was useful in following the severity of lesions. Dousset and colleagues[29] also did some pathological correlation studies. Campi and colleagues[19] and Loevner and colleagues[100] used MTI to show that there were changes seen in MS normal-appearing white matter, suggesting that demyelination or axonal loss occurs remote from the T_2-visible MS lesions. MTI has also been used to show that the MT ratio in the spinal cord may be able to identify significant demyelination and axonal loss.[151b]

Richards[144] and Heide and colleagues[59] both found that diffusion-weighted (DW) MRI could pick up experimental pathological changes that were not seen on the T_2-weighted images, suggesting that subtle changes in large fiber bundles, such as those of the pyramidal tract, can be picked up easily by DW MRI. Richards[145] also showed that in primate EAE, diffusion

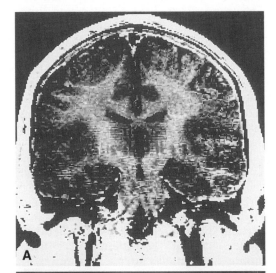

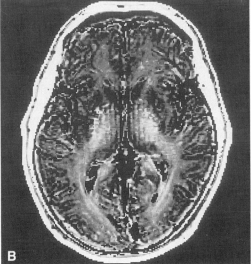

Figure 9–14. These two figures illustrate the myelin map of MacKay in coronal and axial views (see text for explanation). (Courtesy of Dr. Alex MacKay, Department of Physics, University of British Columbia, Magnetic Resonance in Medicine 31:673–677, 1994, p 674–675.)

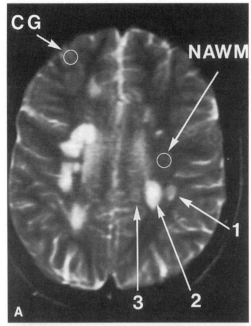

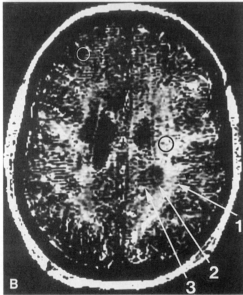

Figure 9–15. (A) A proton-density axial MR scan of a patient with MS showing several typical high-signal lesions. (B) A myelin map (MacKay) from the same patient, obtained on the same day at the same level, showing that three of the lesions seen on the proton-density MR scan have variable loss of the myelin signal. Lesion 1 shows no loss of myelin signal, lesion 2 has severe loss of the myelin signal, and lesion 3 has variable partial loss (see text for explanation). CG = cortical gray matter; NAWM = normal-appearing white matter. (Courtesy of Dr. Alex MacKay, Department of Physics, University of British Columbia, Magnetic Resonance in Medicine 31:673–677, 1994, p 676.)

imaging may help to distinguish between acute monophasic inflammatory lesions and clinical demyelinated ones. Acute lesions were associated with the diffusion-sensitizing gradient in three orthogonal directions, whereas chronic lesions were associated with the diffusion-sensitizing gradient in two orthogonal directions (see Table 9–4). Diffusion imaging may also be helpful in MS.[42]

Armspach and colleagues[1] and Rumbach and associates[150] evaluated T_2 relaxation times in 19 examinations on seven patients. They reported that the T_2 relaxation times in MS lesions were biexponential and that the normal-appearing white matter had abnormal T_2 relaxation times. They proposed that T_2 relaxation analysis could be helpful in differentiating edema from demyelination and gliosis. Others[55,103] have also been able to distinguish between some lesions using T_2 relaxation analysis and automatic segmentation methods.[139a]

Larsson and co-workers[96] looked at the T_2 relaxation times in patients with MS with acute MRI lesions and followed the changes serially. They found that the T_2 was monoexponential in the acute phase and that T_2 became biexponential in most patients after 60 days, with a tendency to revert to monoexponentiality after some time.

Karlik and colleagues[73] looked carefully at the T_1 and T_2 relaxation times in tissue excised from guinea pigs with EAE. They found that the magnetic resonance relaxation times varied with the pathology, but the changes were inconsistent from lesion to lesion. For instance, in some inflammatory lesions, the T_1 relaxation times were prolonged in edematous tissue. However, when a heavy cellular infiltrate was present, the trend was reversed and the T_1 relaxation times were normal.

In a series of studies in primate EAE, Stewart and her colleagues[159] showed that MRI lesions could be seen to develop before the animals showed signs of impairment. In one animal, a delayed relapsing-remitting disease detected by serial MRI followed a single low-dose immunization. The animal was inoculated with an unusually small amount of myelin basic protein in Freund's adjuvant to produce sublethal disease. In that animal, bilateral cerebral MRI lesions developed entirely asymptomatically after an unusual delay (53 days). Those lesions disappeared, but subsequent MRI follow-up showed an asymptomatic new lesion to spontaneously appear at a new anatomical site (93 days). All of the MRI activity came and subsequently resolved without the appearance of impairment in the animal. Pathological examination did not show any evidence for either demyelination or inflammation, suggesting that the lesions seen on MRI were initially inflammatory ones that resolved without any demyelination. If the lesions had been remyelinated, the pathological characteristics of remyelination should have been seen (see Chapter 8). Additional attention to this very mild EAE model in the future should help to better understand the mechanisms involved in the evolution of these transient, presumably inflammatory lesions.

Morrissey and associates[116] looked at 7-Tesla imaging in rats with adoptive transfer EAE both before and after gadolinium injection. They found that MRI findings at high-field strength could detect changes before cellular inflammation could be seen pathologically or clinical signs appeared. They proposed that MRI could distinguish between vasogenic edema and inflammation in this model.

It is exciting that in the future, the use of combined serial MRI, MRS, and relaxation time studies might possibly allow the simultaneous identification of the lesions and the anatomical and chemical changes that occur in the lesions during their evolution. MRS has recently been done on volumes as small as a mouse brain using very high field strengths.[176a] Tables 9–3 and 9–4 list the MR and other pathological variables in MS that may be useful for MRI characterization of pathology in vivo. Figure 9–16 gives an overall schema for the evolution of MS lesions and their investigation. Figure 9–17 illustrates the evolution of a single MS lesion

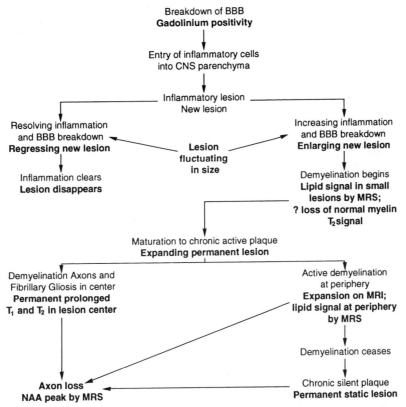

Figure 9–16. Our view of the evolution of a single MS lesion over time and the MR techniques that can reveal the evolving pathology (see text for explanation). NAA = *N*-acetyl aspartate.

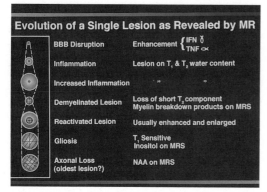

Figure 9–17. Evolution of a single lesion as revealed by magnetic resonance techniques. This cartoon outlines the MR techniques that can help in distinguishing specific pathological changes in the evolution of a single MS lesion. (**See Color Plate IV.**)

and how MR techniques might detect the pathological changes.

SUMMARY AND FUTURE DIRECTIONS

Table 9–5 lists some proposed techniques that have been or soon will be used to study the living pathology of MS. Figure 9–16 illustrates how those techniques can be used in a systematic fashion.

The following points summarize the current relationship between MRI and the detection and characterization of MS lesions:

1. The sectional area, and eventually the volume, of MS lesions seen on MRI scan can be measured with reasonable accuracy.
2. Serial studies have shown that many chronic lesions increase in extent over time. In follow-up, significant increases in size can be measured.
3. Pathological correlation studies in chronic cases have supported the concept that most areas with increased T_2 signal represent demyelination, although there is a component of inflammation as well. Increased T_1 signal may reflect gliosis as well as demyelination. Lesions seen on T_1 and by MTI seem to be those with the most advanced changes. Pathological correlation studies also show that enhancement represents breakdown of the

BBB associated with active inflammation.
4. Many asymptomatic lesions (probably mostly inflammatory) can appear, enlarge, and then shrink in size or occasionally disappear over time. Many of these asymptomatic active lesions are seen in the deep cerebral white matter, which is a different distribution from the commonly seen established periventricular confluent lesions and periventricular demyelination.
5. Of new MRI lesions, 80 percent enhance with gadolinium, indicating active breakdown in the BBB. The BBB disruption occurs early in the evolution of the lesion. In addition, experimental studies show that passage of gadolinium across the BBB is an active metabolic process by vesicular transport. New methods of quantitation of the enhancement will add yet another dimension to our ability to analyze the evolution of the active lesions.
6. Relaxation time studies, using multiexponential T_2 measurements, show a short component of the T_2 signal that may originate from the water trapped in the myelin lamellae that could serve as a marker for normal myelin. Also, new methods of studying lesions, such as MTI and diffusion-weighted imaging,[42] will help to further define the MS lesions in relation to specific pathways and eventually specific pathological characteristics. High-field MRI may also help to distinguish vasogenic edema from inflammation.
7. Magnetic resonance spectroscopy has the ability to detect metabolic changes that seem to be markers for axonal loss (NAA) and active demyelination (neutral fat). However, the NAA level may be reversible in some instances. Persistent changes (confirmed by follow-up) may be a reliable marker for axonal loss.

Based on MRI experience, many investigators believe that new or active MRI lesions develop after a breakdown in the BBB and that initially they are probably purely inflammatory in nature. New or active lesions detected by MRI go through a cycle of waxing or waning over time and only become stable and permanent after some time has

Table 9–5. **MAGNETIC RESONANCE VARIABLES THAT MAY BE HELPFUL IN DETERMINING MULTIPLE SCLEROSIS PATHOLOGY IN VIVO**

Year	Senior Author	Technique	Possible Revealed Tissue Specificity
1988	Paty[130]	T_2-weighted imaging	Extent of disease by morphologic findings.
		Series T_2-weighted imaging	Serial studies show the dynamics of morphologic changes.
1988	Miller[113]	Enhancement	This technique identifies BBB disruption. On serial studies, 10% of active lesions identified only by enhancement.
1986	Barnes[10]	T_2 relaxation analysis	Water, sometimes biexponential.
1988	Barnes[9]	T_1 relaxation analysis	Gliosis, demyelination.
1991	McKay[103]	Short components of T_2 on relaxation analysis	Normal myelin.
1990	Wolinsky[191]	Fat on ^{2}H MRS	Active demyelination
1991	Arnold[2]	NAA peak on ^{2}H MRS	Reduced NAA levels may be a measure of axonal loss; levels can be reduced in pure inflammation as well.
1992	Dousset[31]	Magnetization transfer imaging (MTI)	Experimental study suggests that MTI measures demyelination.
1993	Koopmans[84]	Inositol	Metabolic activity may reflect active gliosis.
1993	Heide[59]	Diffusion imaging (DI)	DI may detect lesions in tracts.
1994	Grossman[50]	MTI	Free water versus immobile water: demyelination and/or axonal loss.
1994	Wolinsky[189]	^{2}H MRS	"Inositol storms" occur in normal-appearing white matter in patients with MS studied serially.
1995	Richards[145]	Diffusion imaging (DI)	May distinguish between inflammation and demyelination.
1996	Morrissey[116]	7-T MRI	Highfield MRI may distinguish between edema (T_1) and inflammation (enhancement).

BBB = blood-brain barrier; ^{2}H = proton; NAA =*N*-acetyl aspartate; ^{31}P = phosphorus.

passed. How much of this dynamic activity is due to fluctuations in the inflammatory infiltrate and the edema of BBB breakdown and how much is due to demyelination followed by remyelination is not known at this point. A given lesion behaves independently of neighboring lesions in its evolution.

We believe that demyelination is present only when the lesion has become permanent on the MRI scan or when it has merged with neighboring lesions to appear confluent. Permanent neurological deficits may develop because of persistent conduction block in demyelinated axons or because of axonal loss. As in pathological studies, the extent of the MRI changes can be more extensive than predicted clinically.[117a]

Recent MRS studies have shown that NAA levels in MS are low, and have rekindled interest in study of the axon in MS. Some investigators[2,132] have suggested that the only permanent loss of function in MS may be due to the loss of axons. A clinical study of the retina[102] showed a loss of the retinal nerve fiber layer in MS. However, the mechanism for this neuronal loss is unknown. Some axonal loss may be due to damage at the time of the intense inflammatory response in acute lesions (bystander effect). It is also possible that neuronal cell loss may occur more slowly as demyelination changes the neuron cell body physiology, perhaps making the cell more vulnerable to otherwise tolerated endogenous or other toxins, such as excitatory amino acids and free radicals.

Systematic study of the phenomenon of neuronal and axonal loss in MS is needed. If the loss of axons is a chronic process following the initial demyelinating injury and is responsible for major components of the clinical neurological impairment, then new therapeutic strategies directed toward neuronal protection must be developed. The relationship between the morphology, physiology, and clinical expression of the MS lesion was discussed further in Chapter 8. As a result of clinical and experimental studies in pathology, neurophysiology, and MRI technology, an emerging concept is that inflammation, demyelination, and axonal loss may be dissociated (at least in time). Demyelination may be secondary, but not an invariable accompaniment secondary to inflammation.

Future research should determine whether the histological features of MS can be resolved by using MRI techniques. Long-term clinical follow-up of serial MRI studies will give some indication of the prognostic importance of the observed levels of MRI activity. Several studies have found that MRI changes at onset predict the neurological impairment at 5 years follow-up. Certainly, the concept of new lesions accumulating over time, eventually determining the clinical evolution of the disease, makes intuitive sense. Consequently, the next few years should provide exciting new insights into pathogenesis, which, in turn, will result in much more accurate assessment of new therapies.

REFERENCES

1. Armspach JP, Gounot D, Rumbach L, and Chambron J: In vivo determination of multiexponential T2 relaxation in the brain of patients with multiple sclerosis. Magn Reson Imaging 9:107–113, 1991.
2. Arnold DL, Matthews PM, Francis GS, and Antel J: Proton MR spectroscopic imaging (SI) for metabolic characterization of the brain plaques of demyelinating disease. Neurology 41(suppl 1):144, 1991.
3. Arnold DL, Matthews PM, Francis GS, O'Connor J, and Antel JP: Proton magnetic resonance spectroscopic imaging for metabolic characteri-

zation of demyelinating plaques. Ann Neurol 31:235–241, 1992.
4. Arnold DL, Matthews PM, Mollevarger L, Luyten P, Francis G, and Antel J: In Vivo–Localized proton magnetic resonance spectroscopy allows plaque characterization in multiple sclerosis. Society of Magnetic Resonance in Medicine, Book of Abstracts, Vol. 1. New York, N.Y. 1990, p 110.
5. Barkhof F: Gadolinium Enhanced Magneti Resonance Imaging in Multiple Sclerosis. Vrije Universiteit University Press, Amsterdam, 1992.
6. Barkhof F, Frequin STFM, Hommes OR, et al: A correlative triad of gadolinium-DTPA MRI, EDSS, and CSF-MBP in relapsing multiple sclerosis patients treated with high-dose intravenous methylprednisolone. Neurology 42:63–67, 1992.
6a. Barkhof F, Scheltens P, Frequin STFM, et al: Relapsing-remitting multiple sclerosis: Sequential enhanced MR imaging vs clinical findings in determining disease activity. AJR 159:1041–1047, 1992.
7. Barkhof F, Valk J, Hommes OR, Scheltens P, and Nauta JJ: Gadopentetate dimeglumine enhancement of multiple sclerosis lesions on long TR spin-echo images at 0.6 T. American Journal of Neuroradiology 13:1257–1259, 1992.
8. Barnes D, du Bolay EG, McDonald WI, Johnson G, and Tofts PS: The NMR signal decay characteristics of cerebral oedema. Acta Radiol Suppl 369:503–506, 1986.
9. Barnes D, McDonald WI, Landon DN, and Johnson G: The characterization of experimental gliosis by quantitative nuclear magnetic resonance imaging. Brain 111:83–94, 1988.
10. Barnes D, McDonald WI, Tofts PS, Johnson G, and Landon DN: Magnetic resonance imaging of experimental cerebral oedema. J Neurol Neurosurg Psychiatry 49:1341–1347, 1986.
11. Barnes D, Munro PM, Youl BD, Prineas JW, and McDonald WI: The longstanding MS lesion: A quantitative MRI and electron microscopic study. Brain 114:1271–1280, 1991.
12. Bastianello S, Pozzilli C, Bernardi S, Bozzao L, Fantozzi LM, Buttinelli C, and Fieschi C: Serial study of gadolinium-DTPA MRI enhancement in multiple sclerosis. Neurology 40:591–595, 1990.
13. Baum K, Nehrig C, Schörner W, and Girke W: Periventricular plaques in multiple sclerosis: irreversible? An MRI follow-up study. Eur Neurol 32:219–221, 1992.
14. Baumhefner RW, Syndulko K, Tourtellotte WW, et al: Multiple sclerosis: Area and circumference correlations of MRI-demonstrated lesions with CSF parameters and measurements of clinical disability. Neurology 41(suppl 1):144, 1991.
15. Bodian D: Pathogenesis and histopathology. In River TM, and Horsfall FL (eds): Viral and Rickettsial Infections of Man, ed 3. Pitman Medical, London, 1959, pp 478–498.
16. Brainin M, Neuhold A, Reisner T, Maida E, Lang S, and Deecke L: Changes within the "normal" cerebral white matter of multiple sclerosis patients during acute attacks and during high-

dose cortisone therapy assessed by means of quantitative MRI. J Neurol Neurosurg Psychiatry 52: 1355–1359, 1989.

17. Brenner RE, Williams SC, Bell JD, et al: The proton NMR spectrum in acute EAE: An in-vivo and in-vitro correlative study. Society of Magnetic Resonance in Medicine, Works in Progress, San Francisco, 1991 and 1994, p 1049.

18. Bruhn H, Frahm J, Merboldt KD, et al: Multiple sclerosis in children: Cerebral metabolic alterations monitored by localized proton magnetic resonance spectroscopy in vivo. Ann Neurol 32:140–150, 1992.

18a. Cadoux-Hudson TAD, Kermode A, Rajagopalan B, et al: Biochemical changes within a multiple sclerosis plaque in vivo. (Short report) J Neurol Neurosurg Psychiatry 54:1004–1006, 1991.

19. Campi A, Filippi M, Dousset V, et al: A magnetization transfer imaging study of normal appearing white matter in multiple sclerosis. 10th Congress of the European Committee for Treatment and Research in Multiple Sclerosis, Book of Abstracts. Athens Greece, 1994, p 47.

20. Capra R, Marcianò N, Vignolo LA, Chiesa A, and Gasparotti R: Gadolinium-pentetic acid magnetic resonance imaging in patients with relapsing-remitting multiple sclerosis. Arch Neurol 49:687- 689, 1992.

21. Comi G, Filippi M, Martinelli V, et al: Brain MRI correlates of cognitive impairment in primary and secondary progressive multiple sclerosis. J Neurol Sci 132:222–227, 1995.

22. Compston DA, Milligan NM, Hughes PJ, et al: A double-blind controlled trial of high dose methylprednisolone in patients with multiple sclerosis. II. Laboratory results. J Neurol Neurosurg Psychiatry 50:517- 522, 1987.

23. Confort-Gouny S, Vion-Dury J, Nicoli F, et al: A multiparametric data analysis showing the potential of localized proton MR spectroscopy of the brain in the metabolic characterization of neurological diseases. J Neurol Sci 118:123–133, 1993.

24. Davie CA, Hawkins CP, Barker GJ, Brennan A, Tofts PS, Miller DH: Detection of myelin breakdown products by proton magnetic resonance spectroscopy. The Lancet 341:630–631, 1993.

25. Davie CA, Barker GJ, Webb S, et al: Persistent functional deficit in multiple sclerosis and autosomal dominant cerebellar ataxia is associated with axon loss. Brain 118:1583–1592, 1995.

26. Davie CA, Hawkins CP, Barker GJ, et al: Serial proton magnetic resonance spectroscopy in acute multiple sclerosis lesions. Brain 117:49–58, 1994.

27. De Stefano N, Matthews PM, Phil D, et al: Chemical pathology of acute demyelinating lesions and its correlation with disability. Ann Neurol 38: 901–909, 1995.

28. De Stefano N, Matthews PM, Arnold DL: Reversible decreases in n-acetylaspartate after acute brain injury. Society of Magnetic Resonance in Medicine Annual Meeting, New York, 1995.

29. Dousset V, Brochet B, Vital A, et al: Histiopathologic correlates of MR, magnetization transfer and diffusion imaging abnormalities of EAE lesions in primates. 10th Congress of the European Committee for Treatment and Research in Multiple Sclerosis, Book of Abstracts, San Francisco, 1994, p 16.

30. Dousset V, Brochet B, Gaillou A, Mieze S, Lafont P, and Caille JM: Longitudinal magnetization transfer study of MS lesions. 10th Congress of the European Committee for Treatment and Research in Multiple Sclerosis, Book of Abstracts, San Francisco, 1994, p 49.

31. Dousset V, Grossman RI, Ramer KN, et al: Experimental allergic encephalomyelitis and multiple sclerosis: Lesion characterization with magnetization transfer imaging. Radiology 182:483–491, 1992.

32. Ebers GC, Vinuela FV, Feasby TE, and Bass B: Multifocal CT enhancement in MS. Neurology 34:341–346, 1984.

33. Estes ML, Rudick RA, Barnett GH, and Ransohoff RM: Stereotactic biopsy of an active multiple sclerosis lesion: Immunocytochemical analysis and neuropathologic correlation with magnetic resonance imaging. Arch Neurol 47:1299–1303, 1990.

34. Filippi M, Barker GJ, Horsfield MA, et al: Benign and secondary progressive multiple sclerosis: A preliminary quantitative MRI study. J Neurol 241:246–251, 1994(a).

35. Filippi M, Horsfield MA, Bressi S, et al: Intra- and inter-observer agreement of brain MRI lesion volume measurements in multiple sclerosis: A comparison of techniques. 10th Congress of the European Committee for Treatment and Research in Multiple Sclerosis, Book of Abstracts, San Francisco, 1994, p 10.

36. Filippi M, Horsfield MA, Morrissey SP, et al: Quantitative brain MRI lesion load predicts the course of clinically isolated syndromes suggestive of multiple sclerosis. Neurology 44:635–641, 1994(b).

37. Filippi M, Campi A, Martinelli V, et al: A brain MRI study of different types of chronic-progressive multiple sclerosis. Acta Neurol Scand 91:231–233, 1995.

38. Filippi M, Horsfield MA, Campi A, Manni S, Pereira C, Comi G: Resolution-dependent estimates of lesion volumes in magnetic resonance imaging studies of the brain in multiple sclerosis. Ann Neurol 38:749–754, 1995.

39. Filippi M, Yousry T, Campi A, et al: Comparison of triple dose versus standard dose gadolinium-DTPA for detection of MRI enhancing lesions in patients with MS. Neurology 46:379–384, 1996.

40. Fisher BJ: Radiation and MS (letter). Neurology 44:1769, 1994.

41. Ford CC, Ceckler TL, Karp J, and Herndon RM: Magnetic resonance imaging of experimental demyelinating lesions. Magnetic Resonance in Medicine 14:461–481, 1990.

42. Forti A, Bydder GM, Hajnal JV, and Young IR: Use of diffusion weighted magnetic resonance imaging in multiple sclerosis. Society of Magnetic Resonance in Medicine, Book of Abstracts, Vol 1, San Francisco, 1991, p 86.

43. Francis GS, Evans AC and Arnold DL: Neuroimaging in multiple sclerosis in neurologic clinics. Multiple Sclerosis 13:(1)147–171, 1995.

44. Frederiksen JL, Larsson HB, Ottovay E, Stigsby B, and Elesen J: Acute optic neuritis with normal visual acuity. Acta Ophthalmol Suppl 69: 357–366, 1991.

45. Genain CP, Nguyen MH, Roberts T, Uccelli A, Moseley M, and Hauser SL: Characterization of changes in cerebral white matter by magnetic resonance imaging and 1H spectroscopy during experimental allergic encephalomyelitis in primates. Neurology 44(suppl 2):A340, 1994.

46. Gonzalez CF, Vinitski S, Seshagiri S, Lublin FD, and Knobler RL: Volumetric regional analysis of MS lesions of the brain using 3D segmentation. Neurology 44(suppl 2):A339, 1994.

47. Goodkin DE, Ross J, Vander Brug-Medendorp S, Konecsni J, and Rudick RA: Magnetic resonance imaging lesion enlargement in multiple sclerosis: Disease-related activity, chance occurrence or measurement artifact? Ann Neurol 30:306, 1991.

48. Grafton ST, Sumi SM, Stimac GK, Alvord EC, Shaw C, and Nochlin D: Comparison of postmortem magnetic resonance imaging and neuropathologic findings in the cerebral white matter. Arch Neurol 48:293–298, 1991.

49. Grimaud J, Lai M, Thorpe JW, et al: Evaluation of a computer assisted quantification of multiple sclerosis lesions in cranial MRI. J Neurol, Neurosurg Psychiatry 59:200–218, 1995.

50. Grossman RI: Magnetization transfer in multiple sclerosis. Ann Neurol 36(suppl):S97-S99,1994.

51. Grossman RI, Braffman BH, Brorson JR, Goldberg HI, Silberg DH, and Gonzalez-Scarano F: Multiple sclerosis: Serial study of Gadolinium-enhanced MR imaging. Radiology 169:117–122, 1988.

52. Grossman RI, Gomori JM, Ramer KN, Lexa FJ, and Schnall MD: Magnetization transfer: Theory and clinical applications in neuroradiology. Radiographics 14:279–290, 1994.

53. Grossman RI, Lenkinski RE, Ramer KN, Gonzalez-Scarano F, and Cohen JA: MR proton spectroscopy in multiple sclerosis. AJNR 13:1535–1543, 1992.

54. Grossman RI, Lisak RP, Macchi PJ, and Joseph PM: MR of acute experimental allergic encephalomyelitis. American Journal of Neuroradiology 8:1045–1048, 1987.

55. Guttmann CR, Mulkern RV, Clain A, Sandor T, and Jolesz FA: Discrimination of white matter lesion subtypes in multiple sclerosis using multiple T2 relaxation parameters. Society of Magnetic Resonance in Medicine, Book of Abstracts, Vol 1, San Francisco, 1991, p 87.

56. Harris JO, Frank JA, Patronas N, McFarlin DE, and McFarland HF: Serial gadolinium-enhanced magnetic resonance imaging scans in patients with early, relapsing-remitting multiple sclerosis: Implications for clinical trials and natural history. Ann Neurol 29:548–555, 1991.

57. Hartung HP, Reiners K, Archelos JJ, et al: Circulating adhesion molecules and tumor necrosis factor receptor in multiple sclerosis: Correlation with magnetic resonance imaging. Ann Neurol 38:186–193, 1995.

58. Hawkins CP, Munro PMG, MacKenzie F, et al: Duration and selectivity of blood-brain barrier breakdown in chronic relapsing experimental allergic encephalomyelitis studied by gadolinium-DTPA and protein markers. Brain 113(pt 2):365–378, 1990.

59. Heide AC, Richards TL, Alvord EC Jr, Peterson J, and Rose LM: Diffusion imaging of experimental allergic encephalomyelitis. Magnetic Imaging in Medicine 29:478–484, 1993.

60. Honer WG, Hurwitz T, Li DKB, Palmer M, and Paty DW: Temporal lobe involvement in multiple sclerosis patients with psychiatric disorders. Arch Neurol 44:187–190, 1987.

61. Hook CC, Kimmel DW, Kvols LK, et al: Multifocal inflammatory leukoencephalopathy with 5-fluorouracil and levamisole. Ann Neurol 31:262–267, 1992.

62. Husted C: Contributions of neuroimaging to diagnosis and monitoring of multiple sclerosis. Curr Opin Neurol 7:234–241, 1994.

63. Husted CA, Goodin DS, Hugg JW, et al: Biochemical alterations in multiple sclerosis lesions and normal-appearing white matter detected by in vivo p and h spectroscopic imaging. Ann Neurol 36:157–165, 1994.

64. Husted CA, Matson GB, Adams DA, Goodin DS, and Weiner MW: In vivo detection of myelin phospholipids in multiple sclerosis with phosphorus magnetic resonance spectroscopic imaging. Ann Neurol 36:239–241, 1994.

65. IFNB Multiple Sclerosis Study Group: Interferon beta-1b in the treatment of multiple sclerosis: Final outcome of the randomized controlled trial. Neurology 45:1277–1285, 1995.

66. Isaac C, Li DKB, Genton M, et al: Multiple sclerosis: A serial study using MRI in relapsing patients. Neurology 38:1511–1515, 1988.

67. Jackson EF, Narayana PA, Wolinsky JS, and Doyle TJ: Accuracy and reproducibility in volumetric analysis of multiple sclerosis lesions. J Comput Assist Tomogr 17:200–205, 1993.

67a. Jacobs LD, Cookfair DL, Rudick RA, et al: Intramuscular interferon beta-1a for disease progression in relapsing multiple sclerosis. Ann Neurol 39:285–294, 1996.

68. Johnson MA, Li DKB, Bryant DJ, and Payne JA: Magnetic resonance imaging: Serial observations in multiple sclerosis. AJNR 5:495–499, 1984.

69. Kamber M, Collins DL, Shinghal R, Francis GS, and Evans AC: Model-based 3D segmentation of multiple sclerosis lesions in dual-echo MRI data. (Proceedings of the International Society for Optical Engineering.) Visualization in Biomedical Computing p 590–600:1992.

70. Kamber M, Collins DL, Narayanan S, Pioro E, Evans AC, and Arnold DL: Tissue probability models in standardized brain space and the classification of MS plaques in MRI. Proceedings of the 12th Annual Scientific Meeting of the Society of Magnetic Resonance in Medicine, New York, 3:1600, 1993.

71. Kapouleas I: Automatic detection of white matter lesions in magnetic resonance brain images.

Comput Methods Programs Biomed 32:17–35, 1990.

72. Kappos L, Städt D, Ratzka M, et al: Magnetic resonance imaging in the evaluation of treatment in multiple sclerosis. Neuroradiology 30:299–302, 1988.

73. Karlik SJ, Gilbert JJ, Wong C, Vandervoort MK, and Noseworthy JH: NMR studies in experimental allergic encephalomyelitis: Factors which contribute to T1 and T2 values. Magn Reson Med 14:1–11, 1990.

74. Karlik SJ, Noseworthy J, Gilbert JJ, St. Louis J, and Strejan G: Nuclear magnetic resonance (NMR) spectroscopy studies in experimental allergic encephalomyelitis (EAE). Proceedings of the Society of Magnetic Resonance in Medicine: Scientific Program Third Annual Meeting. Academic Press, San Diego, 1984, p 399.

75. Karlik SJ, Strejan G, Gilbert JJ, and Noseworthy JH: NMR studies in experimental allergic encephalomyelitis (EAE): Normalization of T1 and T2 with parenchymal cellular infiltration. Neurology 36:1112–1114, 1986.

76. Kastrukoff LF, Oger JJF, Tourtellotte WW, Sacks SL, Berkowitz J, and Paty DW: Systemic lymphoblastoid interferon therapy in chronic progressive multiple sclerosis. II. Immunologic evaluation. Neurology 41:1936–1941, 1991.

77. Katz D, Taubenberger JK, Canella B, McFarlin DE, Raine CS, and McFarland HF: Correlation between magnetic resonance imaging findings and lesion development in chronic, active multiple sclerosis. Ann Neurol 34:661–669, 1993.

78. Kauppinen RA, Williams SR, Busza AL, and van Bruggen N: Applications of magnetic resonance spectroscopy and diffusion-weighted imaging to the study of brain biochemistry and pathology of multiple sclerosis. TINS-Trends in Neuroscience 16:88–95, 1993.

79. Kermode AG, Tofts PS, Thompson AJ, et al: Heterogeneity of blood-brain barrier changes in multiple sclerosis: An MRI study with gadolinium-DTPA enhancement. Neurology 40:229–235, 1990.

80. Khoury SJ, Guttmann CRG, Orav EJ, et al: Longitudinal MRI in multiple sclerosis: Correlation betweeen disability and lesion burden. Neurology 44:2120–2124, 1994.

81. Kidd D, Thompson AJ, Kendall BE, Miller DH, and McDonald WI: Benign form of multiple sclerosis: MRI evidence for less frequent and less inflammatory disease activity. J Neurol Neurosurg Psychiatry 57:1070–1072, 1994.

82. Koopmans RA, Li DKB, Grochowski E, Cutler PJ, and Paty DW: Benign versus chronic progressive multiple sclerosis: Magnetic resonance imaging features. Ann Neurol 25:74–81, 1989.

83. Koopmans RA, Li DKB, Oger JJF, et al: Chronic progressive multiple sclerosis: Serial magnetic resonance brain imaging over six months. Ann Neurol 26:248–256, 1989.

83a. Koopmans RA, Li DKB, Oger JJF, Mayo J and Paty DW: The lesion of multiple sclerosis: Imaging of acute and chronic stages. Neurology 39:959–963, 1989.

84. Koopmans RA, Li DKB, Zhu G, Allen PS, Penn A, and Paty DW: Magnetic resonance spectroscopy of multiple sclerosis: In-vivo detection of myelin breakdown products. The Lancet 341:631–632, 1993.

85. Koopmans RA, Li DKB, Zhao GJ, Redekop WK, and Paty DW: MRI assessment of cyclosporine therapy of MS in a multi-center trial. Neurology 42(suppl 3):210, 1992, in the press, J. of Neuroimaging, 1997.

86. Koopmans RA, Li DKB, Redekop WK, et al: The use of magnetic resonance imaging in monitoring interferon therapy of multiple sclerosis. J Neuroimaging 3:163–168, 1993.

87. Koopmans RA, Zhao GJ, Li DKB, Allen PS, Javidan M, and Paty DW: In-vivo proton MRS of the acute and chronic lesion of multiple sclerosis. Society of Magnetic Resonance in Medicine, Works in Progress 1205, 1990.

88. Koopmans RA, Zhao GJ, Li DKB, et al: Localized proton MR spectroscopy of the evolution of multiple sclerosis. Society of Magnetic Resonance in Medicine, Works in Progress, San Francisco, p 1058, 1991.

89. Koopmans RA, Zhao GJ, Li DKB, Tanton B, Redekop WK, and Paty DW: MR detection of multiple sclerosis activity: Effects of scanning frequency (abstract). Neurology 43(suppl):A183,1993.

90. Kruse B, Barker PB, van Zijl PCM, Duyn JH, Moonen CTW, and Moser HW: Multislice proton magnetic resonance spectroscopic imaging in X-linked adrenoleukodystropy. Ann Neurol 36: 595–608, 1994.

91. Kurtzke JF: The disability status scale for multiple sclerosis: Apologia pro DSS sua. Neurology 39:291–302, 1989.

92. Larsson HBW, Christiansen P, Jensen M, et al: Localized *In Vivo* Proton Spectroscopy in the Brain of Patients with Multiple Sclerosis.

93. Larsson HBW, Christiansen P, Zeeberg I, and Henriksen O: In vivo evaluation of the reproducibility of T1 and T2 measured in the brain of patients with multiple sclerosis. Magn Reson Imaging 10:579–584, 1992.

94. Larsson HBW, Christiansen P, Jensen M, Frederiksen J, Heltberg A, Olesen J, and Henriksen O: Localized in vivo proton spectroscopy in the brain of patients with multiple sclerosis. Magn Reson Med 22:23–31, 1991.

95. Larsson HBW, Frederiksen J, Petersen J, et al: Assessment of demyelination, edema, and gliosis by in vivo determination of T1 and T2 in the brain of patients with acute attack of multiple sclerosis. Magn Res Med 11:337–348, 1989.

96. Larsson HBW, Frederiksen J, Kjaer L, Henriksen O, and Olesen J: In vivo determination of T1 and T2 in the brain of patients with severe but stable multiple sclerosis. Magn Reson Med 7:43–55, 1988.

97. Lenkinski RE, Grossman RI, Ramer KN, Gonzalez F, and Silberberg DH: Proton MRS studies of multiple sclerosis: Correlation with Gd en-

hancement on MRI. Society of Magnetic Resonance in Medicine, Book of Abstracts, Vol 1, San Francisco, 1991, p 84.

98. Levine RA, Gardner JC, Fullerton BC, Stufflebeam SM, Furst M, and Rosen BR: Multiple sclerosis lesions of the auditory pons are not silent. Brain 117:1127–1141, 1994.

99. Li D, Mayo J, Fache S, Robertson WD, Paty D, and Genton M: Early experience in nuclear magnetic resonance imaging of multiple sclerosis. Ann NY Acad Sci 436:483–486, 1984.

100. Loevner LA, Grossman RI, Cohen JA, Lexa FJ, Kessler D, and Kolson DL: Microscopic disease in normal-appearing white matter on conventional MR images in patients with multiple sclerosis: Assessment with magnetization-transfer measurements. Radiology 196:511–515, 1995.

101. Losseff NA, Kingsley FRCR, McDonald WI, Miller DH, and Thompson AJ: Clinical and magnetic resonance imaging predictors of disability in primary and secondary progressive multiple sclerosis, 1996.

101a. Losseff NA, McDonald WI, Miller DH, Thompson AJ, and NMR Research Unit. Institute of Neurology, London, U.K. Multiple Sclerosis 2:28–29, 1996.

101b. Losseff NA, Wang L, Lai M, et al: Institute of Neurology, London, U.K. Multiple Sclerosis 2:29, 1996.

102. MacFadyen DJ, Drance SM, Douglas GR, Airaksinen PJ, Mawson DK, and Paty DW: The retinal nerve fiber layer, neuroretinal rim area, and visual evoked potentials in MS. Neurology 38:1353–1358, 1988.

103. MacKay AL, Whittall KP, Cover KS, Li DKB, and Paty DW: In vivo T2 relaxation measurements of brain may provide myelin concentration. Society of Magnetic Resonance in Medicine, Book of Abstracts, Vol 2, San Francisco, p 917, 1991.

104. Matthews PM, Phil D, Francis GS, Antel JP, and Arnold DL: Proton magnetic resonance spectroscopy for metabolic characterization of plaques in multiple sclerosis. Neurology 41: 1251–1256, 1991.

105. McDonald WI: The pathological and clinical dynamics of multiple sclerosis. J Neuropathol Exp Neurol 53:338–343, 1994.

106. McDonald WI, Miller DH, and Thompson AJ: Are magnetic resonance findings predictive of clinical outcome in therapeutic trials in multiple sclerosis? The dilemma of interferon-beta. Ann Neurol 36:14–18, 1994.

107. McDonald WI, Miller DH, and Barnes D: The pathological evolution of multiple sclerosis. Neuropathol Appl Neurobiol 18:319–334, 1992.

108. McDonald WI, and Miller DH: Spinal cord MRI using multi-array coils and fast spin echo. 2. Findings in multiple sclerosis. Neurology 43: 2632–2637, 1993.

109. Menon DK, Baudoin CJ, Tomlinson D, and Hoyle C: Proton MR spectroscopy and imaging of the brain in AIDS: Evidence of neuronal loss in regions that appear normal with imaging. J Comput Assist Tomogr 14:882–885, 1990.

109a. Miller DH, Albert PS, Barkhof F, et al: Guidelines for the use of magnetic resonance techniques in monitoring the treatment of multiple sclerosis. Ann Neurol 39:6–16, 1996.

110. Miller DH, Barkhof F, and Nauta JJP: Gadolinium enhancement increases the sensitivity of MRI in detecting disease activity in multiple sclerosis. Brain 116(pt 5):1077–1094, 1993.

111. Miller DH, Barkhof F, Berry I, Kappos L, Scotti G, and Thompson AJ: Magnetic resonance imaging in monitoring the treatment of multiple sclerosis: Concerted action guidelines. J Neurol Neurosurg Psychiatry 54:683–688, 1991.

112. Miller DH, Newton MR, van der Poel JC, et al: Magnetic resonance imaging of the optic nerve in optic neuritis. Neurology 38:175–179, 1988.

113. Miller DH, Rudge P, Johnson G, et al: Serial gadolinium enhanced magnetic resonance imaging in multiple sclerosis. Brain 111:927–939, 1988.

114. Minderhoud JM, Mooyaart EL, Kamman RL, et al: In vivo phosphorus magnetic resonance spectroscopy in multiple sclerosis. Arch Neurol 49:161–165, 1992.

115. Mooyaart EL, Kamman RL, Minderhoud JM, Gravenmade EJ, and Hoogstraten C: NMR spectroscopy in patients with multiple sclerosis: A correlation with clinical data. ECTRIMS Conference, Book of Abstracts, Amsterdam, 1989, p 459.

116. Morrissey SP, Stodal H, Zettl U, et al: In vivo MRI and its histological correlates in acute adoptive transfer experimental allergic encephalomyelitis: Quantification of inflammation and oedema. Brain 119:239–248, 1996.

117. Multiple Sclerosis Study Group: Efficacy and toxicity of cyclosporine in chronic progressive multiple sclerosis: A randomized, double-blinded, placebo-controlled clinical trial. Ann Neurol 27:591–605, 1990.

117a. Namerow NS and Thompson LR: Plaques, symptoms, and the remitting course of multiple sclerosis. Neurology 19:765–774, 1969.

118. Narayana PA, Wolinsky JS, Jackson EF, and McCarthy M: Magnetic resonance of multiple sclerosis: Correlation between proton spectroscopy and GdDTPA enhancement. Society of Magnetic Resonance in Medicine, Book of Abstracts, Vol 1, San Francisco, p 82, 1991.

119. Narayana PA, Wolinsky JS, and Fenstermacher MJ: Proton magnetic resonance spectroscopy in multiple sclerosis. Society of Magnetic Resonance Medicine, Book of Abstracts, San Francisco, 1989, p 457.

120. Narayana PA, Wolinsky JS, Jackson EF, and McCarthy M: Proton MR spectroscopy of gadolinium-enhanced multiple sclerosis plaques. J Magn Reson Imaging 2:263–270, 1992.

121. Nesbit GM, Forbes GS, Scheithauer BW, Okazaki H, and Rodriguez M: Histopathologic and MR and/or CT correlation in 37 cases at biopsy and 3 cases at autopsy. Radiology 180: 467–474, 1991.

122. Newcombe J, Hawkins CP, Henderson CL, et al: Histopathology of multiple sclerosis lesions detected by magnetic resonance imaging in unfixed postmortem central nervous system tissue. Brain 114:1013–1023, 1991.

123. Noseworthy JH, Strejan G, Gilbert JJ, and Karlick S: Comparison of in vitro nuclear magnetic resonance (NMR) properties and histopathology in experimental allergic encephalomyelitis (EAE). Neurology 35:135–136, 1985.

124. Oger J, O'Gorman M, Willoughby E, Li DKB, and Paty DW: Changes in immune function in relapsing multiple sclerosis correlate with disease activity as assessed by magnetic resonance imaging. Ann NY Acad Sci 540:597–601, 1988.

125. Orita T, Tsurutani T, and Izumihara A: Coronal MR imaging for visualization of wallerian degeneration of the pyramidal tract. J Comput Assist Tomogr 15:802–804, 1991.

126. Ormerod IEC, Miller DH, McDonald WI, et al: The role of NMR imaging in the assessment of multiple sclerosis and isolated neurological lesions. Brain 110:1579–1616, 1987.

127. Palmer MR, Bergstrom M, Grochowski E, et al: Magnetic resonance imaging (MRI) in multiple sclerosis (MS): Quantitative changes in the size of the lesions over 6 months in the placebo limb of a therapeutic trial. Can J Neurol Sci 13:168, 1986.

128. Palo J, Ketonen L, and Wikström J: A follow-up study of very low field MRI findings and clinical course in multiple sclerosis. J Neurol Sci 84:177–187, 1988.

129. Pannizzo F, Stallmeyer MJB, Friedman J, et al: Quantitative MRI studies for assessment of multiple sclerosis. Magn Reson Med 24:90–99, 1992.

130. Paty DW: Magnetic resonance imaging in the assessment of disease activity in multiple sclerosis. Can J Neurol Sci 15:266–272, 1988.

131. Paty DW: Magnetic resonance in multiple sclerosis. Current Opinion in Neurology and Neurosurgery 6:202–208, 1993.

132. Paty DW: Multiple sclerosis: Assessment of disease progression and effects of treatment (review). Can J Neurol Sci 14(3 suppl):518–520, 1987.

133. Paty DW: Multiple Sclerosis-Functional Neuroimaging. Kelley, RE (ed): Futura Publishing, Armonk, New York, 1994, pp 395–413.

133a. Paty DW, Koopmans RA, Redekop WK, Oger JJF, Kastrukoff LF and Li DKB: Does the MRI activity rate predict the clinical course of MS? Neurology 42 (3 suppl): p 427, 1992.

134. Paty DW, Isaac CD, Grochowski E, et al: Magnetic resonance imaging (MRI) in multiple sclerosis (MS): A serial study in relapsing and remitting patients with quantitative measurements of lesion size (abstract). Neurology 36(suppl 1):1986.

135. Paty DW, Li DKB: UBC MS/MRI Study Group and the IFNB Multiple Sclerosis Study Group. Interferon beta-1b is effective in relapsing-remitting multiple sclerosis. II. MRI analysis results of a multicenter, randomized, double-blind, placebo-controlled trial. Neurology 43: 662–667, 1993.

136. Paty DW, Studney D, Redekop WK, and Lublin FD: MS COSTAR: A computerized patient record adapted for clinical research purposes. Ann Neurol 36 Suppl:S134–135, 1994.

137. Peersman GV, Van de Vyver FL, Lohman JE, et al: High resolution nuclear magnetic resonance imaging of the spinal cord in experimental demyelinating disease. Acta Neuropathol (Berl) 76:628–632, 1988.

138. Peters AR, Geelen JAG, den Boer JA, Prevo RL, Minderhoud JM, and Gravenmade EJ: A study of multiple sclerosis patients with magnetic resonance spectroscopic imaging. Multiple Sclerosis, Vol 1:25–31, 1995.

139. Peterson K, Rosenblum MK, Powers JM, Alvord E, Walker RW, and Posner JB: Effect of brain irradiation on demyelinating lesions. Neurology 43:2105–2112, 1993.

139a. Phillips II WE, Phuphanich S, Velthuizen RP, Silbiger ML: Automatic magnetic tissue characterization for three-dimensional magnetic resonance imaging of the brain. J Neuroimag 5: 171–177, 1995.

140. Pioro EP, Antel JP, Cashman NR, and Arnold DL: Detection of cortical neuron loss in motor neuron disease by proton magnetic resonance spectroscopic imaging in vivo. Neurology 44: 1933–1938, 1994.

141. Prineas JW, Barnard RO, Revesz T, Kwon EE, Sharer L, and Cho ES: Multiple sclerosis: Pathology of recurrent lesions. Brain 116:681–693, 1993.

142. Raine CS: Multiple sclerosis: Immune system molecule expression in the central nervous system. J Neuropathol Exp Neurol 53:328–337, 1994.

143. Revesz T, Kidd D, Thompson AJ, Barnard RO, and McDonald WI: A comparison of the pathology of primary and secondary progressive multiple sclerosis. Brain 117:759–765, 1994.

143a. Richards TL: Proton MR spectroscopy in MS: Value in establishing diagnosis, monitoring progression, and evaluating therapy. AJR 157: 1073–1078, 1991.

144. Richards TL, Heide AC, Tsuruda JS, and Alvord EC Jr: Vector analysis of diffusion images in experiment allergic encephalomyelitis. Society of Magnetic Resonance Imaging, Book of Abstracts, Berlin, Germany, Vol 1, p 412, 1992.

145. Richards TL, Alvord EC, He Y, et al: Experimental allergic encephalomyelitis in non-human primates: diffusion imaging of acute and chronic brain lesions. Multiple Sclerosis, 1:109–117, 1995.

146. Richards TL, Rose LM, Peterson J, Petersen R, and Alvord EC Jr: Changes in brain proton spectra precede the onset of experimental allergic encephalomyelitis in macaques. Society of Magnetic Resonance Imaging, Book of Abstracts, San Francisco, Vol 1. 1991, p 427.

147. Richards TL, Rose LM, Golden RN, and Alvord EC: In vitro proton spectroscopy of the primate brain after induction of experimental allergic encephalomyelitis. Proceedings of the Society of Magnetic Resonance in Medicine. Academic Press, San Diego, 1987, p 64.

148. Robertson WD, Li DK, Mayo JR, Fache JS, and Paty DW: Assessment of multiple sclerosis lesions by magnetic resonance imaging. Can Assoc Radiol J 38:177–182, 1987.

149. Rose LM, Richards TL, Petersen R, Peterson J, Hruby S, and Alvord EC Jr: Remitting-relapsing

EAE in non-human primates: A valid model of multiple sclerosis (review). Clin Immunol Immunopathol 59:1–15, 1991.

150. Rumbach L, Armspach JP, Gounot D, et al: Nuclear magnetic resonance T2 relaxation times in multiple sclerosis. J Neurol Sci 104:176–181, 1991.

151. Sappey-Marinier D: High-resolution NMR spectroscopy of cerebral white matter in multiple sclerosis. Magn Res Med 15:229–239, 1990.

151a. Scheltens PH, Barkhof F, Leys D, Wolters EC, Ravid R, and Kamphorst W: Histopathologic correlates of white matter changes on MRI in Alzheimer's disease and normal aging. Neurology 45:883–888, 1995.

151b. Silver NC, Barker GJ, MacManus DG, and Miller DH: Magnetisation transfer ratio in the cervical cord in multiple sclerosis. Multiple Sclerosis 2:30–31, 1996.

152. Simon JH, and Fonte D: Proton NMR spectroscopy of demyelination in experimental allergic encephalomyelitis. Soc Magn Reson Med Annual Meeting, New York, N.Y., 69, 1988.

153. Smith ME, Martin R, Frank JA, et al: Gadolinium-enhanced magnetic resonance imaging and its correlation with expanded disability status score in multiple sclerosis. Ann Neurol 30:270, 1991.

154. Smith ME, Stone LA, Albert PS, et al: Clinical worsening in multiple sclerosis is associated with increased frequency and area of gadopentetate dimeglumine-enhancing magnetic resonance imaging lesions. Ann Neurol 33:480–489, 1993.

155. Städt D, Kappos L, Rohrbach E, Heun R, and Ratzka M: Occurrence of MRI abnormalities in patients with isolated optic neuritis. Eur Neurol 30:305–309, 1990.

156. Stewart WA: Proton spin relaxation as a means of characterizing the pathology of multiple sclerosis. Dissertation, University of British Columbia, Vancouver, British Columbia, 1989.

157. Stewart WA, Alvord EC, Hruby S, Hall LD, and Paty DW: Early detection of experimental allergic encephalomyelitis by magnetic resonance imaging. The Lancet 2:898, 1985.

158. Stewart WA, and Alvord EC Jr: Magnetic resonance imaging of experimental allergic encephalomyelitis in primates. Brain 114:1069–1096, 1991.

159. Stewart WA, Barwick SE, Whittall KP, Hall LD, and Paty DW: In vitro multi-exponential relaxation in multiple sclerosis and experimental allergic encephalomyelitis. Society of Magnetic Resonance in Medicine, New York, 1988.

160. Stewart WA, Hall LD, Berry K, and Paty DW: Correlation between NMR scan and brain slice: Data in multiple sclerosis. Lancet 2:412, 1984.

161. Stewart WA, Hall LD, Berry K, et al: Magnetic resonance imaging (MRI) in multiple sclerosis (MS): Pathological correlation studies in eight cases. Neurology 36:320, 1986.

162. Stewart WA, MacKay AL, Whittall KP, Moore GRW, and Paty DW: Spin-spin relaxation in experimental allergic encephalomyelitis: Analysis of CPMG data using a non-linear least squares method and linear inverse theory. Magn Reson Med 29:767–775, 1993.

163. Stewart WA, Whittall KP, and Paty DW: Analysis of CPMG data from CNS tissue: A potential method for detecting demyelination in multiple sclerosis. Society of Magnetic Resonance in Medicine, Book of Abstracts, Vol 1, San Francisco, p 85, 1991.

164. Stone L, Smith ME, Frank JA, et al: Incidence of contrast enhancement on MRI over time in MS patients. Neurology 44(suppl 2):A391, 1994.

165. Stone LA, Albert PS, Smith ME, et al: Changes in the amount of diseased white matter over time in patients with relapsing-remitting multiple sclerosis. Neurology 45:1808–1814, 1995.

166. Stone LA, Smith ME, Albert PS, et al: Blood-brain barrier disruption on contrast-enhanced MRI in patients with mild relapsing-remitting multiple sclerosis: Relationship to course, gender, and age. Neurology 45:1122–1126, 1995.

167. Swirsky-Sacchetti T, Mitchell DR, Seward J, et al: Neuropsychological and structural brain lesions in multiple sclerosis: A regional analysis. Neurology 42:1291–1295, 1992.

168. Tas MW, Barkhof F, van Walderveen MAA, et al: Natural disease course on enhanced T1 and T2 MR imaging in 13 multiple sclerosis patients. 10th Congress of the European Committee for Treatment and Research in Multiple Sclerosis, Book of Abstracts, Athens, Greece, p 16, 1994.

169. Thompson AJ, Kermode AG, Wicks D, et al: Major differences in the dynamics of primary and secondary progressive multiple sclerosis. Ann Neurol 29:53–62, 1991.

170. Thompson AJ, Miller D, Youl B, et al: Serial gadolinium-enhanced MRI in relapsing/remitting multiple sclerosis of varying disease duration. Neurology 42:60–63, 1992.

171. Thompson AJ, Youl B, Feinstein A, et al: Serial enhanced MRI in early relapsing/remitting and benign multiple sclerosis. Neurology 41(suppl 1):169, 1991.

172. Thorpe JW, Kidd D, Kendall BE, et al: Spinal cord MRI using multi-array coils and fast spin echo. I. Technical aspects and findings in healthy adults. Neurology 43:2625–2631, 1993.

173. Thorpe JW, Kidd D, Moseley IF, et al: Serial gadolinium-enhanced MRI of the brain and spinal cord in early relapsing-remitting multiple sclerosis. Neurology 46:373–378, 1996.

174. Tofts PS, and Kermode AG: Measurement of the blood-brain barrier permeability and leakage space using dynamic MR imaging: Fundamental concepts. Magn Reson Med 17:357–367, 1991.

175. Tofts PS, Wicks DAG, and Barker GJ: The MRI measurement of NMR and physiological parameters in tissue to study disease process. Prog Clin Biol Res 363:313–325, 1991.

176. Tourtellotte WW, and Parker JA: Some spaces and barriers in postmortem multiple sclerosis. In Lajtha A, and Ford DH (eds): Progress in Brain Research: Brain Barrier Systems, Vol 29. Elsevier, New York, 1968, pp 493–522.

176a. Tracey I, Dunn JF, Parkes HG and Radda GK: An in vivo and in vitro ^{1}H-magnetic resonance spectroscopy study of mdx mouse brain: Abnormal development or neural necrosis? J Neurological Sciences 141:13–18, 1996.

177. Truyen L, Gheuens J, Van de Vyver FL, Parizel PM, Peersman GB, and Martin JJ: Improved correlation of magnetic resonance imaging (MRI) with clinical status in multiple sclerosis (MS) by use of an extensive standardized imaging-protocol. J Neurol Sci 96:173–182, 1990.

178. Truyen L, Gheuens J, Parizel PM, Van de Vyver FL, and Martin JJ: Long term follow-up of multiple sclerosis by standardized, non-contrast-enhanced magnetic resonance imaging. J Neurol Sci 106:35–40, 1991.

179. Uhlenbrock D, Herbe E, Seidel D, and Gehlen W: One-year MR imaging follow-up of patients with multiple sclerosis under cortisone therapy. Neuroradiology 31:3–7, 1989.

180. Van Hecke P, Marchal G, Johannik K, et al: Human brain proton localized NMR spectroscopy in multiple sclerosis. Magn Reson Med 18:199–206, 1991.

181. van Walderveen MAA, Barkhof F, Hommes OR, Polman CH, Frequin STFM, and Valk J: T1 SE more specific than T2 SE in identifying disabling lesions in multiple sclerosis. A quantitative follow-up study. Society of Magnetic Resonance Imaging, Book of Abstracts, Vol 1, San Francisco, p 536, 1994.

182. van Walderveen MAA, Barkhof F, Hommes OR, et al: Correlating MRI and clinical disease activity in multiple sclerosis: Relevance of hypointense lesions on short-TR/short-TE (T1-weighted) spin-echo images. Neurology 45:1684–1690, 1995.

183. Weiner HL, Guttman CRG, Khoury SJ, et al: Correlation of magnetic resonance imaging with immune and clinical measures in 45 MS patients receiving 20–24 MRI scans each over a one year period. Works in Progress (abstract). American Academy of Neurology, San Francisco, p 1, 1995.

184. Weinshenker BG, Gilbert JJ, and Ebers GC: Some clinical and pathologic observations on chronic myelopathy: A variant of multiple sclerosis. J Neurol Neurosurg Psychiatry 53:146–149, 1990.

185. Wicks DAG, Tofts PS, Miller DH, et al: Volume measurement of multiple sclerosis lesions with

magnetic resonance images: A preliminary study. Neuroradiology 34:475–479, 1992.

186. Wiebe S, Lee DH, Karlik SJ, et al: Serial cranial and spinal cord magnetic resonance imaging in multiple sclerosis. Ann Neurol 32:643–650, 1992.

187. Willoughby EW, Grochowski E, Li DKB, Oger J, Kastrukoff LF, and Paty DW: Serial magnetic resonance scanning in multiple sclerosis: A second prospective study in relapsing patients. Ann Neurol 25:43–49, 1989.

188. Wilson R, and Tocher DR: Lipid and fatty acid composition is altered in plaque tissue from multiple sclerosis brain compared with normal brain white matter. Lipids 26:9–15, 1991.

189. Wolinsky JS: "Inositol storms." Comments made at the 10th Congress of European Committee for Treatment and Research in Multiple Sclerosis, Athens, Greece, 1994.

190. Wolinsky JS, Narayana PA, Jackson EF, and McCarthy M: Localized proton magnetic resonance spectroscopy (MRS) in multiple sclerosis (MS): Correlation with gadolinium-DTPA enhanced MRI. Neurology 41(suppl 1):169, 1991.

191. Wolinsky JS, Narayana PA, and Fenstermacher MJ: Proton magnetic resonance spectroscopy in multiple sclerosis. Neurology 40:1764–1769, 1990.

192. Yetkin FZ, Haughton VM, Fischer ME, et al: High-signal foci on MR images of the brain: Observer variability in their quantification. AJR 159:185–188, 1992.

193. Zhao GJ, Li DKB, Tanton BL, and Paty DW: Assessment of activity of the individual lesions in relapsing-remitting multiple sclerosis on magnetic resonance imaging. Ann Neurol 30:270,1991.

194. Zhao GJ, Koopmans RA, Li DIB, Redekop K, Morrison W, Nelson J, and Paty DW: Corticospinal tract lesions in multiple sclerosis: Relationship between MRI activity and clinical course. Neurology 43:246, 1993.

195. Zhu G, Allen PS, Koopmans R, Li DK and Paty DW: A marked elevation of inositol in M.S. lesions. Society of Magnetic Resonance in Medicine, Book of Abstracts, Vol 1, Eleventh Annual Scientific Meeting, Berlin, Germany, p 1948, 1992.

CHAPTER 10

VIROLOGY

Lorne F. Kastrukoff, MD
George P. A. Rice, MD

Despite intensive investigation, the etiology and pathogenesis of MS remains unclear. The complicated interaction of multiple factors likely plays a role in this disease.[3] Infectious agents may be one of the factors involved.[144] Support for the role of an infectious agent in MS originates largely from epidemiological studies[168]; evidence from serological and virological studies is somewhat less compelling.[35] A wide variety of infectious agents, including spirochetes, mycoplasma, mycobacteria, and toxoplasma, have been isolated from the central nervous system (CNS) of patients with MS. These agents have all been implicated in the etiology of MS, as have a variety of viruses, including rabies, herpes simplex virus (HSV), scrapie, parainfluenza 1, measles, chimpanzee cytomegalovirus (CMV), simian viruses (SVs) I and V, coronaviruses (CVs), MS-associated agent,[46] and the bone marrow agent.[207] These agents most likely represent contaminants or adventitious rather than causal agents, but this remains controversial.[143] The role of retroviruses[263] or herpes simplex virus type 6[54] in the development of MS has yet to be determined. If infectious agents do play a role, they likely involve complex mechanisms. Weiner and colleagues[349] have described a number of theoretical mechanisms by which viruses could induce CNS demyelination.

EXPERIMENTAL ANIMAL MODELS OF VIRUS-INDUCED CENTRAL NERVOUS SYSTEM DEMYELINATION

Experimental animal models offer an approach to the study of mechanisms mediating virus-induced CNS demyelination and may provide insight into human demyelinating disease. The ability of a number of viruses, including vesicular stomatitis virus, chandipura virus, and Venezuelan equine encephalomyelitis virus, to induce demyelination has been investigated to varying degrees. These models have been reviewed elsewhere.[68,69,194,279,292] This chapter will focus on six experimental animal models of virus-induced CNS demyelination: Theiler's murine encephalomyelitis virus (TMEV), JHM strain of mouse hepatitis virus (MHV), maedi visna virus (MVV), canine distemper virus (CDV), Semliki Forest virus (SFV), and herpes simplex virus (HSV), emphasizing contributions of the virus, the genetic makeup that may predispose the host to the development of CNS demyelination, the clinical course, CNS pathology, and pathogenesis.

Theiler's Murine Encephalomyelitis Virus

Theiler's murine encephalomyelitis virus, a well-studied model of virus-induced CNS demyelination,[179] is a single-stranded, positive, RNA-containing virus. Originally described by Max Theiler in 1934,[233] when he observed that some mice in his colony developed a flaccid paralysis of their hind limbs,[330] it is a cardiovirus in the family Picornaviridae.[179,254]

Since 1934, a number of different TMEV strains have been identified. All are of the same serotype and cross-neutralize with polyclonal antibodies. The strains can be divided into two subgroups on the basis of different biologic and pathological characteristics. The first subgroup consists of at least four isolates (GDVII, FA, VIE, [145]HTR, and Ask-1) that are highly virulent and cause a rapid and fatal encephalitis.[330] Neurons as well as glial cells (astrocytes and oligodendrocytes) are infected, and the pathological picture is that of an acute polioencephalitis, with necrosis of neurons and neuronophagia in the hippocampus, cerebral cortex, basal ganglia, thalamus, brain stem, and spinal cord. Although the original wild-type TMEV usually produces an asymptomatic enteric infection in mice and rarely encephalomyelitis, the Theiler

original (TO) subgroup, consisting of the Daniels (DA), WW, BeAn, and 10 to 12 other isolates, produces a biphasic disease of the CNS after intracerebral inoculation in susceptible strains of mice.[177] Mice infected with these strains develop a poliomyelitis (early phase) followed by demyelinating disease (late phase) and chronic persistent viral infection.[77] Different strains of the TO subgroup will influence the course of the disease: the WW strain produces a relapsing model,[73] whereas the BeAn strain minimizes the gray matter stage of the disease.[183] Differences in neurovirulence, viral persistence, and the ability to induce demyelination among the different strains of TMEV are being mapped in the viral genome.[280] Different strains of TMEV are approximately 90 percent identical at the nucleotide level and approximately 96 percent at the amino acid level. Fifty percent of the amino acid differences, however, are at the level of VP1, VP2, and VP3.[253] Single nucleotide changes resulting in amino acid substitutions can influence neurovirulence and viral persistence.[141] Neurovirulence has been mapped primarily to the *P1* genomic region encoding the leader and coat proteins.[44,100,197] Viral persistence appears to be related to the sequences encoding VP1.[325,365,366] Thus, mechanisms for the pathogenic properties of neurovirulence and viral persistence appear to involve the exterior of the virus and would implicate immune- or receptor-mediated events as being involved. Multiple gene segments likely influence the number and extent of the demyelinating lesions.[275] The three-dimensional structure of Theiler's virus has been elucidated:[189] The virus has an icosahedral capsid with large star-shaped plateaus at the fivefold axes. Most of the sequence differences between the demyelinating and neurovirulent strains that could play a role in determining pathogenesis appear to map to the surface of this star-shaped plateau.[121]

Host genetic determinants also influence susceptibility and the development of CNS demyelination induced by Theiler's virus.[33,36] Originally, different murine strains were recognized to vary in their degree of susceptibility to TMEV.[178] Strains such as DBA/2 and SJL/J were found to be susceptible, whereas C57BL/6 mice were resistant. Substrain differences, as in Balb/c mice, were also recognized.[225] Susceptibility to demyelination is controlled, in part, by genes linked to the *H-2* complex[180,269] and specifically to the class I locus *H-2d*.[63,269,271] Non-*H-2* genes also appear to influence susceptibility.[33,201] A locus close to the constant gene for the beta chain of the T-cell receptor has been related to susceptibility,[202] whereas another non-*H-2* gene localized on the centromeric end of chromosome 3 near the carbonic anhydrase-2 enzyme (*Car-2* locus) appears to be important for the development of demyelination in some strains.[203] The relative importance of the *H-2* and non-*H-2* genes to determination of susceptibility appears to be dependent on murine strain combinations. In some cases, *H-2* genes play an important role along with non-*H-2* genes,[203] whereas in others, *H-2* genes play little or no role in determining susceptibility.[202] Host determinants also appear to influence viral persistence. Loci close to lfg on chromosome 10 and possibly a second locus near Mbp on chromosome 18 have been implicated in influencing viral persistence.[41] Thus with TMEV, a number of different host gene loci can contribute to susceptibility, depending on the particular strain of mouse that is infected.

The intracerebral inoculation of a TO strain of TMEV in susceptible strains of mice will reliably produce a biphasic neurological disease.[177] Within the first few weeks postinfection, encephalomyelitis develops in 80 percent of infected mice. This phase of the infection, which lasts 1 to 4 weeks, is characterized by virus growth, necrosis of neurons, glial cell proliferation, and minimal lymphocytic inflammation.[71] TMEV is predominantly present in motor neurons of the brain stem and spinal cord, but sensory neurons and glial cells are also infected during this stage.[272] Clinically, mice develop a flaccid paralysis usually of the hind limbs. Most of the animals will recover completely but will develop a chronic inflammatory demyelinating phase of the disease by the second or third week postinfection. One to 5 months postinfection, survivors develop the clinical manifestation of this stage of the disease, gait spasticity.

Intense mononuclear cell (MNC) infiltrates are observed initially in the spinal cord leptomeninges and later in the white matter.[72] At first the MNC infiltrates are largely lymphocytic in nature but later macrophages and plasma cells predominate.[71] With the development of demyelination, MNC are observed to actively strip myelin lamellae from normal-appearing axons or are in contact with myelin sheaths undergoing vesicular disruption.[32,72,272] In the later stages of the disease, remyelination may occur and appears to result from invading Schwann cells.[73]

The pathogenesis of TMEV-induced CNS demyelination is likely multifactorial.[359] Observations that would favor a direct effect of virus include:

- Persistence of infectious virus in the CNS for prolonged periods of time[185] albeit at low titers during the chronic phase[177,181]
- Co-localization of demyelinating lesions with areas of ongoing CNS infection as determined by in situ hybridization and immunochemistry[37,55]
- Studies indicating that nude mice infected with DA strain intracerebrally can develop demyelination after lytic infection of oligodendrocytes (OLs) in the presence of rising titers of virus and in the absence of mature T cells and of anti-TMEV antibody.[282,284]

Other observations would favor an indirect effect of virus. Initially, cells that are most heavily infected during acute demyelination are macrophages and astrocytes,[74] although some OLs can be infected.[10,272] In later stages of demyelination, viral RNA can be identified in both macrophages and glial cells,[39] with infected cells consisting of 10 percent microglia-macrophages, 5 to 10 percent astrocytes, and 40 percent OLs.[10] In immunocompetent mice, the majority of these RNA-positive cells neither produce detectable levels of viral capsid protein nor express viral antigens on the surface of the cell membrane.[50] RNA replication in the persistently infected cells appears to be restricted at the level of negative strand RNA synthesis.[49] Viral replication does appear to occur in macrophages in the CNS, albeit at a highly restricted level.[64] These MNCs are likely responsible for the predominant viral antigen burden in the CNS.[186] These results would suggest that infection of OLs may be only a secondary factor in the process leading to myelin destruction.[72,243,284] Support for this comes from several observations. Recurrent demyelination can develop in areas remyelinated by Schwann cells in the absence of virus in these cells.[75] Furthermore, studies of early demyelination have shown myelin-associated glycoprotein, which is localized to the periaxonal component of myelin, to be preserved, whereas myelin basic protein (MBP), found in central myelin, and PO protein, found in peripheral myelin, were absent.[70] This would suggest that demyelination develops from the outside of the sheath and is consistent with histological observations suggesting an immune-mediated process. It is possible, however, that viral infection of OLs could induce demyelination by interfering with "luxury functions" of the cell.[232]

The immune system also plays an important role in TMEV infection, which was predicted early on the basis of the pathological picture.[72] This impression was supported by studies using different immunosuppressive agents.[182] Studies suggest that the immune system plays a role not only in limiting virus after the initial infection but also in inducing demyelination. A virus-specific humoral response develops during the first week and peaks by 1 to 2 months.[247,285] Most of the antiviral IgG in persistently infected susceptible mice is of the IgG2a subclass, whereas IgG1 is largely present in resistant and immunized mice.[48,247] The early humoral immunity appears to play an important role in mediating resistance among resistant strains of mice.[286] Furthermore, antibody to VP1 may play the major role in limiting viral spread and affecting the survival of the mice.[105] In persistently infected mice, elevated levels of immunoglobulin and oligoclonal banding (OB) are also found in the cerebrospinal fluid (CSF).[48,184] These include antibodies to both virus and myelin components.[273,281] Because CD4+ T cells of the Th1 subset mediate delayed type hypersensitivity (DTH) and regulate IgG2a production via interferon gamma and because T cells of the Th2 subset regulate IgG1 and IgE production via interleukin-4, these results suggest that in susceptible

mice there may be a preferential stimulation of the Th1 subset. In contrast to its role in limiting viral spread, humoral immunity in the development of demyelination is likely unimportant. Although MBP and anti-MBP antibodies appear in both the serum and CSF of persistently infected mice,[264,351] treatment with myelin components does not prevent demyelination, making MBP more likely a marker of demyelination than a target.[172]

Recent studies suggest that cell-mediated immunity plays an important role in TMEV infection. Although some evidence would support a role for nonspecific cellular immunity such as natural killer (NK) cells and their contribution to the protection of acutely infected mice,[242] most studies suggest an important role for T lymphocytes. During the acute stage of infection, H-2-restricted CD8+ cytotoxic T lymphocytes (CTLs) are induced.[286] These cells can be found in the CNS during both the acute and chronic stages of infection.[176] Studies in which CD8+ T cells were depleted in vivo with specific monoclonal antibody (mAb)[15] or using β_2-microglobulin-deficient mice (mice not expressing MHC class I antigen and lacking CD8+ T cells)[94] resulted in a less effective clearance of virus from the CNS. These results would suggest the CD8+ T cells play an important role in limiting the spread of virus but not the only role, because these mice failed to succumb to the infection.[260] At this time, the mechanism by which TMEV evades immune surveillance in the chronic phase of infection is unknown but does not appear to involve antigenic shift.

Cell-mediated immunity also plays a role in the development of demyelination, as was first suggested by the presence of MNC infiltrates in the leptomeninges and spinal cord of persistently infected mice.[69] Subsequently, immunosuppressive studies using a number of different modalities also supported a role for cell-mediated immunity in the development of demyelination.[205] Cells mediating DTH appear within 2 weeks of infection with TMEV and remain elevated for at least 6 months.[62,205] The possible role of this subset of T cells in the development of demyelination was recognized when it was observed that only susceptible murine strains developed a significant level of anti-TMEV DTH response[62,274] mediated by CD4+ cells.[61,204,206] Depletion of these cells in vivo with mAb prior to the demyelinating phase reduced the incidence of demyelination.[351] More rigorous studies involved thymectomy, irradiation, and bone marrow reconstitution along with adoptive transfer of TMEV-specific CD4+ T cells to mice that were then infected with a suboptimal dose of virus. These studies resulted in an increased incidence of demyelination and an accelerated onset of clinical disease.[113] Pretreatment of cells before transfer with anti-CD4 mAb led to a decreased incidence and severity of demyelination. The immunodominant T-cell epitope of the DTH mediating CD4+ cells appears to be a 13-amino acid peptide on VP2 (VP2 74–86) at least in SJL/J mice.[111,112] In contrast, CD8+ cells do not appear to play a direct role in demyelination[15,94,260,270] but may play a role in down regulating the CD4+ T-cell response.[15,260] Although the exact mechanism by which the immune system induces demyelination is unclear, it may be the result of a DTH CD4+-induced macrophage-mediated "innocent bystander" effect.[179] Autoimmune T cells have not been observed to play a role in TMEV-induced demyelination[206] despite the identification of cross-reactivity between TMEV and galactocerebroside.[229]

JHM Strain of Mouse Hepatitis Virus

Coronaviruses have been isolated from the brains of two patients with MS,[42] and CV-like particles have been identified in the brain of an additional patient with MS.[324] The significance of these reports remains unclear because they have not yet been confirmed. JHM and SD, the viruses recovered from the brain of one patient with MS,[42] can induce demyelinating lesions in the CNS of Old and New World monkeys,[212] and the detection of murinelike CV RNA and, to a lesser extent, antigen has been detected in MS brain tissue from two patients with MS.[211] These findings have renewed interest in the possibility that CV may play a role in the development of human demyelinating disease.

Mouse hepatitis virus (MHV) is a member of the family Coronaviridae. It is an enveloped virus with a positive, single-stranded RNA of 31 kb.[174] There are several antigenic and biologically distinguishable strains, three of which (JHM, -S, -A59) can induce CNS demyelination.[16] JHM virus (JHMV), a neurotropic variant of MHV, was originally isolated from a paralyzed mouse in the late 1940s[11,56] and has become a well-studied model of virus-induced CNS demyelination.[239] Viral variants of JHMV, which have arisen spontaneously or were selected based on resistance to neutralization with mAbs, have also been extensively studied.[170] Results would suggest that the S glycoprotein, which forms the peplomers and is involved in attachment to receptors, syncytiogenesis, and elicitation of neutralizing mAbs,[65] plays an important role in pathogenesis. Three distinct antigenic sites have been identified on the S glycoprotein.[323] Despite extensive study, no definitive correlations have been made between specific alterations of S and a neuroattenuated phenotype. Attenuated JHMV variants may, therefore, have a genotype in which S contains point mutations or major deletions,[169,210] or gene amplifications,[321,322] or possesses a conditional-lethal thermosensitive phenotype.[131,158] The inability to identify specific alterations may be partially explained based on neurovirulence being due not to a single unique site but more likely to the interaction of several sites along the molecule.[342] Furthermore, the biologic properties of the JHMV variants are, to some extent, host cell dependent and make interpretation of results difficult.

Information on how the host genetic makeup influences JHM viral infection is limited. Specific strains of mice, such as Balb/c, are recognized to be susceptible to JHM encephalitis, whereas others, such as SJL/J, are resistant.[311] Such observations have suggested that resistance is inherited as a single autosomal recessive trait that is not linked to *H-2*.[157] Differences in resistance to JHMV in rat strains are also known. Lewis rats are susceptible to this virus, whereas Brown Norway rats are resistant.

After infection with JHMV, the clinicopathological disease that is induced is highly variable. Infection can result in the absence of disease, an acute encephalomyelitis, a chronic panencephalitis, a delayed-onset demyelinating encephalomyelitis, or recurrent demyelinating disease.* Outcome depends on a number of variables, including genotypes of the virus and host, dose and route of inoculation, and age and immune competence of the host.† The intracerebral inoculation of JHM strain results in the development of acute fatal encephalitis within 10 days postinfection in newborn to 2-week-old mice, whereas 8- to 12-week-old mice are generally resistant to virus. In 4-week-old mice, a percentage of the animals will survive and develop the demyelinating form of the disease. Clinical signs develop after 14 days postinfection and usually progress to a spastic paralysis.

The pathogenesis of JHM-induced CNS demyelination is likely multifactorial. A number of studies suggest that JHMV has the potential to infect most neuroectodermal cells, including neurons, glia, and ependymal cells. In vivo however, the ability to infect cells appears to be influenced by host factors. Neurons are an important target in vivo in acute encephalomyelitis[40,157,196,236,363] and may act as a repository for virus during persistent infection.[95] Furthermore, infection of neurons appears to be a prerequisite for infection of glia.[240] After intranasal inoculation, JHMV spreads, likely interneuronally, to different CNS regions using specific neuroanatomic tracts such as the olfactory nerve.[13] In the chronic demyelinating form of the disease in both rats and mice, virus persists in the white matter. Early studies indicated that the JHMV had a tropism for OLs, and it was concluded that demyelination was the result of a direct effect of virus on OLs.[24,171,240,357] However, additional studies have shown that astrocytes are also targets of JHMV,‡ and that tropism for OLs is far from unconditional.[24,173,240] Productive infection of OL was even more complicated and dependent on the stage of differentiation of the O-2A lineage cells,[24,25,240,357] because both mitotically ac-

tive progenitor stages and terminally differentiated OLs are nonpermissive targets. In the nonpermissive stages, productive infection is blocked at an early phase before the expression of viral genes.[25] Postnatal myelination, a process under the control of a number of intrinsic and extrinsic factors, is therefore important to the development of JHMV-induced CNS demyelination.[45] It remains unclear if a direct effect of virus on OL is a major factor in the development of JHMV-induced CNS demyelination.

The immune system may also play a role in the development of JHMV-induced CNS demyelination in both mice[343] and rats.[344] Both humoral- and cell-mediated immunity can modulate the outcome of MHV CNS infection by allowing the survival of animals and thus permitting the development of demyelinating disease.[96] Passive immunization of mice with mAbs specific for any of the three viral envelope glycoproteins (S, M, or HE) protects animals from acute lethal encephalitis but not the delayed demyelinating disease. Passive immunization with mAbs specific for the S peplomer is associated with a significant reduction in viral titers in the brain.[40] Viral infection in neurons is affected preferentially, with infection in OLs being unaffected. The mechanism mediating this effect is unknown. Antibody-mediated cytotoxicity may also play a role.[363] T cells appear to play an important role in mediating viral clearance and limiting disease progression. Adoptive transfer of virus-specific CD4+ T-cell clones, mediating class II-restricted DTH response, to C57BL/6 mice prevents the lethal acute encephalitis.[314,315] They do not, however, significantly reduce viral titers in the brain or alter the demyelinating phase of the disease. In a similar fashion to mAbs, the CD4+ T-cell clones alter viral growth in the neurons.[314] Clearance of virus from the CNS is also T-cell–mediated but requires both CD4+ and CD8+ cells.[320,355,356,360] H-2–restricted virus-specific CTLs were postulated to be the T cells mediating clearance of virus from the CNS. After infection with JHMV, Balb/c mice develop a CTL response. Splenocytes recognize S and N proteins but neither M nor HE proteins.[308] In contrast, CTL clones derived from the

---

*References 134, 159, 214, 304, 305, 309, 348, 363.
†References 76, 97, 157, 196, 245, 305, 306, 309, 311, 362.
‡References 173, 195, 240, 244, 357, 363.

brain are directed to the N protein.[313] The cells are directed at a peptide contained in the carboxy-terminal end of the N protein,[312] which has been further mapped to 15 amino acids that encompass the MHV epitope containing the L^d-specific binding motif.[22] Adoptive transfer of these CTLs to the periphery of mice protects them from subsequent viral challenge by reducing viral replication in the CNS.[310] Transfer of these cells to the CNS directly increases the protection 10-fold. The CTL reduces viral replication in ependymal cells, astrocytes, and microglia but not in OLs. Survivors showed minimal viral persistence and no evidence of chronic ongoing demyelination, supporting an important role for CTL in these two areas of the disease. The CTL response appears to be strain-specific, however, as JHMV infection in C57BL/6 mice will induce a CTL response to the S glycoprotein but not to the N protein.[52] These cells have been identified in the brains and spinal cords of both acutely and persistently infected mice but do not appear to be sufficient to prevent demyelination. Similarly, CTLs may also be induced in rats after infection with JHMV.[99]

Although it remains unclear, some evidence would support a role of cell-mediated immunity in the development of demyelinating disease. C57BL/6 mice infected with a neuroattenuated viral variant (2.2-V-1) and then immunosuppressed using whole-body gamma irradiation develop significantly less severe demyelinating disease when compared with control subjects, although viral titers in the brain are higher and infected OLs are more prevalent in the irradiated animals.[343] Adoptive transfer of syngeneic JHMV-immune splenocytes after irradiation results in the development of significant demyelinating disease, which is abrogated if the splenocytes are treated with Thy 1 before transfer.[98] In Lewis rats, experimental allergic encephalomyelitis (EAE)-like lesions can be induced by adoptively transferring T cells from syngeneic animals with coronavirus-induced demyelinating encephalomyelitis,[344] again supporting a role for cell-mediated immunity in the development of JHMV-induced CNS demyelination.

Maedi Visna Virus

In the late 1930s, an epidemic of lentivirus infection in domestic animals was reported in Iceland.[293,294] The viral etiology of this disease was established in 1957 and led to the concept of slow virus diseases.[126,216,218] The epidemic caused by the maedi visna virus (MVV) had two major clinical features: a respiratory disease characterized by a diffuse interstitial pneumonitis (maedi) and a demyelinating leukoencephalomyelitis associated with wasting (visna). The chronic progressive clinical course[295] and the pathological picture of demyelination originally led to MVV being proposed as a model of virus-induced CNS demyelination.* Recent studies have led to a better understanding of this virus and the disease it produces.[198] MVV is a member of the lentivirinae, a nononcogenic subfamily of Retroviridae. The virion is enveloped and approximately 70 to 100 nm. The nucleocapsid contains a positive, single-stranded RNA of approximately 9.3 kb that replicates via a proviral DNA intermediate derived by reverse transcription of the viral genome. The structural genes for gag, pol, and env are organized 5' to 3'. The envelope glycoprotein (gp 135) consists of two parts. The external part (gp 110) is necessary for binding of virus to a cell membrane receptor, whereas the transmembrane glycoprotein (gp 41) is important for cell fusion and syncytia formation. The antigenic plasticity of env and, to a lesser extent, gag allows the development of antibody and T-cell escape mutants during infection. The classic strain used in most studies is K1514; however, the use of more virulent strains will accelerate the course of the disease.[109,190]

Although host genetic factors might influence this disease, little information is currently available.[221,249] Comparison of infection in Icelandic and British sheep shows that CNS lesions are more common in the former and therefore would lend support to the concept that these factors may play a role.[155]

---

*References 57, 80, 127, 128, 217, 221, 364.

After infection of sheep with MVV, early lesions can be found in 50 percent of cases within 2 weeks, but their appearance can continue for years.[218] MNC infiltrates consisting of lymphocytes, macrophages, and plasma cells are present but may be particularly severe in the choroid plexus. Lesions begin typically subependymally in the walls of the lateral ventricles and then extend into the dorsal and lateral columns of the spinal cord. More severe lesions are characterized by foci of demyelination, proliferation of glial cells, and neuronal loss. Both gray and white matter of the brain and spinal cord can be affected, with necrosis and cavitation developing in later stages. Clinically, the animals develop locomotor dysfunctions with progressive hind limb ataxia leading to hind limb paralysis. A second type of lesion, the late lesion, can be identified in long-term studies of up to 11 years.[219] The lesions are characterized by well-demarcated areas of demyelination, axonal sparing, and the presence or absence of inflammatory cell infiltrates. Most often they are seen in the spinal cord.

The pathogenesis of MVV-induced CNS demyelination is unclear but is likely multifactorial. Viral infection appears to progress through four stages: initial exposure to the virus by virus-infected cells, an early acute immune response to the virus, a protracted period of viral persistence, and progressive development of the pathological lesions in organs such as the brain.

How MVV is able to persist in its host is a key question in the understanding of how the virus induces CNS demyelination. Initially, it was proposed that antigenic shift of viral surface glycoproteins during infection allowed persistence by allowing virus to escape antibody neutralization.[219] However, antigenic variants were observed to make up only a small percentage of total virus and did not replace the infecting serotype.[191] It was then suggested that restriction of viral gene expression might be the main explanation for viral persistence.[110,127,129] In vivo, MVV shows a marked tropism for cells of the monocyte-macrophage series.[38] It is likely that MVV, like other lentiviruses, goes through three stages of replication: latent, restricted, and productive.[127] A block in viral transcription appears to exist in infected monocytes. In contrast, macrophages have higher levels of expression of both messenger RNA (mRNA) and viral proteins. This suggests that a switch occurs from the restricted pattern observed in monocytes to the productive infection observed in macrophages. This switch is related to the tissue differentiation of monocytes to macrophages[38] and may involve the interaction of cellular transcription factors with promoter sequences in the long terminal repeat (LTR) segment of MVV.[135] The spread of infection is the result of the dissemination of virus in the cells of the monocyte-macrophage series.[220] The spread of virus to the CNS is unclear but may be due to the localization of infected monocytes and their direct migration across the blood-brain barrier or, alternatively, by cell-to-cell transmission into the CNS from infected cells in the choroid plexus. Once in the CNS, extensive turnover of monocytes to macrophages occurs in the brain with the differentiation of monocytes to macrophages and results in a shift from restricted to productive infection.

The early stage of infection with MVV is characterized by the development of humoral- and cell-mediated responses. Within 48 to 60 days after infection, neutralizing antibody, proliferating CD4$^+$ T cells, and precursor CD8$^+$ CTLs can be detected in the peripheral blood.[30] The antibody response is directed against gag, reverse transcriptase, and env. The predominant response is against gag, the major antigenic component of the virus.

In the protracted period of viral persistence, sheep will develop significant levels of neutralizing antibodies and precursor CTLs in the peripheral blood. These responses fail to control the infection, however, which eventually evolves into the progressive development of pathological lesions.

It remains unclear whether the development of demyelination and neuronal cell destruction is the direct result of the action of virus on cells in the CNS or is secondary to an immune-mediated process. Studies suggest that the *tat* gene of visna may be directly neurotoxic, with its activity the result of a particular amino acid motif that bears similarity to neurotoxic peptides characteristic of venom toxins.[132] This could affect infected OLs[38] directly and compromise their ability to sustain myelin production. Other studies[222,223,250] suggest that immune mechanisms may play a role in the development of demyelination. CD8+ T cells have been implicated in the induction of CNS demyelination.[332] The development of an autoimmune humoral or cell-mediated response does not appear to play a role in this model of virus-induced CNS demyelination.[235]

Canine Distemper Virus

Canine distemper virus is a morbillivirus in the family Paramyxoviridae. It is an enveloped, positive, single-stranded, RNA-containing virus with one large and one small glycoprotein. CDV can induce four separate types of disease: acute encephalopathy, acute encephalitis, subacute to chronic encephalitis with demyelination, and old dog encephalitis.[163] Different viral strains of CDV have been identified that can influence the nature of the infection and the development of either acute or chronic demyelinating disease.[4,199,261,318,358] In vivo, strains A75/17 and CH84-CDV are virulent and capable of producing demyelination, whereas strain SH-CDV, although still virulent, is unable to induce demyelination. Strain OP-CDV is nonvirulent. Despite their differences in vivo, all strains produce OL degeneration when infected in vitro.[367]

The dog is the natural host for CDV, so little information is available on the potential role of host genetic factors in the development of CNS demyelination. Early attempts to adapt the virus to a murine system had only limited success,[114] but more recent studies using mice have been undertaken.[137]

After infection with CDV, CNS infection can be biphasic. The acute phase of infection develops after several weeks of incubation have elapsed.[4] In the natural infection, CNS lesions may be demyelinating or destructive. Early demyelinating lesions are not necessarily associated with inflammatory cell infiltrates.[358] In the chronic phase of the infection, demyelinating lesions are more often associated with inflammatory cell infiltrates.

The pathogenesis of CDV-induced CNS demyelination remains unclear but again may be multifactorial. Viral gene expression is present in demyelinating lesions,[207,358] but the nature of the cells infected is somewhat controversial. Some studies suggest that astrocytes represent the main target for CDV in vivo,[213,338] whereas OLs are not infected.* In contrast, Blakemore and colleagues were able to identify virus in OLs when very early white matter lesions were examined.[31] In vitro, CDV has been identified in OLs in some cases[370] but not in others.[338] In infected mixed cultures, OLs develop lytic changes about 20 days postinfection, and these will be complete in 10 days.[368] These changes could be explained on the basis of a defective infection of OLs without antigen expression or on the basis of toxicity mediated by infected astrocytes.[368,369] The latter possibility is given some support by ultrastructural studies.[117,317] A recent report identified in vivo viral proteins in both neurons and astrocytes after infection with CDV.[2] Furthermore, restricted synthesis of CDV envelope proteins were identified in both the acute and chronic phases of infection.

The role of the immune system in the clearance of virus from the CNS and the development of demyelination is also unclear. Some studies[34,137,267] would support a role for humoral immunity in eliminating virus from the CNS. Macrophages have been suggested to play a role in demyelination possibly by mediating a bystander effect.[124] It is unlikely that an autoimmune mechanism plays a role in the development of CDV-induced CNS demyelination, although MBP has been identified in the CSF of infected dogs at various times after infection.[319]

Semliki Forest Virus

Semliki Forest virus is a nonhuman alphavirus in the family Togaviridae. It is an enveloped, single-stranded, RNA-containing virus with an icosahedral nucleocapsid

---

*References 136, 261, 317, 318, 339, 358.

surrounded by a membrane containing 80 transmembrane trimereic spikes.[340] The virus was originally isolated from mosquitoes in the Semliki Forest of Uganda and when inoculated in mice or rats could induce CNS demyelination.[8,345]

The ability to induce CNS demyelination in mice or rats[59] depends on a number of factors, including the viral strain.[6,7,14] In rats, the L10 strain causes extensive neural damage in the CNS, whereas the A7 or M9 mutant strains induce CNS demyelination.[9] Viral genome determinants affecting neurovirulence are beginning to be mapped,[116] with preliminary studies suggesting that differences in the viral *E2* gene may play an important role in determining virulence.[289]

It is also recognized that differences in mouse or rat strains affect the pathological picture in the CNS.[8,345] Host genetic factors likely contribute to the development of virus-induced CNS demyelination but have not yet been characterized.

The pathological appearance of the CNS after infection with SFV also depends on the route of inoculation. Virus can be given intracerebrally, peripherally (intranasally or subcutaneously), or intraperitoneally. If given peripherally, virus invades the brain via neurons and, at least in early stages of infection, disseminates in the CNS via neurons.[146] After the intranasal inoculation of SFV in adult Balb/c mice, outcome is then determined by the strain of the virus.[12] Virulent SFV4 proves lethal within 4 days, whereas, with the A7 strain, animals appear normal throughout. Neuronal necrosis in the pyriform cortex is present with both strains of virus but develops sooner and is more severe with the SFV4 virus. With SFV4 virus, both neurons and OLs contain viral RNA and viral antigens, whereas, in A7-infected mice, only viral RNA is present in these cells. If given intraperitoneally, infectious virus is present in the brain for up to 14 days. Inflammatory demyelination follows from day 10 to 21 postinfection. In Balb/c mice, demyelination is repaired and does not persist, whereas, in SJL mice, persistent demyelination does occur along with concurrent myelin repair.

The pathogenesis of SFV-induced CNS demyelination remains unclear but is likely multifactorial. Virus can persist in the CNS after SFV infection. Viral E1 is localized in cerebral capillaries, whereas E2 and envelope glycolipids are localized to the cytoplasm of neurons and glia after infection with SFV A7.[156] Viral antigens are present in astrocytes and OLs of infected mice 183 days postinfection. Despite this, it remains unclear if virus may contribute to the development of demyelination either by a direct cytolytic effect, by interfering with luxury functions of the infected cells, or by release of autoantigens with the lysis of the infected cell.

The immune system may play a role in clearance of virus. After infection with SFV, both humoral-[238] and cell-mediated[300] immune responses are identified. The same epitope, the amino acid sequence between 137 and 151, appears to induce both DTH and effector helper T-cell activity for antibody production.[301]

SFV-induced CNS demyelination may also be immune mediated.[89,291] Demyelination and inflammatory cell infiltrates do not develop in immunosuppressed mice,[91,107,108] except those reconstituted with normal spleen cells.[90] Although IgG-positive cells appear in the meninges, choroid plexus, and in the demyelinating lesions of the white matter by day 9 postinfection,[237] it is unlikely that they are the major effector mechanism. More likely, it is a T-cell–mediated effect.[142] Subak-Sharpe and colleagues[316] injected Balb/c mice intraperitoneally with the A7 strain of SFV and then treated the mice with anti-CD4+ or anti-CD8+ mAb. Administration of anti-CD4 resulted in the removal of CD4+ cells from the spleen, prevented the production of antiviral IgG, increased viral titers in the brain, and increased demyelination. In contrast, administration of anti-CD8 resulted in the removal of CD8+ cells from the spleen, did not affect IgG synthesis, did not affect spread of virus, reduced CNS inflammatory response, and abolished demyelinating lesions. These results would suggest an important role for CD8+ cells in the development of demyelination. Although the exact nature of the CD8+ cells is unknown, the results would implicate CTLs as playing an important role.

Autoimmunity also has been suggested to play a role in the development of SFV-induced CNS demyelination. Immune responses to glycolipid[346] and MBP[209] have been identified in mice infected with SFV. Furthermore, EAE has been induced in genetically resistant strains of mice after infection with SFV.[88,208] Although the mechanism by which SFV may assist in the induction of EAE is unclear, it may be by damaging the cerebral microvasculature.[302]

Herpes Simplex Virus

Herpes simplex virus is an enveloped, double-stranded, DNA-containing virus of the family Herpesviridae.[19] The genome, which is linear in the virion but likely circular in the host, contains about 152 kb pairs and a guanine and cytosine content of about 68 percent. It consists of two covalently linked nucleotide sequences designated as the long (L) and short (S) segments, with at least 76 separate open reading frames encoding 73 distinct proteins. The capsid contains 162 capsomeres made from at least seven polypeptides, has icosadeltahedral symmetry, and is about 100 to 110 nm in diameter. The tegument surrounds the capsid and varies in thickness, so that the size of the intact virion ranges from 120 to 300 nm. The tegument contains at least seven polypeptides important in transcriptional regulation. A trilaminar envelope, containing at least 11 viral glycoproteins that play a role in viral attachment, penetration, membrane fusion, envelopment, and egress, surrounds the tegument. It is derived from the host cell as the capsid buds through the nuclear membrane. The epidemiology and clinical characteristics of this human virus have been extensively reviewed.[200,277]

Some evidence would suggest a possible link between HSV and the human demyelinating disease MS. Herpes simplex virus type 1 (HSV-1) has been isolated from the CSF of a patient during the first attack of MS.[23] Furthermore, one study[193] using the polymerase chain reaction (PCR) technique identified viral antigens in glial cells or HSV viral genomes near demyelinating lesions in patients with MS (W.W. Tourtellote, personal communication), but another study[226] did not. These observations remain provocative.

Herpes simplex virus can induce demyelinating lesions in the CNS of experimental animals after peripheral inoculation with virus.[148] As with other models of virus-induced CNS demyelination, differences in viral strains, route of inoculation, size of the inoculum, and the age and strain of the experimental animal significantly affect the clinical and pathological pictures.[147,152]

Virulent strains such as Roizman F and Glasgow 17 viruses give rise to high levels of mortality and necrotizing encephalitis in specific murine strains. In contrast, less virulent strains such as lab strain 2 produce low levels of mortality and the induction of CNS demyelinating lesions.[147] Viral genes that may influence neurovirulence, both neuroinvasiveness and neurogrowth, are under investigation.[276] Preliminary results suggest than specific mutations in the gene specifying glycoprotein D result in the development of highly neuroinvasive mutants, whereas mutations in the thymidine kinase *(tk)* gene and in the gene specifying the infected cell protein 34.5 (*ICP34.5*) will reduce neurogrowth.

Differences in strains of experimental animals also influence HSV infection. Host genetic factors influence resistance to acute and lethal infections[51,187] as well as the development of latency in the peripheral nervous system (PNS).[152] The *H-2* locus appears to influence the severity of HSV infection of the PNS, with the *H-2^k* locus associated with impaired ability to clear virus.[296] In contrast, two independently segregating, non-*H-2* loci appear to influence resistance to virus in the CNS.[188] Similarly, although *H-2* does not appear to determine the development of multifocal CNS demyelination, it will influence the number and morphological appearance of the lesions that develop.[151]

After peripheral inoculation of HSV-1 in mice, virus spreads from the lip to the trigeminal ganglia (TG), most likely by retrograde intra-axonal transport. Beyond the TG, virus appears in the CNS, spreading along nerve fibers and tracts by cell-to-cell extension. During the acute stage (less than 10 to 14 days postinfection), infectious virus can be isolated from the TG, whereas in the latent stage (less than 10 to 14 days), virus can be identified only by cocultivation techniques.[147] In the CNS, infectious virus can be isolated for less than 10 days in the acute phase; in the chronic phase, only viral nucleic acid can be identified by using either in situ hybridization or PCR.[151] Clinically, mice will show signs of encephalitis during the first 10 days; survivors beyond 10 days will appear healthy during the chronic phase of the infection.

In both Swiss and Balb/c mice, CNS demyelination is limited to the trigeminal root entry zone (TREZ) beginning at 5 to 8 days postinfection. The lesions are associated with an inflammatory cell infiltrate, including myelin-laden macrophages.[164,335] Somewhat later, naked axons are observed, which may be followed by remyelination.[164,334] In specific strains of mice, multifocal CNS demyelination can follow infection with HSV-1. A/J mice will develop the sequential appearance of multifocal demyelinating lesions in the brain stem, cerebellum, and cerebral hemispheres following lip inoculation with HSV-1.[149] The lesions are associated with a mononuclear inflammatory cell infiltrate consisting primarily of macrophages and monocytes but with occasional lymphocytes.[148] HSV-1 infection of PL/J mice results in the development of relapsing disease with new demyelinating lesions appearing sporadically in the CNS for at least 28 weeks postinfection.[151]

The mechanisms mediating the development of HSV-1-induced CNS demyelination remain unclear but are likely multifactorial. The focal demyelination that develops at the TREZ during the acute stage is likely the result of a viral effect on CNS cells along with an immune-mediated response to the virus. Viral titration studies have identified a good correlation between viral titers and the severity of the pathology in the brain stem.[149] Immunohistological and electron microscopy studies would support this conclusion but suggest that astrocytes may play a key role because they are infected early and their loss precedes the development of demyelination.[139] The role of the immune system is less clear. Townsend

and Baringer[333,335] observed a decrease in demyelination using nude mice or mice immunosuppressed with cyclophosphamide, and interpreted their results as implicating a role for the host immune system. In contrast, Kristensson and colleagues[165] performed similar experiments with cyclophosphamide but observed increased demyelination. They interpreted their results as indicating an increased spread of virus from the periphery and in support of a direct cytocidal effect of virus.

The mechanisms mediating the development of multifocal and relapsing CNS demyelination are not well understood but also are likely multifactorial. Viral titration studies in the CNS of several different strains of mice have not shown a direct correlation with the development of the multifocal lesions, suggesting that mechanisms other then a direct cytolytic effect of virus are important.[149] The presence of viral nucleic acid in the CNS demyelinating lesions, as determined by in situ hybridization, however, does suggest a role for the virus.[151] Differences in resistance to virus mediated by glial cells derived from different strains of mice may also contribute to the development of demyelination. OLs derived from resistant mice such as C57BL/6J are much more resistant to infection with HSV-1 than OLs derived from susceptible A/J mice.[149] Further studies by Thomas and colleagues[331] suggest that OLs derived from A/J mice are similar to permissive cells, whereas OLs derived from C57BL/6J mice have a replicative block at the level of the cytoplasmic membrane.

Both humoral and cell-mediated immune responses to HSV develop after infection of experimental animals.[153] Immunosuppression studies suggest that the immune system plays an important role in limiting the spread of virus in the PNS.[150] CD8+ T cells are likely the important subset of cells that clear virus in the PNS.[297] Similar studies suggest that the immune system limits the spread of virus in the CNS and that both NK cells and T cells play a role.[150] The role of the immune system in the development of CNS demyelination is less clear,[28] but again, immunosuppression studies would suggest a role for T cells. Autoimmunity also may have a role in the development of HSV-induced CNS demyelination.[29]

Mechanisms of Virus-induced Demyelination

A number of different mechanisms have been postulated by which viruses might induce CNS demyelination.[349] In the models that have been reviewed, the mechanisms mediating demyelination appear to be complex and multifactorial, often involving a number of the postulated mechanisms. Even in those cases where the immune system plays an important role, it often involves different aspects of the immune system as well as, in some cases, autoimmunity. Molecular mimicry has been suggested as a potential mechanism leading to the development of demyelination.[101] MBP and the polymerase protein of hepatitis B, for example, are homologous for six amino acids. Inoculation of the six amino acids in Freund's adjuvant results in pathological lesions that resemble EAE.[102] Increasing awareness of the interaction of virus with CNS cells and the control these cells appear to have over viral replication, often as a function of cell differentiation and maturation, add a new dimension to the future study of pathogenic mechanisms.

Many common factors appear to be present in these models of virus-induced CNS demyelination:

1. CNS demyelination can be induced by many different viruses.
2. Specific strains of virus are more likely to result in CNS demyelination than other strains. Viral genome determinants appear to control this difference, at least in part.
3. Specific strains of animals are more susceptible to the development of CNS demyelination. Host genome determinants appear to control this difference, at least in part.
4. An acute stage of CNS infection occurs before the development of chronic demyelination.
5. Persistence of viral infection, defective viral replication, or viral latency in the CNS appears to be required for the development of CNS demyelination, at least in these models.
6. The immune system is required during the acute stage of infection in most cases; in some, it plays a pivotal role in the development of chronic demyelination.

Despite the inherent complexities of these experimental systems, the major advantage each enjoys is the defined nature of the etiologic agent, a situation that does not exist in MS. For this reason, these models provide a promise of a better understanding of how viruses can induce CNS demyelination. Insight derived from these model systems will be valuable in understanding MS.

HUMAN DISEASES CHARACTERIZED BY VIRUS-INDUCED DEMYELINATION OR VIRUS-ASSOCIATED IMMUNE ACTIVATION

Some myelopathies similar to MS are caused by direct viral infection or immunological perturbations that occur in the wake of viral infection.

HTLV-1 Associated Myelopathy (or Tropical Spastic Paraparesis)

EPIDEMIOLOGY

The clinical features of this chronic progressive myelopathy were consolidated in 1956 by Cruickshank,[67] although similar cases were described in the last century. The myelopathy is common in a number of regions in the world. In Martinique, 78 percent of the patients with this syndrome are seropositive for HTLV-1, compared with a general population prevalence of 4 percent.[341] Japanese patients with this chronic myelopathy are uniformly seropositive for HTLV-1; in the Kii peninsula, the rate of seropositivity is 16 percent in the general population.[231] Although cases are more prominent in some regions of the world,[256,278] geography is no longer an impediment to making the diagnosis. The prevalence of HTLV-1 seropositivity in the United States is estimated to be 0.025 percent. The cases are concentrated among blacks in the eastern United States, especially in intravenous drug users and their sexual partners.[354] Cases have been recently described in aboriginal populations in North America.[84,255]

CLINICAL FEATURES

The average age of onset is 40 years (range, 6 to 75 years). The history reveals insidiously progressive leg weakness and stiffness. Back pain, lower extremity dysesthesias, and bowel and bladder dysfunction are common. Physical examination typically reveals a spastic paraparesis with brisk deep tendon reflexes and extensor plantar responses. Cranial nerve dysfunction (optic neuritis and deafness) is uncommon and sensory findings are less prominent in this form of myelopathy compared with spinal forms of MS. Mild involvement of peripheral nerves has been described and polymyositis may complicate the condition.[119] Cognitive changes are rare.[299]

The natural history of the myelopathy is largely uncharted. Much of the progression appears to occur in the first year or two, followed by long periods of relative stability.[5]

PATHOLOGY

Neuropathological studies have demonstrated demyelination in the dorsal and lateral funiculi and some axonal loss, with variable degrees of vacuolation and inflammation.[268] Demyelination in plaques has not been described. Proviral DNA can be amplified from spinal cord.[175,257,326]

ETIOLOGY

The association of TSP with HTLV-1 was first made by Gessain and his colleagues in 1985.[113a] They demonstrated enzyme-linked immunosorbent assay-reactive antibodies in 10 of 17 Caribbean patients with TSP. The absence of antibody in some patients with the clinical phenotype might represent the inclusion of non-HTLV-1 myelopathies or suboptimal sensitivity of the earlier serological assays. Some patients with retroviral

myelopathies do not have the usual serological markers.

Subsequently the virus was isolated[140] and viral DNA has been amplified from leukocytes and neural tissues of patients with TSP.[26] The identification of the types of cells infected in the CNS is incomplete.

PATHOGENESIS

Although TSP has been linked to infection with HTLV-1 infection, the pathogenesis remains a mystery. It is uncertain whether the nervous system damage is the result of direct virus-induced cytopathic effect or whether the disease involves the immune system. The following observations are of note:

1. The myelopathy appears to be a relatively uncommon manifestation of HTLV-1 infection, occurring in no more than 1 of 100 individuals infected with this virus, although long-term follow-up of infected individuals is lacking.[288]

2. TSP occurs in a different subset of individuals than those predisposed to adult T-cell leukemia. Coincidental cases are only rarely described.[17]

3. The incubation period for development of the myelopathy is variable. The condition can develop as quickly as 18 weeks after infection. Gout and colleagues[120] described a 41-year-old patient who developed a subacute myelopathy as a complication of transfusion during cardiac transplantation. Spinal cord signs developed within 4 weeks of seroconversion, which occurred 14 weeks after the transfusion. Several decades can separate the viral infection and the myelopathy. The maximum latency between infection and myelopathy is unknown.

4. The sequence of viral strains of HTLV-1 that cause the myelopathy does not appear to be different from strains that are leukemogenic. Although this observation requires confirmation, it suggests that the infected host is the principal determinant of pathogenesis.

5. Leukocytes from those who develop the myelopathy appear to support

higher levels of virus replication than leukocytes from those who do not.[361]

6. Occasional familial clusters of TSP have been described, suggesting that host susceptibility is genetically determined.[215]

7. It has been suggested that human leukocyte antigen type is important, but this observation awaits confirmation.[336]

8. Some viral proteins bear some sequence homology to MBP, raising the possibility of molecular mimicry in the disease pathogenesis.[350]

9. Immune activation is suggested by the demonstration of tumor necrosis factor receptor in CSF.[259]

IMPLICATIONS FOR MULTIPLE SCLEROSIS

Tropical spastic paraparesis is arguably the best human "model" for MS. The potential for confusion with MS, especially spinal forms, is obvious and diagnostic criteria for both conditions need revision. Many of the patients with TSP identified in our clinics were referred because they were thought to have MS. Only rarely do patients with TSP have magnetic imaging that would meet diagnostic criteria for MS.[166] Differences between TSP and spinal forms of multiple sclerosis are summarized in Table 10–1.

The first attempts to demonstrate HTLV-1-like sequences in patients with MS have failed. Indeed, viruses of this nature may have little to do with the etiology of MS.

However, it should be remembered that patients with retroviral myelopathies do not always have the standard serological markers. A viral etiology for TSP could not be identified until the advent of the culture techniques required for the preparation of HTLV-1 as an antigen source for immunoassays. Advances in molecular biology, particularly the PCR technique, have greatly facilitated the ability to identify such diseases. New insights into retrovirus biology and better technology for the detection of novel human retroviruses might allow further consideration of this kind of virus in the etiology of MS. In the next few years, we will see the delineation of a new spectrum of neurological disorders caused by other retroviruses. In the last few years, a variety of spinal cord and cerebellar syndromes have been linked to infection with HTLV-2. The complete spectrum has yet to be defined.[138]

Acquired Immunodeficiency Syndrome Myelopathy

EPIDEMIOLOGY

Infection of the CNS has greatly extended the clinical spectrum of acquired immunodeficiency syndrome (AIDS). In 1985, Petito and her colleagues[248] described a progressive myelopathy in patients with AIDS. In her series of 89 consecutive autopsies, pathological evidence of myelopathy was found in 20 of 89 cases. A dementia was

Table 10–1. **COMPARISON OF MS AND TROPICAL SPASTIC PARAPARESIS (TSP)**

	TSP	MS
HTLV-1 serology (ELISA)	Positive	Negative
HTLV-1 gene amplification	Positive	Negative
Affected population	Chiefly blacks from Caribbean basin	Chiefly whites
Sensory findings	Rare	Common
Peripheral nerve and muscle involvement	Common	Absent
Magnetic resonance scan— periventricular T_2 abnormalities	Rare	Common

evident in 70 percent of these patients. Although the syndrome is now commonly recognized and can herald the onset of AIDS,[258] it generally develops much later in the illness, with failing immunocompetence and an increased virus load.

PATHOGENESIS

The myelopathy is likely due to a direct virus-mediated cytopathic effect. The virus gains access to the nervous system by either direct infection through the blood-brain barrier or by prior infection of MNCs and secondary invasion of the CNS.

Virus localization has been reasonably well mapped. Wiley and colleagues[353] used in situ hydridization and immuno-histochemistry to map the distribution of human immunodeficiency virus (HIV)-infected cells in brains studied postmortem. The principal cells infected are the brain monocyte (microglial) and the endothelial cell. Low-level involvement of neurons and astrocytes was seen in a single case with severe CNS involvement. Peudenier and associates[252] adduced some evidence that the infected mononuclear cells of the brain are cells that have crossed the blood-brain barrier, rather than the resident brain macrophages (microglia).[251,252]

The virus receptor in brain may be different from the CD4 molecule on lymphocytes and monocytes. Cells of the mononuclear phagocyte system are the predominant cell producing human immunodeficiency virus type 1 (HIV-1) in most tissues, including the CNS (where it is associated with dementia and neuropathy), lung (with pneumonitis), and skin (with dermatitis). Different HIV-1 isolates vary markedly in their ability to infect mononuclear phagocytes productively. Mononuclear phagocyte infectivity appears to be determined by a 157-amino acid region of the gp 120; significantly, this region is upstream from the CD4-binding domain.[228] The envelope determinants of tropism have been mapped to the V3 loop of gp120, for both macrophages and brain microglia.[290] Although variable amounts of CD4 have been demonstrated on cells of neuroglial origin,[106] these cells appear to be infected by a non-CD4-mediated route. The infection is not blocked by soluble CD4.[58]

Some neuronal cell lines appear to be infected through a galactosyl ceramide receptor that is also expressed on oligodendrocytes.[60,130]

A few neurotropic HIV isolates may preferentially infect the nervous system. Some patients infected with the same neurotropic strain of HIV appear to have pursued the same clinical courses.[162] Several differences in envelope sequence have been identified among strains of HIV that appear to be neurotropic. Weber[347] identified some envelope sequences that were associated with a higher prevalence of CNS disease. Mutational changes in the viral envelope that conferred enhanced neurotropism could be present at the time of infection in some individuals or could develop in the course of the infection in a single patient.[154] It remains an open question whether the development of neurotropic changes in the viral envelope is essential to the development of the encephalopathy.

Most myelopathies develop in the context of failed immunocompetence and a tremendous increase in systemic virus load.[258] The myelopathy is common in patients with HIV infection and relatively uncommon in patients with HTLV-1 infection.

Some individuals appear to be able to tolerate HIV infection for several decades. Evidence for host resistance has not been forthcoming. Some evidence suggests that long survivorship is secondary to deletion in the viral *nef* gene.[82]

Several mechanisms could act in concert in the pathogenesis of the nervous system assault. First of all, although the virus is present in neuroglial cells, the level of viral protein expression varies. In small numbers of patients, Pang and colleagues[234] demonstrated that the presence of HIV encephalitis was associated with the amount of unintegrated viral DNA and not the level of viral antigen expression.

Second, the glycoproteins are neurotoxic:

- The viral glycoprotein can stimulate the release of neurotoxins from monocytes.[115]
- Glycoprotein 120 (gp 120) kills primary cultures of cortical neurons; this appears to be mediated by nitrous oxide. This effect can be blocked by

N-methyl-D-aspartate (NMDA) antagonists.[81]

- A region of gp 120 bears some homology to snake venom neurotoxins and rabies virus glycoprotein (the neurotoxic loop).[303]
- As a result of modulation of astrocytic function by gp 120, the ensuing neuronal depolarization and glutamate exposure could activate both voltage-gated and NMDA-regulated calcium channels, leading to increases in intraneuronal calcium and neuronal death.[20]
- Mice that are manipulated transgenically to express the envelope gene develop neuropathological changes.

Third, viral transactivating proteins are neurotoxic. HIV can transactivate a variety of cellular genes. The tat protein that mediates this transactivation is involved in the physiological upregulation of the expression of HIV RNA by enhancing the prolongation of viral transcripts from the RNA start site. The tat protein acts directly on the HIV LTR segment. This can occur directly within infected cells, or indirectly by passage of tat from one infected cell to another. At concentrations of 10^{-9} to 10^{-10}, the agent appears to bind specifically to synaptosomal membranes.[162] At micromolar concentrations, tat appears to be neurotoxic in a number of functional assays and can be lethal when injected into the brains of mice. Although it is unlikely that tat reaches concentrations in this order within serum or spinal fluid, it could reach this concentration within regions of infected brain. The role of transactivation in the pathogenesis of the AIDS encephalopathy is still undefined.[287]

Fourth, the generation of toxic cytokines may have an effect. Release of cytokines by infected monocytes or lymphocytes can stimulate virus replication in cells[352] and induce class II expression on astrocytes. This could expedite the immune assault on infected neuroglial cells. Elevated levels of tumor necrosis factor-α have been found in the spinal fluid of patients with AIDS. Its presence suggests active infection or inflammation, but it does not discriminate between primary infection by HIV and opportunistic infection.

Finally, cofactorial processes may play a role, but the delineation of cofactorial processes is incomplete. It is likely that HIV can induce the encephalopathy of AIDS by itself. The most important cofactor is probably the extent of the virus-induced immunosuppression, as mentioned above. Another likely cofactor is concomitant infection with viruses known to alter expression of the HIV genome. HIV and other herpes viruses have been identified in the same cells within the nervous system.[224] The immediate early genes of CMV can transactivate the promoter of HIV.[78] The effects of this transactivation may be bidirectional and have been demonstrated in astroglial lines.[86,298]

PATHOLOGY

The posterior and lateral columns of the thoracic cord exhibit the greatest pathology. A vacuolar degeneration of myelin is the prominent light microscopic finding and virions can be identified by microscopy.[230]

IMPLICATIONS FOR MULTIPLE SCLEROSIS

Understanding how HIV interacts with the nervous system will improve our concepts of neurobiology. Individuals with both AIDS and MS have a poor prognosis. HIV-1-mediated immunosuppression does not appear to benefit the disease.[21]

Subacute Sclerosing Panencephalitis

CLINICAL FEATURES

Subacute sclerosing panencephalitis (SSPE) is an unusual manifestation of measles virus infection, which was first described in 1934[79] and later consolidated.[337] It follows natural measles virus infection by a latency of 6 to 8 years; the latency is shorter after vaccination with live-attenuated virus.[87] Children and adolescents are principally affected. The risk for this complication is increased by early natural infection (often before the first 2 years) and is increased by the administration of immunoglobulin.[262] The illness evolves as a progressive dementia, variably punctuated by seizures, myoclonus, ataxia, and chorioretinitis, usually resulting in complete decortication and death in 1 to 3 years. The electroencephalographic pattern is typified by burst suppression. The spinal fluid is laced with oligoclonally restricted immunoglobulin, much of which is specific for measles virus.

PATHOLOGY

Gray and white matter are damaged by a persistent viral infection, resulting in death of neurons and loss of myelin. Viral nucleocapsids appear as typical eosinophilic inclusion bodies. The immune response of the host is evident by perivascular lymphocyte cuffing and fibrous gliosis (i.e., sclerosing encephalitis).

PATHOGENESIS

In uncomplicated measles virus infection, the virus infects a cell (typically respiratory epithelium) and replicates. The mature virions incite the immune response and are subsequently eliminated by immune defenses of the host. The deviations that occur in SSPE are summarized below:

1. The B lymphocyte response of the infected patient is probably normal. Large amounts of measles virus-specific antibody are present in serum and spinal fluid. It had once been thought that patients with SSPE failed to raise antibody to a viral subcomponent (the matrix or M protein), but this more likely relates to the low immunogenicity of this protein. Only small amounts of antibody are raised to this protein in conventional measles virus infections. The one B-cell abnormality is that antibody present before the "infection" can influence the outcome of the infection. SSPE is most prone to occur when the infection occurs in the very young, in whom maternal antibody is likely present, or in those given immune globulin near the time of natural infection or vaccination.
2. Antibody might facilitate infection of cells for which the virus does not have a natural tropism. Culture of measles virus-infected cells in the presence of specific neutralizing antibodies alters the biology of the infection. Expression of surface proteins (hemaglutinin and fusions proteins) and the matrix protein is turned off. The virus remains inside the cell and can elude host defense.[104] The virus is then free to damage the cell.
3. RNA viruses have an incredible predilection for mutation, and selection pressure is increased when infected cells are cultured in the presence of antibodies. This best explains the development of replication-defective strains and perhaps the more neurovirulent strains that have been isolated from SSPE brains.[53] A variety of mutations have been identified in the measles virus genome in patients with SSPE.[27,66]
4. The ability of T lymphocytes from affected patients to lyse measles virus-infected target cells is impaired,[85] at least in established cases. This vital T-cell function has not been measured at the inception of the disease. Measles virus has a direct ability to infect lymphocytes and abrogate their function.[47]

IMPLICATIONS FOR MULTIPLE SCLEROSIS

Subacute sclerosing panencephalitis is a good model for the study of interaction of the nervous and immune systems with measles virus. Measles virus is no longer thought to have an etiologic role in MS (vide infra). Vaccination programs have almost eradicated SSPE except for vaccine-associated cases,[87] and the incidence of MS does not appear to have changed.

Progressive Multifocal Leukoencephalopathy

CLINICAL FEATURES

This rare white matter disease develops insidiously, with multifocal symptoms. Paralysis, visual loss, and sensory abnormalities are common. Cerebellar and isolated spinal cord involvement are less common. The disease has a unique propensity for the iatrogenically or virally immunosuppressed but has rarely been reported in healthy individuals. The disease progresses relentlessly, usually resulting in death within 6 months. If the underlying immunosuppression can be reversed, recovery can occur.[327]

The diagnosis is clinched by imaging techniques, which reveal multifocal demyelination, and by spinal fluid analysis, which is generally normal. Gene amplification of papovavirus sequences from biopsy material has been reported,[122] and papovavirus sequences and antigens can be demonstrated within OLs.

PATHOLOGY

Multifocal areas of demyelination, with loss of OLs and myelin, and relative sparing of axons are the essential features. The OLs are typically enlarged and show intranuclear inclusion bodies. Enlarged astrocytes may show bizarre mitotic figures and unusual nuclear configurations.

PATHOGENESIS

The disorder is caused by direct papovavirus infection, which is very common in the general population (approximately 75 percent have antibody). These endogenous viruses are normally held in check by immune defense. When immune defense fails, the virus expresses its cytopathic effect in a broader range of host tissues, including the nervous system. Damage to the nervous system is likely the sequel of direct virus-induced cytopathic effect in glial cells.

IMPLICATIONS FOR MULTIPLE SCLEROSIS

Papovavirus infection has not been incriminated in the development of multiple sclerosis.

Myelopathies Indirectly Due to Infection

ACUTE DISSEMINATED ENCEPHALOMYELITIS

An acute myelitis or encephalomyelitis can develop in the wake of viral infection or following vaccination. The immune response to a viral infection results in the last two perturbations, B-lymphocyte activation and lymphokine generation.

It has long been recognized that a variety of autoantibodies are generated following viral infection. For example, rheumatoid factor, cryoglobulins, antinuclear antibodies, and red cell-specific antibodies are commonly generated after infections with the CMV. Several mechanisms might be operative in the activation of B lymphocytes. A generalized release of B-cell growth and differentiation factors might have a stimulatory effect on B-cell clones of specificity different from the virus. Up to 4 percent of murine monoclonal antibodies raised against diverse viruses appear to be autoreactive.[307] The sharing of antigenic epitopes between viruses and host tissues might explain the frequent demonstration of such antibodies. For example, the encephalitogenic site of MBP shares sequence with the hepatitis B polymerase. Immunization of rabbits with the viral peptide can induce perivascular inflammation within the CNS similar to that produced by inoculation of myelin basic protein.[103]

A variety of lymphokines are released after viral infection. Release of interleukin-2 is likely involved in the frequent lymphocytosis that accompanies viral infection. Production of interferon gamma has been shown to increase expression of class II antigens on a variety of cells that do not express them constitutively. This might initiate T-cell recognition of previously cloistered antigens. The viral factors that perturb the immune system in the genesis of encephalomyelitis might be similar to those that aggravate MS after viral infection. Most viruses appear to have the ability to induce postinfectious myelopathies. The perturbations are better understood for some than for others.

Clinical Features. Spinal cord symptoms develop acutely, following a latency of 1 to 3 weeks after infection or vaccination. Leg weakness and numbness, pain, neurogenic bladder, and occasionally cerebral symptoms develop over a few days. The constellation of clinical features is usually monophasic. After measles, the nervous system signs develop as the rash clears.

CSF. An MNC pleocytosis and raised protein level, without OBs, are quite typical. Virus cannot be isolated.

Pathology. The findings closely parallel those seen in EAE encephalomyelitis. Periventricular demyelination and meningitic lymphocytic infiltration are the essential features.

Pathogenesis. The best understood myelitis is that which follows measles. The following observations are important:

1. The virus cannot be isolated from the brain or the CSF during the encephalomyelitis.
2. Measles virus can suppress[265] or activate various elements that constitute the immune response.[123] The acute infection induces proliferation of lymphocytes with receptors for the virus. This occurs with release of a soluble receptor for interleukin-2. The effector limbs of the immune response, as measured by the release of soluble CD8, are recruited somewhat later. This coincides with the development of the encephalomyelitis and the disappearance of the rash.[123]
3. Lymphocytes that proliferate on culture with MBP have been demonstrated in those patients with encephalomyelitis. Because virus cannot be isolated at the same time, direct infection is unlikely.
4. The mechanism of recruitment of lymphocytes specific for MBP is not understood. Clones of measles-virus–specific T cells do not appear to be alloreactive.[266]

Similar mechanisms might be deemed operative for other viral infections and after vaccination, but the mechanisms are less well established.

Treatment. Based on encouraging anecdotal reports,[241] steroids are usually given as soon as the diagnosis is suspected. Controlled trials are lacking, however.

POSTVACCINAL ENCEPHALOMYELITIS

The pathophysiology of these myelopathies is likely the same as for the postinfectious myelopathies. The clinical and pathological features are similar. The myelopathy that follows the Semple rabies vaccine is likely secondary to an immune response that develops to CNS antigens in the inoculum. Those who develop the encephalomyelitis appear to raise antibody to MBP.[133]

Implications for MS. Some cases of postinfectious myelitis can be confused with spinal forms of MS. However, the postinfectious forms are generally monophasic and generally negative for OB. Postinfectious myelitis is a better model of acute disseminated encephalomyelitis. Cases of encephalomyelitis can be confused with acute MS. Widespread white matter lesions can develop in both. Greater involvement of deep gray matter structures favors acute disseminated encephalomyelitis.[18]

Measles virus has long been suspected to have a role in MS because most serological studies have suggested an increase in antibody titers of this specificity.[1,227] The significance of this observation is uncertain; an elevated titer is neither sufficient nor essential but might relate to immunogenetic factors operative in populations at risk for the development of MS or circumstances present in the environments in which those populations reside. Vaccination programs have not altered the incidence of MS, but further work is necessary in this area.[145]

THE QUEST FOR A VIRUS IN MULTIPLE SCLEROSIS

Published observations in this field of MS research are rarely reproducible. All claims to isolate a virus and to demonstrate virus footprints (antibody to a virus, viral genetic material, or viral antigen) have failed the test of reproducibility. The iniquitous track record of irreproducibility is an embarrassment to science and greatly tempers the credibility of all emerging publications on the subject. This is unfortunate because scientists at large would welcome the identification of a virus or other pathogen in MS. Epidemiologists have long awaited such an agent to explain the curious geographic distribution of MS and the occasional epidemics.[167] The agents that have been claimed to be causal to MS are listed in

Table 10–2. It is more useful to review the lessons learned from the refutations than to review in detail the various contentions.

1. **Heed the control subjects.** Clinical materials are derived far too commonly from a population with MS in a different geographic area from control subjects. It is important to study patients with other kinds of neurological and autoimmune diseases in addition to the so-called normal control subjects. It is all too easy to collect a few patients with strokes or amyotrophic lateral sclerosis and call them the "control subjects." It is important to include patients with nervous system diseases in which immune activation is a feature. Studies would be welcomed if they included more comprehensive control groups composed of non-affected siblings, discordant dizygotic and monozygotic twins, and parents of patients with MS. Every study that has neglected these controls has evaded reproducibility.

2. **Has the investigator been blinded?** We have been led astray many times by unblinded investigators who invariably examine the MS sample with a level of scrutiny different from that used to examine the controls. The process of coding samples is usually undertaken by those who refute claims of isolation.

3. **Beware of laboratory contamination.** Many investigators have hastened to publish the "discovery" of agents growing in their own laboratory as common contaminants. This may be the best explanation for the reports of Simian CMV,[283] HTLV-1,[161] and measles virus.[246]

4. **Be skeptical of marginal differences.** Many of the assays used to implicate a virus have been cumbersome to perform, have had substantial intrinsic variability, and have had ranges for normal values with remarkable overlap with that seen for control subjects. Claims based on marginal differences have been disproved.

5. **Beware of new technology.** Because the conventional approaches have been exhausted, the identification of a virus in MS will likely require some innovative technology. When new reagents or technologies are applied to the study of MS, investigators commonly find "differences" between patients and control subjects. When the shortfalls of such reagents and technologies are later understood, others fail to find the same "differences." This phenomenon has been borne out by recent experience with gene amplification techniques in the pursuit of viral sequences related to HTLV-1.[83,161]

Table 10–2. CLAIMS OF VIRUS ISOLATIONS IN MULTIPLE SCLEROSIS

Virus	Year	Senior Investigator
Rabies	1946	Mangolis[192]
Herpes simplex	1964	Gudnadottir[125]
Scrapie-like agent	1966	Field[92]
Measles	1972	Field[93]
Parainfluenza 1	1972	Ter Meulen[328]
Carp agent	1972	Carp[46]
MS agent	1975	Koldovsky[160]
Paramyxovirus	1976	Pertschuk[246]
Simian CMV	1979	Rorke[283]
Coronavirus	1979	Burks[43]
Simian virus V	1987	Goswami[118]
HTLV-1	1985	Koprowski[161] H, DeFreitas EC, Harper ME

CMV = cytomegalovirus.

SUMMARY

Although a virus has not yet been incriminated in the pathogenesis of MS, our general understanding of virus–nervous system interaction has improved. Insights from the study of retrovirus biology will undoubtedly reveal new means by which viruses can cause disease. The elucidation of genetic factors of the host and virulence factors in the virus will be particularly revealing in TSP. This science will be interesting to watch.

REFERENCES

1. Adams JM, and Imagawa DT: Measles virus antibodies in multiple sclerosis. Proc Soc Exp Biol Med 111:562, 1962.
2. Alldinger S, Baumgartner W, and Orvell C: Restricted expression of viral surface proteins in canine distemper encephalitis. Acta Neuropathol (Berl) 85:635, 1993.
3. Allen I, and Brankin B: Pathogenesis of multiple sclerosis: The immune diathesis and the role of viruses. J Neuropathol Exp Neurol 52:95, 1993.
4. Appel MJG: Pathogenesis of canine distemper. Am J Vet Res 30:1167, 1969.
5. Araujo AQ, Leite AC, Dultra SV, and Andrada-Serpa MJ: Progression of neurological disability in HTLV-1 associated myelopathy/tropical spastic paraparesis. J Neurol Sci. 129:147–151, 1995.
6. Atkins GJ: The avirulent A7 strain of Semliki Forest virus has reduced cytopathogenicity for neuroblastoma cells compared to the virulent L10 strain. J Gen Virol 64:1401, 1983.
7. Atkins GJ, and Sheahan BJ: Semliki Forest virus neurovirulence mutants have altered cytopathogenicity for CNS cells. Infect Immun 36:333, 1982.
8. Atkins GJ, Sheahan BJ, and Dimock NJ: Semliki Forest virus infection of mice: A model for genetic and molecular analysis of viral pathogenicity (review article). J Gen Virol 66:395, 1985.
9. Atkins GJ, Sheahan BJ, and Mooney DA: Pathogenicity of Semliki Forest virus for the rat CNS and primary rat neural cell cultures: Possible implications for the pathogenesis of multiple sclerosis. Neuropathol Appl Neurobiol 16:57, 1990.
10. Aubert C, Chamorro M, and Brahic M: Identification of Theiler's virus infected cells in the central nervous system of the mouse during demyelinating disease. Microb Pathog 3:319, 1987.
11. Bailey OT, Pappenheimer AM, Cheever FS, and Daniels JB: A murine virus (JHM) causing disseminated encephalomyelitis with extensive destruction of myelin. II. Pathology. J Exp Med 90:195, 1949.
12. Balluz IM, Glasgow GM, Killen HM, Mabrok MJ, Sheaban BJ, and Atkins GJ: Virulent and avirulent strains of Semliki Forest virus show similar cell tropism for the murine central nervous system but differ in the severity and rate of induction of cytolytic damage. Neuropathol Appl Neurobiol 19:233, 1993.
13. Barnett EM, and Perlman S: The olfactory nerve and not the trigeminal nerve is the major site of CNS entry for mouse hepatitis virus strain JHM. Virology 194:185, 1993.
14. Barrett PN, Sheahan BJ, and Atkins GJ: Isolation and preliminary characterization of Semliki Forest virus mutants with altered virulence. J Gen Virol 49:141, 1980.
15. Barrow P, Tonks P, Welsh CJ, and Nash AA: The role of CD8+ T cells in the acute and chronic phases of Theiler's murine encephalomyelitis virus induced disease in mice. J Gen Virol 73:1861, 1992.
16. Barthold SW: Research complications and state of knowledge of rodent coronaviruses. In Hamm TE (ed): Complications of Viral and Mycoplasmal Infections in Rodents to Toxicology Research and Testing. Hemisphere Publishing, Washington, DC, 1986, p 53.
17. Bartholomew C, Cleghorn F, Wavenay C, et al: HTLV-1 and tropical spastic paraparesis. The Lancet ii:99–100, 1986.
18. Baum PA, Barkovich AJ, Koch TK, et al: Deep gray involvement in children with acute disseminated encephalomyelitis. AJNR 15:1275–1283, 1994.
19. Beers DR, Henkel JS, and Stroop WG: Herpes simplex virus. In McKendall RR, and Stroop WG (eds): Handbook of Neurovirology. Marcel Dekker, New York, 1994, p 225.
20. Benos DJ, Hahn BH, Bubien JK, et al: Envelope glycoprotein gp120 of human immunodeficiency virus type 1 alters ion transport in astrocytes: Implications for AIDS dementia complex. Proc Natl Acad Sci USA 91:494–48, 1994.
21. Berger JR, Shermata WA, Resnick L, Atherton S, Fletcher MA, and Norenberg M: Multiple sclerosis-like illness occurring with human immunodeficiency virus infection. Neurology 39:324–329, 1989.
22. Bergmann C, McMillan M, and Stohlman S: Characterization of the Ld restricted cytotoxic T lymphocyte epitope in the mouse hepatitis virus nucleocapsid protein. J Virol 67:7041, 1993.
23. Bergstrom T, Anderson O, and Vahlne A: Isolation of herpes simplex virus type 1 during first attack of multiple sclerosis. Ann Neurol 26:283, 1989.
24. Beushausen S, and Dales S: In vivo and in vitro models of demyelinating disease XI. Tropism and differentiation regulate the infectious process of coronavirus in primary explants of the rat CNS. Virology 141:89, 1985.
25. Beushausen S, Narindrasorasak S, Sanwal BD, and Dales S: In vivo and in vitro models of demyelinating disease: Activation of the adenylate cyclase system influences JHM virus expression in explanted rat oligodendrocytes. J Virol 61:3795, 1987.
26. Bhagavati S, Ehrlich G, Kula RW, et al: Detection of human t-cell lymphoma/leukemia virus type I DNA and antigen in spinal fluid and blood of patients with chronic progressive myelopathy. N Engl J Med 318:1141–1147, 1988.

27. Billeter MA, Cattaneo R, Spielhofer P, et al: Generation and properties of measles virus mutations typically associated with subacute sclerosing panencephalitis. Ann NY Acad Sci 724:367–377, 1994.

28. Bishop SA, and Hill TJ: Herpes simplex virus infection and damage in the central nervous system: Immunomodulation with adjunct, cyclophosphamide, and cyclosporin A. Arch Virol 116:57, 1991.

29. Bishop SA, and Hill TJ: Herpes simplex virus infection and damage in the central nervous system: Immune response to myelin basic protein. J Neurol Sci 91:109, 1989.

30. Blacklaws B, Bird P, Allen D, and McConnell I: Circulating cytoxic T-lymphocyte precursors in maedi-visna virus infected sheep. J Gen Virol 75:1589, 1994.

31. Blakemore WF, Summers BA, and Appell MG: Evidence of oligodendrocyte infection and degeneration in canine distemper encephalomyelitis. Acta Neuropathol (Berl) 77:550, 1989.

32. Blakemore WF, Welsh CJR, Tonks P, and Nash AA: Observations on demyelinating lesions induced by Theiler's virus in CBA mice. Acta Neuropathol (Berl) 76:581, 1988.

33. Blankenhorn FP, and Stranford SA: Genetic factors in demyelinating diseases: Genes that control demyelination due to experimental allergic encephalomyelitis (EAE) and Theiler's murine encephalitis virus. Reg Immunol 4:331, 1992.

34. Bollo E, Zurbriggen A, Vandevelde M, and Fankhauser R: Canine distemper virus clearance in chronic inflammatory demyelination. Acta Neuropathol (Berl) 72:69, 1986.

35. Booss J, and Kim JH: Evidence for a viral etiology of Multiple Sclerosis. In Cook SD (ed): Handbook of Multiple Sclerosis. Marcel Dekker, New York, 1990, p 41.

36. Brahic M, Bureau JF, and McAllister A: Genetic determinants of the demyelinating disease caused by Theiler's virus. Microb Pathog 11:77, 1991.

37. Brahic M, Haase AT, and Cash E: Simultaneous in-situ detection of viral RNA and antigens. Proc Natl Acad Sci USA 81:5445, 1984.

38. Brahic M, Stowring L, Ventura P, and Haase AT: Gene expression in visna virus infection in sheep. Nature 292:240, 1981.

39. Brahic M, Stroop WG, and Baringer JR: Theiler's virus persists in glial cells during demyelinating disease. Cell 26:123, 1981.

40. Buchmeier MJ, Lewicki HA, Talbot PJ, and Knobler RL: Murine hepatitis virus-4 (strain JHM) induced neurologic disease is modulated in vivo by monoclonal antibody. Virology 132:261, 1984.

41. Bureau JF, Montagutelli X, Bihl F, Lefebvre S, Guenet JL, and Brahic M: Mapping loci influencing the persistence of Theiler's virus in the murine central nervous system. Nat Genet 5:87, 1993.

42. Burks JS, DeVald BL, Jankovsky LD, and Gerdes JC: Two coronaviruses isolated from central nervous system tissue of two multiple sclerosis patients. Science 209:933, 1980.

43. Burks JS, Devald-Macmillan B, Jankovsky L, et al: Characterization of coronaviruses isolated using multiple sclerosis autopsy brain material. Neurology 29:547, 1979.

44. Calenoff MA, Faaberg KS, and Lipton HL: Genomic regions of neurovirulence and attenuation in Theiler murine encephalomyelitis virus. Proc Natl Acad Sci USA 87:978, 1990.

45. Cameron RS, and Rakic P: Glial cell lineage in the cerebral cortex: A review and synthesis. Glia 4:124, 1991.

46. Carp RI, Licursi PC, Merz PA, and Merz GS: Decreased percentage of polymorphonuclear neutrophils in mouse peripheral blood after inoculation with material from multiple sclerosis patients. J Exp Med 136:618–629, 1972.

47. Casali P, Rice GPA, and Oldstone MBA: Viruses disrupt functions of human lymphocytes: Effects of measles virus and influenza virus on lymphocyte mediated killing and antibody production. J Exp Med 159:1322–1337, 1984.

48. Cash E, Bandeira A, Chirinian S, and Brahic M: Characterization of B lymphocytes present in the demyelinating lesions induced by Theiler's virus. Immunology 143:984, 1989.

49. Cash E, Chamorro M, Brahic M: Minus-strand RNA synthesis in the spinal cords of mice persistently infected with Theiler's virus. J Virol 62:1824, 1988.

50. Cash E, Chamorro M, and Brahic M: Quantitation, with a new assay, of Theiler's virus capsid protein in the central nervous system of mice. J Virol 60:558, 1986.

51. Caspary L, Schindling B, Dundarov S, and Falke D: Infections of susceptible and resistant mouse strains with herpes simplex virus types 1 and 2. Arch Virol 65:219, 1980.

52. Castro RF, Evans GD, Jaszewski A, and Perlman S: Coronavirus induced demyelination occurs in the presence of virus specific cytotoxic T-cells. Virology 200:733, 1994.

53. Cattaneo R, Schmid A, Spielhofer P, et al. Mutated and hypermutated genes of persistent measles viruses which caused lethal human brain diseases. Virology 173:415–425, 1989.

54. Challoner PB, Smith KT, Parker JD, et al: Plaque-associated expression of human herpesvirus 6 in multiple sclerosis. Proc Natl Acad Sci USA 92: 7440, 1995.

55. Chamorro M, Aubert C, and Brahic M: Demyelinating lesions due to Theiler's virus are associated with ongoing central nervous system infection. J Virol 57:992, 1986.

56. Cheever FS, Daniels JB, Pappenheimer AM, and Bailey OT: A murine virus (JHM) causing disseminated encephalomyelitis with extensive destruction of myelin 1: Isolation and biological properties of the virus. J Exp Med 90:181, 1949.

57. Cheevers WP, and McGurie TC: The lentiviruses: Maedi/visna, caprine arthritis-encephalitis, and equine infectious anemia. Adv Virus Res 34:189, 1988.

58. Chesebro B, Buller R, Portis J, and Wherly K: Failure of human immunodeficiency virus entry and infection in CD4 positive human brain and skin cells. J Virol 64:215–221, 1990.

59. Chew-Lim M, Suckling AJ, and Webb HE: Demyelination in mice after two or three infec-

tions with avirulent Semliki Forest virus. Vet Pathol 14:62, 1977.

60. Clapham PR, Weber JN, Whitby D, et al: Soluble CD4 blocks the infectivity of diverse strains of HIV and SIV for T cells and monocytes but not for brain and muscle cells. Nature 337:68–70, 1989.

61. Clatch RJ, Lipton HL, and Miller SD: Characterization of Theiler's murine encephalomyelitis virus (TMEV) specific delayed type hypersensitivity responses in TMEV-induced demyelinating disease: Correlation with clinical signs. J Immunol 136:920, 1986.

62. Clatch RJ, Melvold RW, Dal Canto MC, Miller SD, and Lipton HL: The Theiler's murine encephalomyelitis virus (TMEV) model for multiple sclerosis shows a strong influence of the murine equivalents of HLA-A, B, and C. J Neuroimmunol 15:121, 1987.

63. Clatch RJ, Melvold RW, Miller SD, and Lipton HL: Theiler's murine encephalomyelitis virus (TMEV)-induced demyelinating disease in mice is influenced by the H-2 D region: Correlation with TMEV-specific delayed type hypersensitivity. J Immunol 135:1408, 1985.

64. Clatch RJ, Miller SD, Metzner R, Dal Canto MC, and Lipton HL: Monocytes/macrophages isolated from the mouse central nervous system contain infectious Theiler's murine encephalomyelitis virus (TMEV). Virology 176:244, 1990.

65. Collins AR, Knobler RL, Powell H, and Buchmeier MJ: Monoclonal antibodies to murine hepatitis virus-4 (Strain JHM) define the viral glycoprotein responsible for attachment and cell-cell fusion. Virology 119:358, 1982.

66. Crowlry J, Lowenthal A, Karcher D, et al: Defective measles virus in human subacute sclerosing panencephalitis brain. Virology 202:631–641, 1994.

67. Cruickshank EK: A neuropathic syndrome of uncertain origin: A review of 100 cases. West Indian Med J 5:147–158, 1956.

68. Dal Canto MC: Uncoupled relationship between demyelination and primary infection of myelinating cells in Theiler's virus encephalomyelitis. Infect Immun 35:1133, 1982.

69. Dal Canto MC: Experimental models of virus-induced demyelination. In Cook SD (ed): Handbook of Multiple Sclerosis. Marcel Dekker, New York, 1990, p 63.

70. Dal Canto MC, and Barbano RL: Immunocytochemical localization of MAG, MBP, and PO protein in acute and relapsing demyelinating lesions of Theiler's virus infection. J Neuroimmunol 10:129, 1985.

71. Dal Canto MC, and Lipton HL: Multiple sclerosis. Animal model: Theiler's virus infection in mice. Am J Pathol 88:497–500, 1977.

72. Dal Canto MC, and Lipton HL: Primary demyelination in Theiler's virus infection: An ultrastructural study. Lab Invest 33:626, 1975.

73. Dal Canto MC, and Lipton HL: Schwann cell remyelination and recurrent demyelination in the central nervous system of mice infected with attenuated Theiler's virus. Am J Pathol 98:101, 1980.

74. Dal Canto MC, and Lipton HL: Ultrastructural immunohistochemical localization of virus in acute and chronic demyelinating Theiler's virus infection. Am J Pathol 106:20, 1982.

75. Dal Canto MC, and Rabinowitz SG: Experimental models of virus-induced demyelination of the central nervous system. Ann Neurol 11:109, 1982.

76. Dalziel RG, Lampert PW, Talbot PJ, and Buchmeier MJ: Site-specific alteration of murine hepatitis virus type 4 peplomer glycoprotein E2 results in reduced neurovirulence. J Virol 59:463, 1986.

77. Daniels JB, Pappenheimer AM, and Richardson S: Observations on encephalomyelitis of mice (DA strain). J Exp Med 96:517, 1952.

78. Davis M, Kenney S, Kamine J, Pagano JS, and Huang E: Immediate early gene region of human cytomegalovirus trans-activates the promotor of human immunodeficiency virus. Proc Natl Acad Sci U.S.A. 84:8642–8646, 1987.

79. Dawson J: Cellular inclusions in cerebral lesions of epidemic encephalitis. Archives of Neurology and Psychiatry 31:685, 1934.

80. Dawson M: Pathogenesis of maedi-visna. Vet Rec 120:451, 1987.

81. Dawson VL, Dawson TM, Uhl GR, and Snyder SH: Human immunodeficiency virus type 1 coat protein neurotoxicity mediated by nitric oxide in primary cortical cultures. Proc Natl Acad Sci USA 90:3256–3259, 1994.

82. Deacon NJ, Tsykin A, Solomon A, et al: Genomic structure of an attenuated quasi species of HIV-1 from a blood transfusion and recipients. Science 270:988–991, 1995.

83. Dekaban G, and Rice G: Retroviruses in multiple sclerosis. II. Failure of gene amplification techniques to detect viral sequences unique to the disease. Neurology 40:1254–1258, 1990.

84. Dekaban GA, Oger JJF, Foti D, et al: HTLV-1 infection associated with disease in aboriginal Indians from British Columbia: A serological and PCR analysis. Clinical and Diagnostic Virology 2:67–68, 1994.

85. Dhib-Jalbut S, Jacobson S, McFarlin DE, and McFarland HF: Impaired human leukocyte antigen-restricted measles virus specific cytotoxic T-cell response in subacute sclerosing panencephalitis. Ann Neurol 25:272–280, 1989.

86. Duclos H, Elfassi E, Michelson S, et al: Cutomegalovirus infection and trans-activation of HIV-1 and HIV-2 LTRs in human astrocytoma cells (published erratum appears in AIDS Res Hum Retroviruses, Oct;5(5):555, 1989). AIDS Res Hum Retroviruses 5:217–224, 1989.

87. Dyken PR, Cunningham SC, and Ward LC: Changing character of subacute sclerosing panencephalitis in the United States. Pediatr Neurol 5:339–341, 1989.

88. Eralinna JP, Soila-Hanninen M, Roytla M, et al: Facilitation of experimental allergic encephalomyelitis by irradiation and virus infection: Role of inflammatory cells. J Neuroimmunol 55:81, 1994.

89. Fazakerley JK, Amor S, and Webb HE: Reconstitution of Simliki Forest virus infected mice induces immune mediated pathological changes in the CNS. Clin Exp Immunol 52:115, 1983.

90. Fazakerley JK, and Webb HE: Semliki Forest virus-induced, immune-mediated demyelination: Adoptive transfer studies and viral persistence in nude mice. J Gen Virol 68:377, 1987.

91. Fazakerley JK, and Webb HE: Semliki Forest virus- induced, immune mediated demyelination: the effect of radiation. British Journal of Experimental Pathology 68:101, 1987.

92. Field EJ: Transmission experiments with multiple sclerosis. An interim report. BMJ 2:564–565, 1966.

93. Field EJ, Cowshall S, Narang HK, and Bell TM: Viruses in multiple sclerosis? The Lancet 2:280–281, 1972.

94. Fiette L, Aubert C, Brahic M, and Rossi CP: Theiler's virus infection of beta-2 microglobulin deficient mice. J Virol 67:589, 1993.

95. Fishman PS, Gass JS, Swoveland PT, Lavi E, Highkin MK, and Weiss SR: Infection of the basal ganglia by a murine coronavirus. Science 229:877, 1985.

96. Fleming JO, Shubin RA, Sussman MA, Casteel N, and Stohlman SA: Monoclonal antibodies to the matrix (E1) glycoprotein of mouse hepatitis virus protect mice from encephalitis. Virology 168: 162, 1989.

97. Fleming JO, Trousdale MD, El-Zaatari FA, Stohlman SA, Weiner LP: Pathogenicity of antigenic variants of murine coronavirus JHM selected with monoclonal antibodies. J Virol 58: 869, 1986.

98. Fleming JO, Wand F-I, Trousdale MD, Hinton DR, and Stohlman SA: Interaction of immune and central nervous systems: Contribution of anti-viral Thy 1+ cells to demyelination induced by coronavirus JHM. Reg Immunol 5:37, 1993.

99. Flory E, Pfleiderer M, Stuhler A, and Wege H: Induction of protective immunity against coronavirus induced encephalomyelitis: Evidence for an important role of CD8+ T cells in vivo. Eur J Immunol 23:1757, 1993.

100. Fu JL, Stein S, Rosenstein L, et al: Neurovirulence determinants of genetically engineered Theiler's viruses. Proc Natl Acad Sci USA 87:4125, 1990.

101. Fujinami RS: Molecular mimicry: virus modulation of the immune response. In McKendall RR, and Stroop WG (eds): Handbook of Neurovirology. Marcel Dekker, New York, 1994, p 103.

102. Fujinami RS, and Oldstone MBA: Amino acid homology and immune responses between the encephalitogenic site of myelin basic protein and virus: A mechanism for autoimmunity. Science 230:1043–1045, 1985.

103. Fujinami RS, and Oldstone MBA: Amino acid homology between the encephalitogenic site of myelin basic protein and virus: Mechanism for autoimmunity. Science 230:1043, 1985.

104. Fujinami RS, and Oldstone MBA: Antiviral antibody reacting on the plasma membrane alters measles virus expression inside the cell. Nature 279:529–530, 1979.

105. Fujinami RS, Rosenthal A, Lampert PW, Zurbriggen A, and Yamada M: Survival of athymic (nu/nu) mice after Theiler's murine encephalomyelitis virus infection by passive administration of neutralizing monoclonal antibody. J Virol 63:2081, 1989.

106. Funke I, Hahn A, Rieber EP, Weiss E, and Reithmuller G: The cellular receptor (CD4) of the human immunodeficiency virus is expressed on neurons and glial cells in human brain. J Exp Med 165:1230–1235, 1987.

107. Gates MC, Sheahan BJ, and Atkins GJ: The pathogenicity of the M9 mutant Semliki Forest virus in immune-compromised mice. J Gen Virol 65: 73, 1984.

108. Gates MC, Sheahan BJ, O'Sullivan MA, and Atkins GJ: The pathogenicity of the A7, M9, and L10 strains of Semliki Forest virus for weanling mice and primary mouse brain cell cultures. J Gen Virol 66:2365, 1985.

109. Georgsson G, Houwers DJ, Palsson PA, and Petursson G: Expression of viral antigens in the CNS of visna-infected sheep: An immunohistochemical study on experimental visna induced by virus strains of increased neurovirulence. Acta Neuropathol 77:299, 1989.

110. Georgsson G, Palsson PA, and Petursson G: Pathogenesis of visna. In Serlup-Crescenzi E (ed): A Multidisciplinary Approach to Myelin Diseases. Plenum, New York, 1987, p 303.

111. Gerety SJ, Clatch RJ, Lipton HL, Goswami RG, Rundell MK, and Miller SD: Class II-restricted T cell responses in Theiler's murine encephomyelitis virus induced demyelinating disease. IV. Identification of an immunodominant T cell determinant on the N-terminal end of the VP2 capsid protein in susceptible SJL/J mice. J Immunol 146:2401–2408, 1991.

112. Gerety SJ, Karpus WJ, Cubbon AR, et al: Class II restricted T cell responses in Theiler's murine encephalomyelitis virus-induced demyelinating disease V. Mapping of a dominant immunopathologic VP2 T cell epitope in susceptible SJL/J mice. J Immunol 152:908, 1994.

113. Gerety SJ, Rundell MK, Dal Canto MC, and Miller SD: Class II-restricted T cell responses in Theiler's murine encephalomyelitis virus induced demyelinating disease. VI. Potentiation of demyelination and characterization of an immunopathologic CD4+ T cell line specific for an immunodominant VP2 epitope. J Immunol 152:919, 1994.

113a. Gessain A, Barin F, Vernant JC, et al: Antibodies to human T-lymphotropic virus type-I in patients with tropical spastic paraparesis. The Lancet 2:407–410, 1985.

114. Gilden DH, Welsh M, Rorke LB, and Wroblewska Z: Canine distemper virus infection of weanling mice: Pathogenesis of CNS disease. J Neurol Sci 52:327, 1981.

115. Giulian D, Wendt E, Vaca KK, and Noonan CA: The envelope glycoprotein of human immunodeficiency virus type 1 stimulates release of neurotoxins from monocytes. Proc Natl Acad Sci USA 90:2769–2772, 1994.

116. Glasgow GM, Killem HM, Liljestrom P, Sheahen BJ, and Atkins GJ: A single amino acid change in the E2 spike protein of a virulent strain of Semliki Forest virus attenuates pathogenicity. J Gen Virol 75:663, 1994.

117. Glaus T, Griot C, Richard A, Althaus U, Herschkowitz U, and Vanderelde M: Ultra structural

and biochemical findings in brain cell cultures infected with canine distemper virus. Acta Neuropathol 80:59, 1990.

118. Goswami KKA, Randall RE, Lange LS, and Russell WC: Antibodies against the paramyxovirus SV5 in the cerebrospinal fluids of some multiple sclerosis patients. Nature 327:244–247, 1987.

119. Goudreau G, Karpati G, and Carpenter S: Inflammatory myopathy in association with chronic myelopathy in HTLV-1 seropositive patients. Neurology 38(suppl):206, 1988.

120. Gout O, Baulac, Gessin A, et al: Rapid development of myelopathy after HTLV-1 infection acquired by transfusion during cardiac transplantation. N Engl J Med 322:383–388, 1990.

121. Grant RA, Filman DJ, Fujinami RS, Icenogle JP, and Hogle JM: Three-dimensional structure of Theiler virus. Proc Natl Acad Sci USA 89:2061, 1992.

122. Grenlee JE: Progressive multifocal leukoencephalopathy. Curr Clin Top Infect Dis 10: 140–156, 1989.

123. Griffin DE, Ward BJ, Jaurequi E, et al: Immune activation in measles. N Engl J Med 320: 1667–1672, 1989.

124. Griot C, Burge T, Vandeveide M, and Peterhons E: Antibody induced generation of reactive oxygen redicals by brain macrophages in canine distemper encephalitis: a mechanism for bystander demyelination. Acta Neuropathol (Berl) 78:396, 1989.

125. Gudnadóttir M, Helgadóttir H, and Bjarnason O: Virus isolated from the brain of a patient with multiple sclerosis. Exp Neurol 9:85–95, 1964.

126. Gudnadottir M, and Palsson PA: Short virus interaction in visna infected sheep. J Immunol 95: 1116, 1966.

127. Haase AT: Pathogenesis of lentivirus infections. Nature 322:130, 1986.

128. Haase AT: The pathogenesis of slow virus infections: Molecular analysis. J Infect Dis 153:441, 1986.

129. Haase AT, Stowring L, Narayan O, Griffin D, and Price D: Slow persistent infection caused by visna virus: Role of host restriction. Science 195:175, 1977.

130. Harouse JM, Bhat S, Spitalnick SL, et al: Inhibition of entry of HIV-1 in neural cell lines by antibodies against galactosyl ceramide. Science 253:320–322, 1991.

131. Haspel MV, Lampert PW, and Oldstone MBA: Temperature-sensitive mutants of mouse hepatitis virus produce a high incidence of demyelination. Proc Natl Acad Sci USA 75:4033, 1978.

132. Hayman M, Arbuthnott G, Harkiss G, et al: Neurotoxicity of peptide analogues of the transactivating protein tat from maedi-visna virus and human immunodeficiency virus. Neuroscience 53:1, 1993.

133. Hemachudha T, Griffin DE, Giffels JJ, Johnson RT, Moser AB, and Phanuphak P: Myelin basic protein as an encephalitogen in encephalomyelitis and polyneuritis following rabies vaccination. N Eng J Med 316:369–374, 1987.

134. Herndon RM, Griffin DE, McCormic U, and Weiner LP: Mouse hepatitis virus-induced recurrent demyelination. Arch Neurol 32:32, 1975.

135. Hess JL, Small JA, and Clements JE: Sequences in the visna virus long terminal repeat that control transcriptional activity and respond to viral trans-activation: Involvement of AP-1 sites in basal activity and trans-activation. J Virol 63: 3001, 1989.

136. Higgins RJ, Krakowka SG, Metzler A, and Koestner A: Primary demyelination in experimental canine distemper virus induced encephalomyelitis in gnotobiotic dogs: Sequential immunologic and morphologic findings. Acta Neuropathol (Berl) 58:1, 1982.

137. Hirayama N, Senda M, Nakashima N, et al: Protective effects of monoclonal antibodies against lethal canine distemper virus infection in mice. J Gen Virol 72:2827, 1991.

138. Hjelle B, Appenzeller O, Mills R, et al: Chronic neurodegenerative disease associated with HTLV II. The Lancet 339:645–646, 1992.

139. Itoyama Y, Sekizawa T, Openshaw H, Kogur K, and Goto I: Early loss of astrocytes in herpes simplex virus induced central nervous system demyelination. Ann Neurol 29:285, 1991.

140. Jacobson S, Raine CS, Mingioli ES, and McFarlin DE. Isolation of an HTLV-1 like retrovirus from patients with tropical spastic paraparesis. Nature 331:540, 1988.

141. Jarousse N, Grant RA, Hogle JM, et al: A single amino acid change determines persistence of a chimeric Theiler's virus. J Virol 68:3364, 1994.

142. Jenkins MG, Tansey EM, Macefield F, and Ikeda H: Evidence for a T-cell related factor as the cause of demyelination in mice following Semliki Forest virus infection. Brain Res 459:145, 1988.

143. Johnson RT: Viral Infections of the Nervous System. Raven Press, New York, p 237, 1982.

144. Johnson RT: The virology of demyelinating diseases. Ann Neurol 36 (suppl):S54, 1994.

145. Jordan JR: Measles immunization: Remaining needs for research. Rev Inf Dis 5:612–618, 1983.

146. Kaluza G, Lell G, Reinacher M, Stitz L, and Willems WR: Neurogenic spread of Semliki Forest virus in mice. Arch Virol 93:97, 1987.

147. Kastrukoff LF, Hamada T, Schumacher U, Long C, Doherty PC, and Koprowski H: Central nervous system infection and immune response in mice inoculated into the lip with Herpes simplex virus type 1. J Neuroimmunol 2:295, 1982.

148. Kastrukoff LF, Lau A, Osborne D, and Kim SU: Herpes simplex virus type 1 (HSV I): A murine model of virus induced central nervous system demyelination. In Kim SU (ed): Myelination and Demyelination: Implications for MS. Plenum, New York, p 153, 1989.

149. Kastrukoff LF, Lau AS, and Kim SU: Multifocal CNS demyelination following peripheral inoculation with Herpes simplex virus type I. Ann Neurol 22:52, 1987.

150. Kastrukoff LF, Lau AS, Leung GY, and Thomas EE: Contrasting effects of immunosuppression on herpes simplex virus type I (HSV I) induced central nervous system (CNS) demyelination in mice. J Neurol Sci 117:148, 1993.

151. Kastrukoff LF, Lau AS, Leung GY, Walker D, and Thomas EE: Herpes simplex virus type I

(HSV I)-induced multifocal central nervous system (CNS) demyelination in mice. J Neuropathol Exp Neurol 51:432, 1992.

152. Kastrukoff LF, Lau AS, and Puterman ML: Genetics of natural resistance of Herpes simplex virus type I latent infection of the peripheral nervous system in mice. J Gen Virol 67:613, 1986.

153. Kastrukoff LF, Long C, and Koprowski H: Herpes simplex virus immune system interaction in a murine model. In Nahmias AJ, Dowdle WR, and Schinazi RF (eds): The Human Herpesviruses: An Inter-disciplinary Perspective. Elsevier Biomedical, New York, p 320, 1981.

154. Keating JA, Griffiths PD, and Weis RA: HIV susceptibility conferred to human fibroblasts by cytomegalovirus-induced receptor. Nature 343:659–661, 1990.

155. Kennedy PG: Neurological aspects of lentiviral infections in animals. Baillieres Clinical Neurology, Vol 1. p 41–59, 1992.

156. Khalili-Shirazi A, Gregson N, and Webb HE: Immunocytochemical evidence for Semliki Forest virus antigen persistence in mouse brain. J Neurol Sci 85:17, 1988.

157. Knobler RL, Haspel MV, and Oldstone MBA: Mouse hepatitis virus type 4 (JHM) strain-induced fatal central nervous system disease. I. Genetic control and the murine neuron as the susceptible site of disease. J Exp Med 153:832, 1981.

158. Knobler RL, Lampert PW, and Oldstone MBA: Virus persistence and recurring demyelination produced by a temperature-sensitive mutant of MHV-4. Nature 298:279, 1982.

159. Koga M, Wege H, and ter Meulen V: Sequence of murine coronavirus JHM induced neuropathological changes in rats. Neuropath Appl Neurobiol 10:173, 1984.

160. Kolodovsky V, Koldovsky P, Henle G, Henle W, Ackermann R, and Haase G: Multiple sclerosis-associated agent: Transmission to animals and some properties of the agent. Infect Immun 12:1355–1366, 1975.

161. Koprowski H, DeFreitas EC, Harper ME, et al: Multiple sclerosis and human T-cell lymphotropic retroviruses. Nature 318:154–160, 1985.

162. Koyanagi Y, Miles S, Mitsuyasu RT, Merrill JE, and Vinters HV: Dual infection of the central nervous system by AIDS viruses with distinct cellular tropisms. Science 236:819–822, 1987.

163. Krakowka S, Axthelm MK, Johnson GC: Canine distemper virus. In Olsen RG, Krakowka S, and Blakeslee JB (eds): Comparative Pathobiology of Viral Diseases, Vol 2. CRC Press, Boca Raton, p 137, 1985.

164. Kristensson K, Svennerholm B, Persson L, Vahlne A, and Lycke E: Latent Herpes simplex virus trigeminal ganglionic infection in mice and demyelination in the central nervous system. J Neurol Sci 43:253, 1979.

165. Kristensson K, Svennerholm B, Vahlne A, Nilheden E, Persson L, and Lycke E: Virus-induced demyelination in Herpes simplex virus-infected mice. J Neurol Sci 53:205, 1982.

166. Kuroda Y, Matsui M, Yukitake M, et al: Assessment of MRI criteria for MS in Japanese MS and HAM/TSP. Neurology 45:30–33, 1995.

167. Kurtzke JF: Epidemiological contributions to multiple sclerosis: An overview. Neurology 30:61–80, 1980.

168. Kurtzke JF: Epidemiologic evidence for multiple sclerosis as an infection. Clin Microbiol Rev 6:382, 1993.

169. La Monica N, Banner LR, Morris VL, and Lai MMC: Localization of extensive deletions in the structural genes of two neurotropic variants of murine coronavirus JHM. Virology 182:883, 1991.

170. Lai MMC, and Stohlman SA: Molecular basis of neuropathogenicity of mouse hepatitis virus. In Roos EP (ed): Molecular Neurovirology: Pathogenesis of Viral CNS Infections. Humana Press, Totowa, NJ, p 319, 1992.

171. Lampert PW, Sims JK, and Kniazeff AJ: Mechanism of demyelination in JHM virus encephalomyelitis. Acta Neuropath (Berl) 24:76, 1973.

172. Lang W, Wiley C, and Lampert P: Theiler's virus encephalomyelitis is unaffected by treatment with myelin components. J Neuroimmunol 9:109, 1985.

173. Lavi E, Suzumura A, Hirayama M, et al: Coronavirus mouse hepatitis virus (MHV)-A59 causes a persistent, productive infection in primary glial cell cultures. Microb Pathol 3:379, 1987.

174. Lee H-J, Shieh C-K, Gorbalenya AE, et al: The complete sequence (22 kilobases) of murine coronavirus gene 1 encoding the putative proteases and RNA polymerase. Virology 180:567, 1991.

175. Lehky TJ, Fox CH, Koenig S, et al: Detection of human T-lymphotropic virus Type I (HTLV-I) tax RNA in the central nervous system of HTLV-I-associated myelopathy/tropical spastic paraparesis patients by in situ hybridization. Ann Neurol 37:167–175, 1995.

176. Lindsley MD, Thiemann R, and Rodriguez M: Cytotoxic T cells isolated from the central nervous system of mice infected with Theiler's virus. J Virol 65:6612, 1991.

177. Lipton HL: Theiler's virus infection in mice: An unusual biphasic disease process leading to demyelination. Infect Immun 11:1147, 1975.

178. Lipton HL: Persistent Theiler's murine encephalomyelitis virus infection in mice depends on plaque size. J Gen Virol 46:169, 1980.

179. Lipton HL: Theiler's murine encephalomyelitis virus: Animal models. In McKendall RR, and Stroop WG (eds): Handbook of Neurovirology. Marcel Dekker, New York, p 521, 1994.

180. Lipton HL, and Melvold R: Genetic analysis of susceptibility to Theiler's virus-induced demyelinating disease in mice. J Immunol 132:1821, 1984.

181. Lipton HL, and Dal Canto MC: Chronic neurologic disease in Theiler's virus infection of SJL/J mice. J Neurol Sci 30:201, 1976.

182. Lipton HL, and Dal Canto MC: Theiler's virus induced demyelination: prevention by immunosuppression. Science 192:62, 1976.

183. Lipton HL, and Dal Canto MC: The TO strain of Theiler's viruses cause "slow virus like" infection in mice. Ann Neurol 6:25, 1979.

184. Lipton HL, and Gonzalez-Scarano F: Central nervous system immunity in mice infected with

Theiler's virus. I. Local neutralizing antibody response. J Infect Dis 137:145, 1978.

185. Lipton HL, Kratochvil J, Sehti P, and Dal Canto MC: Theiler's virus antigen detected in mouse spinal cord two and one-half years after infection. Neurology 34:1117, 1984.

186. Lipton HL, Twaddle G, and Jelachich ML: The predominent virus antigenic burden is present in macrophages in Theiler's murine encephalomyelitis virus induced demyelinating disease. J Virol 69:2525, 1995.

187. Lopez C: Genetics of natural resistance to herpesvirus infections in mice. Nature 258:152, 1975.

188. Lopez C: Resistance to HSV I in the mouse is governed by two major, independently segregating, non H-2 loci. Immunogenetics 11:87, 1980.

189. Luo M, He C, Toth KS, Zhang CX, and Lipton HL: Three-dimensional structure of Theiler's murine encephalomyelitis virus (BeAn strain). Proc Natl Acad Sci USA 89:2409, 1992.

190. Lutley R, Petursson G, Georgsson G, Palsson PA, and Nathanson N: Strains of visna virus with increased neurovirulence. In Sharp JM, and Hoff-Jorgensen R (eds): Slow viruses in sheep, goats, and cattle. Commission of the European Communities, Luxembourg, p 45, 1985.

191. Lutley R, Petursson G, Palsson PA, Georgsson G, Klein J, and Nathanson N: Antigenic drift in visna: Virus variation during long term infection of Icelandic sheep. J Gen Virol 71:1433, 1983.

192. Mangolis MS, Soloviev VD, and Schubladze AK: Aetiology and pathogenesis of acute sporadic encephalomyelitis and multiple sclerosis. J. Neurol Neurosurg Psychiatry 9:63–64, 1946.

193. Martin JR, Holt RK, and Webster HD: Herpes simplex related antigen in human demyelinating disease and encephalitis. Acta Neuropathol (Berl) Vol 76(4)325–337, 1988.

194. Martin JR, and Nathanson N: Animal models of virus-induced demyelination. Prog Neuropathol 4:27, 1979.

195. Massa PT, Wege H, and ter Meulen V: Analysis of murine hepatitis virus (JHM) strain tropism toward Lewis rat glial cells in vitro. Lab Invest 55:318, 1986.

196. Matsubara Y, Watanabe R, and Taguschi F: Neurovirulence of six murine coronavirus JHMV variants for rats. Virus Res 20:45, 1991.

197. McAllister A, Tangy F, Aubert C, and Brahic M: Genetic mapping of the ability of Theiler's virus to persist and demyelinate. J Virol 64:4252, 1990.

198. McConnell I, and Watt NJ: Maedi Visna Virus. In McKendall RR, and Stroop WG (eds): Handbook of Neurovirology. Marcel Dekker, New York, p 773, 1994.

199. McCullough B, Krakowka S, and Koestner A: Experimental canine distemper virus-induced demyelination. Lab Invest 31:216, 1974.

200. McKendall RR: Herpes simplex virus diseases. In McKendall RR, and Stroop WG (eds): Handbook of Neurovirology. Marcel Dekker, New York, p 253, 1994.

201. Melvold RW, Jokinen DM, Knobler R, and Lipton HL: Variations in genetic control of susceptibility to Theiler's murine encephalomyelitis virus (TMEV) induced demyelinating disease. I.

Differences between susceptible SJL/J and resistant Balb/c strains map near the T cell B-chain constant genes on chromosome 6. J Immunol 138:1429, 1987.

202. Melvold RW, Jokinen DM, Miller SD, Dal Canto MC, and Lipton HL: H-2 genes in TMEV-induced demyelination, a model for multiple sclerosis. In David CS (ed): Antigens. Plenum, New York, p 735, 1987.

203. Melvold RW, Jokinen DM, Miller SD, Dal Canto MC, and Lipton HL: Identification of a locus on mouse chromosome 3 involved in differential susceptibility to Theiler's murine encephalomyelitis virus-induced demyelinating disease. J Virol 64:686, 1990.

204. Miller SD, Clatch RJ, Pevear DC, Trotter JL, and Lipton HL: Class II restricted T cell responses in Theiler's murine encephalomyelitis virus (TMEV)-induced demyelinating disease. I. Cross-specificity among TMEV substrains and related picornaviruses, but not myelin proteins. J Immunol 138:3776, 1987.

205. Miller SD, and Gerety SJ: Immunologic aspects of Theiler's murine encephalomyelitis virus (TMEV)-induced demyelinating disease. Seminars in Virology 1:263, 1990.

206. Miller SD, Gerety SJ, Kennedy MK, et al: Class II-restricted T cell responses in Theiler's murine encephalomyelitis virus (TMEV)-induced demyelinating disease III. Failure of neuroantigen-specific immune tolerance to affect the clinical course of demyelination. J Neuroimmunol 26:9, 1990.

207. Mitchell WJ, Summers BA, and Appel MJA: Viral expression in experimental canine distemper demyelinating encephalitis. J Comp Pathol 104:77, 1991.

208. Mokhtarian F, Shi Y, Zhu PF, and Grib D: Immune responses and autoimmune outcome during virus infection of the central nervous system. Cell Immunol 157:195–210, 1994.

209. Mokhtarian F, and Swoveland P: Predisposition to EAE induction in resistant mice by prior infection with Semliki Forest virus. J Immunol 138: 3264, 1987.

210. Morris VL, Tieszer C, MacKinnon J, and Percy D: Characterization of coronavirus JHM variants isolated from Wistar Furth rats with a viral-induced demyelinating disease. Virology 169: 127, 1989.

211. Murray RS, Brown B, Brian D, and Cabirac GF: Detection of coronavirus RNA and antigen in multiple sclerosis brain. Ann Neurol 31:525, 1992.

212. Murray RS, Cai G-Y, Hoel K, Zhang J-Y, Soike KF, and Cabirac GF: Coronavirus infects and causes demyelination in primate central nervous system. Virology 188:274, 1992.

213. Mutinelli F, Vandevelde M, Griot C, and Richard A: Astrocytic infection in canine distemper virus induced demyelination. Acta Neuropathol 77: 333, 1988.

214. Nagashima K, Wege H, Meyermann R, and ter Meulen V: Corona virus induced subacute demyelinating encephalomyelitis in rats: A morphologic analysis. Acta Neuropathol 44:63, 1978.

215. Nakamura T, Matsuo H, Shirabe S, et al: Familial clusters of human T-cell lymphotropic virus type 1-associated myelopathy. Arch Neurol 46:250–251, 1989.

216. Narayan O, and Clements JE: Lentiviruses. In Fields BN, Knipe DM, Chanock RM, et al (eds): Fields Virology, Vol 2. Raven Press, New York, p 1571, 1990.

217. Narayan O, Clements J, Kennedy-Stoskopf S, Sheffer D, and Royal W: Mechanisms of escape of visna lentivirus from immunological control. Contrib Microbiol Immunol 8:60, 1987.

218. Narayan O, and Cork LC: Lentiviral diseases of sheep and goats: Chronic pneumonia, leukoencephalomyelitis and arthritis. Review Infectious Diseases 7:89, 1985.

219. Narayan O, Griffin DE, and Chase J: Antigenic shift of visna virus in persistently infected sheep. Science 197:376, 1977

220. Narayan O, Wolinshy HS, Clements JE, Strandberg JD, Griffin DE, and Cork LC: Slow virus replication: The role of macrophages in the persistence and expression of visna viruses of sheep and goats. J Gen Virol 59:345, 1982.

221. Nathanson N, Georgsson G, Palsson PA, Najjar JA, Lustley R, and Petursson G: Experimental visna in Icelandic sheep: The prototype Lentiviral infection. Review Infectious Diseases 7:75, 1985.

222. Nathanson N, Martin JR, Georgsson G, Palsson PA, Lutley RE, and Petursson G: The effect of post infection immunization on the severity of experimental visna. J Comp Pathol 91:185, 1981.

223. Nathanson N, Panitch H, Palsson PA, Petursson, G, and Georgsson G: Pathogenesis of visna. II. Effect of immunosuppression upon early central nervous system lesions. Lab Invest 35:444, 1976.

224. Nelson JA, Reynolds Kohler C, Oldstone MB, and Wiley CA: HIV and HCMV coinfect brain cells in patients with AIDS. Virology 165:286–290, 1988.

225. Nicholson SM, Peterson JD, Miller SD, Wang K, Dal Canto MC, and Melvold RW: Balb/c substrain differences in susceptibility to Theiler's murine encephalomyelitis virus-induced demyelinating disease. J Neuroimmunol 52:19, 1994.

226. Nicoll JA, Kinrade E, and Love S: PCR mediated search for Herpes Simplex virus DNA in sections of brain from patients with multiple sclerosis and other neurological disorders. J Neurol Sci 113:144, 1992.

227. Norrby E: Viral antibodies in multiple sclerosis. Prog Med Virol. 24:1–39, 1978.

228. O'Brien WA, Koyanagi Y, Namazie A, et al: HIV-1 tropism for mononuclear phagocytes can be determined by regions of gp120 outside the CD4-binding domain. Nature 348:69–73, 1990.

229. Oldstone MBA, and Notkins AL. Molecular mimicry. In Notkins AL, and Oldstone MBA (eds): Concepts in Viral Pathogenesis II. Springer-Verlag, New York, p 185, 1986.

230. Orenstein JM, and Janotta F: HIV and papovavirus infections in acquired immunodeficiency syndrome: An ultrastructural study. Hum Pathol 19:350–361, 1988.

231. Osame M, Matsamuto M, Usuka K, et al: Chronic progressive myelopathy associated with elevated antibodies to HTLV-1 and adult T-cell leukemia-like cells. Ann Neurol 21:117–122, 1987.

232. Ozden S, Aubert C, Gonzalez-Dunia D, and Brahic M: In-situ analysis of proteolipid protein gene transcripts during persistent Theiler's virus infection. J Histochem Cyotchem 39:1305, 1991.

233. Ozden S, Tangy F, Chamorro M, and Brahic M: Theiler's virus genome is closely related to that of encephalomyocarditis virus the prototype cardiovirus. J Virol 60:1163, 1986.

234. Pang S, Koyanagi Y, Miles S, Wiley C, Vinters HV, and Chen ISY: High levels of unintegrated HIV-1 DNA in brain tissues of AIDS dementia patients. Nature 343:85–89, 1990.

235. Panitch H, Petursson G, Georgsson G, Palsson PA, and Nathanson N: Pathogenesis of visna. III. Immune responses to central nervous system antigens in experimental allergic encephalomyelitis and visna. Lab Invest 35:452, 1976.

236. Parham D, Tereba A, Talbot PJ, Jackson DP, and Morris VL: Analysis of JHM central nervous system infections in rats. Arch Neurol 43:702, 1986.

237. Parsons LM, and Webb HE: Identification of immunoglobulin-containing cells in the central nervous system of the mouse following infection with the demyelinating strain of Semliki Forest virus. Br J Exp Pathol 70:247, 1989.

238. Parsons LM, and Webb HE: IgG subclass response in brain and serum in Semliki forest virus demyelinating encephalitis. Neuropathol Appl Neurobiol 18:351, 1992.

239. Pasick J, and Dales S: Coronavirus diseases. In McKendall RR, and Stroop WG (eds): Handbook of Neurovirology. Marcel Dekker, New York, p 649, 1994.

240. Pasick JMM, and Dales S: Infection by coronavirus JHM or rat neurons and oligodendrocyte type-2 astrocyte lineage cells during distinct developmental stages. J Virol 65:5013, 1991.

241. Pasternak JF, DeVivo DC, and Prensky AL: Steroid responsive encephalomyelitis in childhood. Neurology 30:481–486, 1980.

242. Paya CV, Patick AK, Leibson PJ, and Rodriguez M: Role of natural killer cells as immune effectors in encephalitis and demyelination induced by Theiler's virus. J Immunol 143:95, 1989.

243. Penney JB, and Wolinsky JS: Neuronal and oligodendroglial infection by the WW strain of Theiler's virus. Lab Invest 40:324, 1979.

244. Perlman S, and Ries D: The astrocyte is a target cell in mice persistently infected with mouse hepatitis virus, strain JHM. Microb Pathog 3:309, 1987.

245. Perlman S, Schelper R, Bolger E, and Ries D: Late onset, symptomatic, demyelinating encephalomyelitis in mice infected with MHV-JHM in the presence of maternal antibody. Microb Pathog 3:185, 1987.

246. Pertschuk LP, Cook AW, and Gupta J: Measles antigen multiple sclerosis: Identification in the jejunum by immunofluorescence. Life Sci 19:1603–1608, 1976.

247. Peterson JD, Waltenbaugh C, and Miller SD: IgG subclass responses to Theiler's murine encephalomyelitis virus infection and immunization suggest a dominant role for Th1 cells in susceptible mouse strains. Immunology 75:652, 1992.

248. Petito CK, Navia BA, Cho ES, Jordan BD, George DC, and Price RW: Vaculolar myelopathy pathologically resembling subacute combined degeneration in patients with the acquired immunodeficiency syndrome. N Engl J Med 312:874–879, 1985.

249. Petursson G, Nathanson N, Georgsson G, Panitch H, and Palsson PA: Pathogenesis of visna. I. Sequential virologic, serologic, and pathologic studies. Lab Invest 35:402, 1976.

250. Petursson G, Nathanson N, Palsson PA, Martin J, and Georgsson G: Immunopathogenesis of visna: A slow virus disease of the central nervous system. Acta Neurol Scand 57(suppl 67):205, 1978.

251. Peudenier S, Hery C, Montagnier L, and Tardieu M: Human microglial cells: Characterization in cerebral tissue and in primary culture, and study of their suspectibility to HIV-1 infection. Ann Neurol 29:152–161, 1991.

252. Peudenier S, Hery C, Ng KH, and Tardieu M: HIV receptors within the brain: a study of CD4 and MHC-II on human neurons, astrocytes and microglial cells. Res Virol 142:145–149, 1991.

253. Pevear DC, Borkowski J, Calenoff M, Oh CK, Ostrowski B, and Lipton HL: Insights into Theiler's virus neurovirulence based on a genomic comparison of the neurovirulent GDVII and less virulent BeAn strains. Virology 165:1, 1988.

254. Pevear DC, Calenoff M, Rozhon E, and Lipton HL: Analysis of the complete nucleotide sequence of the picornavirus Theiler's murine encephalomyelitis virus indicates that it is closely related to cardioviruses. J Virol 61:1507, 1987.

255. Picard FJ, Coulthart MB, Ojer J, et al: Human T-lymphotropic virus type 1 in coastal natives of British Columbia. Phylogenetics, affinities and possible origins. J Virol 69: 7248–7256, 1995.

256. Power C, Weinshenker BG, Dekaban GA, et al: HTLV-1 associated myelopathy in Canada. Can J Neurol Sci. 16:330–335, 1989.

257. Power C, Weinshenker BG, Dekaban GA, Kaufmann JCE, and Rice GPA: Pathological and molecular biological features of a myelopathy associated with HTLV-1 infection. Can J Neurol Sci 18:352–355, 1991.

258. Price RW, Brew B, Sidtis J, et al: The brain in AIDS: Central nervous system HIV-1 infection and AIDS dementia complex. Science 239: 586–592, 1988.

259. Puccioni-Sohler M, Rieckmann P, Kitze B, et al: A soluble form of tumor necrosis factor receptor in cerebrospinal fluid and serum of human T-lymphotropic virus type 1 associated myelopathy and other neurological diseases. J Neurol 242:239–242, 1995.

260. Pullen LC, Miller SD, Dal Canto MC, and Kim BS: Class I deficient resistant mice intracerebrally inoculated with Theiler's virus show an increased T cell response to viral antigens and susceptibility to demyelination. Eur J Immunol 23:2287, 1993.

261. Raine CS: On the development of CNS lesions in natural canine distemper encephalomyelitis. J Neurol Sci 30:13, 1976.

262. Rammohan KW, McFarland HF, and McFarlin DE. Subacute sclerosing panencephalitis after passive immunization and natural measles infection: Role of antibody in persistence of measles virus. Neurology 32:390–394, 1982.

263. Rassmussen HB, Perron H, and Clausen J: Do endogenous retroviruses have etiological implications in inflammatory and degenerative nervous system diseases? Acta Neurol Scand 88:190, 1993.

264. Rauch H, Montgomery IN, Hinmann CL, Harb W, and Benjamins JA: Chronic Theiler's virus infection in mice: Appearance of myelin basic protein in cerebrospinal fluid and serum antibody directed against MBP. J Neuroimmunol 14:35, 1987.

265. Rice GPA, Schrier RD, Southern PJ, Nelson J, Casali P, and Oldstone MBA: Cytomegalovirus and measles virus: In vitro models for virus-mediated immunosuppression. Viral Mechanisms of Immunosuppression. Eds: Gilmore N, Wainberg MA; Publisher: Alan R. Liss, New York, N.Y. pp 15–28, 1985.

266. Richert JR, Robinson ED, Reuben-Burnside CA, et al: Measles virus specific human T cell clones: Studies of alloreactivity and antigenic cross reactivity. J Neuroimmunol 19:68–69, 1988.

267. Rima BK, Duffy N, Mitchell WJ, Summers BA, and Appell MJ: Correlation between humoral immune responses and presence of virus in the CNS in dogs experimentally infected canine distemper virus. Arch Virol 121:1, 1991.

268. Robertson WB, and Cruickshank EK: Jamaican (tropical) myeloneuropathy. In Minkler J (ed) Pathology of the Nervous System, Vol 3, ed 3. McGraw, New York, pp 2466–2476, 1972.

269. Rodriguez M, and David CS: Demyelination induced by Theiler's virus: Influence of the H-2 haplotype. J Immunol 135:2145, 1985.

270. Rodriguez M, Dunkel AJ, Thiemann RL, Leibowitz J, Ziglstra M, and Jaenisch R: Abrogation of resistance to Theiler's virus induced demyelination in H-2b mice deficient in beta-2 microglobulin. J Immunol 151:266, 1993.

271. Rodriguez M, Leibowitz J, and David CS: Susceptibility to Theiler's virus induced demyelination. J Exp Med 163:620, 1986.

272. Rodriguez M, Leibowitz JL, Lampert PW: Persistent infection of oligodendrocytes in Theiler's virus-induced encephalomyelitis. Ann Neurol 13:426, 1983.

273. Rodriguez M, Lucchinetti CF, Clark RJ, Yakash TL, Markowitz H, and Lennon VA: Immunoglobulins and complement in demyelination induced in mice by Theiler's virus. J Immunol 140:800, 1988.

274. Rodriguez M, Oleszak E, and Leibowitz J: Theiler's murine encephalomyelitis: A model of demyelination and persistence of virus. Crit Rev Immunol 7:325, 1987.

275. Rodriguez M, and Roos RP: Pathogenesis of early and late disease in mice infected with Theiler's virus, using intratypic recombinant GDVII/DA viruses. J Virol 66:217, 1992.

276. Roizman B, and Kaplan LJ: Herpes simplex viruses, central nervous system, and encephalitis. In Roos RB (ed): Molecular Neurovirology: Pathogenesis of Viral CNS Infections. Humana Press, Totowa, NJ, p 3, 1992.

277. Roizman B, and Lopez C: The Herpesviruses, Vols 1–4. Roizmas B (ed) Plenum, New York, 1985.

278. Roman GC: The neuroepidemiology of tropical spastic paraparesis. Ann Neurol 23 (suppl): S113-S120, 1988.

279. Roos RP: Viruses and demyelinating disease of the central nervous system. Neurol Clin 1:681, 1983

280. Roos RP, and Casteel N: Determinants of neurological disease induced by Theiler's murine encephalomyelitis virus. In Roos RP (ed): Molecular Neurovirology: Pathogenesis of Viral CNS Infections. Humana Press, Totowa, NJ, p 283, 1992.

281. Roos RP, Nalefski EA, Nitayaphan S, Variakajis R, and Singh KK: An isoelectric focusing overlay study of the humoral immune response in Theiler's virus demyelinating disease. J Neuroimmunol 13:305, 1987.

282. Roos RP, and Wollmann R: DA strain of Theiler's murine encephalomyelitis virus induces demyelination in nude mice. Ann Neurol 15:494, 1984.

283. Rorke LB, Iwasaki Y, Koprowski H, et al: Acute demyelinating disease in a chimpanzee three years after inoculation of brain cells from a patient with MS. Ann Neurol 5:89–94, 1979.

284. Rosenthal A, Fujinami RS, and Lampert PW: Mechanism of Theiler's virus-induced demyelination in nude mice. Lab Invest 54:515, 1986.

285. Rossi CP, Cash E, Aubert C, and Coutinho A: Role of the humoral immune response in resistance to Theiler's virus infection. J Virol 65:3895, 1991.

286. Rossi CP, McAllister A, Fiette L, and Brahic M: Theiler's virus infection induced a specific cytotoxic T lymphocyte response. Cell Immunol 138:341, 1991.

287. Sabatier JM, Vives E, Mabrouk K, et al: Evidence of neurotoxic activity of tat from human immunodeficiency virus type 1. J Virol 65:961–967, 1991.

288. Saida T: HTLV-1 associated myelopathy in Japan. Paper presented at the International Symposium on Retrovirus in Multiple Sclerosis and Related Disease, Copenhagen, 1988.

289. Santagati MB, Maata JA, Itaranta PV, Salmi AA, and Hinkkanen AE: The Semliki Forest virus E2 gene as a virulence determinant. J Gen Virol 76:47, 1995.

290. Sharpless NE, Obrien WE, Verdin E, Kufta CV, and Chen ISY: HIV I tropism for brain microglial cells is determined by a region of the env glycoprotein that also controls macrophage tropism. Journal of Virology 66:2588–2593, 1992.

291. Sheahan BJ, Gates MC, Caffrey JF, and Atkins GJ: Oligodendrocyte infection and demyelination produced in mice by the M9 mutant of Semliki forest virus. Acta Neuropathol (Berl) 60:257, 1983.

292. Shubin RA, Weiner LP: Viruses and demyelination. In Kim SU (ed): Myelination and demyelination: Implications for Multiple Sclerosis. Plenum, New York, p 129, 1989.

293. Sigurdsson B: Maedi: A slow progressive pneumonia of sheep—An epizoological and a pathological study. Br Vet J 110:254, 1954.

294. Sigurdsson B: Rida: A chronic encephalitis of sheep. Br Vet J 110:341, 1954.

295. Sigurdsson B, and Palsson PA: Visna of sheep: A slow, demyelinating infection. British Journal of Experimental Pathology 39:519, 1958.

296. Simmons A: H-2 linked genes influence the severity of Herpes Simplex virus infection of the peripheral nervous system. J Exp Med 169:1503, 1989.

297. Simmons A, and Tschovke DC: Anti-CD8 impairs clearance of Herpes Simplex virus from the nervous system: implications for the future of virally infected neurons. J Exp Med 175:1337, 1992.

298. Skolnik PR, Kosloff BR, and Hirsch MS: Bidirectional interactions between human immunodeficiency virus type 1 and cytomegalovirus. J Infect Dis 157:508–514, 1988.

299. Smith CS, Dickson D, and Samkoff L: Recurrent encephalopathy and seizures in a US native with HTLV-1 associated myelopathy/tropical spastic paraparesis: A clinicopathological study. Neurology 42:658–661, 1992.

300. Snijders A, Benaissa-Trouw BJ, Oosting JD, Snippe H, and Kraaijeveld CA: Identification of a DTH inducing T-cell epitope on the E2 membrane protein of Semliki Forest virus. Cell Immunol 123:23, 1989.

301. Snijders A, Benaissa-Trouw BJ, Visser-Vernooy HJ, Fernandez I, Snippe H, and Kraaijeveld CA: A delayed type hypersensitivity inducing T-cell epitope of Semliki Forest virus mediates effector T-helper activity for antibody production. Immunology 77:322, 1992.

302. Soila-Hanninan M, Evalinna JP, and Hakkanen V: Semliki Forest virus infects brain endothelial cells and causes blood-brain barrier damage. J Virol 68:6291, 1994.

303. Sonnerborg A, and Johansson B: The neurotoxin-like sequence of human immunodeficiency virus gp120: A comparison of sequence data from patients with and without neurological symptoms. Virus Genes 7:23–31, 1993.

304. Sorensen O, Dugre R, Percy D, and Dales S: In vivo and in-vitro models of demyelinating disease: Endogenous factors influencing demyelinating disease caused by mouse hepatitis virus in rats and mice. Infect Immun 37:1248, 1982.

305. Sorensen O, Percy D, and Dales S: In vivo and in-vitro models of demyelinating diseases. III. JHM virus infection of rats. Arch Neurol 37:478, 1980.

306. Sorensen O, Saravani A, and Dales S: In vivo and in vitro models of demyelinating disease. XVII. The infectious process in athymic rats inoculated with JHM virus. Microb Pathog 2:79, 1987.

307. Srinivasappa J, Saegusa J, Prabhakar BS, et al: Molecular mimicry: Frequency of reactivity of monoclonal antiviral antibodies with normal tissues. J Virol 57:397–401, 1986.

308. Stohlman S, Bergmann C, La Monica N, Lai M, Yeh J, and Kyuwa S: JHM virus specific cytotoxic T cells derived from the central nervous system. Adv Exp Med Biol 342:419, 1993.

309. Stohlman S, and Weiner LP: Chronic central nervous system demyelination in mice after JHM virus infection. Neurology 31:38, 1981.

310. Stohlman SA, Bergmann CC, van der Veen RC, and Hinton DR: Mouse hepatitis virus specific cytotoxic T lymphocytes protect from lethal infection without eliminating virus from the central nervous system. J Virol 69:684, 1995.

311. Stohlman SA, and Frelinger JA: Resistance to fatal central nervous system disease by mouse hepatitis virus, strain JHM I: Genetic analysis. Immunogenetics 6:277, 1978.

312. Stohlman SA, Kyuwa S, Cohen M, et al: Mouse hepatitis virus nucleocapsid protein specific cytotoxic T lymphocytes are L^d restricted and specific for the carboxy terminus. Virology 189:217, 1992.

313. Stohlman SA, Kyuwa S, Polo J, Brady D, Lai M, and Bergmann C: Characterization of mouse hepatitis virus specific cytotoxic T cells derived from the central nervous system of mice infected with the JHM strain. J Virol 67:7050, 1993.

314. Stohlman SA, Matsushima GKL, Casteel N, and Weiner LP: In vivo effects of coronavirus specific T cell clones: DTH inducer cells prevent a lethal infection but do not inhibit virus replication. J Immunol 136:3052, 1986.

315. Stohlman SA, Sussman MA, Matsushima GK, Shubin RA, and Erlish SS: Delayed type hypersensitivity reponse in the central nervous system during JHM virus infection requires viral specificity for protection. J Neuroimmunol 19:255, 1988.

316. Subak-Sharpe I, Dyson H, and Fazakerley J: In-vivo depletion of CD8+ T cells prevents lesions of demyelination in Semliki Forest virus infection. J Virol 67:7629, 1993.

317. Summers BA, and Appel MJG: Demyelination in canine distemper encephalomyelitis: An ultrastructural analysis. J Neurocytol 16:871, 1987.

318. Summers BA, Greisen HA, and Appel MJG: Early events in canine distemper demyelinating encephalomyelitis. Acta Neuropathol (Berl) 46:1, 1979.

319. Summers BA, Whitaker JN, and Appel MJG: Demyelinating canine distemper encephalomyelitis: measurement of myelin basic protein in cerebrospinal fluid. J Neuroimmunol 14:227, 1987.

320. Sussman MA, Shubin RA, Kyuva S, and Stohlman SA: T-cell mediated clearance of mouse hepatitis virus strain JHM from the central nervous system. J Virol 63:3051, 1989.

321. Taguchi F, Massa PT, and ter Meulen V: Characterization of a variant virus isolated from neural cell culture after infection of mouse coronavirus JHMV. Virology 155:267, 1986.

322. Taguchi F, Siddell SG, Wege H, and ter Meulen V: Characterization of a variant virus selected in rat brains after infection by coronavirus mouse hepatitis virus JHM. J Virol 54:429, 1985.

323. Talbot PJ, Salmi AA, Knobler RL, and Buchmeier MJ: Topographical mapping of epitopes on the glycoproteins of murine hepatitis virus-4 (strain JHM): Correlation with biological activities. Virology 132:250, 1984.

324. Tanaka R, Iwasaki Y, and Koprowsi H: Ultrastructural studies of perivascular cuffing cells in multiple sclerosis brain. American Journal of Pathology 81:467, 1975.

325. Tangy F, McAllister A, Aubert C, and Brahic M: Determinants of persistence and demyelination of the DA strain of Theiler's virus are found only in the VP1 gene. Virology 65:1616, 1991.

326. Tangy F, Vernant JC, Coscoy L, et al: A search for human T-cell leukemia virus type I in the lesions of patients with tropical spastic paraparesis and polymyositis. Ann Neurol 38:454–460, 1995.

327. Telenti A, Aksamit AJ Jr, Proper J, and Smith TE: Detection of JC virus DNA by polymerase chain reaction in patients with progressive multifocal leukoencephalopathy. J. Infect Dis 162:858–861, 1990.

328. ter Meulen V, Koprowski H, Iwasaki Y, Käckell YM, and Müller D: Fusion of cultured multiple sclerosis brain cells with indicator cells: Presence of nucleocapsids and virions and isolation of parainfluenza type virus. The Lancet 2:1–5, 1972.

329. Theiler M: Spontaneous encephalomyelitis of mice: A new virus disease. Science 80:122, 1934.

330. Theiler M: Spontaneous encephalomyelitis of mice: A new virus disease. J Exp Med 65:705, 1937.

331. Thomas EE, Lau AS, Kim SU, Osborne D, and Kastrukoff LF: Variation in resistance to herpes simplex virus type I of oligodendrocytes derived from inbred strains of mice. J Gen Virol 72:2051, 1991.

332. Torsteinsdottir S, Georgsson G, Gisladotti E, Rafner B, Palsson PA, and Petursson G: Pathogenesis of central nervous system lesions in visna cell mediated immunity and lymphocyte subsets in blood, brain, and cerebrospinal fluid. Ann NY Acad Sci 724:159, 1994.

333. Townsend JJ: The demyelinating effect of corneal HSV infections in normal and nude (athymic) mice. J Neurol Sci 50:435, 1981.

334. Townsend JJ: Schwann cell remyelination in experimental Herpes simplex encephalitis at the trigeminal root entry zone. J Neuropathol Exp Neurol 42:529, 1983.

335. Townsend JJ, and Baringer JR: Morphology of central nervous system disease in immunosuppressed mice after peripheral herpes simplex virus inoculation. Lab Invest 40:178, 1979.

336. Usuku K, Sonoda S, Osame M, et al: HLA haplotype-linked high immune responsiveness against HTLV-1 in HTLV-1 associated myelopathy: comparison with adult T-cell leukemia/lymphoma. Ann Neurol 23(suppl) S143-S150, 1988.

337. Van Bogaert L: Une leuco-encephalite sclerosante subaigue. J Neurol Neurosurg Psychiatry 8: 101, 1945.

338. Vandevelde M, Zurbriggen A, Dumas M, and Palmer D: Canine distemper virus does not infect oligodendrocytes in-vitro. J Neurol Sci 69:133, 1985.

339. Vandevelde M, Zurbriggen A, Higgins RJ, and Palmer D: Spread and distribution of viral anti-

gen in nervous canine distemper. Acta Neuropathol (Berl) 67:211, 1985.

340. Venien-Bryan C, and Fuller SD: The organization of the spike complex of Semliki Forest virus. J Mol Biol 236:572, 1994.

341. Vernant JC, Maurs L, Gessain A, et al: Endemic tropical spastic paraparesis associated with human T-lymphotropic virus type I: A clinical seroepidemiological study of 25 cases. Ann Neurol 21:123–130, 1987.

342. Wang F-I, Fleming JO, and Lai MMC: Sequence analysis of the spike protein gene of murine coronavirus variants: Study of genetic sites affecting neuropathogenicity. Virology 186:742, 1992.

343. Wang F-I, Stohlman SA, and Fleming JO: Demyelination induced by murine hepatitis virus JHM strain (MHV-4) is immunologically mediated. J Neuroimmunol 30:31, 1990.

344. Watanabe R, Wege H, and ter Meulen V: Adoptive transfer of EAE-like lesions from rats with coronavirus-induced demyelinating encephalomyelitis. Nature 305:150, 1983.

345. Webb HE, Chew-Lim M, Jagelman S, et al: Semliki Forest virus infections in mice as a model for studying acute and chronic central nervous system virus infections in man. In Rose C (ed): Clinical Neuroimmunology. Blackwell Scientific, Oxford, 1979, p 369.

346. Webb HE, Mehta S, Gregson NA, and Leibowitz S: Immunological reaction of the demyelinating Semliki Forest virus with immune serum to glycolipids and its possible importance to central nervous system viral auto-immune disease. Neuropathol Appl Neurobiol 10:77, 1984.

347. Weber I: DNA sequence analysis identifies regions likely responsible for neurotropism of HIV-1: Int. Conf. AIDS 9:18, 1993.

348. Weiner LP: Pathogenesis of demyelination induced by mouse hepatitis virus (JHM virus). Arch Neurol 28:298, 1973.

349. Weiner LP, Johnson RT, and Herndon RM: Viral infections and demyelinating diseases. N Engl J Med 288:1103, 1973.

350. Weinshenker BG, and Rice GPA: Retroviral diseases of the nervous system. In Kim S (ed): Myelination and Demyelination: Implications of MS. Plenum, New York, pp 145–152, 1988.

351. Welsh CJR, Tonks P, Nash AA, and Blakemore WF: The effect of L3T4 T cell depletion on the pathogenesis of Theiler's murine encephalomyelitis virus infection in CBA mice. J Gen Virol 68:1659, 1987.

352. Wiley CA, Masliah E, Morey M, et al: Neocortical damage during HIV infection. Ann Neurol 29:651–667, 1991.

353. Wiley CA, Schrier RD, Nelson JA, Lampert PW, and Oldstone MBA: Cellular localization of human immunodeficiency virus within the brains of acquired immunodeficiency patients. Proc Natl Acad Sci USA 83:7089–7093, 1986.

354. Williams AE, Fang CE, Slamon DJ, et al: Seroprevalence and epidemiological correlates of HTLV-1 infection in U.S. blood donors. Science 240:643–646, 1988.

355. Williamson JSP, and Stohlman SA: Effective clearance of mouse hepatitis virus from the central nervous system requires both CD4+ and CD8+ T cells. J Virol 64:4589, 1990.

356. Williamson JSP, Sykes KC, and Stohlman SA: Characterization of brain infiltrating mononuclear cells during infection with mouse hepatitis virus strain JHM. J Neuroimmunol 32:199, 1991.

357. Wilson GAR, Beushausen S, and Dales S: In vivo and in vitro models of demyelinating disease. XV. Differentiation influences the regulation of coronavirus infection in primary explants of mouse CNS. Virology 151:253, 1986.

358. Wisniewski H, Raine CS, and Kay WJ: Observations on viral demyelinating encephalomyelitis: Canine distemper virus. Lab Invest 26:589, 1972.

359. Yamada M, Zurbriggen A, and Fujinami RS: Pathogenesis of Theiler's murine encephalomyelitis virus. Adv Virus Res 39:291, 1991.

360. Yamaguchi K, Goto N, Kyuwa S, Hayami M, and Toyoda Y: Protection of mice from a lethal coronavirus infection in the central nervous system by adoptive transfer of virus-specific T cell clones. J Neuroimmunol 32:1, 1991.

361. Yoshida M, Osame M, Kawai H, et al: Increased replication of HTLV-1 in HTLV-1 associated myelopathy. Ann Neurol 26:331–335, 1989.

362. Zimmer MJ, and Dales S: In vivo and in vitro models of demyelinating diseases. XXIV. The infectious process in cyclosporin A treated Wistar Lewis rats inoculated with JHM virus. Microb Pathog 6:7, 1989.

363. Zimprich F, Wionter J, Wege H, and Lassmann H: Coronavirus induced primary demyelination: Indications for the involvement of a humoral immune response. Neuropathol Appl Neurobiol 17:469, 1991.

364. Zink MC, Narayan O, Kennedy PGE, and Clements JE: Pathogenesis of Visna/Maedi and Caprine arthritis-encephalitis: New leads on the mechanism of restricted virus replication and persistent infection. Vet Immunol Immunopathol 15:167, 1987.

365. Zurbriggen A, Hogle JM, and Fujinami RS: Alteration of amino acid 101 within capsid protein VP-1 changes the pathogenicity of Theiler's murine encephalomyelitis virus. J Exp Med 170:2037, 1989.

366. Zurbriggen A, Thomas C, Yamada M, Roos RP, and Fujinami RS: Direct evidence of a role for amino acid 101 of VP1 in central nervous system disease in Theiler's murine encephalomyelitis virus infection. J Virol 65:1929–1937, 1991.

367. Zurbriggen A, Vandevelde M, and Bollo E: Demyelinating, nondemyelinating and attenuated canine distemper virus strains induce oligodendroglial cytolysis in vitro. J Neurol Sci 79:33, 1987.

368. Zurbriggen A, Vandevelde M, and Dumas M: Secondary degeneration of oligodendrocytes in canine distemper virus infection in vitro. Lab Invest 54:424, 1986.

369. Zurbriggen A, Vandevelde M, Dumas M, Griot C, and Bollo E: Oligodendroglial pathology in canine distemper virus infection in vitro. Acta Neuropathol (Berl) 74:366, 1987.

370. Zurbriggen A, Yamawaki M, and Vandevelde M: Restricted canine distemper virus infection of oligodendrocytes. Lab Invest 68:277, 1993

CHAPTER 11

IMMUNOLOGY

George C. Ebers, MD

All reasoning is analogizing.–Emerson

Lack of understanding about the cause of MS has generated a remarkable variety of hypotheses over the last century. Few mechanisms have not been proposed to explain the bewildering phenomena associated with this disease. Currently evolving concepts of etiology and pathogenesis, though not consensual, strongly support the view that MS is an autoimmune disease. Pathological studies that have shown the abundant immune cells and their secretory products in the presence of injury consistent with immunologic damage have been for many the "smoking gun" of forensic science (see Chapter 8). Regardless of how compelling the evidence, the data that attribute the pathogenesis of MS to organ-specific tissue injury by the immune system remain largely circumstantial. Unfortunately, whether these immunologic phenomena represent primary events or are secondary or reactive to some other process has not yet been resolved. Many researchers continue to draw strong analogies between MS and other conditions in which immunologic injury is clearly the primary pathogenic event. One such analogy is between MS in humans and experimentally induced MS in animals, both of which resemble one another pathologically.

More than a generation ago, the insightful immunologist, E. Witebsky, proposed some criteria modeled on Koch's postulates to establish the autoimmune nature of human diseases.[131] They required the demonstration of specific autoantibody, the identification of the corresponding antigen, and the induction of an analogous immune response in an experimental animal. It could be argued that these criteria have been satisfied for MS, yet the context has changed. Contemporary concepts of autoimmunity recognize that autoreactive cells and antibody are normal phenomena, and reactivity against several autoantigens can be found in normal MS and in other diseases. Finally, experimental autoimmunity resembling MS can also be induced with more than one autoantigen.

The literature dealing with immune function in MS is extensive. Although it is beyond the scope of this chapter to cover this area definitively, it does present some general background and a subjective review of the most important observations.

OBSERVATIONS ON THE NATURAL HISTORY OF MULTIPLE SCLEROSIS THAT SUPPORT THE CONCEPT OF AUTOIMMUNITY

Female Predominance

The well-known sex predominance in females that characterizes MS parallels similar observations in most human autoimmune disorders. A female predominance is seen, for example, in rheumatoid arthritis, Sjögren's syndrome, and Graves' disease and is especially marked in systemic lupus erythematosus. Two exceptions to this generalization are the equal gender risk in juvenile diabetes and the marked male predominance in ankylosing spondylitis.

A large variety of spontaneous and induced experimental autoimmune disorders in mice and rats (including murine non-obese diabetes, NOD,[121] and experimental allergic encephalitis, EAE) demonstrate the same female predilection (see Chapter 3). In many of these animal models, experimental evidence shows clearly that susceptibility is determined by female hormones. As proof, female or male castration and the exogenous administration of estrogens or androgens can substitute for the effect of chromosomally determined gender. Similar data are more difficult to come by for humans, although there appears to be an increased frequency of lupus in Klinefelter's syndrome and a lowered androgen level in lupus females.[76] The effects of hormonal factors on susceptibility to MS and to autoimmunity have been discussed in two recent reviews.[32,162]

Age of Onset

The age-of-onset curve in MS (see Chapter 5) finds no ready explanation, but it is compatible with the gradual cumulative selection of a small group of individuals with age-related risk out of the total population who bear a developmentally regulated and genetically based susceptibility. Exactly how selection might occur is problematic. The reduction in incidence past the third decade could be an age-related event, could reflect a diminishing at-risk birth cohort as susceptible, or more likely results from a combination of both factors. Possible selection factors that determine those in the susceptible population who will be diagnosed are discussed in Chapter 3. Relative age restriction for the induction of disease may also be seen in some models.[94,166]

Relapses and Remissions

The relapsing-remitting character typifying early MS suggests a dynamic or phasic process that ordinarily occurs in equilibrium. Many human diseases that are thought to be autoimmune in nature also have relapses and remissions as a characteristic feature of their natural history. These include myasthenia gravis, systemic lupus erythematosus, and rheumatoid arthritis. In psoriasis and vitiligo, the evolution of exacerbations is particularly accessible to the naked eye.[20] Events that precipitate relapses in these disorders are not any better understood than they are in MS. Relapse and one remission is also known to be common even in juvenile diabetes, where remission was intially thought to be rare because preclinical trial efforts to withdraw insulin occurred infrequently. Recent studies of immunosuppressive therapy have resulted in a more careful evaluation of the frequency with which patients lose their insulin requirement shortly after onset. Control subjects from these studies have led to the recognition that remissive phases ("honeymoons") may occur in up to half the patients in the months after onset.[167]

Triggering Events

Although, for most patients, neither onset attack nor subsequent relapses bear a clear temporal relationship to any consistent event, consensus suggests that the most common identifiable precipitant of relapse is an upper respiratory infection, an event associated with activation of the immune system (see Chapter 5). On the other hand, a clear association of relapse with vaccination has not been identified, but it is a question perhaps worth re-examination using magnetic resonance imaging (MRI) scans after vaccination with a variety of viral and bacterial vaccines. A stronger association exists between the monophasic demyelinating disorder, acute disseminated encephalomyelitis, and either vaccination or preceding viral infection. Unfortunately, no spontaneous form of EAE is recognized in experimental laboratory animals.

Clinical Course

Assuredly, the early relapsing-remitting course that evolves into a chronic progressive disorder so characteristic of the prototypical patient is not unique to MS and is exhibited by some other human autoimmune conditions. This pattern of evolution is well recognized, for example, in uveitis, where 31 percent of patients will run a relapsing course and 59 percent a chronic progressive course.[141]

Effect of Pregnancy

Pregnancy is a special kind of immunosuppressed state in which it is remarkable that the mother fails to reject the fetus. This phenomenon represents a form of allograft that bears paternal antigens to which only a limited and apparently beneficial immunologic response is made by the mother. Accordingly, diseases autoimmune in nature should ameliorate during pregnancy,[162] and some evidence suggests that this is the case in MS. The exacerbation rate in prospectively studied patients appears to diminish in the second and third trimesters. Consistent with this finding, limited evidence also suggests amelioration during pregnancy of systemic lupus erythematosus, myasthenia gravis, and autoimmune thyroid disease, although a worsening of these conditions may also occur.[24,51,124,151]

Association with Major Histocompatibility Complex Antigen

Many other organ-specific and putatively autoimmune disorders in humans share with MS an association between susceptibility and specific alleles of the major histocompatibility complex (MHC) antigen,[106] with some exceptions. The finding of a human leukocyte antigen (HLA) association is not decisively in favor of autoimmunity for several reasons. Among these, a number of sequelae of viral infections in experimental animals also demonstrate an association of susceptibility with the MHC antigen. However, in this situation, interactions of the immune system in limiting spread of the virus or influencing persistence may lead to the association. Furthermore, many genes in or near the MHC antigen code for proteins are not directly involved in immune activation and not enough is known about MS to rule out a non–immune-related reason for an MHC antigen association, although this seems improbable. The role of class II genes in antigen presentation makes them good candidates for being susceptibility loci themselves. The apparent upregulation of class II antigen expression at the site of autoimmune attack also supports a direct role,[21] but in no way proves it. Recent evidence indicates that knockout mice having a genetic defect leading to upregulation of MHC antigen (as in deletion of tumor growth factor-β, TGF-β, an important immunomodulator) are highly prone to autoimmunity.

Response to Immunosuppressive Drugs

Patients undergoing organ transplant and those treated for malignant disease have provided many of the data and much of the empirical knowledge on the use and complications of cytotoxic and immunosuppressive medications. Hard-won experience gained by the study of such disorders, where uniform mortality is the expectation, has been applied by analogy to human autoimmunity. Nevertheless, these two situations are not exactly parallel. In the early posttransplant period, the opportunity exists to interfere with the development of the primary immune response by giving therapy concomitant with, or even before, the administration of the immunogens. Experimentally, it has been much easier to prevent a primary immune response than to abolish an ongoing secondary or anamestic reaction. In contrast, an ongoing autoimmune process, such as that which occurs in MS, would be most certainly a secondary one and, therefore, not analogous to the situation for organ transplant.

Some have suggested that the "response" of patients with MS to immunosuppressive drugs demonstrates that the disease is autoimmune in nature. Drugs that suppress organ transplant rejection have had extensive trials in MS. Only a modest benefit has been found with azathioprine, and any benefit for cyclosporine and cyclophosphamide may be relatively nonexistent. Cyclophosphamide may actually be deleterious in the long term for patients with MS. However, the notion that immunosuppressive drugs should necessarily improve autoimmune disorders does not take into account many observed paradoxes. It is improbable that a therapy directed against

dividing cells could entirely ignore the phase of the disease when the therapy is given. Under a number of experimental circumstances, alkylating agents, such as cyclophosphamide, can actually enhance the immune response.[77] For example, cyclophosphamide can increase the penetrance of spontaneous autoimmune diabetes in the NOD mouse. Moreover, low-dose cyclosporine can convert acute uniphasic EAE to chronic relapsing EAE.[120] A recent trial of the highest tolerable doses of this drug in patients with inflammatory bowel disease led to the premature cessation of the trial because the patients with Crohn's disease who were stable at the time of institution of cyclosporine therapy were made significantly worse by the treatment.[37] Similar paradoxes occur in the BB rat, where the reconstitution of lymphopenia prevents the diabetes and where monoclonal antibodies to T cells produce an increased penetrance.

In the clinical setting, we have observed a male patient who had both Hodgkin's disease and successful renal transplant who later developed MS while receiving treatment with immunosuppressant drugs. We also have treated two female patients who have developed MS in the setting of adequate and successful immunosuppression for orthotopic liver transplants. A number of suspected autoimmune phenomena have been described in acquired immunodeficiency syndrome (AIDS), and putative autoimmune disorders such as psoriasis have been markedly exacerbated in the setting of acquired immunosuppression. In the acute measles infection, an autoimmune postinfectious encephalomyelitis may emerge despite the evidence of depression of cell-mediated immunity. These anecdotal observations prove nothing, but they do complement experimental data indicating that autoimmunity occurs in the setting of a dynamic interplay of both enhancing and suppressive factors, which may be affected neither selectively nor predictably by cytotoxic drugs or diseases that "suppress" the immune system. Given these considerations, we do not believe that available data on responsiveness to nonspecific alkylating agents or immunosuppressive drugs can be comfortably taken as evidence for or against autoimmunity. Furthermore, the use of such agents must be considered to be empirical until appropriate clinical trials are carried out.

SELECTED ASPECTS OF NORMAL IMMUNITY

Development of the Immune Repertoire

CLONAL SELECTION AND TOLERANCE INDUCTION

T cells are selected for reactivity with MHC self-antigen in the thymus;[16] those T cells lacking this reactivity are largely deleted.[70] This leaves the organism with a T-cell repertoire that recognizes antigen in the context of MHC. This is a form of positive selection in that thymic T-cell–MHC antigen interaction presumably delivers a signal preventing the apoptotic cell death that befalls T cells not capable of this interaction.

CLONAL DELETION

In contrast to positive selection, T cells reactive with self-antigens other than MHC are largely deleted in the thymus (negative selection). The process by which self-reactive cells are deleted is still incompletely understood. Although it seems clear that this phenomenon occurs within the thymus, it has not been determined how antigens from distant organs would reach or are expressed in the thymus to deliver a deletion signal. This is particularly puzzling for antigens that are developmentally regulated and may be associated with late expression. However, recent evidence suggests that some of these antigens are indeed expressed in the thymus at least transiently.

PERIPHERAL TOLERANCE

Clearly, autoreactive T cells are detectable in peripheral blood, lymph nodes, and spleen. The mechanism by which these autoreactive cells remain "peripherally tolerant" is uncertain, although the term *clonal anergy* has been applied to this phe-nomenon. The present status of "suppressor cells" is uncertain. The in vitro phenomena of suppression are unequivocal, but many of the mechanisms remain uncertain. T cells with the postulated characteristics of suppressor cells have not been identified in transgenic mouse experiments characterized by highly restricted T-cell repertoires. Furthermore, in suppressor T-cell hybridomas there has been no expression or rearrangement of T-cell *V*-region genes.[56] Some suggest that suppressor effects may originate, in part, from T cells that are cytotoxic to other T effector cells.[18,19]

A variety of in vitro manipulations can demonstrate that antigen-specific autoreactive T cells are active in carrying out effector functions.[13] Furthermore, this self-reactivity is not restricted to hidden antigens or self-antigens but includes reactivity to determinants on readily accessible molecules. Clearly, tolerance is a complex process with several mechanisms, which may result in autoimmunity when dysfunctional.

Antigen Processing and Major Histocompatibility Complex Restriction

Antigen-reactive T cells are presented with small peptides processed within antigen-presenting cells (i.e., dendritic cells, macrophages, and B cells). Specific transport mechanisms, which result in intracellular assembly of MHC polypeptide chains in conjunction with antigenic peptides and subsequent insertion of these complexes into the cell membrane, have been identified. Occupied peptide-binding clefts in class II molecules have been identified at a crystallographic level. It is quite clear that MHC class II molecules can bind a large variety of peptides and effectively present them to T cells; indeed, this process is necessary for adequate protection of the organism. T cells recognize antigen epitopes presented in the context of MHC self-antigen because of thymic selection. CD8+ cytotoxic T cells recognize cell-associated antigens in the context of MHC class I molecules, whereas CD4+ helper cells recognize antigens in the context of class II molecules. There are also some cytotoxic T cells that use class II molecules as a restricting element. Epitope recognition takes place when the T-cell receptor complex that contains several gene products encounters the antigen contained in the MHC cleft. For most T cells, the two variable regions of the alpha and beta chains constitute the key portion for antigen recognition.[103]

A large segment of chromosome 6p, comprising some 4.5 megabases of DNA, constitutes the MHC molecule. It can be divided into three regions,[6,156] which contain the MHC class I, class II, and class III antigens, although they contain a number of unrelated genes as well. The class II region, in addition to the HLA-DP, DR, and DQ loci, is also known to harbor at least two additional class II gene loci. Each class II molecule consists of two polypeptide chains, alpha and beta, the latter accounting for polymorphism at this locus. The class III region contains some 36 genes, including several complement loci (*C4, C2, Bf*), and the cytokines known as tumor necrosis factor-α (TNF-α) and TNF-β. It also contains the gene for heat shock protein 70 (hsp 70). There are also several other genes with no known relevance to the immune system, including the steroid 21-hydroxylase gene. In the class I region, which is less well-studied, several homologous class I genes have been recognized, including the well-known *A, B,* and *C* loci. Each class I molecule consists of the invariant smaller chain (β_2-microglobulin) and a second highly polymorphic polypeptide chain that influences antigen association.

Activation of the Immune System and Effector

HELPER T CELLS (TH1, TH2) AND CYTOTOXIC T CELLS

As already mentioned, histocompatibility molecules are proteins that bind peptides and present them to T cells. Class I molecules bind peptides derived from endogenous proteins, including viruses. In addition, class II molecules can present peptides from endocytosed (exogenous) antigen.

Binding of peptides by histocompatibility molecules is a function of their assembly, intracellular trafficking, and endocytosis. For class I molecules, assembly appears to be a most important step for peptide acquisition.

On the face of the class I molecule is a peptide-binding groove formed by two alpha helices lying parallel on a beta-pleated sheet, which is available for binding by a T-cell receptor. A similar binding site, which could accommodate peptides of 10 to 20 amino acids, is characteristic of class II molecules. The specificity of T-cell receptor recognition is influenced both by polymorphic residues in the antigen-binding groove and by the primary sequence of the bound antigen-derived peptide. T-cell receptors on CD8+ cytotoxic T cells are recognized by antigen peptides bound to MHC class I molecules, whereas class II peptide complexes are recognized by CD4+ helper cells. Helper cells can be divided into two types, Th1 and Th2, based on the pattern of cytokine secretion. Th1 cells secrete interleukin-2 (IL-2), interferon gamma, and lymphotoxin (LT) in response to antigen, whereas Th2 cells secrete interleukins 4, 5, 6, and 10. TNF-α is secreted by both types. Th1 cells are primarily involved in cellular immunity and inflammatory responses by activating cytotoxic T cells and macrophages via IL-2 and interferon gamma. Th2 cells produce cytokines that induce B-cell differentiation and growth. There are also effects of Th1 and Th2 cells on each other via cytokine secretion; for example, the interleukin (IL-10) secreted by Th2 cells inhibits the interferon gamma produced by Th1 cells.

Cytotoxic T cells lyse their targets through the release of cell mediators known as perforins, which produce holes in cell membranes and subsequently lead to cell death. The recognition that T cells may also deliver a signal that induces apoptotic cell death has contributed an added dimension to our understanding of cytotoxicity.

NATURAL KILLER CELLS

Natural killer (NK) cells can lyse virally infected cells, tumor cells, and allogeneic or parental marrow stem cells. They appear to play an important role in tumor surveillance. No clear role in autoimmunity has been recognized. NK cell deficiency characterizes patients with Chédiak-Higashi syndrome.

B CELLS

B cells carry immunoglobulin molecules on their surface, with antigen specificity being determined by the combination of *V*-region genes expressed on the immunoglobulin receptor for antigen. Stimulation of these cells by antigen results in cell maturation and differentiation to plasma cells and the production of specific antibodies, initially IgM and subsequently one of the four subclasses of IgG as the predominant isotype.

ANTIBODIES

These circulatory B-cell products exert their effects by aggregation, blockade, stimulation, opsonization, complement fixation, sensitization to the action of effector cells, direct enzymatic action, or indirect sensitization of a target molecule to other enzymatic action. However, the presence of autoantibodies can be pathogenic, be secondary and harmless, or be secondary and contributory to pathogenesis.[104] Autoantibodies to some self-antigens are normally present in the circulation. Their avidity and affinity are low. It is not easy to determine if detectable autoantibodies play a pathogenic role, and a number of criteria have been suggested to help in resolving this question. There is good evidence that antibodies play a complementary role in the demyelination seen in some forms of EAE, but their role in MS is not yet clear.

MACROPHAGES

Macrophages play an important role both in antigen processing and presentation to T cells. They also provide essential functions as scavengers and secrete a variety of lymphokines and complement factors. Evidence from pathological studies suggests that macrophages may be impor-

tant effector cells in MS (see Chapter 8) and perhaps the first at the site of an MS lesion. Dendritic cells have a particularly important role in antigen presentation.[62]

COMPLEMENT

The complement system is composed of a complex group of molecules with specific enzymatic activities. They interact with each other in serial cascades to form a terminal attack complex consisting of the C7–9. This complex produces cell lysis, and the molecules bear similarity to the perforins secreted by cytotoxic T cells.[28]

Cytokines and Adhesion Molecules

A variety of cytokines are released by activated T cells and macrophages. They play an important role in immunoregulation. TNF, interleukins 1 through 13, and the leukotrienes, among others, are included in this class of molecule. Many play an intermediary role in tissue injury. The number of these molecules is bewilderingly large, and the field is growing very fast. The similarity of uncharacterized sequences in DNA libraries to known cytokines suggests that many more will be found. The demonstration that interferon gamma may exacerbate MS and that interferon beta may be beneficial (see Chapter 12) has drawn greater attention to the role of these molecules in MS research. The presence of numerous cytokines at the site of MS lesions has been well documented (see Chapter 8). The potential interactions among these molecules is great. Some are suppressive in nature, such as IL-10, which can delay the onset of spontaneous autoimmunity in mice.[65] The complexity of interaction is further underscored by the fact that monoclonal antibodies to interferon gamma suppress the spontaneous autoimmune diabetes that develop in the NOD mouse but can exacerbate acute EAE.[17,25]

Not only has the number of known cytokines greatly expanded, but the variety of in vivo and in vitro actions they exhibit is great and overlapping. The roles of cytokines that have been known longer have been more comprehensively studied. More recently studied chemokines may play important roles in the inflammatory process of autoimmune disease.

The mechanism whereby inflammatory cells stick to vascular endothelium in the area of inflammation or tissue injury is complex. T lymphocytes appear to stick to vascular endothelium via the expression of E selection, vascular adhesion molecule-1 (VCAM-1), and intercellular adhesion molecule-1 (ICAM-1) via their own ligands. These include lymphocyte function-associated antigen-14 (LFA-14), ICAM-1, and very late activation antigen-4 (VLA-4) for VCAM-1. These molecules are inducible on the surface of leukocytes by chemokines such as interleukin-8.

IMMUNOLOGIC ABNORMALITIES IN MULTIPLE SCLEROSIS

From early histopathological observations, it was clear that MS lesions contained cells that would later be recognized as essential parts of the immune system. Furthermore, experimental observations such as the production of EAE in primates after the injection of spinal cord with adjuvant and the subsequent demonstration of large amounts of immunoglobulin in the spinal fluid of patients with MS directed investigators to search for immunopathological mechanisms in this disease. Surprisingly, however, this research has added little to our understanding that has not been directly derived by analogizing with developments in basic immunology and in autoimmune diseases in animals. Even if it is accepted that MS lesions resemble those known to be experimentally produced by T cells, fundamental questions remain that are common to most human autoimmune diseases. Is the immune reaction in MS cause or effect and, if cause, is it a specific antigen, cell, tissue, or organ to which this response is directed? What are the effector mechanisms leading to tissue injury and the cellular pathology resulting in lack of recovery?

Certainly one of the most lengthy and unfinished chapters in the history of MS research has been the search for the postulated "immune defect" believed to cause MS. In an attempt to leave no stone unturned, few immunologic phenomena have not been studied by comparing patients with MS and control subjects. These studies are difficult, time consuming, technically demanding, and bedeviled by problems of reproducibility. Differences between patients with MS and the normal population have often been found, but interpretation of these differences is more difficult. Failure to control for factors subsequently found to influence assays can be a problem, and many findings on functional assays are found to be nonspecific to MS. Other neurological diseases or putative autoimmune disorders represent additional important control conditions that have increasingly been used. It is sobering to realize that despite decades of cellular immunologic research of the survey type, no specific abnormality that characterizes or defines MS has been identified. Neither has any observation in this field achieved even adjunctive diagnostic value on a widespread basis, with the notable exception of the oligoclonal banding pattern in cerebrospinal fluid (CSF). Of course, this state of affairs is equally true for most of the other putative autoimmune disorders in which the antigens serving as the focus for immune attack remain at large. It can be appreciated why the status of the autoimmune hemolytic anemias and myasthenia gravis (in which the acetylcholine receptor is implicated with virtual certainty as a target antigen) would be viewed with some envy by MS investigators.

It might be anticipated a priori that for any exquisitely organ-specific autoimmune disorder, it would be unlikely that any generalized defect in immune function would be recognized as the primary factor underlying pathogenesis. Indeed, abundant epidemiological evidence has accumulated against any generalizable immune dysfunction in patients with MS. No evidence exists for increased risk of cancer, increased risk of other autoimmune diseases (see following discussion), immune complex disease, or systemic amyloidosis. In contrast, patients with MS seem characterized by relatively good health in organ systems other than those affected directly and indirectly by their central nervous system (CNS) disease process. Patients are successful in dealing with local or systemic bacterial and fungal infections and seem to differ little from the normal population or from those with traumatic paraplegia in this regard. These general observations have not discouraged numerous investigators from evaluating nonspecific immune functions in patients with MS in the hope that some abnormality would provide a clue as to the nature of the underlying disease process. These studies have yielded persuasive evidence that immune activation is present in MS, but little in the way of abnormalities that can confidently be concluded to be primary or to account for tissue specificity.

A precedence has been established for the operation of generalized lymphoproliferative abnormalities as complementing factors in organ-specific animal models of autoimmunity,[140] yet there is little such evidence in MS. Postulated lacunes in the immune apparatus commonly characterized as "inadequate suppression"[8,27] might reasonably be expected to result in a more generalized autoimmunity, a feature clearly lacking in MS. On the other hand, immunodeficiency, excepting a selective variety, might be expected to be associated with abnormal susceptibility to infection and cancer. Similarly, defects in NK cell function, T-cell function, and B-cell function would be directly relevant to the pathogenesis only if an additional factor, which determines organ specificity, could be incorporated. I am not persuaded that the oft-repeated statement that MS is a disease of "disordered immunoregulation"[46] entails any greater understanding than traditional concepts of autoreactivity popular decades ago.

Cellular Immunology of Multiple Sclerosis

The division of the immune system into many functional components, including specific cellular types and subtypes by quantitative and functional assays, has led to extensive studies in patients with MS. These studies have often aimed to demonstrate differences between patients with MS and control subjects and were in some way at the root of a postulated fundamental defect characterizing the immune system in patients with MS that resulted in the disease. Findings have not been uniform. In fact, the more spectacular the result,[123] the more likely it has been to encounter difficulty with reproducibility or to later find the postulated defect to be nonspecific.[102,125,130] The general approach of surveying each immune function, enumerating each lymphocyte subset,[7,72] and measuring each cytokine level in MS, although arguably necessary, has not been highly rewarding to date. One reason is that it has not been easy to select the ideal control patients with a dynamic and organ-specific disease (see following discussion).

Homogeneity

The comparison of patients to control subjects presupposes some homogeneity in unselected populations of patients. Potential factors that could result in heterogeneity of an MS population and therefore limit the power of detecting meaningful differences using any functional bioassay include gender, age, mood, nutrition, hormonal status, diurnal variation, recent and past medication history, presence or absence of bacterial infection, and physical activity, among others. Many of these factors are well known to influence many biologic variables, including measures of immune responsiveness in experimental circumstances. More specific to a disease with relapsing-remitting and progressive types is the timing of the assay in relation to disease activity, because the disorder is notoriously phasic.

Furthermore, the fact that subclinical activity often greatly exceeds that which results in symptoms makes the clinical determination of disease quiescence hazardous at best. Studies carried out in conjunction with MRI-based determinations of disease activity seem to represent a potentially valuable advance.[111]

Control Subjects

Among functional or quantitative immunologic assays developed in the last two decades—some of which have been said to discriminate between patients with MS and control subjects—relatively few have first been thoroughly evaluated in normal persons. Presumably, this method could aid in identifying factors that need to be controlled in any study evaluating diseased patients. If a convincing and reproducible difference could be found between patients with MS and control subjects, it would remain a difficult task to determine if any abnormality is causal or results from the disease process. Nonspecific consequences or perturbations associated with inflammation might also be expected to occur in other suspected autoimmune disorders. Control subjects of this type have generally been underutilized.[27] Seemingly, in vitro changes that are the result of immune activation or inflammation could be recognized in normal individuals who are studied before and after vaccinations or concurrent viral or bacterial infections. Certainly inflammatory processes entail a complex variety of humoral or secretory and cellular interactions.

Immune Abnormalities

Hundreds of studies have documented quests for non–antigen-specific abnormalities of immune function in MS. Noteworthy among these were early studies indicating that systemic immune cellular abnormalities were present in active MS.[4,45,110] From these studies, a general belief that "something is awry with immune function in MS" has emerged.[96,122] This notion has not yet greatly extended early pathological observations based on the presence of lymphocytes, plasma cells, and macrophages in MS tissue. Mounting evidence that the immune system may be activated during exacerbations[2,52,137] has supported a causal role for immune effector cells. Helper T, suppressor, and suppressor and inducer cells have been found many times in stable and relapsing patients. Initial claims that suppressor cells disappear during attacks[123] were not reproduced. A number of studies have reported more modest alterations;[60,61,72,102,130,152] these may be secondary phenomena. Numerous indicators of T-cell activation are detectable,[49] including elevated

levels of IL-2 receptors[2] and soluble CD8 levels,[95] among others (see following discussion). The T-cell repertoire found in MS lesions has been evaluated, and the notion that T-cell infiltrates would have restriction in repertoire seemed unlikely a priori. The diverse T-cell receptor cell usage in EAE seemed to belie such a notion. Evidence that T-cell receptor genes or combinations of T-cell and MHC gene products[109] determine MS susceptibility at a germline level[144] has largely gone unsupported.[34,59] Some found reduced NK cell activity in MS,[15,54,63,97,105] including in CSF.[97]

An elevation of serum and CSF levels of several cytokines correlates modestly with clinical activity, although none is predictably altered. Elevated levels of ICAM-1 have also been reported.[158] These include interleukin-6 (IL-6),[42] IL-2, and TNF-α.[155] LT and TNF are also present in MS lesions.[139] In sum, if a specific primary abnormality of the immune system exists in MS, it may be relatively subtle. Perhaps the phasic nature of the disease has helped it escape detection.

Because it has not yet been possible to confirm a specific antigen that serves as a target for T-cell–mediated tissue injury, several investigators have examined the T-cell repertoire in MS spinal fluid and in brain lesions. Initial claims that T cells in CSF are oligoclonal[48] have not been confirmed.[126,133] Similarly, initial claims that brain-derived T cells predominantly express specific V-region genes (a finding pointing to antigen-specific T-cell infiltration) also needed confirmation and also seem a priori very unlikely if the heterogeneity of T-cell infiltration at sites of antigen-specific delayed hypersensitivity reactions is any indication.

IMMUNOLOGY OF CANDIDATE ANTIGENS IN MULTIPLE SCLEROSIS

One assumption has been that if MS were autoimmune in nature, a specific antigen (and epitope) would be the focal point of attack, resulting in tissue injury. This notion finds much support in induced EAE, where the pathological process can be initiated using T-cell clones with very discrete reactivity to small myelin protein peptides. Furthermore, the concept of molecular mimicry,[43] in which autoimmunity results from a cross-reaction between an exogenous antigen and self, implies an extremely narrow specificity for a peptide sequence shared by antigen and self. On the contrary, pathological features resembling MS appear to be more readily produced in EAE by the injection of whole spinal cord tissue than by specific proteins or peptides. No specific MS antigen or epitope has been identified.

Further support for the existence of an MS antigen comes from the observation of oligoclonal banding in MS spinal fluid, a phenomenon often seen in antigen-specific, as opposed to nonspecific, immune reactions. The antigenic specificity for even a single one of the major oligoclonal bands in any individual patient with MS has yet to be found. Although reactivity to myelin and viral antigens is readily demonstrable, these specificities constitute a tiny fraction of the overall antibody present in the oligoclonal bands.

Although these findings have been tantalizing, extensive search for specific antigens to which patients with MS develop unique reactivity has been unsuccessful. Nor has success been forthcoming in searches for antigens specific to MS tissue that would then represent an exogenous epitope to which immunity develops. In contrast, reactivity to a wide range of endogenous CNS and exogenous viral antigens is found in patients with MS as well as in control subjects.

Although myelin antigens remain likely candidates for harboring epitopes for auto-aggressive pathogenic T cells in MS, cellular infiltration also characterizes the retinal sheathing seen in MS, where myelin is not present. It must be conceded that these phenomena could also be secondary. There are likely many more proteins as yet uncharacterized, and accordingly unstudied, that could serve as the site for autoimmune attack.

Unfortunately, in vitro tests of T-cell reactivities are not necessarily decisive. The modification that many proteins undergo after transcription or perhaps even during membrane turnover may generate a critical epitope identified by T cells. Furthermore, there is clearly heterogeneity of behavior among T cells after exposure to specific antigens. Initial studies with a variety of antigens have been ambiguous at the cellular level. Considerable discrepancy exists between proliferation, as measured by thymidine incorporation, and cytokine secretion, as measured by the single-cell spot assay, for interferon gamma production.[116]

Despite these considerations, it remains unclear why no antigen reactivity that uniquely characterizes MS has been found. A quantitative difference may exist within a qualitative similarity. The single-T-cell and single-B-cell assays developed by Olsson and colleagues[41,113] are the most direct and powerful means available for answering this question. These authors readily acknowledge that the data are short of proof that any of the specific antigens they have tested are the focus of autoimmune attack. Unfortunately it still remains possible that all of the immunologic changes seen could be secondary modifications of immune function, rather than primary pathogenic markers.[111]

Even though myelin basic protein constitutes some 30 percent of the total protein in myelin and is an effective autoimmunogen, there is good reason to consider the possibility of other proteins or antigens that may have a more important or perhaps crucial role in the development of MS. The protein target for autoimmune attack could be a small component of the total protein in the tissue, such as exemplified by the acetylcholine receptor in muscle in myasthenia gravis and perhaps still unrecognized. Alternatively, the epitope to which autoimmunity is directed could be destroyed during the process of isolation, or the conformational change that takes place during the isolation of proteins may destroy some high-order structure that is recognized in vivo by T cells, B cells, or antibody. Finally, the lesson derived from the protein abnormality in Duchenne's muscular dystrophy may be relevant. The abnormality in dystrophin that ought to have been demonstrable by simple electrophoresis (because many patients carry huge deletions in the dystrophin molecule) was not readily recognized. This failure was due to the molecule being so large that it did not penetrate the usual gels used to separate abnormal proteins from control and dystrophic muscle.

Pathological and pathophysiological studies leave little doubt that most of the pathological change in MS occurs in the white matter. Although this finding does not prove that a myelin antigen is being specifically targeted, it has nevertheless focused efforts on the specific components of white matter. It must be kept in mind, however, that tissue injury may occur as part of a bystander effect and that myelin could be injured as the result of an immune reaction to a nonmyelin antigen. The bystander effect has been well studied in TNF and interferon transgenic models.[58] In the S-100 model of EAE, bystander demyelination was found to be absent.[165] Many myelin proteins have been purified and their genes cloned and sequenced both in small laboratory animals and in humans. This effort has provided material for the development of immunologic assays that evaluate antigen-specific reactivity, in contrast to those summarized in Table 11–1.

Table 11–1. A SUGGESTED APPROACH TO THE EVALUATION OF IMMUNOLOGIC FUNCTION IN MULTIPLE SCLEROSIS

I. Assay
  A Well defined
  B. Reproducible
  C. Evaluated for potential influences of:
    1. Diurnal variation
    2. Age
    3. Gender
    4. Physical activity
    5. Commonly used medications
    6. Common coincident illnesses
  D. Blinded evaluators
II. Control subjects
  A. Normal individuals
  B. Other neurological diseases matched for disability
  C. Other putative autoimmune disorders matched for phase of activity
  D. Prevaccination and postvaccination or upper respiratory infection
III. MS Specificity
  A. Relationship to disease activity: clinical and/or gadolinium enhancement of MRI
  B. Concordant monozygotic twins
  C. Discordant monozygotic twins
  D. Concordant siblings

Myelin Basic Protein

The myelin component that has received the most attention has been MBP. This small planar molecule is the major protein component of myelin (30 percent by weight) and has the capacity to induce EAE when given along with adjuvant to susceptible laboratory animal strains. The application of in vitro methods of detection of antigen-specific proliferation to the role of MBP in MS initially suggested some reactivity was present.[11,91] Ideal control conditions, however, were not always available, and it was found that reactivity was not specific to MS but could be found in other disorders of the CNS.

More recently, the candidacy of MBP as an MS antigen has been supported by the identification of T cells that react specifically with MBP in patients with MS. Unfortunately, such T cells are also commonly, if not universally, found in the peripheral blood of normal individuals.[41,66,119] Because of this observation, it is untenable to postulate that the MHC antigen is a restricting element for the development of an anti-MBP T-cell response. However, the presence or absence of anti-MBP T-cell–mediated tissue injury could hinge on factors such as cell numbers, affinity, and pattern of cytokine release secondary to encountering antigen. The methodology of production of T-cell lines using antigen-driven proliferation has made approaches to quantitation less than straightforward. The search for antigen-specific T cells in MS has been dogged by the low numbers of reactive cells in peripheral blood and CSF, the latter making proliferation assays most difficult. However, recently a number of clever assays have surmounted some of these difficulties.

It was anticipated that the development of assays that could enumerate antigen-specific or epitope-specific T cells would shed considerable light on the long-standing conundra of MS autoimmunity. Specifically, candidate antigens could be evaluated and the number of T cells reactive with these antigens was expected to differentiate among them. A further step would take these evaluations past simple enumeration of antigen-reactive cells to the identification of cells that undergo specific functional consequences of activation, such as the production of interferon gamma and the cytokines. This would be especially important because the pattern of cytokine production resulting from antigen stimulation plays an important role in shaping the immune response.[55] A further refinement would be to identify interferon-specific or interleukin-specific messenger RNA (mRNA) production in specific T cells by in situ hybridization. These aims have been achieved by a productive and reliable group of investigators in Stockholm led by Olsson and Link.

Olsson and his collaborators have used methodologies that enumerate immunologic cells (both B and T) reactive with specific MBP epitopes (peptides), both in peripheral blood lymphocytes and CSF. Cells stimulated with MBP are identified by a spot assay that measures individual cells producing interferon gamma.[114] Their data seem to establish unequivocally a marked expansion of the MBP-specific T-cell pool both in the systemic and CSF compartments in patients with MS as compared with normal control subjects. This expansion is not MS specific, however; similar numbers of MBP-reactive T-cells can also be found in other conditions such as Lyme disease and stroke.[164] At present, their role in the pathogenesis of MS is uncertain, but MBP reasonably remains a leading candidate for MS-specific T-cell–mediated autoreactivity. When several MBP peptides were used as antigen stimulators, responses showed no preference for specific peptide sequences, nor was response correlated with HLA-DR.[142] It is perhaps surprising to learn that the elevation of MBP-reactive cells is not only seen in many other disorders where there is CNS injury (e.g., stroke), but that their numbers also rise in response to experimental peripheral nerve injury.[115] Thus, the dual vexing problems of specificity and of cause versus effect still remain. Cord blood has MBP-antigen–specific T cells in numbers even greater than in MS, although the significance of this phenomenon remains relatively unexplained.[40] The same investigators, using parallel techniques, have also demonstrated that MBP-specific antibody-producing cells are simi-

larly found to be increased in patients with MS as compared with control subjects.[116]

These sophisticated assays, although clearly dependent on antigen-specific recognition and blocked by antibodies to MHC class II antigens, have demonstrated discordance between T-cell proliferation and cytokine release. They have the added advantages of allowing the enumeration of cells secreting specific patterns of cytokines in response to antigen and thus providing insight into T-cell heterogeneity that is not detectable using cell surface markers.[116] This methodology, therefore, has considerable potential for use in screening candidate antigens in patients with MS.

Other Candidate Antigens

PROTEOLIPID PROTEIN

Proteolipid protein (PLP) can also induce EAE and constitutes some 50 percent of myelin by weight. No direct evidence links this protein to MS by activity, although PLP-reactive T and B cells are present in patients with MS in numbers far exceeding those in normal control subjects and a 40-fold to 50-fold enrichment is found in CSF over peripheral blood.[147]

MYELIN-ASSOCIATED GLYCOPROTEIN AND MYELIN-OLIGODENDROCYTE GLYCOPROTEIN

Two minor components of myelin, myelin-associated glycoprotein (MAG) and myelin-oligodendrocyte glycoprotein (MOG), are also plausible candidates. However, little information implicates them as autoantigens. T and B cells that recognize MOG and MAG epitopes have been identified in numbers similar to MBP and PLP and are enriched 100-fold in CSF versus blood.[9,146]

Studies involving myasthenia gravis help put these results in context. In myasthenia, where the acetylcholine receptor is almost certainly the primary autoantigen, α-subunit-specific responses are found by immunospot assays in 73 percent of the patients with MS and in 14 percent of control subjects.[85] Studies of cytokine-specific activation may be informative and could serve as a type of positive control in that the pattern of antigen-specific cytokine production to acetylcholine receptor may be characteristic of active disease.[56,88] Similar studies would be of interest in other diseases where strong candidate autoantigens are known, such as the Lambert-Eaton and Miller-Fisher syndromes.

Data similar to that described for T cells have been found for both B cells and antibody so that parallel detection of antigen-reactive B cells and antibody has been commonly found in patients with MS for all these myelin antigens.[85,87,89,90] Again, these frequencies substantially exceed those for normal control subjects and some other neurological diseases. Although they may be common in inflammatory non-MS CNS disorders, the cells and antibody tend not to persist. This finding is in contrast to what is found in MS.[83]

These observations seem to indicate that the presence of antigen-reactive T cells and B cells can be the result of nervous system injury in humans and in experimental animals (the latter is well demonstrated by Olsson's findings after sural nerve section). Nevertheless, they do not weigh heavily against an important role in pathogenesis for myelin-reactive B and T cells. Examination of patients with optic neuritis demonstrates that these responses are present early in the disease[142] and that finding them in the MRI-negative unaffected offspring of conjugal pairs raises the possibility that they may even antedate the biologic onset of CNS disease.[40]

Preliminary evidence from the same group indicates that T-cell mRNA positive for TGF-β RNA, a cytokine which downregulates both T-cell and B-cell immunity, is found to be elevated in patients with mild disease and depressed in patients with progressive MS, suggesting a possible role for this molecule in the regulation of disease activity.

Expression of ICAM may be essential for the egress of antigen-specific T cells from the intravascular compartment into the CNS. Circulating levels of these molecules can be detected in inflammatory processes, although there is no strong reason nor data to support the idea that these alterations are in any way disease specific.[44,53] Adhesion molecules (e.g., VLA) on circulating T cells[57] may interact with endothelial integrins to result in the initial step leading to diapedesis. Highly charged molecules such as heparan appear to block this interaction.[64] It has been demonstrated that monoclonal antibodies directed against ICAM-1 can suppress EAE.[5]

HUMORAL IMMUNITY IN MULTIPLE SCLEROSIS

Measurements of serum proteins in MS have shown no characteristic abnormalities. However, a small proportion of patients will show a mild systemic hypergammaglobulinemia (see following discussion). On the other hand, evidence that immune activation is present is further supported by the finding of elevated levels of cytokines on their receptors in active MS. As mentioned previously, IL-2 receptor levels are increased in active MS, as are the plasma IL-6 levels.[42]

Viral Antibodies

Some epidemiological evidence (see Chapter 2), which has implicated a specific viral infection in the pathogenesis of MS, has led to a large number of serological studies measuring the antibody responses of patients with MS to almost every known virus. This line of investigation was given added impetus by the then-emerging concept that MS resulted from an age-specific viral infection, as had been demonstrated for poliomyelitis. The poliomyelitis analogy was derived from the observation that infection with poliovirus early in life led to nonparalytic disease, whereas delayed (later in life) infection by the virus was much more likely to lead to neuronal loss and paralysis (neurotropism). Common childhood infections underwent careful scrutiny, and it soon became apparent that antibodies to measles virus were modestly elevated in patients with MS as compared with controls. Although the titers were not nearly as high as in lupus or in chronic active hepatitis, this finding caused considerable enthusiasm for the idea that measles were somehow responsible for MS. Almost simultaneously, it became clear that subacute sclerosing panencephalitis (SSPE) resulted from the persistence of measles virus infection in the CNS. Extensive studies, however, failed to demonstrate any evidence for measles virus persistence in MS brains, or at least not in such a way to distinguish patients with MS from control subjects.

Apparently, patients with MS carry elevated levels of antibody against a number of viruses. However, these findings have been substantiated only in population studies where comparisons are based on mean levels in groups of patients and control subjects. In addition, the elevated antibody levels are found mostly in women, suggesting that high antibody levels are related to the sex of patients with MS. In addition, in this group, there may be some MHC antigen control exerted on antibody levels. The subsequent identification of patients with MS who had never had measles or who had been successfully vaccinated against measles has dampened the enthusiasm for the virus as the cause of MS.

One explanation for the elevated antibody level to viruses in MS is the presence of mild background immunologic stimulation. These antibody elevations may also indicate more about the nature of the virus than about MS.[108]

Complement

No consistent abnormality of serum or CSF complement has been found in MS. Two reports found terminal C9 levels to be normal in CSF,[50,129] and another one found elevated levels of the terminal attack complex.[101] Both MS and hereditary C2 deficiency are associated with the MHC class II antigen DR2. Occasional patients may have both MS and C2 deficiency, but they are relatively rare and no causal connection is apparent.

Role of Cytokines in Multiple Sclerosis

Cytokines are secretory products of the immune cells that constitute a large variety of molecules playing an important role in differentiation and regulation of the immune system.[10,23] The presence of cytokines in MS serum, CSF, and pathological lesions has been evaluated by a number of investigators.[139] Elevated levels of TNF-α in serum and CSF have been found in some patients by most investigators. Similarly elevated levels of IL-2 and an increase in the number of IL-2 receptors have been found. None of these findings are in any way specific for MS; they do not seem to be sensitive measures of disease activity and might be expected to occur in a variety of other inflammatory disorders. Much attention has been focused on the role of interferon gamma. It upregulates MHC class II antigen expression on antigen-presenting cells, and it is downregulated by interferon beta and IL-10. Its secretion plays an important role in activating macrophages. Among the many molecules secreted by activated macrophages is IL-1, which acts on the brain to induce sleep and perhaps fatigue.[31]

Findings in MS research to some extent depend on the methodology used. In situ measurement of cytokines within lesions may be particularly sensitive to the age of the lesion examined. No systematic pattern has emerged that definitively characterizes the age of the MS lesion or the lesion itself other than identifying it as the site of an inflammatory process. This is reviewed in more detail in Chapter 8; however, the secretion of TNF-α[139] may be particularly important as an effector mechanism. The potential role of cytokine receptors in the brain is of interest,[30] although beyond the scope of this chapter. A number of transgenic mice deficient in specific cytokines (e.g., IL-10, IL-2) developed chronic inflammatory diseases, especially of the bowel,[75,135] and mice in whom the gene for TGF-β has been deleted developed a propensity for autoimmunity. Although it is unclear why this occurs,[100,145] chronic local infection is a possibility. Expression of class II molecules in the oligodendrocytes of mice transgenic for class II gene produces dis-demyelination,[159] which may be a nonspecific way of causing cellular pathology.

Cerebrospinal Fluid

The study of CSF has a long history in MS research. The analysis of CSF continues to be useful for diagnosis. Although advances in modern imaging have made it less often used than previously, many mysteries about the immunologic features of CSF in MS remain unsolved.[29,82]

CELLS

The CSF cell count is normal (equal or less than 5 cells per cubic millimeter) in 66 percent of patients with MS and is equal to or less than 15 cells per cubic millimeter in 95 percent.[153] These cells have been extensively characterized by cytologic methods and by use of cell surface marker detection. The great majority of CSF cells are T lymphocytes bearing CD4.[112,133,134,136,138] T cells in MS CSF do not appear to be demonstrably oligoclonal. Variable but relatively small numbers of macrophages and plasma cells are also detectable and an increase in the number of cells bearing CD5 has been found.[99] This B-cell subpopulation tends to produce autoantibodies, and CD5-bearing B cells do not undergo somatic mutation. Adhesion molecules are detectable on the surface of CSF T cells and may play a role in recruitment.[149]

The specificity of T cells and B cells remains largely unknown although a surprising number are reactive against proteins of the "heat shock" category.[168]

PROTEINS

Cerebrospinal fluid represents a kind of plasma ultrafiltrate because of the blood-brain CSF barriers.[38,39] Small proteins, such as β_2-microglobulin, as well as β and γ trace proteins, are relatively concentrated in CSF.[80]

The protein level is normal in 77 percent of patients and is equal to or less then 890 mg per deciliter in 95 percent.[153] A characteristic feature of CSF has been the presence of elevated levels of IgG, first demonstrated by Kabat and colleagues in 1948.[67] This elevation occurs in the presence of normal levels of other CSF proteins such as albumin, serving to distinguish the IgG elevation in MS from that seen when there is breakdown of the blood-brain barrier. A modest degree of barrier leakage is present in some patients with MS. The topic of quantitative changes in CSF proteins has

been extensively reviewed by Tourtellotte[153] and Link,[81] among others. Formulas designed to calculate the rate of IgG synthesis have been developed by Tourtellotte and are diagnostically useful[154] because they can correct for the modest blood-brain barrier leakage occurring in some patients. A scholarly account of this area is given in a monograph on CSF.[150]

ANTIBODIES

The elevated IgG levels found by Kabat[67] were later discovered to have restricted heterogeneity when subjected to electrophoresis.[79,92] This phenomenon, called *oligoclonal banding,* has been found to be present in many antigen-specific immune responses.[117] It is readily demonstrable in SSPE, where specificity of the bands to measles has been shown. Oligoclonal banding has also been demonstrated in EAE.

Accordingly, the presence of oligoclonal bands in the spinal fluid of over 90 percent of patients with MS[150] has been a stimulus for extensive searches for the antigen to which these antibodies are directed.[93] This search has largely been unsuccessful, although small amounts of the antibody have been found to be directed against a variety of common viral antigens.[107] Not a single oligoclonal band visible with standard techniques of CSF electrophoresis has been identified as to its antigen specificity. The restricted nature of these antibodies has been demonstrable in several ways. First, there is an abnormal light-chain ratio with an excess of kappa over lambda chains.[86] Second, the antibodies are predominantly of the IgG I subclass.[161] Third, oligoclonal bands are predominately cathodally migrating. The pattern of bands, once established, tends to remain constant,[163] although not invariably so. Free light chains are frequently present in MS CSF, although they are also found in other disorders with local CNS antibody production[35,134] and have no increased specificity for MS. Clinicopathological correlation of autopsy material with and without bands indicates that plasma cells are absent in the plaque and meninges of patients lacking CSF bands, while numerous in those in which oligoclonal bands are present.[36] No clear correlation of outcome can be associated with the presence or absence of bands, nor with the degree of abnormality of CSF immunoglobulin derangements.

Abundant evidence suggests that bands are locally synthesized and that the production of an oligoclonal banding pattern by cultured CSF cells matching that of CSF has been reported. Although IgG is the predominant immunoglobulin isotype in both normal and MS CSF, a small amount of IgM and IgA is also present. Their significance remains unclear. The question of whether oligoclonal bands in MS CSF represent specific or nonspecific B-cell activation is difficult to resolve. CSF certainly demonstrates the latter, but the presence of the former is difficult to exclude. Nonetheless, the presence of IgG bands in MS CSF remains diagnostically useful[84] (see Chapter 4).

CYTOKINES

It might be expected that CSF from patients with MS and ongoing inflammation would show a variety of humoral abnormalities resulting from the inflammatory process, such as circulating cytokine levels. TNF levels have been found to be elevated by some observers, as have levels of TNF receptor and ICAM-1.[157]

EXPERIMENTAL ALLERGIC ENCEPHALOMYELITIS

Experimental allergic encephalomyelitis is the most intensively studied animal model of MS, and many believe the best. A recent Medlar search revealed more than 7000 papers published on this topic! (H. Bauer, personal communication 1993). Acute EAE was first observed in the experimental animal by Rivers and colleagues,[127,128] after repeated injection of a primate with spinal cord material. It was Kabat[68,69] who suggested that EAE may have an autoimmune etiology and that the appropriate autoantigen was located in the white matter. He shrewdly observed that injection of fetal CNS tissue (before myelination) did not cause EAE. How he knew it was not induced by an ontogenetically late-developing antigen is unclear.

This model has evolved considerably over the last few decades, and a number of new developments have made it increasingly relevant to MS. The initial EAE model was uniphasic and resembled acute disseminated encephalomyelitis more than it did MS. The more recent demonstration of the production of chronic progressive and relapsing-remitting disease in small laboratory animals such as the guinea pig,[166] the SJL mouse,[94] and the Lewis rat[143] and the production of MBP-antigen–specific T-cell lines,[14] which can transfer the disease into naive recipients, has provided an enormous stimulus towards understanding the immunopathogenesis of this condition (reviewed by Turnley and colleagues[159]). EAE can be produced in monkeys, mice, rats, guinea pigs and rabbits using a variety of antigen preparations, including whole spinal cord, MBP, PLP,[137] and peptides of these proteins.[96] In most EAE models, inflammation considerably exceeds demyelination, although this is not always made clear. One adoptive transfer model,[165] in which both massive inflammation and demyelination are seen, uses MBP-specific T-cell lines and the simultaneous injection of MOG antibodies.[78]

An increasing number of parallels with MS are evident in these animal models. These include some age restriction for induction, a lowering of the threshold by female hormones, and an association with MHC antigen. Various background genes are clearly important, and these have been mapped.[148] Experimental conditions in which EAE can be relapsing-remitting have been identified. This was initially demonstrated in the SJL strain of mouse by Lublin and colleagues[94] and appears to be related to genetic factors in this strain. Relapses have been seen in strains not usually showing them when the CD8 gene has been "knocked out" by homologous recombination.[73,74] EAE has also been produced in mice lacking CD3 and CD8.[118] The experimental control possible in the small laboratory animal, coupled with advances in laboratory in vitro study T cells, has led to the recognition that MHC-restricted CD4+ cloned T-cell lines specific for MBP or PLP[137,170,171] can adoptively transfer the disease. These experiments unequivocally demonstrate that EAE is T-cell–mediated and have allowed for further exploration of the fine specificities of this T-cell–mediated disorder. One study in which spontaneous EAE was said to develop in transgenic mice bearing only T-cell receptors specific for MBP is difficult to interpret.[47] The pathology was modest and its relation to human disease seems unclear. Although this model seems "unphysiological" and perhaps remote from any naturally occurring circumstance, it has produced interesting information on the effect of environmental factors.

The onset and severity of EAE adoptively transferred with T cells depends on the number of T cells injected. When fewer T cells are injected, the clinical course is milder and of later onset. Some animals injected with small numbers of cells developed relapsing paralysis, whereas other animals suffered a more chronic, unremitting paraplegia.

Encephalitogenic T-cell lines or clones were found to be MHC-restricted and their specificity (the portion of MBP serving as epitope) differed from strain to strain. The question of T-cell receptor usage in EAE induced by MBP has been studied by several groups. Although in some experimental conditions, T-cell receptor usage may be restricted,[1,169] this phenomenon does not appear to be the case among all susceptible strains. Moreover, T-cell receptor usage by effector T cells typically broadens over the period of disease, even in strains where T-cell restriction is said to be present.

These observations on EAE make it less promising that some form of T-cell–specific immunotherapy will be effective in MS. Based on preliminary evidence that T-cell receptor usage in MBP-reactive clones is restricted in patients with MS, attempts have been made to vaccinate patients with MS with T-cell receptor peptides.[160] This program may be premature because not only have other investigators been unable to find common V-region gene usage among patients with MS, but even in highly controlled and short-term experiments with inbred mouse strains, a wide variety of results have been reported. The highly reliable findings of Wekerle and colleagues[165] found no restriction of T-cell receptor usage among MBP-reactive T-cell lines from pa-

tients with MS. Because the T cells of both patients with MS and control subjects appear to react to MBP, it is difficult to understand how the MHC could account for truly restrictive antigen recognition, because individuals have yet to be identified who do not bear MBP-reactive T cells.

EAE has also been a convenient model to study the role of inflammatory cytokines. Cytokine effects and interactions are complex, and the lack of complete understanding of the role and regulation of these molecules is highlighted by the unexpected results not rarely seen in EAE when their levels are altered. For example, one group[17] found that the administration of antibodies to interferon gamma exacerbated EAE instead of producing the expected amelioration, although recent studies from the same group suggest that these antibodies may actually increase the secretion of interferon gamma (A. Billiau, personal communication, 1994).

The availability of EAE as an experimental model has attracted much interest from investigators wishing to screen potential therapeutic agents in this condition. Clinicians treating patients with MS must envy the small animal population, which seems to be readily delivered of their EAE by scores of seemingly unrelated therapies. Molecular dissection of the pathogenesis of EAE has led to a large number of rational and increasingly specific immunologic interventions aimed at interfering with specific steps in the pathway leading to T-cell–mediated tissue injury.[12] However, among the many strategies employed, a bewildering variety of specific and nonspecific therapies are included. These immunotherapies have included monoclonal antibodies against T cells,[22] their subsets, MHC class II antigen, antigen-presenting cells, cytokines, and others. Specific vaccinations with T cells and T-cell lines[13] have worked, but so does immunization with Freund's adjuvant. Many immunomodulators are effective, including interferons, mitogens, and linoleic acid. It seems that all cytotoxic drugs can be effective depending on dosage. However, prostaglandin inhibitors, hormones, physicochemical therapies such as hyperbaric oxygen, coagulation modifiers, dietary manipulations, and many other agents have been shown to be effective in some studies. Indeed, the ease with which EAE can be suppressed contrasts starkly with the modest inroads made by available MS therapies. Nevertheless, several of the therapies first shown to be effective in EAE are completing or beginning human trials.[33,71]

Bemoaning the ubiquity of EAE suppression, a colleague once suggested that even his "Granny's knickers could suppress EAE." It is sobering to realize that not one of the large number of agents that suppress EAE have been shown to alter substantially the long-term natural history of MS.

VIRAL MODELS OF MULTIPLE SCLEROSIS

Viral models of MS are discussed in Chapter 10. Some of these models entail a significant component of the host immune process.[3] Evidence from non-EAE viral infections has demonstrated strong genetic regulation of virus-host interactions.[26] The best characterized of these models is that of Theiler's murine encephalomyelitis virus (TMEV), a picornavirus similar to human poliovirus. After intracerebral innoculation, some susceptible animals develop a progressive demyelinating myelopathy. Susceptibility to the disease correlates with strong delayed-type hypersensitivity mediated by class-II–restricted TMEV-specific T cells. Late demyelination can be prevented by administering cyclophosphamide. This disorder is mediated by both T cells and humoral mechanisms as part of a bystander-induced demyelination.[98]

SUMMARY

The circumstantial and analogical evidence that MS is an autoimmune disease is very strong. The similarity of some EAE models to MS has become increasingly striking, yet a spontaneous model of MS does not exist. Evidence that MS can be transferred by bone marrow cells to immune-deficient mice (SCID), if confirmed, would be the strongest evidence to date that MS is an autoimmune disease, but researchers have had difficulty confirming this finding. Although prevailing concepts of an organ-specific or antigen-specific disease caused by T-cell–mediated injury to myelin-forming cells are short of being proven, they are increasingly supportable.

REFERENCES

1. Acha-Orbea H, Mitchell DJ, Timmerman L, et al: Limited heterogeneity of T cell receptors from receptors from lymphocytes mediating experimental autoimmune encephalomyelitis allows specific immune intervention. Cell 54:263–273, 1988.
2. Adachi K, Kumamoto T, and Araki S: Elevated soluble interleukin-2 receptor levels in patients with active multiple sclerosis. Ann Neurol 28:687–691, 1990.
3. Allen I, and Brankin B: Pathogenesis of multiple sclerosis: The immune diathesis and the role of viruses. J Neuropathol Exp Neurol 5:95–105, 1993.
4. Antel JP, Arnason BGW, and Medof ME: Suppressor cell function in multiple sclerosis: Correlation with clinical disease activity. Ann Neurol 5:338–342, 1979.
5. Archelos JJ, Jung S, Maurer M, et al: Inhibition of experimental autoimmune encephalomyelitis by an antibody to the intercellular adhesion molecule ICAM-1. Ann Neurol 34:145–154, 1993.
6. Arnaiz-Villena A: MHC research: Fast forward. Immunol Today 14:3–5, 1993.
7. Bach MA, Martin C, Cesaro P, Eizenbaum JF, and Degos JD: T cell subsets in multiple sclerosis. A longitudinal study of exacerbating-remitting cases. J Neuroimmunol 7:331–343, 1985.
8. Bach MA, Phan-Dinh-Tuy F, and Tournier E: Deficit of suppressor T cells in active multiple sclerosis. The Lancet 2:1221–1223, 1980.
9. Baig S, Olsson T, Yu-Ping J, Höjeberg B, Cruz M, and Link H: Multiple sclerosis: Cells secreting antibodies against myelin-associated glycoprotein are present in cerebral spinal fluid. Scand J Immunol 33:73–79, 1991.
10. Balkwill F: Cytokines in health and disease. Immunol Today 14:4:149–150, 1993.
11. Baxevanis CN, Reclos GJ, Servis C, et al: Peptides of myelin basic protein stimulate T lymphocytes from patients with multiple sclerosis. J Neuroimmunol 22:23–30, 1989.
12. Bell RB, and Steinman L: Trimolecular interactions in experimental autoimmune demyelinating disease and prospects for immunotherapy. Semin Immunol 3:237–245, 1991.
13. Ben-Nun A, Wekerle H, and Cohen IR: The rapid isolation of clonable antigen specific T-lymphocyte lines capable of mediating autoimmune encephalomyelitis. Eur J Immunol 11:195–199, 1981.
14. Ben-Nun A, Wekerle H, and Cohen IR: Vaccination against autoimmune encephalomyelitis with T-lymphocyte line cells reactive against myelin basic protein. Nature 292:181–183, 1981.

15. Benczur M, Petranyi GG, Palffy G, et al: Dysfunction of natural killer cells in multiple sclerosis: A possible pathogenetic factor. Clin Exp Immunol 39:657–666, 1980.

16. Benoist C, and Mathis D: Positive selection of the T cell repertoire: Where and when does it occur? Cell 58:1027–1033, 1989.

17. Billiau A, Heremans H, Vanderkerckhove F, et al: Enhancement of experimental allergic encephalomyelitis in mice by antibodies against IFN-γ. J Immunol 140:1506–1510, 1988.

18. Bloom BR, Modlin RL, and Salgame P: Stigma variations: Observations on suppressor T-cells and leprosy. Ann Rev Immunol 10:453–488, 1992.

19. Bloom BR, Salgame P, and Diamond B: Revisiting and revising suppressor T-cell. Immunol Today 13:131–136, 1992.

20. Bos JD, and Kapsenberg ML: The skin immune system: Progress in cutaneous biology. Immunol Today 14:2:75–78, 1993.

21. Bottazzo GF, Dean BM, McNally JM, MacKay EH, Swift PGF, and Gamble DR: In situ characterization of autoimmune phenomena and expression of HLA molecules in the pancreas in diabetic insulitis. N Engl J Med 313:353–360, 1985.

22. Brostoff SW, and Mason PW: Experimental allergic encephalomyelitis: Successful treatment in vitro with a monoclonal antibody that recognizes T helper cells. J Immunol 133:1938–1942, 1984.

23. Burke F, Naylor MS, Davies B, and Balkwill F: The cytokine wall chart. Immunol Today 14:165–170, 1993.

24. Burrow GN: Maternal-fetal consideration in hyperthyroidism. Clinics in Endocrinology and Metabolism 7:115–125, 1978.

25. Campbell IL, Kay TW, Oxbrow L, and Harrison LC: Essential role for interferon-gamma and interleukin-6 in autoimmune insulin-dependent diabetes in NOD/Wehi mice. J Clin Invest 87:739–742, 1991.

26. Chesebro B, Miyazawa M, and Britt WJ: Host genetic control of spontaneous and induced immunity to friend murine retrovirus infection. Ann Rev Immunol 8:477–499, 1990.

27. Chofflon M, Weiner HL, Morimoto C, and Hafler DA: Decrease of suppressor inducer (CD4 + 2H4+) T cells in multiple sclerosis cerebrospinal fluid. Ann Neurol 25:494–499, 1989.

28. Colten HR, and Rosen FS: Complement deficiencies (review article). Ann Rev Immunol 10: 809–834, 1992.

29. Cruz M, Olsson T, Ernerudh J, Höjeberg B, and Link H: Immunoblot detection of oligoclonal anti-myelin basic protein IgG antibodies in cerebrospinal fluid in multiple sclerosis. Neurology 37:1987.

30. Cunningham ET Jr, and de Souza EB: Interleukin 1 receptors in the brain and endocrine tissues. Immnol Today 14:171–176, 1993.

31. Dinanrello C: Modalities for reducing interleukin 1 in disease. Immunol Today 14:260–264, 1993.

32. Duqeutte P: Hormonal factors in susceptibility to multiple sclerosis. Current Opinion in Neurology and Neurosurgery 6:195–201, 1993.

33. Ebers GC: Treatment of multiple sclerosis. The Lancet 343:275–279, 1994.

34. Ebers GC, and Sadovnick AD: The role of genetic factors in multiple sclerosis susceptibility: A critical review. J Neuroimmunol 54:1–17, 1994.

35. Fagnart OC, Sindic CJM, and Laterre C: Free kappa and lambda light chain levels in the cerebrospinal fluid of patients with multiple sclerosis and other neurological diseases. J Neuroimmunol 19:119–132, 1988.

36. Farrell MA, Kaufmann JCE, Gilbert JJ, Noseworthy JH, Armstrong HA, and Ebers GC: Oligoclonal bands in multiple sclerosis: Clinical-pathologic correlation. Neurology 35:212–218, 1985.

37. Feagan BG, McDonald JW, Rochon J, et al: Low dose cyclosporine for the treatment of Crohn's disease. N Engl J Med 330:1846–1851, 1994.

38. Felgenhauer K: Protein filtration and secretion at human body fluid barriers. Pflugers Arch 384: 9–17, 1980.

39. Felgenhauer K: The blood-brain barrier redefined. J Neurol 233:193–194, 1986.

40. Fredrickson S, Michelsberg J, Hillert J, et al: Conjugal multiple sclerosis: Immunogenetic characterization and analysis of T and B cell reactivity to myelin proteins. Neurology 42:577–582, 1992.

41. Frederickson S, Sun JB, Huang WX, Li BL, Olssons T, and Link H: Cord blood contains high numbers of autoimmune T-cells recognizing multiple myelin proteins and acetylcholine receptor. J Immunol 151:2217–2224, 1993.

42. Frei K, Fredrikson S, Fontana A, and Link H: Interleukin-6 is elevated in plasma in multiple sclerosis. J Neuroimmunol 31:147–153, 1990.

43. Fujinami RS, and Oldstone MBA: Amino acid homology between the encephalitogenic site of myelin basic protein and virus: Mechanism for autoimmunity. Science 230:1043–1045, 1985.

44. Gearing AJH, and Newman W: Circulating adhesion molecules in disease. Immunol Today 14: 506–512, 1993.

45. Golaz J, Steck A, and Moretta L: Activated T lymphocytes in patients with multiple sclerosis. Neurology 33:1371–1373, 1983.

46. Goust JM, Hoffmann PM, Pryjma J, Hogan EL, and Fudenberg HH: Defective immunoregulation in multiple sclerosis. Ann Neurol 8:526–533, 1980.

47. Goverman J, Woods A, Larson L, Weiner LP, Hood L, and Zaller DM: Transgenic mice that express a myelin basic protein-specific T cell receptor develop spontaneous autoimmunity. Cell 72: 551–560, 1993.

48. Hafler DA, Duby AD, Lee SJ, Benjamin D, Seideman JG, and Weiner HL: Oligoclonal T lymphocytes in the cerebrospinal fluid of patients with multiple sclerosis. J Exp Med 167:1313–1322, 1988.

49. Hafler DA, Fox DA, Manning ME, Schlossman SF, Reinherz EL, and Weiner HL: In vivo activated T lymphocytes in the peripheral blood and cerebrospinal fluid of patients with multiple sclerosis. N Engl J Med 312:1405–1411, 1988.

50. Halawa I, Lolli F, and Link H: Terminal component of complement C9 in CSF and plasma of patients with MS and aseptic meningitis. Acta Neurol Scand 80:130–135, 1989.

51. Hanson GC, and Ghosh S: Systemic lupus erythematosus and pregnancy. BMJ 2:1227, 1965.

52. Hartung HP, Hughes RAC, Taylor WA, Heininger K, Reiners K, and Toyka KV: T cell activation in Guillain-Barré syndrome and in MS: elevated serum levels of soluble IL-2 receptors. Neurology 40:215–218, 1990.

53. Hartung HP, Michels M, Reiners K, Seeldrayers P, Archelos JJ, and Toyka KV: Soluble ICAM-1 serum levels in multiple sclerosis and viral encephalitis. Neurology 43:2331–2335, 1993.

54. Hauser SL, Ault KA, Levin MJ, Garovoy MR, and Weiner HL: Natural killer cell activity in multiple sclerosis. J Immun 127:1114–1117, 1981.

55. Hayglass K, and Stefura W: Anti-interferon-gamma treatment blocks the ability of glutaraldehyde-polymerized allergens to inhibit IgE responses. J Exp Med 173:279–285, 1991.

56. Hedrick SM, Germain RN, Bevan MJ, et al: Rearrangement and transcription of a T-cell receptor β-chain gene in different T-cell subsets. Proc Nat Acad Sci USA 82:531–535, 1985.

57. Hemler ME: VLA proteins in the integrin family: Structures, functions, and their role on leukocytes. Ann Rev Immunol 8:365–380, 1990.

58. Higuchi Y, Herrera P, Muniesa P, et al: Expression of a tumor necrosis factor-transgene in murine pancreatic β cells results in severe and permanent insulitis without evolution toward diabetes. J Exp Med 176:1719–1731, 1992.

59. Hillert J, and Olerup O: Germ-line polymorphism of TCR genes and disease susceptibility: Fact or hypothesis? Immunol Today 13:47–49, 1992.

60. Huddlestone JR, and Oldstone MBA: T suppressor (Tg) lymphocytes fluctuate in parallel with changes in the clinical course of patients with multiple sclerosis. J Immunol 123:1615–1618, 1979.

61. Huddlestone JR, and Oldstone MBA: Suppressor T cells are activated in vivo in patients with multiple sclerosis coinciding with remission from acute attack. J Immunol 129:915–917, 1982.

62. Ibrahim MA, Chain BM, and Katz DR: The injured cell: The role of the dendritic cell system as a sentinel receptor pathway (review article). Immunol Today 16:181–186, 1995.

63. Ilonen J, Nurmi T, Reunanen M, and Salmi A: NK activity and NK-like non-specific cytolysis after PPD, rubella and measles antigen stimulation in multiple sclerosis. J Neurol Sci 77:77–85, 1987.

64. Inrcke NS, Wrenshall LE, Lindman BJ, and Platt JL: Role of heparan sulfate in immune system-blood vessel interactions. Immunol Today 14:500–505, 1993.

65. Ishida H, Muchamuel T, Sakaguchi S, Andrade S, Menon S, and Howard M: Continuous administration of anti-interleukin 10 antibodies delays onset of autoimmunity in NZB/W F1 mice. J Exp Med 179:305–310, 1994.

66. Jingwu Z, Medaer R, Hashim GA, Chin Y, van den Berg-Loonen E, and Raus JCM: Myelin basic protein-specific T lymphocytes in multiple sclerosis and controls: precursor frequency, fine specificity, and cyotoxicity. Ann Neurol 32:330–338, 1992.

67. Kabat EA, Glusman M, and Knaub V: Quantitative estimation of the albumin and gamma globulin in normal and pathologic cerebrospinal fluid by immunochemical methods. Am J Med 4:653–662, 1948.

68. Kabat EA, Wolf A, and Bezer AE: The rapid production of acute disseminated encephalomyelitis in Rhesus monkeys by injection of brain tissue with adjuvants. Science 104:362–363, 1946.

69. Kabat EA, Wolf A, and Bezer AE: The rapid production of acute disseminated encephalomyelitis in Rheusus monkeys by injection of heterozygous and homologous brain tissue with adjuvants. J Exp Med 85:117–129, 1947.

70. Kappler JW, Roehm N, and Marrack P: T cell tolerance by clonal elimination in the thymus. Cell 49:273–280, 1987.

71. Karussis DM, Lehmann D, Slavin S, et al: Inhibition of acute, experimental autoimmune encephalomyelitis by the synthetic immunomodulator linomide. Ann Neurol 34:654–660, 1993.

72. Kastrukoff LE, and Paty DW: A serial study of peripheral blood T lymphocyte subsets in relapsing-remitting multiple sclerosis. Ann Neurol 15:250–256, 1984.

73. Koh DR, Ho A, Ramentulla A, Peninger J, and Mak TW: Experimental allergic encephalomyelitis (EAE) in mice lacking CD4 and T cells. Eur J Immunol 24:2250–2253, 1994.

74. Koh DR, Fung-Leung WP, Ho A, Gray D, Acha-Orbea H, and Mak TW: Less mortality but more relapses in EAE in Cd8 -/- mice. Science 256:1210–1213, 1992.

75. Kühn R, Löhler J, Rennick D, Rajewsky K, and Müller W: Interleukin-10 deficient mice develop chronic enterocolitis. Cell 75:263–274, 1993.

76. Lahita RG, Bradlaw HL, Ginzler E, Pang S, and New M: Low plasma androgen in women with systemic lupus erythematosus. Arthritis Rheum 30:241–248, 1987.

77. Lando Z, Teitelbaum P, and Arnon R: Effect of cyclophosphamide on suppressor cell activity in mice unresponsive to EAE. J Immunol 123:2156–2160, 1979.

78. Lassmann H, Brunner C, Bradl M, and Linington C: Experimental allergic encephalomyelitis: The balance between encephalitogenic T lymphocytes and demyelinating antibodies determines size and structure of demyelinated lesions. Acta Neuropathol (Berl) 75:566–576, 1988.

79. Laterre EC: Les proteines du liquid cephalo-rachidien a l'etat normal et pathologique. Brussels, Edition Arscia, 1965.

80. Link H: Immunoglobulin G and low molecular weight proteins in human cerebrospinal fluid: Chemical and immunological characterization with special reference to multiple sclerosis. Acta Neurol Scand 43(suppl 28):1–136, 1967.

81. Link H: CSF IgG and its congeners. In Thompson EJ (ed): Advances in CSF Protein Research and Diagnosis. MTP Press, Lancaster, England, 1987.

82. Link H: Immunological abnormalities in the cerebrospinal fluid in multiple sclerosis. Current Opinion in Neurology and Neurosurgery 3:199–203, 1990.

83. Link H, Baig S, Olsson O, Yu-Ping J, Höjeberg B, and Olsson T: Persistent anti-myelin basic protein IgG antibody response in multiple sclerosis

cerebrospinal fluid. J Neuroimmunol 28:237–248, 1990.

84. Link H, and Kostulas V: Utility of isoelectric focusing of cerebrospinal fluid and serum on agarose evaluated for neurological patients. Clin Chem 29:810–825, 1983.

85. Link H, Olsson O, Sun JB, et al: Acetycholine receptor-reactive T and B cells in myasthenia gravis and controls. J Clin Invest 87:2191–2196, 1991.

86. Link H, and Zettervall O: Multiple sclerosis: Disturbed kappa-lambda chain ratio of immunoglobulin G in cerebrospinal fluid. Clin Exp Immunol 6:435–438, 1970.

87. Link J, He B, Navikas V, et al: Transforming growth factor-beta 1 suppresses auto-antigen induced expression of proinflammatory cytokines but not of interleukin-10 in multiple sclerosis and myasthenia gravis. J Neuroimmunol 58: 21–35, 1995.

88. Link J, Navikas V, Yu M, Fredrikson S, Osterman P, and Link H: Augmented interferon-gamma, interleukin-4, and transforming growth factor beta RNA expression in blood mononuclear cells in myasthenia gravis. J Neuroimmunol 51:185–192, 1994.

89. Link J, Söderström L, Ljungdahl A, et al: Organspecific autoantigens induce IFN-γ and IL-4 mRNA expression in mononuclear cells in multiple sclerosis and myasthenia gravis. Neurology 44:728–734, 1994.

90. Link J, Söderström M, Olsson T, et al: Increased transforming growth factor-beta, interleukin-4 and interferon-gamma in multiple sclerosis. Ann Neurol 36:379–386, 1994.

91. Lisak RP, and Zweiman B: In vitro cell-mediated immunity of cerebrospinal fluid lymphocytes to myelin basic protein in primary demyelinating diseases. N Engl J Med 297:850–853, 1977.

92. Lowenthal A, Van Sande M, and Karcher D: The differential diagnosis of neurological diseases by fractionating electrophoretically the CSF gamma globulins. J Neurochem 6:51–56, 1960.

93. Lubetzki C, Lombrail P, Hauw JJ, and Zalc B: Multiple sclerosis: rat and human oligodendrocytes are not the target for CSF immunoglobulins. Neurology 36:524–528, 1986.

94. Lublin FD, Maurer PH, Berry RG, and Tippett D: Delayed relapsing experimental allergic encephalomyelitis in mice. J Immunol 126:819–822, 1981.

95. Maimone D, and Reder AT: Soluble CD8 levels in the CSF and serum of patients with multiple sclerosis. Neurology 41:851–854, 1991.

96. Martin R, McFarland HF, and McFarlin DL: Immunological aspects of demyelinating diseases. Annu Rev Immunol 10:153–187, 1992.

97. Merrill J, Jondal M, Seeley J, Ullberg M, and Siden A: Decreased NK killing in patients with multiple sclerosis: An analysis on the level of the single effector cell in peripheral blood and cerebrospinal fluid in relation to the activity of the disease. Clin Exp Immunol 47:419–430, 1982.

98. Miller SD, Gerety SJ, Kennedy MK, et al: Class II-restricted T cell responses in Theiler's murine encephalomyelitis virus (TMEV)-induced demyelinating disease. III. Failure of neuroantigen-specific immune tolerance to affect the clinical course of demyelination. J Neuroimmunol 26:9–23, 1990.

99. Mix E, Olsson T, Correale J, et al: B cells expressing CD5 are increased in cerebrospinal fluid of patients with multiple sclerosis. Clin Exp Immunol 79:21–27, 1990.

100. Mombaerts P, Mizoguchi E, Grusby MJ, Glimcher LH, Bhan AK, and Tonegawa S: Spontaneous development of inflammatory bowel disease in T cell receptor mutant mice. Cell 75:275–282, 1993.

101. Morgan BP, Campbell AK, and Compston DAS: Terminal component of complement (C9) in cerebrospinal fluid of patients with multiple sclerosis. The Lancet 2:251–254, 1984.

102. Morimoto C, Hafler DA, Weiner HL, et al: Selective loss of the suppressor-induced T-cell subset in progressive multiple sclerosis: Analysis with anti-2H4 monoclonal antibody. N Engl J Med 316:67–72, 1987.

103. Moss PA, Rosenberg WM, and Bell J: The human T-cell receptor in health and disease. Annu Rev Immunol 10:71–96, 1992.

104. Naparstek Y, and Platz PH: The role of autoantibodies in autoimmune disease. Annu Rev Immunol 11:79–104, 1993.

105. Neighbour PA, Grayzel AI, and Miller AE: Endogenous and interferon-augmented natural killer cell activity of human peripheral blood mononuclear cells in vitro: Studies of patients with multiple sclerosis, systemic lupus erythematosus or rheumatoid arthritis. Clin Exp Immunol 49:11–21, 1982.

106. Nepom GT, and Erlich H: MHC Class II molecules and autoimmunity. Annu Rev Immunol 9:493–525, 1991.

107. Nordal HJ, Vandvik B, and Norrby E: Demonstration of electrophoretically restricted virus-specific antibodies in serum and cerebrospinal fluid by imprint electroimmunofixation. Scand J Immunol 7:381–388, 1978.

108. Norrby E: Viral antibodies in multiple sclerosis. Prog Med Virol 24:1–39, 1978.

109. Nygard NR, McCarthy DM, Schiffenbauer J, and Schwartz BD: Mixed haplotypes and autoimmunity. Immunol Today 14:2:53–56, 1993.

110. Oger JJF, Arnason BGW, Wray SH, and Kistler JP: A study of B and T cells in multiple sclerosis. Neurology 25:444–447, 1975.

111. Oger JJF, Kastrukoff L, Li DKB, et al: Multiple sclerosis: In relapsing-remitting patients immune functions vary with disease activity as assessed by MRI. Neurology 38:1739–1744, 1988.

112. Oger J, Antel JP, and Arnason BGW: Studies of immune regulation in MS using mAb against T cell subsets. In Kuroiwa Y and Kurhand LT (ed): Multiple Sclerosis: East and West. Kyushu University Press, Fukuoka, 1982.

113. Olsson T: Immunology of multiple sclerosis. Current Opinion Neurology Neurosurgery 5:195–202, 1992.

114. Olsson T, Baig S, Höjeberg B, and Link H: Antimyelin basic protein and antimyelin antibody-producing cells in multiple sclerosis. Ann Neurol 27:132–136, 1990.

115. Olsson T, Sun JB, Solders G, et al: Autoreactive T and B cell responses to myelin antigens after diagnostic sural nerve biopsy. J Neurol Sci 117(1–2):130–139, 1993.

116. Olsson T, Zhi WW, Höjeberg B, et al: Autoreactive T lymphocytes in multiple sclerosis determined by antigen-induced secretion of interferon-gamma. J Clin Invest 86:981–985, 1990.

117. Osterland CK, Miller EJ, Karakawa WW, and Krause RM: Characteristics of streptococcal group-specific antibody isolated from hyperimmune rabbits. J Exp Med 123:599–614, 1966.

118. Penninger JM, Neu N, Timms E, et al: Induction of experimental autoimmune myocarditis in mice lacking CD3 or CD3 molecules. J Exp Med 178:1837–1842, 1993.

119. Pette M, Fujita K, Kitze B, et al: Myelin basic protein-specific T lymphocyte lines from MS patients and healthy individuals. Neurology 40:1770–1776, 1990.

120. Polman CH, Matthaei I, de Groot CJA, Koetsier JC, Sminia T, and Dijkstra CD: Low-dose cyclosporin A induces relapsing-remitting experimental allergic encephalomyelitis in the Lewis rat. J Neuroimmun 17:209–216, 1988.

121. Pozzilli P, Signore A, Williams AJK, and Beales PE: NOD mouse colonies around the world: Recent facts and figures. Immunol Today 14: 193–196, 1993.

122. Reder AT, and Arnason BGW. Immunology of multiple sclerosis. In Koetsier JC (ed): Handbook of Clinical Neurology, Vol 47, Demyelinating Diseases. Elsevier, New York, 1985.

123. Reinherz EL, Weiner HL, Hauser SL, Cohen JA, Distaso JA, and Schlossman SF: Loss of suppressor T cells in active multiple sclerosis. N Engl J Med 303:125–129, 1980.

124. Repke J, and Klein V: Myasthenia gravis in pregnancy. In Goldstein PJ (ed): Neurological Disorders of Pregnancy. Futura Publishing, Mt Kisco, New York, 1986.

125. Rice GPA, Finney D, Braheny SL, Knobler RL, Sipe JC, and Oldstone MBA: Disease activity markers in multiple sclerosis: Another look at suppressor cells defined by monoclonal antibodies OKT4, OKT5 and OKT8. J Neuroimmunol 6:75–84, 1984.

126. Richert JR, Robinson ED, Johnson AH, et al: Heterogeneity of the T-cell receptor β gene rearrangements generated in myelin basic protein-specific T-cell clones isolated from a patient with multiple sclerosis. Ann Neurol 29:299–306, 1991.

127. Rivers TM, and Schwentker FF: Encephalomyelitis accompanied by myelin destruction experimentally produced in monkeys. J Exp Med 61:689–702, 1935.

128. Rivers TM, Sprunt DH, and Berry GP: Observations on attempts to produce acute disseminated encephalomyelitis in monkeys. J Exp Med 58:39–53, 1933.

129. Rodriguez M, Wynn DR, Kimlinger TK, and Katzmann JA: Terminal component of complement (C9) in the cerebrospinal fluid of patients with multiple sclerosis and neurologic controls. Neurology 40:855–857, 1990.

130. Rohowsky-Kochan C, Eiman D, Troiano R, et al: Decreased suppressor-inducer T lymphocytes in multiple sclerosis and other neurological diseases. J Neuroimmunol 28:161–166, 1990.

131. Rose NR, and Bona C: Defining criteria for autoimmune diseases (Witebsky's postulates revisited). Immunol Today 14:426–430, 1993.

132. Rotteveel FTM, Kokkelink I, van Walbeek HK, Polman CH, van Dongen JJM, and Lucas CJ: Analysis of T cell receptor-gene rearrangement in T cells from the cerebrospinal fluid of patients with multiple sclerosis. J Neuroimmunol 15:243–249, 1987.

133. Rotteveel FTM, Kuenen B, Kokkelink I, Meager A, and Lucas CJ: Relative increase of inflammatory CD4+ T cells in the cerebrospinal fluid of multiple sclerosis patients and control individuals. Clin Exp Immunol 79:15–20, 1990.

134. Rudick RA, Peter DR, Bidlack JM, and Knutson DW: Multiple sclerosis: Free light chains in cerebrospinal fluid. Neurology 35:1443–1449, 1985.

135. Sadlack B, Merz H, Schorle H, Schimpl A, Feller AC, and Horak I: Ulcerative colitis-like disease in mice with a disrupted interleukin-2 gene. Cell 75: 253–261, 1993.

136. Salonen R, Illonen J, Jageroos H, Syrjala H, Nurmi T, and Reunanen M: Lymphocyte subsets in the cerebrospinal fluid in active multiple sclerosis. Ann Neurol 25:500–502, 1989.

137. Satoh J, Sakai K, Endoh M, et al: Experimental allergic encephalomyelitis mediated by murine encephalitogenic T cell lines specific for myelin proteolipid apoprotein. J Immunol 138:179–184, 1987.

138. Scolozzi R, Boccafogli A, Tola M, et al: T-cell phenotypic profiles in the cerebrospinal fluid and peripheral blood of multiple sclerosis patients. J Neurol Sci 108:93–98, 1992.

139. Selmaj K, Raine CS, Cannella B, and Brosnan CF: Identification of lymphotoxin and tumor necrosis factor in multiple sclerosis lesions. J Clin Invest 87:949–954, 1991.

140. Smith HR, and Steinberg AD: Autoimmunity: A perspective. Annu Rev Immunol 1:175–210, 1984.

141. Smith RE, Godfrey WA, and Kimura SJ: Chronic cyclites. I. Course and visual prognosis. Transactions of the American Academy of Ophthalmology and Otolaryngology 77:760–768, 1973.

142. Söderström M, Link H, Sun JB, et al: T cells recognizing multiple peptides of myelin basic protein are found in blood and enriched in cerebrospinal fluid in optic neuritis and multiple sclerosis. Scand J Immunol 37:355–368, 1993.

143. Stanley GP, and Pender MP: The pathophysiology of chronic relapsing experimental allergic encephalomyelitis in the Lewis rat. Brain 114: 1827–1853, 1991.

144. Steinman L, Oksenberg JR, and Bernard CCA: Association of susceptibility to multiple sclerosis with TCR genes. Immunol Today 13:49–51, 1992.

145. Strober W, and Ehrhardt RO: Chronic intestinal inflammation: an unexpected outcome in cytokine or T cell receptor mutant mice. Cell 75: 203–205, 1993.

146. Sun JB, Olsson T, Wang WZ, et al: Autoreactive T and B cells responding to proteolipid protein in

multiple sclerosis and controls. Eur J Immunol 21:1461–1468, 1991.

147. Sun J, Link H, Olsson T, et al: T and B cell responses to myelin-oligodendrocyte glycoprotein in multiple sclerosis. J Immunology 146:1490–1495, 1991.

148. Sundvall M, Jirholt J, Yang HT, et al: Identification of murine loci associated with susceptibility to chronic experimental autoimmune encephalomyelitis. Nat Genet 10:313–317, 1995.

149. Svenningsson A, Hansson GK, Andersen O, Andersson R, Patarroyo M, and Stemme S: Adhesion molecule expression on cerebrospinal fluid T lymphocytes: Evidence for common recruitment mechanisms in multiple sclerosis, aseptic meningitis, and normal controls. Ann Neurol 34:155–161, 1993.

150. Thompson EJ (ed): Advances in CSF protein research and diagnosis. MTP Press, Lancaster, England, 1987.

151. Tincani A, Balestrieri G, Faden D, and DiMario C: Systemic lupus erythematosus in pregnancy. The Lancet 2:756–757, 1991.

152. Tjernlund U, Cesaro P, Tournier E, Degos JD, Bach JF, and Bach MA: T cell subsets in multiple sclerosis: A comparative study between cell surface antigens and function. Clin Immunol Immunopath 32:185–197, 1984.

153. Tourtellotte WW: The cerebrospinal fluid in multiple sclerosis. In Koetsier JC (ed): Handbook of Clinical Neurology, Vol 47, Demyelinating diseases. New York, Elsevier, 1985.

154. Tourtellotte WW, Potvin AR, Flemming JO, et al: Multiple sclerosis: Measurement and validation of central nervous system IgG synthesis rate. Neurology 30:240–244, 1980.

155. Trotter JL, Collins KG, and van der Veen RC: Serum cytokine levels in chronic progressive multiple sclerosis: Interleukin 2 levels parallel tumor necrosis factor-alpha levels. J. Neuroimmunol 33:29–36, 1991.

156. Trowsdale J, Ragoussis J, and Campbell RD: Map of the human MHC. Immunol Today 12:443–446, 1991.

157. Tsukada N, Matsuda M, Miyagi K, and Yanagisawa N: Increased levels of intercellular adhesion molecule-1 (ICAM-1) and tumor necrosis factor receptor in the cerebrospinal fluid of patients with multiple sclerosis. Neurology 43:2679–2682, 1993.

158. Tsukada N, Miyagi K, Matsuda M, and Yanagisawa N: Increased levels of circulating intercellular adhesion molecule-1 in multiple sclerosis and human T-lymphotropic virus type 1-associated myelopathy. Ann Neurol 33:646–649, 1993.

159. Turnley AM, Morahan G, Okano H, et al: Dysmyelination in transgenic mice resulting from expression of class I histocompatibility molecules in oligodendrocytes. Nature 353:566–569, 1991.

160. Vandenbark A, Hashim G, and Offner H: Immunization with synthetic T cell receptor V-region peptide protects against experimental autoimmune encephalomyelitis. Nature 341:541–544, 1989.

161. Vandvik B, Natvig JB, and Wiger D: IgGl subclass restriction of oligoclonal IgG from cerebrospinal fluid and brain extracts in patients with multiple sclerosis and subacute encephalitides. Scand J Immunol 5:427–436, 1976.

162. Varner MW: Autoimmune disorders and pregnancy. Semin Perinatol 15:238–250, 1991.

163. Walsh MJ, and Tourtellotte WW: Temporal invariance and clonal uniformity of brain and cerebrospinal IgG, IgA, and IgM in multiple sclerosis. J Exp Med 163:41–53, 1986.

164. Wang WZ, Olsson T, Kostulas V, Höjeberg B, Erke HP, and Link H: Myelin antigen reactive T cells in cerebrovascular disease. Clin Exp Immunol 88:157–162, 1992.

165. Wekerle H, Kojima K, Lannes-Vieira J, Lassmann H, and Linington C: Animal models (review article). Ann Neurol 36(suppl):S47–S53, 1994.

166. Wisniewski HM, and Madrid RE: Chronic progressive experimental allergic encephalomyelitis (EAE) in adult guinea pigs. J Neuropathol Exp Neurol 42:243–255, 1983.

167. Yki-Jarvinen H, and Koivisto VA: Natural course of insulin resistance in type I diabetes. N Engl J Med 315:224–230, 1986.

168. Young RA: Stress proteins and immunology. Annu Rev Immunol 8:401–420, 1990.

169. Zamvil SS, Mitchell DJ, Lee NE, et al: Predominant expression of a T cell receptor VB gene subfamily in autoimmune encephalomyelitis. J Exp Med 167:1586–1596, 1988.

170. Zamvil SS, Nelson P, Mitchell D, Knobler R, Fritz R, and Steinman L: Encephalitogenic T-cell clones specific for myelin basic protein: An unusual bias in antigen recognition. J Exp Med 162:2107–2124, 1985.

171. Zamvil SS, Nelson P, Trotter J, Mitchell D, Knobler R, and Fritz R: T-cell clones specific for myelin basic protein induce chronic relapsing paralysis and demyelination. Nature 317:355–358, 1985.

CHAPTER 12

MANAGEMENT OF MULTIPLE SCLEROSIS AND INTERPRETATION OF CLINICAL TRIALS

Donald W. Paty, MD
Stanley A. Hashimoto, MD
George C. Ebers, MD

PRINCIPLES OF MANAGEMENT

Few diseases provide a greater challenge to the intellectual and humanitarian resources of the physician than the long-term management of MS. In this chapter, we outline our present approach to caring for patients with this disease and review some recent therapeutic trials. Recent developments have changed the perception of MS from a nontreatable to a partially treatable disease, making this time an optimistic one for MS in general.

Conveying the Diagnosis

Receiving the diagnosis of MS represents a seminal moment in a patient's life. The

427

manner in which the diagnosis is conveyed has important long-term consequences for the patient's relationship with the individual physician and often with the medical profession in general. Furthermore, it influences the patient's attitudes toward living with the disease in the future. It is a particularly challenging task because of the spectrum of approaches demanded by the innate variability of human behavior. We propose certain guidelines based on both our experience and on formal surveys of patients with MS.

Proper management of MS of course presupposes an accurate diagnosis (see Chapter 4). If the physician is certain of the diagnosis, patients consistently state their desire to know the diagnosis and to understand its implications. Even if the diagnosis of MS is only suspected, 70 percent of patients wish to know the diagnosis.[213] When patients do not directly ask about their diagnosis, it is often because of fear and anticipation, and these patients should be offered the opportunity to obtain this information. What is said and how it is said can tax the skill of the wisest practitioner of the art of medicine.

Awareness of the patient's personality, circumstance, and background are critical. The way the physician approaches the patient with the possible diagnosis of MS will depend on factors such as age, psychological state, marital status, and future plans regarding career and family. The following examples illustrate two of the problems that can be encountered:

CASE HISTORY: Long-Term Consequences of Not Being Told the Diagnosis

A 20-year-old male community college student developed remitting diplopia and a numb leg. Examination showed an internuclear ophthalmoplegia and extensor plantar response. He was told that he had "a virus" and would get better, which indeed he did. However, in his dictated report, the examining neurologist made a diagnosis of MS. In the meantime, the student pursued his studies in watchmaking. Seven years later when the second attack of optic neuritis (ON) left him with unremitting visual loss, he was told that he had MS and that his initial attack 7 years previously had been his first symptom of the dis-

ease. He was angry and litigious because he said if he had known the diagnosis and implications of MS, he would never have become a watchmaker, a task requiring excellent optic nerve and sensory/motor function of the upper extremities. This story ends on a happy note, however, with the patient finding employment in a nearby Mennonite community, selling and repairing old-style clocks with large movements.

CASE HISTORY: Long-Term Consequences of Being Told the Diagnosis Early

A 40-year-old nurse had had a remitting useless hand syndrome 8 years previously and was seen complaining of weakness in the left foot extensor of several weeks' duration. Physical examination and further investigation supported a diagnosis of MS. The patient seemed to accept this diagnosis with equanimity. Unfortunately, the woman developed a severe depression with persistent fears and images of being bedridden and confined to a nursing home. The depression was unresponsive to antidepressants. She became anhedonic, her marriage floundered, and it took her almost 5 years to recover from this uncharacteristic decline. When seen 5 years later, she had no neurological signs but continued to be troubled by fears of incontinence, nursing home placement, and other phobic preoccupations. Her premorbid personality, according to her family, gave little indication of this outcome, although the family had informed her physicians that she had cared for a bedridden patient with MS as a private-duty nurse for 1 year. She and her husband were particularly distressed that she had been told of her MS, the knowledge of which "ruined several healthy years of my life."

Although these case histories illustrate two extremes, they demonstrate the difficulty in posing absolute rules on how to approach the difficult issue of when to reveal the diagnosis. Not all patients' rights advocates, who demand full disclosure of every patient's illness, realize that conveying a diagnosis of MS in the absence of disability may lead to a reduction in quality of life equal to moderate physical disability.

In general, patients wish to be told their diagnosis by their neurologist in private without the presence of other patients or house staff. Many patients are so shocked that they can later recall nothing of the interview. For this reason, patients should be asked at a later date what they recall about the initial interview. A spouse, family member, or friend should be present at the first and subsequent meetings. Patients should also be asked what they know about MS because experience has shown that any prior exposure or knowledge heavily influences their subsequent attitude toward the disease. The physician should give the information in an honest and compassionate way and convey the feeling of having as much time as the patient needs. A subsequent interview with a medical social worker or a nurse knowledgeable about MS may also help to clear up many issues that later come to patients' minds. It allows the patients to ask questions that they may be reluctant to ask the physician. The physician should caution patients that only some literature on MS provided by the MS Society and other sources is appropriate for the newly diagnosed patient with little disability. Written literature should never substitute for the personal interview. The physician should give patients hope that their individual outlook may be benign, that research will eventually find a cure, and that a good chance exists that major advances will occur before their offspring are at signifi-

cant risk (see Chapter 3). We often tell patients that the first 6 to 12 months are the most difficult because most patients interpret every slip, stagger, clumsy act, or episode of numbness as a sign that "the axe is falling." Usually after a year or so, most patients stop paying undue attention to such symptoms and can adjust to getting on with their life.

Counseling the Patient

Education is the critical component of patient management in the early stages of MS. From the first discussion onward, the physician has the responsibility to give clear and factual information both to the patient and to the family. This approach encourages the patient and family to ask questions and to participate in discussions about the disease. It also protects the patient by providing information about medical and nonmedical aspects and ramifications of having MS.

The most frequently asked questions about MS relate to prognosis, genetic influence, possible infectivity, precipitating events for relapses, effects of heat, effects of pregnancy, and the advisability of immunizations (Table 12–1). Patients may feel uncomfortable posing fundamental ques-

Table 12–1. COMMON QUESTIONS PATIENTS ASK ABOUT MULTIPLE SCLEROSIS*

Prognosis:	What can I expect for my future in terms of life span, quality of life, employability, and new symptoms?
Genetics:	Can I pass MS on to my children?
Pregnancy:	What are the effects of pregnancy on my MS?
Possible infectivity:	Can others—my husband, for example—catch MS from me?
Precipitating events for relapses:	What must I avoid to minimize relapses?
Heat sensitivity:	Why do I get so weak on hot days or after a hot shower or bath?
Immunizations:	Should I have vaccinations or other immunizations?
Diet and lifestyle:	Should I follow any particular diet or lifestyle?
Treatment:	Should I take interferon beta? If so, which form?

*See text discussion for answers.

tions related to their future, such as the potential impact of MS on their job and career, long-term impairment, health insurance, and mortgage and life insurance. Patients should be warned about the types of concerns and feelings that may be experienced by their parents, spouse, and children. Another important topic is how to deal with solicited and unsolicited advice from nonprofessionals. Taking time to address patients' concerns about MS will build a strong foundation for effective long-term patient management.

The diagnosis of MS can engender considerable anger and guilt in patients and their families, and frequently, this emotion is directed at the physician. Some patients may seize on any inconsistency between what is said and what they hear from other sources to illustrate the incompetence of certain physicians (usually those who saw the patient before the diagnosis). It is often best to deal with this kind of behavior in an understanding, rather than a confrontational, manner, without reinforcing negative views of other practitioners. Often the best strategy is to allow patients to vent their anger even though the target may be undeserving.

A proactive, factual discussion about the vexingly frequent "cures" and "breakthroughs" reported in the press will be of value to the patient and their family. The physician should point out that the recovery potential from each relapse of MS is quite good. When an attack occurs, there is a 70 percent chance of spontaneous recovery.[533] Therefore, to be effective, any treatment must have a therapeutic effect greater than 70 percent. Both patients and unsophisticated clinicians should be alerted to the common mistake of crediting the treatment given with recovery after relapse. Accordingly, patients willingly take many therapies because recovery due to the natural tendency of the disease is often attributed to that treatment.[568]

PROGNOSIS

As discussed in Chapter 6, MS has a much more profound effect on quality of life than on long-term survival. Only a few individuals die early from MS complications (causes of death are considered in Chapter 5). Although the nature and severity of MS are unpredictable, some general rules, based on an individual patient's previous history, suggest prognosis. If the disease has remained mild or relatively benign after 5 to 10 years, it is, on the whole, likely to remain relatively benign for the next 5 to 10 years.[333] Similarly, the more severely disabling form of MS is usually recognizable within the first 5 to 10 years. Rapidly disabling MS is usually marked by major residual deficits after relapses, early motor or cerebellar signs, or the onset of a chronic progressive clinical course. A longer period of observation increases the accuracy of the prognosis. As a general rule, a young woman with a sensory onset and a relapsing-remitting course who lacks any disabling residual motor or cerebellar signs tends

Table 12–2. GENERAL PROGNOSTIC GUIDES IN EARLY MULTIPLE SCLEROSIS*

Factor	Relatively Good Prognosis	Relatively Poor Prognosis
Sex:	Female	Male
Age at onset:	Young (<25 yr)	Older (>40 yr)
Onset symptoms:	Sensory	Motor
Clinical course:	Relapsing	Chronic progressive
Time to EDSS 3†	Long	Short
Relapse rate in first 2 yr:	Low	High

*These data are mostly from references 114, 488, 512, 659, 661.
†Extended Disability Status Scale (EDSS) data are from reference 329.

Table 12–3. **EMPIRICAL RECURRENCE RISK FOR DEVELOPING MULTIPLE SCLEROSIS FOR FAMILY MEMBERS OF A PROBAND WITH MULTIPLE SCLEROSIS**[*]

Degree of Relatedness	Empirical Recurrence Risk
I°	2.8% males, 5.6% females
II°	0.2% to 1.8%
III°	0.5%**

Source: Sadovnick AD, and Macleod PM,[550] p 1039–1041, with permission.
*See Chapter 3 for details.
**Revised

to have a more benign prognosis. In early interviews, the possibility of benign disease should be emphasized. However, for those patients demanding to know overall odds, the physician can explain that after 15 years, on average, some 50 percent of patients are still walking and some 40 percent are still working.[154] Table 12–2 lists some prognostic indicators.

Recent studies of coronary disease have shown that survival is best in those patients with strong support systems such as spouse or partner, other close family and good friends, and adequate financial resources. In MS, many times these support systems fail; in addition, economic worries may mount. The same factors that operate to prolong life in coronary heart disease patients also greatly affect quality of life and perhaps survival in patients with MS.

GENETICS

Recent studies of the relatives of patients with MS show that the overall rate for familial occurrence is approximately 20 percent (see Chapter 3). Empirical recurrence risks (ERR) for developing MS are presented in Table 12–3, which should be useful for advising families.[547,550] As shown, the ERR is 2.8 percent for male siblings and 5.6 percent for female siblings. Table 12–4 shows the concordance rate for dizygotic twins is 2.3 percent.[156] In contrast, the clinical concordance rate for monozygotic twins is almost 30 percent and some additional unaffected monozygotic twins have multiple asymptomatic magnetic resonance imaging (MRI) abnormalities, or cerebrospinal fluid (CSF) oligoclonal banding.[156] In addition, approximately 11 percent of asympto-

matic first-degree family members have asymptomatic MRI lesions.[621] It is unknown whether family members with asymptomatic MRI abnormalities will develop clinical MS.

REPRODUCTIVE COUNSELING

As noted in Chapter 3, reproductive counseling is a complex issue, and it is unwise to recommend either pregnancy or termination of pregnancy. The physician should present facts and discuss potential problems but leave decisions concerning pregnancy to the patient and spouse.

The physician can counsel patients on the lifelong risks of their children developing MS, which, based on the results of genetic studies (see Chapter 3), are 30-fold to 50-fold greater for patients with MS than among the general population. This risk is

Table 12–4. **CLINICAL CONCORDANCE AND MAGNETIC RESONANCE IMAGING ABNORMALITIES IN TWINS, ONE OF WHOM HAS MULTIPLE SCLEROSIS**[*]

Type of Twin	Clinical Concordance	Percent MRI Positive in Clinically Unaffected Twin
Monozygotic	26% (7/27)	Up to 40%
Dizygotic	2.3% (1/43)	0

Source: Adapted from Ebers GC, Bulman DE, Sadovnick AD, et al,[156] p 1638–1642.
MRI = magnetic resonance imaging.
*See Chapter 3 for details.

similar to that for serious trauma injury. No evidence suggests a greater risk of miscarriage of congenital defects among children born to parents with MS. The clinical course of MS in an offspring cannot be predicted from the pattern or severity of MS as seen in the parent or other affected relatives.[659]

Data conflict regarding the effect of pregnancy on the course of the disease. Retrospective studies, including our own, have shown an increase in the relapse rate in the first trimester and within the 3 months after delivery.[551] However, a recent careful prospective study by Sadovnick and her colleagues[549] failed to show the expected increase in postpartum relapses. Less confusion exists about the long-term consequences of pregnancy. The physician can tell the patient, with some confidence, that pregnancy will not influence the overall course of the disease or its eventual outcome.

Careful evaluation of many factors should enter into the patient's decision to have a child. The desire for a child should be balanced against the possibility that MS-related impairment may prevent the patient from carrying out some expected functions of a parent. Social factors could be the most important in determining the success or failure of parenting in patients with MS. The impact of MS on employment and earned income may be considerable, as can the potential effect on child care. Many times, a reversal occurs in the traditional roles of mother and father. The relative strength of family support systems, the caring and concern of the extended family, such as in-laws, and the family's economic status should be carefully evaluated.

POSSIBLE INFECTIVITY

No convincing evidence indicates that MS is a transmissible disease despite claims to the contrary by Kurtzke (see Chapter 2).[330] The rarity of conjugal MS, which occurs at the same rate as would be expected by chance in the population (about 1:1000 in British Columbia and Ontario) is one of several lines of evidence that support the concept of noninfectivity and is worth telling worried spouses of newly diagnosed patients. Sexual transmission would ordinarily bias susceptibility toward a lower socioeconomic group and promiscuous patients, neither of which have been shown in MS. Nevertheless, we think that it is prudent for patients to avoid blood donation until the question of transmissibility by blood products has been systematically evaluated.

PRECIPITATING EVENTS FOR RELAPSES

As reported in Chapter 5, retrospective studies have suggested that infections are significant precipitating events for relapses (Table 12–5). A prospective study by Sibley and his colleagues[569] showed that 27 percent of relapses were preceded by upper respiratory infections, and our experience supports these findings. Although relapses are occasionally associated with trauma or surgery, this association does not occur frequently enough to imply causality. Nevertheless, we recommend to our patients that only essential surgery should be done, and if possible, a general anesthetic should not be used. Stressful events have also been associated with both the onset of MS and relapse[649]; in particular, stress has been shown to affect the immune system.[103] Despite these findings, few prospective studies have shown a convincing role for stress as a precipitant of relapse. Nonetheless, most neurologists would counsel patients to avoid highly and continually stressful situations, although stress may produce little more than temporary symptomatic worsening. The controversial possible relationship between trauma and the activation of MS is discussed fully in Chapter 5.

Table 12–5. POSSIBLE PRECIPITATING EVENTS FOR RELAPSES

Likely	Unlikely
Viral infections[569]	Trauma[570]
Delivery of a child[551]	Surgery[570]
	Pregnancy[551]
	Stressful events[215,649]

EFFECTS OF HEAT AND LATITUDE

Neurological function may temporarily deteriorate after exercise, with increased body temperature (fever), and with increased ambient temperature (see Chapter 2). The physiological explanation for this phenomenon is covered in sections on pathophysiology in Chapters 5 and 8. The phenomenon of deterioration associated with heat or fever can be so dramatic as to produce a "pseudorelapse."

Patients who worsen with heat and fever usually respond well to cooling the body or reducing the ambient temperature. For example, cold showers can have a temporary beneficial effect in some patients. Air conditioning is definitely helpful for patients who live in warm, humid environments and should be considered a medical expense under those circumstances. The physician should reassure patients that no permanent damage is done to the nervous system by exposure to heat and increased body temperature. The physician can confidently tell patients that the long-term prognosis of MS is unaffected by climate. (See the following discussion of 4-aminopyridine.)

IMMUNIZATION

If MS is an autoimmune disorder (see Chapters 8, 9 and 10), one could reasonably expect that immunizations that activate the immune system would activate the autoimmune process. As discussed previously, the most well-documented precipitant of relapse is viral infections (upper respiratory).[569] Although immunizations are occasionally followed by exacerbations,[237] some of them severe, a clear relationship has not been documented. For example, a study of influenza vaccination[431] has shown no evidence for neurological deterioration after vaccination.

Because the data on the effect of immunizations on patients with MS remain unclear, only essential vaccinations should be administered. For example, vaccination with tetanus, which is solely for the patient's protection, should be given. Influenza vaccination should be given to disabled patients. Amantadine provides an alternative for in-fluenza prophylaxis and may also reduce symptoms of fatigue.

In some reports, the immune response to vaccination of patients with MS appears normal, but again, the data are inconsistent. Some investigators have found abnormally low levels of antibodies toward common vaccination proteins such as tetanus. In contrast, many studies have shown that naturally occurring antibody levels to measles and other viruses tend to be high.[267] Immunoglobulin secretion also tends to be higher in patients with MS than in control subjects, particularly in active (chronic progressive) MS.[464,465]

SOCIOECONOMIC FACTORS

Chronic and disabling disorders predictably create socioeconomic problems. Counseling in this regard for patients and their immediate families should occur early, so that potential problems are anticipated and possibly offset. If the patient is working outside the home, it is generally advised that he or she continue for as long as possible. In addition to generating income and increasing self-esteem, employment may provide disability coverage and other benefits, such as health insurance. Quitting a job because of fatigue or physical disability may terminate disability and health insurance coverage. Experienced social workers can be of great assistance in dealing with disability benefits, housing, and discrimination. Physicians should become knowledgeable about problems with insurance coverage and make their knowledge available to their patients. Insurance companies often approach MS-related impairment in the same manner as that resulting from trauma or surgical disease, such as head injury, fractures, or loss of limbs, which either stabilize or decrease with time. The worsening nature of MS appears to be misunderstood or reluctantly accepted by some insurance companies. Patients often find it frustrating to receive repeated suggestions for rehabilitation. Patients with MS should be well informed about tax reliefs, disability allowances, and the legal rights of the disabled. Local Multiple Sclerosis Society chapters are a valuable resource for such information. Employability in MS may rely more on cognitive features than on neurological impairment.

DIET

Patients with a chronic disease like MS often find themselves irresistibly drawn to any therapy that promises some control over their illness. Accordingly, dietary modifications may hold some attraction for these patients. Sibley's book on therapeutic claims in MS[568] covers a number of proposed diets, none of which have been shown to be effective. One widely used diet is low in animal fats and dairy products.[605] Claims have surfaced that the diet benefits patients who consume it for a long time. Swank and Dugan[605] described a positive effect in 144 patients who used a low-fat diet for 34 years. Unfortunately, this study suffers from the lack of a control group and the follow-up of only selected patients. When asked for advice on diet, we tell patients that there is no proven influence of diet on MS, but that low-fat diets are not harmful and may have general health benefits.

LIFESTYLE

As with diet, lifestyle alterations have not been proved to have either a positive or a negative impact on long-term outcome in MS. However, lifestyle choices can have an impact on patients' ability to cope with this disease and quality-of-life changes. Patients should be counseled to have realistic expectations about their future and to consider the limitations that may be imposed by neurological deficits. However, even more important, patients should be counseled as to ways in which they can expand and enrich their lives by stretching in areas where they anticipate no limitations.

Supportive Therapy: General Principles

Supportive therapy is critical in any chronic illness; this is particularly true for patients with MS who experience relentlessly progressive disease and a corresponding increase in socioeconomic problems. Evidence suggests that a multidisciplinary health-care team approach may be more effective than standard medical care in providing long-term care for patients with MS.[70] Like anyone else, patients with MS respond to encouragement and to success in meeting life's demands. If a patient's disease is steadily worsening, designing a program in which patients can realize their maximum potential and can successfully accomplish goals can be very important.[410] The following elements are important in this kind of supportive therapy.

OPEN COMMUNICATION

Open communication is essential and involves a two-way process between patients and their families, and between patients and physicians. Patients should know that although little is available at this time that can influence their final outcome, the physician has a great deal of knowledge about their disease and resources that can specifically deal with many symptoms and problems. Moreover, new medical therapies hold great promise for future impact.

VENTING OF EMOTIONS

Patients and families must learn to vent their emotions in a nondestructive way. Commonly, family members become resentful and angry at having to provide special consideration to a patient with MS. Often this anger is repressed and produces guilt, and severe emotional stress and strains can develop. Counseling patients and their families to anticipate feelings of resentment and rage and to accept these emotions as valid and appropriate can minimize threats to family stability. If open discussion of emotions is recognized as a desirable element in relationships, patients and family will generally adjust much better to this most frustrating of diseases.

POSITIVE ATTITUDE

Patients and families must be encouraged to adopt a positive attitude. For the family, a positive attitude involves accepting the diagnosis but not allowing excessively dependent relationships to develop. Patients should be expected to carry out their responsibilities, with appropriate allowances for physical disabilities and fatigue. For the patient, it means learning to accept and adapt to the disability, for example, by pacing oneself according to one's physical abilities. Cooperation among the patient, physicians, and other caregivers must be stressed. In addition, the patient and the caregivers should set attainable goals. They should avoid setting goals that are either too high or too low; goals that are too high are impossible for patients to reach and result in frustration and lowered self-esteem, and goals that are too low do not challenge patients to reach their maximum abilities. Patients may have a tendency to stress lost skills and to grieve excessively. Therefore, the motto should be to "do the best with what you've got." With increasing impairment, goals should be reassessed and new ones established.

Some investigators have also found that promoting socialization with able-bodied persons, as opposed to restricting contact to other disabled persons, helps to create and maintain a positive attitude. Physicians should encourage patients with MS to develop and maximize hobbies; to emphasize humor in their relationships, even under the most trying of circumstances; and to master some sort of recreational activity commensurate with their level of impairment. The patient must accept responsibility for work and decision making; the family can encourage the patient by emphasizing the value of the patient's contribution to the family and to society.

COPING WITH MULTIPLE SCLEROSIS

Communication and understanding are at the core of all adaptation mechanisms.[349] However, negative reinforcement can be a factor in the relationship between disabled patients and their caregivers, and the physician should watch for such negative factors. Patients must be aware that their reaction to the disease can be worse than the disease itself. All of us have seen patients who develop a regression to dependency considerably out of proportion to their loss of physical abilities. These patients uniformly do poorly, and they produce anger, hostility,

and mistrust in themselves as well as in their families and friends. Therefore, patients are well advised to avoid the natural tendency to become paranoid and to withdraw. Denial may also be a counterproductive tool for coping with MS. Some patients who use excessive denial manifest periods of frantic overactivity to prove to themselves and to others that they have no serious disabilities. This pattern is just as detrimental for patients as is withdrawal into self-pity and dependency. Quality of life in MS has been shown to improve after entering a comprehensive coping/support program.[588a]

In recent years, self-help support groups, which can be helpful to both patients and their families, have been formed. Support groups are available for the early diagnosed, for marital partners, for children, for long-term patients, and for patients with sexual dysfunction. Psychotherapy can be helpful as well.[411]

The healthy adjustment process has been described as progressing in the following stages:

1. **Denial:** Denial is often the first reaction to being informed of a serious diagnosis such as MS. Although a natural tendency, denial is a dangerous mechanism if allowed to exist for longer than a few months. The defense mechanisms involved in denial can be very fragile, so that when reality intrudes by either relapses or progressive disability, the patient is left with no effective coping mechanism. Therefore, the use of denial should be discouraged in both the patient and the family.

2. **Intellectualization:** Intellectualization is a form of denial. Instead of dealing directly with the problems and implications of the disease, the patient and family take a step back, depersonalize the situation, and approach it as an intellectual game. They look at the MS as a most interesting disease and seek to discuss it only in the third person. Highly educated persons tend to take this approach, which does not provide for successful long-term emotional coping.

3. **Resistance:** Resistance develops at a time when the patient says, "Well, per-

haps I have got it, but I don't like it and I am going to fight it." Sometimes the emotional expense of the resistance process can be disabling in itself, while the accompanying physical activity is often excessive and harmful.

4. **Information:** In the information phase, patients realize that they must face the situation realistically. Although they do not like the fact that they have a chronic and potentially disabling disorder, with a realistic approach to the disease, the patient can begin the process of adjustment and coping. Realistic discussions concerning impact and prognosis can have their greatest success at this point.

5. **Integration:** The integration phase occurs when patients come to terms with their disease and decide to make the most of it. Patients who adapt the best learn how to emphasize what they "can do" as opposed to emphasizing what they "can't do." Patients in this stage of adjustment can be of great help to others with MS by serving as role models and peer counselors.

Boyle and her colleagues[71] have recently described four distinctive coping styles in MS: "depression," "denial," "exaggerated somatic," and "severity related." It is appropriate for patients to experience anger and frustration, and they need to express these feelings. Unfortunately, the anger and frustration are usually directed toward the family or other caregivers, who, in the long run, carry most of the physical and emotional burdens of this disease. The physician should recognize the need for patients to express these feelings and be willing to act as a surrogate for the family, in turn contributing in a small way toward enhancing the quality of life for the family and the patient. The physician should not express anger in return, a task that can occasionally be formidable. Anger from the doctor can alienate the doctor-patient relationship and contribute nothing towards helping the family. If the goal is to keep the patient home as long as possible, the family's needs in this context must be addressed. If possible, the physician should encourage the patient to channel the energy of rage into constructive activities.

Long-Term Medical Management: The Team Approach

Multiple sclerosis is such a complex disorder that simple models of care managed by isolated health-care providers are inadequate. MS requires comprehensive care managed by a multidisciplinary team. The cornerstone of the team approach is adherence to the principles of research, education, and comprehensive patient care. The team can comprise many experts with specialized knowledge in particular problems or few experts with broad knowledge who know how to mobilize the most appropriate resources. Team members often include the physician, occupational therapist (OT), physical therapist (PT), nurses, and social worker. Both the patient and the family must be considered focal team members and, with the help of the physician and nurse, should participate in the selection of team members. Attention to correct diagnosis of each of the patient's problems is a team responsibility. The MS medical care team then must not only educate the patient and family but also coordinate services in community facilities in mental health, advocacy, therapeutic recreation, and respite care. Moreover, the patient and family should be able to obtain advice from various team members as needed. Advantages to this centralized team approach include: (1) enhanced experience and expertise of the team members, (2) enhanced communication and peer education of the team members, (3) expedited and smooth referral among team members, and (4) enhanced opportunity for research because of the scope of the experience and the rapid accumulation of data from prospective follow-up.

The comprehensive team approach also has a number of drawbacks. The major drawback is less direct communication with the family caregivers than would occur in home-based care. Another drawback is that boredom and alienation can occur for team members without adequate intellectual stimulation and positive feedback. Many team members respond better to the long-term problems of chronic patient management and care if each is expected to contribute toward research in their specific area of expertise. Finally, therapeutic programs for patients would be better individualized if patients were seen in the home, but then the patient would not get out into the social setting of group therapy. A combination of comprehensive institutional outpatient care and home visits would probably address this disadvantage.

The natural history of an individual patient with MS, which is characterized by unpredictability, varied and multiple symptoms, and progressive deterioration, offers a unique challenge to successful rehabilitation strategies. Unlike many other chronic diseases, deterioration may occur repeatedly and relentlessly after variable periods of stabilization. Another challenge to rehabilitation in MS is fatigue: how does one rehabilitate and maintain a patient with a progressive disease in which a dominant symptom is fatigue, a limiting factor in any rehabilitation program? Cognitive impairment, which is variable in each patient, and its corollary, a decrease in ambition and mental energy, are further challenges to rehabilitation. The interaction of cognitive deficits and fatigue demand an extremely specialized approach to maintenance therapy and will sometimes prevent a positive response.

Perhaps the best strategy for successful rehabilitation is to make the patient aware that as physical or mental deficits increase over time, expectations must be lowered in a realistic way. At the same time, consistent encouragement and positive reinforcement of the patient's achievements, no matter how small, must be maintained. The contraction of expectations in this situation is similar to that in adapting to the aging process. In both situations, positive accomplishments are critical, but the difficulty of the achievement must be commensurate with the ability of the patient. To this goal, each patient will require an individualized management program that recognizes and integrates social, environmental, emotional, cognitive, physical, and financial factors crucial to compliance, performance, and success. Moreover, these factors need to be continually monitored and program modifications made as necessary. Long-term care for the younger disabled is not adequate anywhere[127] but is improving.

Symptomatic Therapies

While MS is not medically curable,[580] it is manageable.[580] Available treatments are directed at relief of symptoms* and quality-of-life improvements. Sibley and his colleagues[568] have published a helpful monograph entitled *Therapeutic Claims in MS.* Schapiro[553] and Smith and colleagues[580] have also recently reviewed advances in symptomatic management (see Chapter 5 for a full discussion of the symptoms described).

NEED FOR SLEEP

Many patients with MS do not sleep well. The factors that interfere with sleep are nocturnal spasms, nocturia, pain, and depression. Each of these factors must be treated individually to prevent sleep deprivation and to promote daytime activity. Nocturnal spasms may be reduced by baclofen, diazepam, or other benzodiazepines. Nocturia can be reduced by administration of anticholinergics, self-catheterization, or both, or by administration of intranasal Pitressin (vasopressin (DDAVP)) just before bedtime.[306] Pain control is difficult but can be helped with carbamazepine (Tegretol), a tricyclic antidepressant, or both. Depression can be treated in many ways, but most effectively by the use of tricyclic antidepressants, which may also improve bladder dysfunction by their anticholinergic side effects.

It should not be forgotten that caregivers may lose sleep as well. A recent study by Spackman and colleagues[587] found that 70 percent of caregivers to patients with MS were awakened at least once per night.

FATIGUE AND WEAKNESS

Fatigue ranks at or near the top among symptoms that impair quality of life for patients with MS. A considerable gap can exist between the degree of neurological deficit and the degree of subjective fatigue experienced. Severe fatigue may be present in otherwise mildly affected patients.

---

*Many of the clinical features that require symptomatic therapy are more fully discussed in the Chapters 4 and 5.

There are two forms of fatigue in MS. The first is a persistent sense of tiredness, often associated with nonrestorative sleep. It prevents patients from doing anything except the most trivial physical activity. This lassitude is also seen in depression and other chronic conditions. Patients with the symptom of persistent tiredness should be screened for depression and may respond to antidepressant therapy. However, this form of fatigue in MS can also be associated with poor nocturnal sleep patterns. Amantadine reduces the fatigue in 50 to 60 percent of these patients, often for a limited period of time.[88,106,324a,427,537] The usual dose is 100 mg twice a day. Side effects include insomnia, irritability, livedo reticularis, and rarely hallucinations and encephalopathy. When insomnia occurs, the dose can be reduced to 100 mg in the morning or the entire 200 mg can be taken in the morning. The mechanism for amantadine's benefit may be via the dopamine or the beta endorphin–beta lipotropin pathway. Pemoline (Cylert) may help fatigue in some patients.[662] Tachyphylaxis can be limited by using amantadine or pemoline for only 4 to 5 days out of the week.

The second form of fatigue in MS is more appropriately called fatigability. This is a focal muscle fatigue that occurs after persistence in some focal physical activity. It is most commonly experienced in the legs. Patients may observe that after walking a predictable distance their legs will give out. This fatigability is probably due to the physiological characteristics of demyelinated nerve fibers (see Chapter 8). Patients with fatigability usually find that a short rest will improve their strength.

Treatment of fatigability has not been very rewarding. Strategies directed at limiting rises in body temperature, such as pacing activities over the course of the day, the use of air conditioning in warm climates, and job site modification to minimize heat exposure can be effective. Some patients find that even short immersion in cool water can increase strength and endurance. Energy-saving measures such as using motorized wheelchairs or scooters for mobility may greatly improve the patient's overall activity and productivity levels and therefore quality of life.

At present, pharmacological management is experimental, although 4-aminopyridine (4-AP) and 3,4-diaminopyridine (potassium channel blockers) appear to hold some promise. Dohrn[140] first described the excitatory effects of 4-AP on the central nervous system (CNS), and Davis and colleagues first tried it in humans.[132] Stefoski and colleagues[589] reported on 13 of 17 temperature-sensitive patients who improved significantly in motor and visual function after 4-AP therapy.[313] Polman and colleagues[503–505] and van Diemen and colleagues[637] performed a double-blind crossover study using 4-AP in 70 patients, many of whom were heat sensitive. They found that 20 to 30 mg per day of 4-AP produced a significant benefit in neurological function in 18 patients over a 12-week period of therapy. The heat-sensitive patients were the most likely to improve on 4-AP, and the drug was well tolerated. There is a trend for improvement in cognitive function as well.[585] Bever and colleagues[56a,57,62] also reported both 4-AP and 3, 4-diaminopyridine to be effective. Complications of therapy include seizures and other neurological symptoms. Our own experience with 4-AP is that some patients respond quite well, but the effect may be short-lived. In one patient for whom dysesthetic pain was a predominant feature, one dose of 10 mg of 4-AP dramatically increased the pain, suggesting a pharmacological effect on the transmission of pain impulses. Kaji and colleagues[270] showed that neurological symptoms and presumably conduction block can be temporarily improved by intravenous (IV) digitalis.

SPASTICITY

Spasticity can be both phasic (spasms) and tonic (constant stiffness) and can usually be relieved to some degree. Flexor and extensor spasms can occur at any time but are often most troublesome at night, disturbing sleep and adding to fatigue. Spasms can also upset posture, even in wheelchair-bound patients, and can be very painful. In ambulatory patients, spasticity in the form of tonic increased tone in both agonists and antagonists can interfere with walking, and in bedridden patients, spasticity can interfere with hygiene and nursing care.

In evaluating spasticity, it is important to assess function, not just the stiffness. In some patients, spasticity aids walking, standing, and transferring. Reduction in spasticity in such patients may actually interfere with function. Therefore, in using an antispasticity drug, the dose should be adjusted carefully to meet the individualized needs of the patient. An overdose in this setting usually means that the drug is actually increasing or unmasking weakness, in addition to reducing spasticity. Probably because of a sense of increasing weakness, only about one-half of the patients who are treated with antispasticity drugs continue long-term therapy. In this setting, the patient is often the best judge.

Antispasticity drugs are most helpful (Table 12–6) in those relatively few patients in whom spasticity interferes with walking but who also have near-normal strength. Baclofen is the most frequently used of these drugs and generally the most effective.[75,247] It was developed as an analogue of γ-aminobutyric acid (GABA). It may act by reducing GABA receptors.[324] Azouvi and colleagues[28] found that its main effect is probably postsynaptic inhibition of the H-reflex. It also depresses the activity of spinal interneurons. Common dose-limiting symptoms are weakness, drowsiness, and less often, nausea and vomiting. These symptoms can be minimized by using small dose increments and by taking the drug only with food. Smith and associates[581] reviewed their experience with high-dose oral baclofen (greater than 80 mg/day). Taking a high dose was not associated with discontinuing treatment. Because there has been one report of prolonged seizure activity af-

Table 12–6. **ANTISPASTICITY DRUGS: USE AND SIDE EFFECTS**

Drug	Trade Name	Action	Use	Side Effects
Baclofen (oral)	Lioresal	GABA agonist? It reduces presynaptic inhibition on interneurons.	To reduce tonic co-contraction	GI upset, weakness, encephalopathy, rash
Baclofen (intrathecal)	Lioresal	GABA agonist? It reduces presynaptic inhibition on interneurons.	Intrathecal	Fatigue, sleepiness, weakness
Tizanidine	Sirdalud	It inhibits polysynaptic motor unit activation.	Same as baclofen	Weakness, dry mouth, somnolence, spasms
Dantrolene	Dantrium	Direct action on muscle decreases Ca^{2+} effect on the T system.	To reduce severe spasticity	Weakness, hepatitis (0.3%)
Botulinum toxin	Botox	It produces neuromuscular blockade.	To reduce severe adductor spasm	None
Marijuana	—	?	To reduce spasticity and pain (reported anecdotally)	Euphoric state
Phenol (intrathecal)	—	It destroys nerve roots.	To reduce severe spasticity, especially paraplegia in flexion	Loss of reflexes and tone, headaches, incontinence, leg pains, sensory loss, allergic reactions

Ca^{2+} = calcium; GABA = γ-aminobutyric acid; GI = gastrointestinal.

ter baclofen withdrawal,[314] the drug should not be stopped abruptly.[187,222]

Other drugs used in treating spasticity are dantrolene and tizanidine.[37,113,578,634] Diazepam is used less than before because of the success of other agents. Threonine has also been reported as showing some antispasticity effect.[228] Each drug is effective in only a portion of patients, and the responding populations overlap. The search for an effective antispasticity drug for individual patients involves some trial and error.

Benzodiazepines are particularly useful in reducing nocturnal spasms. They not only reduce the number and severity of nocturnal flexor spasms but can help maintain sleep. Interruption of sleep due to flexor and extensor spasms is a frequent problem in MS and can be a major factor for patients with fatigue. Because the energy reserves in MS are low and easily depleted, adequate sleep must be a priority. Using shorter-acting benzodiazepines may avoid the morning sluggishness that occurs in some patients with longer-acting drugs.

Corticosteroids are highly effective against spasticity; however, their side effects preclude their use in standard therapy. Occasionally they can be useful in temporarily reducing severe spasticity. Severe spasticity has also been treated by intrathecal baclofen.[463] Several recent studies* have reported excellent results. Implantable reservoir pumps can deliver a constant flow of drug intrathecally without a high risk of complications or discomfort. Both muscle tone and spasms were decreased in short-term and long-term studies. However, one case of reversible coma has been described.[530] Botulinum toxin injections may be a promising method of decreasing spasms mainly in the lower extremities.[586] The large dose of toxin needed for such big muscles and the possibility of developing antibodies to the toxin are the limiting factors for its use.

Intrathecal phenol injections can be effective in reducing spasticity and usually provide temporary relief from spasms, especially in nonambulatory patients. Occasionally, surgical therapy must be used, including dorsal root section, dorsal column stimulation,[210] dorsal root entry zone lesions, Bischoff's myelotomy, or even cordectomy. Physical therapy with stretching exercises may also be effective[75] for reduction of pain, stiffness, and contracture, but has little effect in reducing spasticity.

TREMOR

Tremor is a common and disabling feature in MS. It is usually seen in action or intention, and in severe cases, it may be present at rest or simply with postural adjustments (a rubral tremor). Occasionally, extrapyramidal movement disorders such as resting tremor, paroxysmal chorea, athetosis or dystonia, or hemiballismus can be seen. These movements may respond to a benzodiazepine or carbamazepine.

Several drugs have been used in an effort to reduce cerebellar tremor in MS, but none is satisfactory. Isoniazid can have some modest, but usually temporary, effect in reducing intention tremor when used in large doses (600 to 1200 mg/day) along with pyridoxine.[72,146,218,545] Carbamazepine has also been reported to be helpful,[559] perhaps through inhibition of GABA aminotransferase and subsequent increase of GABA levels in the brain. Clonazepam and primidone may also be of value.[482] Propranolol may reduce the action component of the tremor. Glutethimide has also been reported as helpful in intention tremor.[5] Six of eight patients with disabling cerebellar or rubral tremor or both refractory to propranolol and other drugs were improved by taking glutethimide. The primary side effect was sedation. Recently, ondansetron has been found to be effective in an open trial. It is now being studied in a controlled way (G. Rice, personal communication, 1996).

Intention tremors can also be dampened by loading the limbs with weights. This method of therapy reduces tremors, but most patients discard the weights because of the added work involved in making purposeful movements. Thalamotomy or chronic thalamic stimulation has also been used in an effort to reduce tremor.[124,188] Some have claimed a high degree of success. In order to be effective, the patients

---

*References 52a, 251, 252, 434a, 497–499.

must have tremor as the only major manifestation in the arm. Bilateral lesions are associated with a high complication rate. In our experience, the high risk of hemorrhage causing hemiplegia, aphasia, pseudobulbar palsy, or all three outweighs the benefits of thalamotomy for most patients who are considered eligible. Thalamic stimulation has not been tried in many centers and should receive further evaluation.

POSITIONAL DIZZINESS AND OSCILLOPSIA

Even though no truly effective treatments are available for positional dizziness and oscillopsia, oral diazepam, lorazepam, scopolamine dermal patches, and mexiletine have all been reported to have some modest level of benefit.

SEIZURES

Seizures, which occur in approximately 5 percent of cases, can be focal, generalized, or both. In approximately one-half of the patients, seizures are coincidental.[308] In other patients, seizures are probably due to MS lesions in or near the gray matter of the cerebral cortex. When convulsive seizures are seen in MS, the patient should have a full work-up to uncover the cause. Seizures in MS are usually easily controlled with standard anticonvulsants, most appropriately carbamazepine. However, symptomatic CNS side effects from anticonvulsants affect patients with MS more than patients without MS.[379,579]

PAROXYSMAL SYMPTOMS OTHER THAN SEIZURES

Paroxysmal symptoms can be dramatic and frightening. They can usually be controlled by small doses of carbamazepine or a benzodiazepine, but in most patients, they are so minor, self-limiting, or both that therapy is unnecessary. It is important to reassure the patient that these symptoms are not of serious prognostic import and will usually stop spontaneously. Occasionally, Lhermitte's phenomenon can become so persistent or disturbing that it is disabling.

In that case, small doses of carbamazepine or benzodiazepines can reduce the frequency and severity of the symptom. Okada and colleagues[466] reported on two cases of painful tonic seizures and dysesthesia that were improved after treatment with mexiletine. Ibuprofen has also been reported effective in paroxysmal symptoms.[295]

BLADDER DYSFUNCTION

Bladder symptoms are very common in MS. Blaivas and colleagues[64,99] reviewed bladder care in MS and discussed the two most common forms of bladder dysfunction: *failure to empty* and *failure to store*. Many patients unfortunately have a combination of failure to empty and failure to store due to bladder sphincter dyssynergia (Table 12–7). The symptoms listed in Table 12–7 are suggestive of specific bladder physiologies, but often inappropriate therapy can result in worsening of symptoms rather than in improvement. Blaivas and his colleagues found that treatment based on history and physical examination alone was inappropriate in more than 50 percent of patients. Therefore, it may be necessary to refer patients to a urologist knowledgeable about the neurogenic bladder. There has been a recent consensus report from Europe on treatment of urinary symptoms for MS.[176]

In failure to store, the bladder neck sphincter is probably normal, but the bladder wall musculature is both irritable and noncompliant. The most frequent early bladder disturbance in MS, this problem results from bilateral upper motor neuron dysfunction. The resulting symptoms of urgency and frequency can respond well to anticholinergic drugs such as belladonna alkaloids, propantheline, or oxybutynin (Ditropan). Today oxybutynin is the preferred drug. It acts as an anticholinergic agent and as a smooth muscle relaxant. Dicyclomine (Bentylol) and the tricyclic antidepressants can be helpful as well. However, any of these drugs may induce urinary retention or increase the tendency for infection.[139] Anticholinergic drugs are probably best used intermittently or combined with intermittent catheterization.

Table 12–7. **TYPES OF BLADDER DISTURBANCES SEEN IN MULTIPLE SCLEROSIS**

Most Common Symptoms	Type of Bladder Disturbance	Bladder Neck Sphincter	Bladder Wall Muscle	Appropriate Treatment
Irritative—frequency, urgency, incontinence	Failure to store (spastic bladder)	Normal	Spastic	Anticholinergics
Obstructive—hesitancy, retention	Failure to empty (atonic bladder)	Spastic	Flaccid	1. bethanechol 2. intermittent catheterization, phenoxybenzamine, anticholinesterase 3. baclofen
Combination urgency, hesitancy, retention, and incontinence	Both (detrusor-sphincter dyssynergia)	Variable	Variable	Mixture of anti-cholinergics and intermittent catheterization

Failure to empty usually develops late in the course of MS. It can be due to contraction of the external sphincter, inactivity of the detrusor muscle, or both. This condition often follows the stage of failure to store and may be aggravated by chronic infection. However, many patients voluntarily restrict their fluid intake and pass concentrated, foul smelling urine as a result even in the absence of infection.

Most patients with MS have a combination problem, usually referred to as detrusor-sphincter dyssynergia. In this condition, the bladder and the sphincter are at odds and a mixed physiological picture results. Many patients with dyssynergia will require a mixture of anticholinergics and intermittent catheterization for satisfactory bladder control and bladder emptying. Betts and colleagues[56] found that more than half of 170 patients with MS had a raised residual volume and that the severity of urinary involvement correlated with pyramidal involvement.

Intermittent self-catheterization (ISC) may be the best management for failure to empty.[233,337,338] However, the patient must have the manual dexterity and leg mobility necessary to accomplish the catheterization or must have a caregiver who can do it for them. ISC can be quite effective in reducing bladder symptoms, which in turn can significantly improve a patient's mobility and social life. Kornhuber and Schutz[323] used a combination of ultrasound and ISC to manage high residual urine volumes (RUV). They found that appropriately monitored ISC could reduce the residual urine from an average of 113 to 28 mL, showing that complicated urodynamic studies may not be necessary. The authors were able to remove indwelling catheters in a number of their patients. In addition, they found that a high RUV (750 mL) was associated with an increased frequency of bacteriuria (three times) over a low RUV (less than 50 mL).

If incontinence is the major problem, males can wear condom drainage to great social and hygienic advantage. Females must wear removable external pads to absorb the urine. In addition, administration of baclofen may reduce tone in the external bladder sphincter to help improve emptying. O'Riordan and colleagues[470] used indoramin (20 mg twice a day), a selective α_1-adrenergic receptor agonist, to improve bladder emptying. They found a 41 percent improvement in peak urine flow rate compared with 7.4 percent in placebo patients ($P<.05$). Residual volume did not change, but urinary symptoms were improved. Mechanical aid to catheterization along with bladder neck closure may also be helpful.[102]

Cholinergic drugs such as bethanechol (Urecholine) can improve detrusor contractions and therefore reduce hesitancy and retention. Phenoxybenzamine or anticholinesterase drugs such as pyridostigmine (Mestinon) can relax the bladder neck. Unfortunately, phenoxybenzamine can also produce orthostatic hypotension, and its effects on the bladder are usually modest. Antidiuretic hormone (desmopressin, DDAVP) may be helpful to control nocturnal incontinence.[238,306,636a]

In the occasional patient with chronic incontinence, a urinary diversion procedure may be necessary. Urinary diversion with urethral-jejunal anastomosis is usually done in females. The result of urinary diversion can be very satisfying in eliminating incontinence. The major complication of urinary diversion is acute or chronic infection, which can be more severe than in the nondiverted urinary tract. Electrolyte imbalance may occur following the procedure. In males, bladder neck resection combined with condom drainage may be the solution to incomplete emptying and recurrent infection. Although chronic implantation of a urethral or suprapubic catheter should be avoided if possible, at times it is an acceptable solution if other methods are ineffective.

URINARY TRACT INFECTION

Urinary tract infection (UTI) is very common in MS, especially in those patients with high residual bladder volumes. However, ISC if done properly does not increase the risk of infection. Some UTIs present with systemic symptoms only, such as increased fatigue, low-grade fever, and weakness. In patients with known high residual bladder volumes, it is wise to periodically culture the urine. It may be necessary to accept asymptomatic bacteriuria. Chronic infection is very common in MS and can cause major complications, especially in disabled patients. The control of UTI is very important. Patients must be encouraged to maintain good urine flow. A lack of urinary obstruction and better urine flow allow for less of the pooling that promotes bacterial growth. Obstruction to flow, such as bladder neck obstruction, should be relieved and stones removed. The usual urinary tract bacteria grow best in alkaline substrate, so urine should be kept acid by drinking cranberry juice and taking vitamin C (ascorbic acid) or mandelamine. Fi-

nally, antibiotic treatment or suppression of infection should be undertaken only after identification of the antibiotic sensitivities of the organisms. If chronic suppression is to be undertaken, it would be wise to rotate among three suppression regimens on a monthly schedule. The treatment of UTIs was reviewed by Stamm and Hooton[588] and Fowler and colleagues.[176]

BOWEL DYSFUNCTION

Constipation is the most common bowel symptom in MS. Patients should be convinced that it is unnecessary to have a bowel movement once a day; once every 3 to 4 days is adequate for many. Constipation is usually easily treated by dietary manipulation and increasing fluid intake. Increased fiber content in the diet is important for all of us, but especially for the patient with MS. Increasing fluid intake may be difficult in patients with MS because of bladder dysfunction. Varying combinations of fiber, stool softeners, and peristaltic stimulants are usually needed. A few patients (5 percent) will develop urgency and incontinence of bowels, especially in association with increased peristalsis from any cause. Some of these patients may have primary bowel disorders such as colitis, gluten enteropathy, or celiac disease. In disabled patients, fecal incontinence can occur around an impaction, requiring enemas or manual disimpaction to clear the obstruction. One recent study[239] has shown that bowel transit time is frequently abnormal in MS.

SEXUAL DYSFUNCTION

More than half of patients with MS have some sort of sexual dysfunction.[138,354,413,591,609] The diagnosis and treatment of sexual dysfunction has been reviewed.[373a,612a] In males, failure to achieve or maintain erection is the most common complaint, although both failure to ejaculate and retrograde ejaculation are seen. These complaints usually occur in patients with bilateral corticospinal abnormalities. Patients with sexual dysfunction may also have genital sensory loss, spasticity, ataxia, or bladder incontinence alone or in combination. Depression, fatigue, anxiety, marital maladjustment, and drug effects also contribute considerably to sexual dysfunction. Attention to drug and psychological effects becomes important, because these factors can be adjusted. "Organic" impotence due to spinal cord disease is the usual culprit in males and can produce a situation in which psychogenic erection is difficult or impossible but where reflex erection (due to manipulation of the genitalia) is still possible. Rarely, hypogonadism may result from hypothalamic disease, and we have seen several patients with coincidental prolactinomas, some of whom responded to prolactin suppression with bromocriptine.

Female sexual dysfunction can manifest as decreased libido, inability to achieve orgasm, sensory loss, or pain with intercourse. Fear of pregnancy can be a major contributing factor. Adequate birth control and frank discussion of the problems involved can be very helpful. Most large medical centers now have sexual medicine units experienced in the evaluation and treatment of sexual dysfunction in the physically disabled, and many patients appreciate referral to such a unit.

Treatment. Treatment encompasses psychological counseling, physical devices, surgical implantation, and medical approaches.[138,271,591,609] For counseling to work, both partners must participate. The therapist must show an accepting attitude and present an organized approach to gain rapport. Sexual and genital hygiene becomes important because many of these patients have urinary incontinence, urinary tract infection, and occasionally bowel incontinence. Some couples can develop satisfactory sexual encounter methods that do not depend on penetration.

If impotence is thought to be largely psychogenic, professional psychological counseling should be obtained for both the patient and partner. In males in whom counseling has failed and who have normal sensation, a penile prosthetic device might be used,[232,372] such as a Silastic prosthesis (inflatable or noninflatable). The inflatable type provides a more natural state for the penis but is associated with more complications than is the permanent (noninflatable) type. Other instrumentation is available.[562] Vacuum penile tumescence-constriction therapy has also been tried as a noninvasive method.[232] Fifty percent of men in whom it was tried continued to use it and had a statistically significant increase in the frequency of satisfactory intercourse.

The use of penile prosthetic devices is a destructive procedure and has largely been replaced by intracorporeal injections of papaverine (a smooth muscle relaxant), papaverine-phentolamine (an α-adrenergic blocking agent), or prostaglandin E_1 (PGE_1) (a vasodilator and relaxant). One recent study[101] used a mixture of papaverine, phentolamine mesylate, and alprostadil. This regimen should be used with caution, however, because of a report of priapism and lethal pulmonary embolus after a second (nonprescribed) injection of phentolamine and papaverine.[224] Hatzichristou and colleagues[225] studied 79 male patients with neurogenic erectile dysfunction (26 with MS) and found that 18 percent used PGE alone, 71 percent used two agents (papaverine and phentolamine), and 11 percent used three agents (papaverine, phentolamine, and PGE). Complications were 12 episodes of prolonged erection and 5 occurrences of fibrotic nodules. Manual stimulation by the partner or using a vibrator also may help in achieving erection.

An overall approach to treating sexual dysfunction should take into consideration the following issues:

1. **Genitourinary hygiene:** Patients must try to avoid UTIs. Emptying the bladder before intercourse reduces the likelihood of incontinence. Intermittent self-catheterization or catheterization by the patient's partner might be helpful. Fluid intake can be reduced for 3 hours before intercourse. For patients with an indwelling catheter, alternate positions can be useful.

2. **Proper lubrication:** Sterile lubricants (K-Y jelly) can provide a satisfactory solution.

3. **Spasticity:** Experimentation with a variety of positions can be helpful.

4. **Fatigue:** General energy conservation measures, such as motorized scooters and daytime naps, can help to reduce fatigue. One solution is to arrange sexual activity at the best time of day (usually the mornings).

5. **Medications:** Benzodiazepines, antidepressants, antihypertensives, and anti-

spasticity drugs can all decrease the ability to reach orgasm.[2]

6. **Birth control:** Proper use of birth control method should be considered to reduce fears about pregnancy.

7. **Psychosocial factors,** such as:

a. **Caretaking and sex:** The person who performs the caretaker role may not be able to readjust to the sexual partner role easily. The gender role in the relationship may be switched because of disability and therefore undermine a normal sexual relationship. The dependent partner many times learns to control the relationship through use of guilt or other manipulations. Such behavior is bound to change the emotional relationship so that normal sexual activity would be almost impossible.

b. **Fear of hurting or "catching MS":** The partner must be reassured that sexual activity will not hurt the person with MS. In addition, the partner must be reassured that MS cannot be "caught" through sexual activity.

c. **Stressful aspects of financial problems and alienation:** Full communication between partners can help to reduce stress in the relationship.

A guide to understanding sexual dysfunction for patients and families is found in Kalb and colleagues' chapter.[271] Boller and Frank[66] have also written a monograph on sexual dysfunction in neurological disorders that includes many practical suggestions.

In a 5-year follow-up of participants in their sexual dysfunction study, Stenager and colleagues[592] found that sexual dysfunction increased in those patients with increasing physical disability. In addition, only a few patients had received medical treatment for their sexual dysfunction, and only 25 percent (1 of 4) continued to use the medical therapy. The authors concluded that sexual dysfunction was frequent and successful treatment options were limited.

PAIN

In the older literature, MS was referred to as a painless disease. That concept is clearly false (Table 12–8). Recent surveys[105,425] have shown that as many as one-half of patients experience pain or discomfort at some time during their illness. Common aches and pains that affect the general population, such as migraine, tension headache, rheumatic pains, and backache, are probably more frequent in patients with MS than in nonaffected individuals. For example, musculoskeletal pain in MS can be due to muscular weakness, spasticity, and imbalance. Moderately disabled patients may have back pain because of improper seating (wheelchair or otherwise) or incorrect posture while walking. Other sources of somatic pain are osteoporosis secondary to immobility; compression fractures of vertebral bodies; and osteoarthritis of hips, back, and neck. Contractures associated with weakness and spasticity can also be painful. The management of this pain is the same as in non-MS settings.

Musculoskeletal pain, paroxysmal pain (trigeminal neuralgia), and chronic neurogenic pain are thought to be secondary to MS. Treatment of musculoskeletal pain should aim to correct the cause, before consideration of analgesics. Chronic analgesic therapy in this form of chronic pain can be associated with drug dependency. If correction of posture and other musculoskeletal imbalance problems is not effective, low doses of aspirin or acetaminophen can be used without much harm. The nonsteroidal anti-inflammatory drugs (NSAIDs) are also widely used. However, we have not found that NSAIDs are of much help in this situation.

Paroxysmal pains are seen in 5 to 10 percent of patients, of which the most characteristic is tic douloureux (trigeminal neuralgia). When tic occurs in an otherwise normal young person (younger than 55 years), MS must be suspected as a cause. Tic usually responds to carbamazepine or possibly other anticonvulsant therapy. Care must be taken in using carbamazepine, which reportedly has caused encephalopathy,[379,579,600] aseptic meningitis,[574] and leukopenia. If drugs fail, percutaneous trigeminal rhizotomy can be very successful.[76,315]

Chronic neurogenic pain is the most common, distressing, and refractory of the pain syndromes in MS. This pain is vague yet intense, likened to a toothache, and usually occurs in the legs. The pain is de-

Table 12–8. **PAIN SYNDROMES: THEIR CAUSE AND TREATMENT**

Type of Pain	Description	Cause	Frequency	Treatment
Acute (paroxysmal)	Trigeminal neuralgia	MS	9%	Carbamazepine
	Painful tonic spasms	MS	Common	Benzodiazepines, carbamazepine, or baclofen
	Dysesthetic radicular pains	MS	Low	Benzodiazepines or carbamazepine
Chronic	Dysesthetic extremity pain	MS	29%	Carbamazepine and/or tricyclic antidepressants
	Back pain	Lack of movement	14%	Positioning and exercise
	Painful spasms and spasticity	MS	13%	Baclofen
	Abdominal pain	Multiple (e.g., radicular pain or intra-abdominal pathology such as urinary tract infection)	2%	Treatment of the cause
Frozen shoulder		Lack of movement	Common	Physiotherapy
Iatrogenic	Compression fracture	Corticosteroids	Uncommon	Conservative
	Aseptic necrosis of hip	Corticosteroids	Uncommon	Hip replacement
	Hemorrhagic cystitis	Immunosuppressants	Uncommon	Fluid infusion

scribed as constant, boring, burning, or tingling intensely. It is often associated with posterior column findings, but not with major spinothalamic impairment. Most patients have evidence of myelopathy, but not necessarily a severe motor disability. This type of pain is much more common in females than males and does not correlate with disease duration. The mechanism could be due to spontaneous activity in deafferented neurons, ephaptic transmission, or sympathetic activation. Therapy is often unsatisfactory. Carbamazepine, valproate, or clonazepam can be effective in some patients, but in our experience, tricyclic antidepressants are the most effective drugs in reducing pain severity. Fluoxetine (Prozac) has also been reported as helpful. Occasionally the pains will spontaneously remit after persisting for months. Narcotic analgesics may also be necessary and should not be withheld if no other mea-

sures are effective. In this setting, we have only rarely encountered patients who have developed narcotic dependency that interfered with function.

Some patients with MS develop paroxysmal or chronic pains in a radicular or even funicular distribution. These pains are often not recognized to be of MS origin and can mimic root compression syndromes, such as that seen with disk protrusion. When such pains occur in a root commonly entrapped by disk protrusion (C5–6, C6–7 or L4–5, L5–S1), they can easily be misdiagnosed as root entrapment. Although patients with MS may have laminectomy scars as a result of this phenomenon, root entrapment due to disk protrusion does commonly occur in MS; therefore, such pains should be appropriately investigated, especially when mechanical signs are present. Lumbar disk disease can be precipitated by asymmetrical weakness or spasticity and is not uncommon. Relief of mechanical root compression can occasionally provide dramatic reduction of spasticity. Severe specifically distributed root pain, unrelated to entrapment, gradually gets less severe and better tolerated with time.

AUTONOMIC CHANGES

Even though the recent literature has clearly documented nonbladder autonomic changes in MS,[685] therapy is usually not required. For example, even though postural hypotension occurs, it is rarely clinically significant. Some of the heart rate abnormalities seen can be symptomatically troublesome but usually require reassurance only. Neurogenic pulmonary edema is rare and life-threatening or fatal but can be self-limiting or can be successfully treated with positive pressure ventilation. Hiccup and loss of involuntary ventilatory drive are also rare complications that are prone to spontaneous recovery.

COGNITIVE AND PSYCHIATRIC DISTURBANCES

As MS advances, memory, word finding, abstract thinking, and speed of thought can become impaired.[48,511] Frank dementia is unusual but can be seen in the most advanced and physically disabled patients. However, cognitive dysfunction must be identified in mildly and moderately disabled patients because designing an appropriate rehabilitation program depends on the cognitive state of the patient. Rehabilitation is difficult for those patients with significant cognitive impairment whether the goal is job placement or improvement of wheelchair function. Because patients frequently can be depressed as well as cognitively impaired, a full neuropsychological or psychiatric evaluation or both may be necessary. When depression occurs, it is often treatable with standard antidepressants (tricyclics or monoamine oxidase inhibitors). When cognitive deficits underlie a depression, the patient's response to drugs is less predictable than when depression is primary; nevertheless, most depressed patients respond to antidepressant drugs regardless of the underlying cognitive state.

Recent studies have shown that as many as 50 percent of patients with MS may have subtle cognitive deficits[104] and that another 25 percent may have psychiatric disorders.[411] The exact neuropsychological correlates of periventricular lesions have yet to be precisely identified, although the frequently seen disinhibition of emotionality control would be consistent with the presence of lesions in limbic circuits. At some point, as many as 75 percent of patients may require some sort of emotional or antidepressant therapy. Psychiatric counseling for the patient, family, or both may be helpful for adjustment problems and for insight into behavioral difficulty. Antidepressants can also be remarkably beneficial. Desipramine (Pertofrane) may be the most effective antidepressant in this setting. Shafey[563] suggested that fluoxetine (Prozac) may be more effective than most other antidepressants in MS. Emotional lability and incontinence manifested by uncontrollable crying and weeping can be extremely distressing for relatives and may respond to low doses of amitriptyline.[556] However, as with intellectual decline, an explanation of the "organic" nature of the problem to both patient and caregiver can be beneficial in itself. Ron and Feinstein[532] wrote a short but informative editorial review.

An association between MS and manic-depressive (bipolar) disorder has been suggested. A preliminary survey at the University of British Columbia (UBC) MS Clinic found a 38 percent incidence of bipolar disease or depression in the nondisabled MS population. Lithium and carbamazepine can be helpful in controlling mania. Psychotherapy may be helpful as well.[412] Corticosteroids can trigger manic attacks in some patients, probably because patients with MS are mania prone. Caution should therefore be exercised in the use of corticosteroids in such patients.[412] Concomitant administration of haloperidol has been useful in controlling the steroid-induced mania.

When a cognitive disturbance, a primary or secondary depression, or both occur, it is important to involve the family and other caregivers in the treatment process. When psychological or cognitive problems produce behavior changes, the caregiver may misinterpret them. The lack of understanding of the consequences of cognitive deficits can produce increasing stress in an already stressful situation. Once caregivers have been informed about the origins and mechanisms underlying the patient's behavior, they will usually be much more sympathetic and supportive than when left to interpret disruptive behavior as willful in origin. The physician must also consider the high rate of suicide in patients with MS. Sadovnick and her colleagues[548] found that 26 percent of deaths not directly caused by MS were due to suicide. Those patients prone to depression or suicide should be identified, and appropriate treatments and support systems provided.

PSYCHOPHYSIOLOGICAL (HYSTERICAL) PHENOMENA

Patients with MS are under enormous stress, having been told that they have a potentially disabling disease that is both incurable and unpredictable. Under these circumstances, it is not surprising that emotional factors might sometimes predominate as the cause of neurological symptoms. As in epilepsy, where pseudo-seizures are common, psychophysiological phenomena in MS can be mixed with the "true" organic MS symptoms. It can be difficult to distinguish with certainty between symptoms that are psychophysiological in origin and those that are due to new MS lesions. Serial MRI studies have shown that the underlying disease activity detected by MRI scan is at least five times more frequent than is clinical activity.[484] Therefore, some of the symptoms previously interpreted as being psychological in origin may actually be organic, due to otherwise neurologically asymptomatic brain lesions (see Chapter 9).

Therapy for suspected psychophysiological events should be directed at minimizing stressful situations and helping the patient to develop insight into behavior.[21] In the presence of psychophysiological symptoms, the authors have found that a sympathetic rather than confrontational approach promotes acceptance of such information. If patients are told that their current symptoms may result from psychological factors, they may interpret that statement to mean that the problems are all in their head or they are crazy. Patients need to be told that such symptoms are a natural human response to stress that can develop in anyone, including their physician. In addition, explaining that hypertension, ulcers, and seizures can be caused by stress and emotional responses to stress makes the patient much more amenable to psychologically directed therapy.

REHABILITATION

Schapiro and Langer[553] and others[336a] have written extensively on the rehabilitation approach to the management of MS. Ketelar and Battaglia[294] have also edited a recent book on rehabilitation in MS. Physical and occupational therapists can be invaluable in the management of patients with MS. These professionals are expert at motivating patients to do continued range-of-motion exercises to prevent contractures and to use aids for activities of daily living (ADL). PTs also evaluate the gait, strength, and sensory function of patients and give guidance for regular therapy directed at spasticity and incoordination, and can oversee gait training and orthotics. However, care must be taken that the chosen therapist is familiar with the fatigue factor seen in MS. Physical therapy in MS cannot be approached in the same way as in a spinal cord injury. If the PT is too energetic with patients with MS, the pace of therapy may exhaust them and be counterproductive. If exhausted regularly, they will lose motivation and stop therapy altogether.

At present, the management of fatigue is best handled by energy conservation and a paced approach to physical activity. Schapiro has shown that in spite of the fatigue factor, patients with MS can be conditioned physically without a negative impact on their disease course (R. Schapiro, personal communication 1993).

The OT can conduct a home survey and give advice on the optimal layout to help the patient with moderate or severe disabilities. The physician should not hesitate to refer patients to these professionals and to encourage long-term contact for maintenance of function. The OT and PT can also serve as a major part of the support system for disabled patients. Maintenance therapy can be helpful not only for prevention of contractures, maintenance of strength, and adaptation to the problems of ADL, but also for emotional support of both patient and family. The PT can be particularly helpful in this regard. The very nature of the profession involves the "laying on of hands," a time-honored and effective technique used in the long-term management of chronic illness.

For a patient refractory to an outpatient approach to therapy, an inpatient stay in a specialized MS-oriented rehabilitation facility can often be beneficial to both the patient and the family. When the patient is removed from the daily routine of home and encouraged to focus on the best way to approach ADL, a considerable degree of adaptation and adjustment can occur, which in turn can have an immediate impact on the quality of life of both patients and caregivers.

In addition, the OT and PT can introduce the patient to valuable living aids, both for mobility (braces, walkers, scooters) and for communication (home computers). Many disabled persons find home computers helpful in the management of finances, communication, and mobility control and even for gainful employment. Special computer programs have been developed for the disabled that can have a major impact on the quality of their lives.

When using paramedical staff in an intensive program for helping patients with MS, both professional and family caregivers require special attention to their needs. The physical and psychological stress on these caregivers can lead to such serious problems as burnout and loss of excellent workers from the system. Anticipation of potential problems can have significant benefits toward the long-term success of any chronic care program.

SOCIAL WORK

Social workers are invaluable in the management of socioeconomic problems of patients with MS and their families. Their skills can be used to educate and to help pa-tients and families develop coping mechanisms for emotional upset. They also function well in their traditional role of patient and family advocate, identifying and securing housing, income, and community resources so vital for effective long-term management.

THERAPEUTIC TRIALS

Choosing What to Measure

Patients with chronic diseases prone to spontaneous improvement and worsening either have tried or have heard about a remarkably large number of therapies. Many of these treatments are enthusiastically proposed, shine briefly, and then fade. *Therapeutic Claims in MS*[568] places MS in an invaluable historical perspective, comments dispassionately on many different therapeutic claims, and clearly sets out the difficulties involved in evaluating treatments in a spontaneously relapsing-remitting and unpredictable disorder. Rudick and Goodkin[541] also published a monograph on MS treatment that covers a number of topics important in the evaluation of therapies in MS.

In evaluating the findings of any therapeutic study, it is important to ask "what is being treated?"[155,166] Some therapies have been used to treat individual relapses while others are given in the hope of suppressing relapses. Relapse suppression or treatment studies require quantitation of relapses and the awareness that relapse rates decline over time (see Chapter 6 for discussion on the impact of natural history on the evaluation of therapeutic trials). The problem with this measure is that the outcome in MS may be only modestly related to relapse frequency.[659,660,661] In some clinical trials, relapse rate was apparently reduced by the therapy, but progression of the disability was not altered. A more meaningful goal (other than relapse suppression) for therapeutic trials would be to slow down or prevent the development of any new neurological deficits. Brown and colleagues[82] published a detailed guide to the design of clinical trials. The handling of the placebo group turns out to be of primary importance.[661a]

After reviewing a number of therapeutic trials, Myers and Ellison[428,429] wrote a thoughtful critique on the interpretation of trial results in MS. In addition, Weiss and Stadlan[665] wrote a thoughtful and practical guide to design and statistical issues that must be considered in planning and interpreting therapeutic trials in MS. In that article, they advocate using one primary clinical outcome measure, usually the Expanded Disability Status Scale (EDSS), and suggest that the measure should be "time to an event." They defined an event as one full point change on the EDSS score. Kurtzke[330] also reviewed the topic of outcome measures in clinical trials. Whitaker wrote two editorials on clinical trial strategy in MS. In one,[667] he discusses the impact of investigational new drugs (INDs) on clinical trials. The IND is a mechanism providing greater access to "promising new therapies that are under investigation in controlled studies for patients with immediately life threatening or serious diseases for which satisfactory alternate treatment is not available." Although these procedures are providing greater drug access, they may slow down the actual proof of efficacy by reducing the patient accrual rate and promoting dropouts from placebo-controlled trials. In the second, he supports the concept of testing putative MS treatments in experimental allergic encephalitis (EAE).[672] Several meetings on MS clinical trials have refined the approach to evaluation of new therapies.[236,657,671]

Many trials in recent years have been directed at influencing the chronic progressive phase of MS. The pathological characteristics of MS lesions suggest that persistent disability may result from a combination of several mechanisms, including demyelination, inflammation, gliosis, and loss of axons. Although both clinical progression and disability result from continued activity of the inflammatory process with secondary effects on myelin, glial cells, and axons, this concept has not been proved. Several investigators[173,483] have emphasized the possible role of gliosis and axonal loss as significant factors in the increasing impairment seen in chronic progressive disease. In addition, Compston[112] and Zajicek and Compston[689a] have made a number of proposals concerning possible new strategies for future therapeutic trials in MS.

Clinical trials should include a laboratory measure that reflects the biologic activity of the particular therapy being tested.[668,673] If the therapeutic strategy is immunosuppression, there should be an objective demonstration that immunosuppression has in fact been achieved. For example, if loss of suppressor cell function (if indeed suppressor cells exist) were known to be a critical factor in pathogenesis, a measure of the effect of the therapy on suppressor cell function would be necessary. On the basis of this premise, Myers and colleagues[433] administered increasing amounts of cyclophosphamide in an attempt to reduce B-cell levels or to change the "helper/suppressor" ratio. The cyclophosphamide dose required to produce significant laboratory changes was intolerable, resulting in toxic side effects unacceptable for chronic therapy.

Unfortunately, no known laboratory test directly reflects the pathogenic mechanisms in MS. Several distinct immune functions can be measured, but given the current lack of knowledge, there is no guarantee that the "relevant" immune test will be measured. In addition, monitoring specific immune functions is expensive, time consuming, and so far, remarkably uninformative. However, when the alteration of immune function is the mechanism by which a possible therapy "works," the monitoring of specific immune tests should result in a more precise conclusion about the biologic effect achieved. The opposite is also true, as illustrated by several trials that resulted in an ineffective level of immunosuppression. Interestingly, the strongest association yet claimed between therapeutic effect and "immune function" was the reduction in the absolute lymphocyte counts of the "responding" subgroup in the recent total lymphoid irradiation study.[121]

A method for assessing multiple clinical trials has emerged, called *meta-analysis*.[546] Perhaps this method, which allows pooling of previous studies, will help in making sense of the many conflicting and confusing clinical studies in MS. Clinicians still must exercise caution when interpreting the results of pooled studies,[281] as well as when planning and interpreting the statistics used in clinical trials.[209,567]

Need for Control Measures

Because there is no generally recognized effective long-term therapy for MS, it has been axiomatic to say that therapeutic trials should involve simultaneously treated randomized placebo-controlled subjects evaluated in a double blind fashion.[451,454] A placebo effect in MS is known to occur,[240] and the incidence of spontaneous improvement in acute relapses is at least 70 percent.[533] Studies relying upon historical or nonsystematic control trials find little acceptance today, nor should they warrant funding. Studies lacking appropriate controls continue to appear.

Other elements that must be defined specifically and clearly in therapeutic trials are the standard for diagnosis, standards for identifying and quantifying relapses, and the neurological methods of assessing disease activity such as clinical impairment scales.[663] Investigators should decide on endpoints when the trial is planned and should resist the temptation to sift the data for the "responsive subgroup," a term that has appropriately taken on a pejorative connotation. It is hoped that the move toward standardization of data[114,604] will aid in the performance of clinical trials in the future.

Noseworthy and associates[454] have reviewed the impact of blinding on the Canadian Cooperative trial of cyclophosphamide in MS. They found that the unblinded neurologists in that trial found an apparent treatment effect that the blinded neurologist did not. These authors point out that without the blinding, that trial would have made a type I error (false-positive).

Determining Disease Activity and Outcome (Monitoring)

CLINICAL STATUS

Many neurological scales for the rating of neurological impairment in MS (Table

12–9) have been proposed over the past 35 years. Considerable innate variability exists in what is being measured, regardless of the scale used. Patients may vary in their function considerably over the course of a single day and can be affected by stress, fatigue, changes in ambient temperature, and other factors. The Disability Status Scale (DSS) (see Table 12–9)[328,331] and the EDSS (see Table 12–9)[329] are probably the most useful scales for rating impairment. They offer the advantage of the familiarity that comes from their prolonged use. However, the EDSS scale does not measure disability as defined by the World Health Organization (WHO). The dysfunction classifications developed by the WHO as applied to neurological disorders are:

1. **Impairment:** clinical signs and symptoms produced by damage to the nervous system
2. **Disability:** personal limitations imposed on the ADL by the neurological impairment
3. **Handicap:** social and environmental effects of the disability

A scale of impairment can be used to measure disease severity or aid in disease classification. Measures of impairment as defined by neurological signs on examination are at best a very inexact measure of the pathological extent of MS but are clinically relevant. The dissociation between neurological impairment detectable on clinical examination and the pathological burden of the disease has been emphasized in recent years by the increased use of MRI as a measure of disease extent and activity.[484] Impairment in MS may be measured by the standard neurological examination, using both the symptoms described by the patient and the signs detected by the examiner.[456] In most scales, neurological signs based on the standard neurological examination are used as a measure of impairment, but symptoms may be incorporated into the scale, particularly for some functional systems such as bladder or bowel function that are difficult to grade on examination. Quantitative tests of neurological function (a measure of disability) have been studied in detail by Potvin and colleagues.[507,608a] In general, a scale devised as an aid to classification is unlikely to be as

Table 12–9. CLINICAL METHODS FOR QUANTITATING DISEASE SEVERITY

Scale	Authors	Ref. No.	Addition of Subscores	Limbs Scored Separately	Weighted	Comments
EDSS	Kurtzke (1983)	329	No	No	No	Depends heavily on ambulation in higher grades
Illness Severity Score	Mickey et al. (1984)	388	Yes	No	Yes	Is very complicated
Neurological Rating Scale	Sipe et al. (1984)	575	Yes	Yes	Yes	Decreases with increasing severity
—	Patzold et al. (1978)	494	Yes	Yes	No	Has unusual subcategories
—	Fog et al. (1978)	174	Yes	Yes	No	Is computerized, but original standards apparently lost
Quantitative Neurological Examination	Potvin and Tourellotte (1981)	507	Yes	Yes	No	Consists of tests that are timed and reported as percentage of normal function
Ambulation Index	Hauser et al. (1983)	227	No	No	No	Grades ambulation only
Auto DSS	Redekop (1991)	512	No	No	No	Uses computer to assign FS and EDSS scores
Upper Extremity Scale	Goodkin et al. (1988)	203	No	Yes	No	Uses pegs and blocks to measure function

DDS = Disability Status Scale; EDSS = Extended Disability Status Scale; FS = Functional Status.

precise in the assessment of disease severity as one that relies solely on neurological signs. On the other hand, a scale that rates impairment strictly on neurological signs at a given time will not be as clinically useful in classifying MS as one that incorporates aspects of the history of the illness.

In addition to the scoring of impairment, disability and handicap must be measured in some standardized way. Quantitative neuroperformance measures are one approach.[608a] The International Federation of MS Societies (IFMSS) has attempted to bring together the diverse methods of scoring these deficits in a helpful monograph called *The Minimal Record of Disability.*[340,577] Some investigators have adapted the Minimal Record of Disability to a self-assessment format.[14] If reliable and validated, this method would be very helpful in future clinical trials as an additional outcome measure. Computerized clinical databases will also be helpful in future clinical trials.[114,513,604] Several guides to clinical outcome measures have been published recently.[175,540a,566a,671]

THE DISABILITY STATUS SCALE, EXTENDED DISABILITY STATUS SCALE, AND FUNCTIONAL STATUS SCALES

Kurtzke[326] introduced the 10-step DSS in 1955 as a relatively simple scale that could be used to follow the progress of patients over time. In 1961, it was expanded by the incorporation of a complementary set of scales for eight "functional groups" of impairment[327]: pyramidal, cerebellar, brain stem, sensory, bowel and bladder, visual, mental, and "other." The functional groups were later called functional systems (FS). The grades assigned to each functional group could be subsequently used to place the patient in the appropriate grade on the DSS, which remained essentially unchanged and distinct from the functional groups. Dr. Kurtzke does not think it is appropriate to simply add the scores in the different functional groups to obtain a total disability score, and we agree.

The EDSS was introduced in 1983[329] because of criticism that the DSS scale lacked sensitivity, particularly in its middle range.

This scale divided each of the former nine steps into two. From grades one through three, the additional steps were defined by variations in grades in the functional systems. From grades four and above, the steps, as in the earlier scale, largely depended on dysfunction in ambulation.

Several important conceptual and practical problems with the EDSS (and DSS) limit its application as a precise neurological measurement.[682] First, it mixes symptoms and signs to produce a graded system, even in the evaluation of walking. The midportion of the scale almost solely depends on assessment of the patient's ability to walk. Second, the functional systems are also not anatomically independent measures. For example, both brain stem and pyramidal function can be impaired by brain stem lesions. Third, the EDSS is quite insensitive to important changes in the neurological examination unrelated to ambulation. For example, patients with severe neurological deficits (such as blindness) that do not impair their ability to walk may actually be more impaired and functionally disabled than is suggested by their EDSS scores. Fourth, the written guidelines for interpreting the test results are vague and can be interpreted quite differently by experienced neurologists. It is sobering to realize that the correlation for EDSS by independent examiners[448,461] is only moderately good, with a κ value of 0.6, which varies somewhat over the length of the scale. Lastly, the distribution of patients over the scale is neither smoothly cumulative nor Gaussian (Fig. 12–1). In addition, cognitive function is not adequately measured in the EDSS.

Francis and colleagues[177] found that the EDSS was more subject to observer error than was the ambulation index. Even so, they endorsed the use of the EDSS and suggested that the way to correct for the apparent inherent variability was to increase the number of patients in the trial rather than to try to reduce observer error.

Amato and associates[13] did an analysis of interobserver reliability of the EDSS, confirming Kuzma and colleagues' observation[334] that the reliability was reasonably good. However, in a later study[12] the same group found low interobserver agreement.

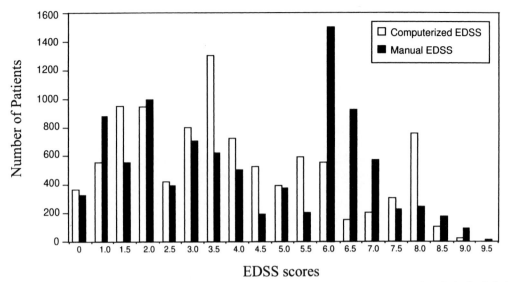

Figure 12–1. This graph shows the distribution of manual and computerized EDSS scores for clinically definite patients on their visits to the Vancouver MS Clinic. Note the bimodal distribution with high frequencies at EDSS 1.0 to 2.0 and EDSS 6.0 to 7.0 for the manual EDSS scores, with the only high frequency at EDSS 3.5 for the computerized EDSS scores and low frequency at 6.5 and 7.0.

They concluded that a two-point change on the EDSS was reliable. They suggested specific training for raters for a specific clinical trial. Verdier-Taillefer and colleagues[643] also found that interobserver agreement was lowest at the low end of the scale (less than five), and in 34 percent of cases, the variability could be as high as at least one DSS point. Because of this high degree of variability, they suggested that at least a two-point change should be considered as the threshold for significant change. Like Amato and associates, they suggested that specific training of neurologists might improve the reliability.

Kurtzke[331,332] wrote an elegant defense of the EDSS scale, which should be read by anyone trying to interpret these scales. Goodkin and his colleagues[202] tested the validity of the EDSS in patients with mild to moderate impairment and found that changes of 0.5 points could be due to instrument variability (intraobserver and interobserver variability), particularly at the midrange of the scale (four to five). At the lower end of the scale, different observers disagreed by one point 40 percent of the time! To improve consistency, they advised that the same examiner be used for evaluating each patient throughout any clinical study, particularly clinical trials. At a 1987

meeting (Jekyll Island) of MS specialists, treatment failure, as defined by at least a one-point progression in EDSS, was considered a clinically significant outcome measure.[459]

None of the recently proposed scales resolves the problems with the EDSS. The Illness Severity Score[388] is a modified form of the DSS with a complicated weighting system stressing pyramidal and cerebellar dysfunction and incorporating additional aspects of disease activity and type of course. The Neurologic Rating Scale (NRS) has the advantage of simplicity in scoring motor and sensory functions separately in each of the limbs but lacks precision in defining the degrees of impairment.[575] An additional problem is a technical one: the score decreases with increasing impairment from a normal total score of 100. The scale proposed by Patzold and colleagues[494] is more idiosyncratic, and a number of the subcategories of dysfunction (e.g., impaired consciousness, astasia, and abasia) that have relatively heavy weighting are of little relevance in most patients with MS. The details of the Patzold scale have been published only in German. The Fog scale has essentially been abandoned.[174] Potvin and colleagues[507] have worked for years on a functional system that expresses inability to perform as a percent of normal function.[608,608a] Unfortunately, the system is cumbersome, requires a trained technician to implement and is time consuming and therefore expensive. Panzer and colleagues[479] evaluated a system of computerized dynamic posturography (CDP) by comparing it with clinical and MRI activity markers. They found that CDP was sensitive enough to pick up activity that was seen on MRI but not picked up by the standard neurological examination. Troiano and colleagues[627] and others[241a] have developed yet other scales to measure impairment.

Rehabilitation outcomes probably measure what is of most importance to the patient.[613] Goldberger[193] provided a patient perspective on the concept of outcome measures, arguing that investigators must be sensitive to patients' concerns when claiming "significant" results. Noseworthy and colleagues[456] cautioned that when assessing strength, neurologists may underestimate weakness. Hutchinson and Hutchinson[252a] have devised a Functional Limitations Profile that may be a helpful measure of disability in clinical trials. Measurement of psychosocial outcomes is also important.[339]

It is hoped that quantitative serial MRI assessment will aid in objective assessment of pathological extent and activity. However, a reproducible measure of neurological deficits will always be necessary as the final endpoint in clinical trials.

Despite the limitations of the EDSS scale, it remains the most widely accepted and validated scale. Therefore, we believe it is pragmatic to recognize its limitations and correct them. There should be a clear description of grades within each "functional system." Selection of functional systems should be based primarily on the ease, reliability, and reproducibility of clinical assessment. Increasing impairment should be accompanied by an increasing score, and the method of combining the subscales to form an overall scale should be clear and simple. Goodkin and colleagues[203] devised an upper extremity scale that may improve the sensitivity of assessment outcome.[543]

Although it is debatable whether a more appropriate scale than the DSS or EDSS could be constructed, the scale could benefit from modification. Redekop and Paty[512]

developed a computerized method of assigning both the functional status (FS) and EDSS scores. The goal is for the computer to use the raw neurological data to assign FS scores based on an empirical set of neurological standards. The "AutoDSS" score is then assigned by the computer based on the FS scores to minimize subjective elements in the assignment of the score. The final score, assigned on a one to nine scale, is still ordinal but is based primarily on neurological impairment, is less dependent upon ambulation, and is also less biased by subjective factors. Figure 12–1 illustrates the distribution of the AutoDSS and the observed EDSS in the same group of patients. The AutoDSS system is based on the MS-COSTAR computerized medical record developed at UBC, using standards for recording the neurological examination that were developed by the neurologists of the UBC MS Clinic.[604] Quality of life scales are becoming widely used as outcome measures.[82a,93a,136a,499a] Their usefulness is yet to be determined. Certainly cognitive[37a] and fatigue[642a] evaluations also have a place as outcome measures.

PARACLINICAL TESTS

The many attempts to develop objective methods for assessing disease activity in MS (Tables 12–10 and 12–11) have included paraclinical tests (see Table 12–10) such as evoked potentials (EPs).[17] Serial studies of EPs have shown worsening with time, and in at least one trial[53,462] EPs significantly

Table 12–10. **PARACLINICAL METHODS FOR MONITORING DISEASE SEVERITY AND ACTIVITY**

Evoked potentials[53,462]

Cognitive function[511]

CT[158]

MRI:

    Quantitative area measurements[484]

    Visual and planimetric assessment[277]

    Frequent serial scans looking for new and active lesions*

*References 39, 221, 257, 292, 316, 318, 401, 583, 617, 681.

Table 12–11. LABORATORY METHODS FOR MONITORING DISEASE ACTIVITY

Measurement	Activity
Immunoglobulins	Serum: immunoglobulins and antibodies[73,136]
	CSF: IgG and antibodies[90,625]
Immunoglobulin production	B cells[19,214,290,465]
Lymphocyte populations	Bibliography[45]
	Activated cells[144,117b]
	Lymphocyte count[121]
	Lymphocyte phenotypes (acute relapse, correlated)[29,30,226,250,515]
	Lymphocyte phenotypes (acute relapse, not correlated)[467,490,518,689]
	Lymphocyte phenotypes (acute relapse, may be correlated)[109,287]
	Lymphocyte phenotypes (low in CPMS)[422,490]
	Suppressor cell function[18]
	NK cells[284]
	CSF: T cells[8]
Cytokine measurements	TNF-α[222a,419a,565]
	IL-6[419a]
	Lymphokine production[419a,561]
Tissue breakdown products and reactions	Prostaglandin release[142]
	MBP: CSF and urine[666,669,670]
	MBP and Anti-MBP[647]
Miscellaneous	Zinc[241]
	Neopterin[180]
	Cortisol[85]
	GFAP in CSF[538]

CSF = cerebrospinal fluid; CPMS = chronic progressive MS; GFAP = Glial fibrillary acidic protein; IFN = interferon; IL-6 = interleukin-6; MBP = myelin basic protein; NK = natural killer; TNF-α = tumor necrosis factor alpha.

distinguished between treated and control groups, even though no clinical benefit was noted. Aminoff and his colleagues[15,16] studied serial changes in EPs in 12 patients, each tested five times in 12 months. They found excessive variability in the EP that was not seen clinically and concluded that EP studies were not reliable monitors of disease activity. Another interpretation of their findings, however, might be that EP studies are more sensitive to change than clinical measures, so that they are providing information not accessible to clinical monitoring. Giesser and associates[189] and Smith and colleagues[584] proposed that EPs can be used as an outcome measure in MS therapeutic trials. The problem so far in multicenter trials has been the lack of both standardized measures and a system for central monitoring. Several recent studies have found cytokines to fluctuate with disease activity[222a, 419a,651a] but measurement of levels has not found acceptance in clinical trial outcomes.

Recent studies of cognitive deficits in MS[37a] have shown not only that these functions can be quantitated but that MRI serial evaluation may provide a means of measuring the disease effects on brain function from involvement of large areas of the nervous system that do not produce motor, sensory, or coordination deficits.[543b] As fully discussed in Chapters 6 and 9, advances in imaging, particularly in MRI, may have finally provided an objective, quantifiable measure of disease activity that can be used as an outcome measure. Quantitative MRI techniques enable the measurement of the extent of the pathological process and, by serial examinations, also give an objective assessment of the level of dynamic disease activity.[399,486] Tissue characterization of the pathological changes detected by MRI may soon be possible. Advances in magnetic resonance spectroscopy (MRS), MRI quantitation, and other magnetic resonance techniques such as the analysis of the multiexponential components of the T_2 signal should help identify specific pathological changes in MS, such as edema, inflammation, demyelination, gliosis, and axonal loss as they occur in vivo. (See Chapter 9.)

Rationale for Using Magnetic Resonance Imaging as an Outcome Measurement

The introduction of MRI provides a powerful tool to quantitate the morbid pathology of MS objectively, as fully discussed in Chapter 9. Proton magnetic resonance images reflect primarily the water content of tissue. However, MRI images also reflect alterations in local populations of cells and their aggregate biochemically defined constituents, particularly their lipid content and composition. For example, the water signal from different reservoirs, such as normal myelin, may be different from that which comes from cell cytoplasm.[358,594,596] These differences in water content and chemical condition between cerebral white and gray matter determine the exquisite anatomical definition of MR images of brain. Evolving data from comparative pathological, biochemical, and MRI and MRS studies of acute and chronic EAE in animals (as well as postmortem studies of MS in man) will likely, in the near future, define the relative contribution of pathological tissue changes to the magnetic resonance signal.

In 1984, Ebers and colleagues[158] suggested that enhancement on CT could be used as an outcome measure in clinical trials. Unfortunately, the exposure to ionizing radia-

tion precludes multiple exposures, but MRI can be used safely at frequent intervals.

Currently used imaging standards, which are appropriately T_2 weighted, exquisitely define MS lesions above the level of the mid-cervical spinal cord, and diagnostically abnormal scans are seen in approximately 90 percent of patients with clinically definite MS (CDMS)[376] (Fig. 12–2). Analysis of early postmortem cadaver magnetic resonance scans and subsequent pathological examination has provided support for using MRI as a measure of the extent of demyelination.[471,595,597,598] Fast spin-echo may be as reliable as conventional spin-echo,[619] but that finding is yet to be validated in quantitative studies in clinical trials. Thompson and colleagues[617] found that primary chronic progressive MS (CPMS) has a different MRI pattern from that seen in relapsing MS or in secondary progressive MS. Koopmans and his colleagues[316,318] found that fluctuations in size of MRI lesions can be quite persistent. Primary progressive MS probably has a different pathology as well.[517] However, MRI scan findings do not correlate well with clinical status in individual patients.

Several groups[39,401] observed that serial imaging of individual patients often shows

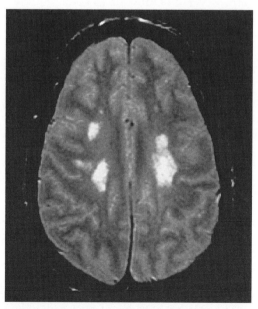

Figure 12–2. An axial proton density image taken from just above the level of the ventricles prior to quantitation.

the asymptomatic appearance of new lesions and the enlargement of previously seen stable lesions with time. MRI methods of detection of new and active lesions will likely provide an objective measure of disease activity that is somewhat independent of changes in clinical neurological status. Spinal cord imaging does not seem to help the strength of the correlation.[303,393,620,626,678] The rate of MRI activity can be 5 to 10 times the rate of clinical activity. The disparity between clinical and MRI activity may be even greater in chronic secondary progressive patients than in other categories. Harris and his colleagues[221] followed up six patients with monthly gadolinium-enhanced and nonenhanced MRI scans for 8 to 11 months. Four of the six had one or more enhancing lesions present on each examination. The duration of enhancement was usually brief (less than 1 month). Smith and associates,[582] in a related study, found that bursts of MRI activity occurred many times without individual clinical correlations. However, 10 of 13 clinical exacerbations occurred in association with bursts of increased MRI activity. Serial MRI studies not only will detect asymptomatic activity but will provide objective supportive data for clinically documented stabilization or improvement of function as well.

A study at UBC[491a] has suggested that, on average, patients with high rates of MRI activity tend to develop more severe neurological worsening than do patients with lesser degrees of MRI activity. However, a great deal of overlap occurred in this study, so that the information was not helpful in individual patients.

The concerted action guidelines published by a European committee on the use of MRI in MS clinical trials[399] have recommended that monthly gadolinium-enhanced scans be performed together with clinical evaluations in clinical trials for at least 6 months. Statistical factors have also been carefully determined.[437] Other guidelines have been prepared by a committee of the National MS Society of the USA.[398a] In recent years many trials have used MRI to monitor treatment.[220,398,407a,453,680]

The method of frequent MRI and quantitative MRI studies has been shown in a large multicenter clinical trial[492] to be more sensitive than clinical measures in detecting treatment effects (see the later section on Interferon Beta). Figures 12–3 and 12–4 illustrate how the quantitative MRI measures are done (see Chapter 9).

The rationale for using MRI as a primary outcome measure in clinical trials can now be stated clearly because of the information available from follow-up studies. The following categories clearly explain the correlations that are seen between MRI and clinical features of MS:

DIAGNOSIS

The fact that most MRI lesions are clinically silent makes MRI scanning helpful in the diagnosis of MS.[493] The clinical-MRI correlation in diagnosis is 90 percent. Multiple lesions and lesion loads at onset predict the risk for diagnosis[424] and the time to diagnosis. The ON treatment trial[50,52] follow-up shows clearly that the number of lesions on MRI scans at onset of ON predicts the diagnosis of MS at 2 years.

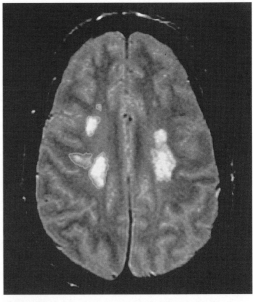

Figure 12–3. The same image as in Figure 12–2, except the lesions in the left cerebral hemispheres have been outlined for the purposes of quantitation.

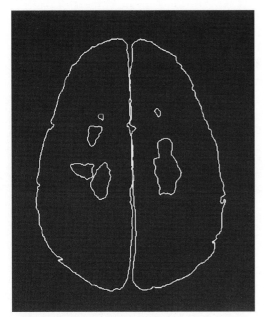

Figure 12–4. The outlining profiles of all the lesions in the MRI slice shown in Figure 12–2.

PATHOLOGY

Correlation studies show that:

1. Single isolated MRI lesions correlate well with pathology.[597]
2. Enhancement in vivo is correlated with inflammation at autopsy.[289]
3. MRI scans probably overestimate the extent of disease, although in one study, MRI scans underestimated the extent of demyelination.[593]
4. New MRI techniques such as T_2 relaxation analysis and spectroscopy have the potential to characterize pathological tissue changes in vivo (see Chapter 9).[24,216,358,414,520]

ISOLATED CLINICAL SYNDROMES

These clinical features have all been correlated with appropriately located lesions on the MRI scan:

- ON[400,471,618a,687]
- Myelopathy[471]
- Propriospinal monoclonus[272]
- Neurogenic pulmonary edema[417,574]
- Acute brain stem syndromes[26,65,117]
- Auditory loss[126]
- Intractable hiccup[100]

- Hemifacial spasm[3a]
- Hemiparesis

NEUROPSYCHOLOGICAL CORRELATES

Many studies of neuropsychological features of MS have shown correlation with the MRI scan as follows:

1. Atrophy of the corpus callosum (particularly the anterior part) correlates with dementia.[508]
2. Poor visual memory correlates with MRI lesion load.[364]
3. Periventricular lesion load correlates with poor concept formation, reasoning, and verbal memory.[20]
4. Periventricular lesion load correlates with overall cognitive impairment.*
5. Patients with isolated symptoms and multiple MRI lesions have subtle cognitive abnormalities.[164]
6. Ventricular enlargement and MRI lesion load correlate with cognitive deficits but not depression.[104]
7. Psychiatric syndromes in MS correlate with temporal lobe involvement on the MRI scan.[245]

NEUROLOGICAL STATUS

Even though the extent of MRI abnormalities and the degree of neurological impairment do not correlate well in individual patients, many studies have shown a significant though not robust correlation in groups of patients.[678]

1. Disabled patients have a much heavier disease burden than do patients with benign disease matched for age, sex, and duration of disease.[317]
2. The overall burden of disease (BOD) does not correlate very well in individual patients, but there is an overall group correlation with disease severity: $(P = 0.01 - 0.001)$[159,209,302,373,632] T_1 abnormalities may correlate better with neurological impairment than do the standard T_2 MRI changes.[640]

---

*References 44, 108a, 179, 258, 380, 509, 516.

3. The overall BOD increases with duration of disease (r value = 0.66, P = 0.0001).[168,285,319]

4. In the interferon beta-1b trial (the Interferon Beta MS Study Group),[256] the patients with the highest relapse rates (greater than 1.5 relapses per patient per year) had a significantly greater increase in MRI-detected BOD than did the patients with low relapse rates (less than 0.5 relapses per patient per year). The same correlation was found for the relationship between relapse rate and increases in EDSS. The final outcome correlations are in Table 12–12.

5. Enhancing lesions and clinical activity correlate with immunological changes.[222a,651a]

6. Magnetic transfer imaging[400] may correlate better with neurological impairment than does standard T_2 MRI. MRS findings correlate with clinical features.[130a,133a]

7. Some of the lack of correlation may be due to the insensitivity of clinical methods. Levine and colleagues[342] performed neurophysiological investigations of patients with brain stem lesions on MRI scan and found evidence for clinically asymptomatic lesions.

MAGNETIC RESONANCE IMAGING ACTIVITY RATE

The MRI activity rate is generally predictive of the future clinical course:

1. A high MRI activity rate is associated with a worse clinical outcome.[491] High MRI activity rates were usually seen in patients who eventually became much worse clinically, but the associations have not been statistically significant because of the small numbers of patients studied. High MRI activity was seen more often in progressive patients with superimposed relapses[302a] rather than in those without such relapses.

2. The clinical courses of relapsing-remitting and primary chronic progressive disease have different MRI patterns.[166a,351a,362,617] Patients with primary CPMS had fewer new lesions and fewer enhancing lesions than did patients with secondary progressive disease.

3. Patients with benign MS and those with early relapsing-remitting MS seem to have different MRI patterns.[302,616,620a] Patients with early relapsing-remitting disease had more activity than did patients with benign disease of longer duration. Spinal and corticospinal tract lesions found on MRI scan are the most likely to be associated with appropriate symptoms.[620a,690a]

Table 12–12. **CORRELATIONS BETWEEN OUTCOME MEASURES IN THE INTERFERON BETA-1b TRIAL**[*]

	Spearman Rank Correlation[*]
Baseline EDSS vs baseline MRI area	0.218
Endpoint EDSS vs endpoint MRI area	0.257
Change in EDSS vs change in MRI area	0.229
Baseline NRS vs baseline MRI area	−0.249
Endpoint NRS vs endpoint MRI area	−0.277
Change in NRS vs change in MRI area	−0.213
Baseline NRS vs baseline EDSS	−0.835
Baseline NRS vs endpoint EDSS	−0.899
Change in NRS vs change in EDSS	−0.709
Exacerbation rate vs change in MRI area	0.203
Exacerbation rate vs change in EDSS	0.252
Exacerbation rate vs change in NRS	−0.301

Source: Adapted from Neurology V45, p 1283, 1995, by permission of Little, Brown and Company (Inc.).

EDSS = Extended Disability Status Scale; MRI = magnetic resonance imaging; NRS = Neurologic Rating Scale.

[*]All correlations significant (P=0.001).

4. Periods of clinical activity and MRI activity have been correlated in some studies.[221,582,583,602a,678] Even though new MRI lesions are frequently neurologically silent (Ratio of at least 7 to 1), when scans are taken over a period of weeks, flurries of MRI activity are usually associated with some evidence of clinical activity. Specific relapse syndromes are not that commonly seen, but corticospinal tract lesions are likely to be symptomatic.[690a]

5. Gadolinium enhanced scans are more sensitive than unenhanced scans for measuring activity[70a,400a,620a] and correlate with biological markers.[189a] However, unenhanced scans are less invasive and may be adequate for monitoring.[40a,492] The FLAIR technique is quick and may replace standard T_2 imaging.[187a]

QUANTITATIVE BURDEN OF DISEASE (BOD)

The BOD also seems to predict clinical course. A follow-up study with MRI scans at onset, and 5 and 10 year points[470a] showed that patients with the highest lesion load at onset were more likely to develop CDMS by a factor of 140 times over patients with a normal MRI scan at onset. In addition, those same patients developed MS earlier.[168,169] The change in lesion load over 5 years correlated with the extent of lesion load at onset ($P = 0.0001$). Clinical impairment score (EDSS) and the brain MRI lesion load at 5 years were also correlated in patients who developed MS ($P = 0.0002$). The lesion load at onset and change in lesion load were both correlated with clinical impairment at 5 years ($P = 0.0001$). Baumhefner and colleagues[44] found that MRI lesion area above the spinal cord correlated with clinical and neuroperformance outcome assessments in chronic progressive MS. Khoury and colleagues[299a] reported a significant correlation between change in MRI lesion burden and change in disability in 18 patients followed up over 1 year with repeated MRI and clinical evaluations. Cerebral and spinal cord atrophy may also be excellent ways to monitor the long term outcome of therapy.[146a,351b,351c] Another study found that T_1 "black holes" correlated with the clinical progression rate.[632a]

THERAPEUTIC TRIAL CORRELATIONS WITH MAGNETIC RESONANCE IMAGING

A number of therapeutic trials have been monitored with MRI. It is obvious that the MRI lesion load and clinical disability both increase predictably over time.

Three early treatment trials monitored by MRI showed no clearly effective clinical or therapeutic effect.[277,278,282,319,321] However, in both studies in which quantitative measurement of BOD was done, a clear-cut increase in average disease burden of approximately 20 percent occurred over 2 years. In addition, in the placebo limb of the interferon beta-1b clinical trial, a 20 percent increase occurred in MRI-detected burden of disease over 3 years.[492] The final report showed a number of correlations between MRI and clinical outcome measures (Table 12–12).[256]

A steroid effect in decreasing enhancing lesions correlates with clinical improvement.[33,84,402]

SUMMARY AND COMMENTS

Follow-up studies in several different institutions clearly show that MRI activity, as defined by the number of lesions and overall BOD, is predictive of the clinical outcome. A number of specific correlations also exist between MRI lesions and specific symptoms. Clearly MRI is not only an objective measure of the extent of in-vivo pathology, but it is more sensitive to treatment effects than are the usual clinical methods. The increased sensitivity and objectivity of MRI scan makes it the preferred method for monitoring therapeutic trials in MS, particularly in monitoring the effects of promising and as yet untested therapeutic agents. Long-term clinical studies will always be needed to show clinical efficacy, but in the relapsing-remitting phase of MS, it may be unprofitable to expend time, patients, and other resources on therapeutic agents that show no effect on early systematic MRI monitoring.

Is it really warranted to discard the use of therapeutic agents that do not show an effect on the MRI scan? Pathological features, such as axonal loss, are not well explained by the specific autoimmune reaction in the usual concepts of the demyelination model. In addition, axonal loss and other pathological features of severity of the lesion are not well monitored by current MRI activity measures. MRS or other methods of measuring tissue-specific severity (i.e., *N*-acetylaspartate, estimate of axonal integrity)[24] may give a measure[377] of active demyelination[320] and of axonal loss.[23] Therefore, we need to expand our methodology in conjunction with currently used methods to develop the degree of specificity necessary to monitor multiple pathological changes in vivo. In addition, volumetric methods will probably provide more accurate and reproducible measures of the extent of MS pathology in the future. However, present automated volumetric methods are probably too insensitive for routine use.[200,259,601,607,677]

For clinical trials, MRI has become necessary and helpful as an outcome measure. However, there are many pitfalls. Any new approaches to the analysis of MRI data must be carefully validated. The results must be reproducible and centrally analysed for any specific clinical trial.

Although gadolinium enhancement may not be necessary for all trials,[493] its use greatly increases the number of active lesions detected.[400a] One caution, however: Recent studies[32,84] have shown that intravenous corticosteroids will reduce enhancement without affecting the lesions seen on T_2-weighted lesion evaluation. Therefore, a correction must be made for this effect. In addition, although endothelial disruption and enhancement may be an important first step in the primary MS lesion, subsequent disruption may be less significant (see Chapter 9).

Goodkin and his colleagues[207,208] caution those enthusiasts of MRI monitoring to be careful that they are not falsely identifying lesions as morphologically active. They point out that some of the changes seen, especially with small lesions, may actually be artifacts caused by technical factors such as poor positioning. Yetkin and colleagues[684] studied observer variability on MRI quantitation and advised caution because of wide variation. Filippi and colleagues[167] looked at two methods of measuring the "brain lesion volume" and concluded that even though the standard is manual tracking of lesions,[492] a semiautomatic thresholding method may be more reproducible and faster.[677] Spectroscopy may also be helpful in the future.[131]

Cobalt-55 positron emission tomography may also be helpful in evaluating the clinical course of MS.[267a]

In summary, therapeutic trials today should include one or both of the following MRI measures:

- A quantitative analysis of the extent of BOD at both entry and exit should be obtained in a blinded fashion in a significant cohort of control and treated patients.
- Frequent serial MRI scans should be performed to assess the development of new and active lesions. Doing frequent and carefully repositioned MRI scans can detect asymptomatic and dynamic changes that cannot be detected by another means. Routine gadolinium enhancement may be necessary in some studies.

Biologic Measures of Disease Activity

Many investigators have tried counting lymphocyte subsets as a way of monitoring disease activity (Table 12–11). Compston[109] found that many factors influenced these measurements, including time of scan and viral infections. Most people have discarded these measures as a reliable indicator of disease activity.[689] However, T-cell activation markers may be helpful as an indicator of activity in chronic progressive patients.[117b,586a]

Whitaker and his colleagues[666,670] studied CSF and urine as possible ways of monitoring disease activity. They reported that an elevated level of myelin basic protein (MBP) in the CSF appears to be a measure of disease activity. In one study,[674] urinary MBP appeared to correlate with the onset of progressive disease. The CSF MBP level may also predict the response to glucocorticoid therapy. Warren and his collaborators,[647] who also studied MBP and antibody to MBP in the CSF as a monitor of disease activity, showed that free MBP and antibody to MBP both increase during clinical attacks of MS. Unfortunately, they did not do MRI monitoring so that the effect of asymptomatic MRI activity on their measurements is unknown.

An interesting cytokine molecule, tumor necrosis factor (TNF), has been implicated as a factor in oligodendrocyte and myelin toxicity.[691] It has also been reported to increase during relapses[222a] and with chronic progressive disease activity.[565] Therapy directed at blockade of TNF seems a promising new avenue. However, caution should be advised because of potential disease activation.[639a] Interleukin-2 (IL-2) and soluble IL-2 receptor have also been proposed as biologic markers for MS activity.[566] Lymphocyte IL-2 receptors may fluctuate with clinical MRI activity.[692]

Looking at serum levels of galactosylceramide (Gal C) in MS, Lubetzki and colleagues[352] found a correlation between elevated levels of Gal C and clinical relapses. If confirmed, this measure could be a good adjunct measure for assessment of disease activity in clinical studies. Antiganglioside antibodies have also been suggested as a way to monitor MS activity,[418] as have T-cell subsets, but the changes they identify are probably nonspecific.[489] Also, soluble vascular adhesion molecules ICAM-1 and VCAM-1 levels fluctuate in correlation with MRI activity.[189a,222a]

Several groups have also attempted to use CSF IgG levels as a way to monitor therapy.[45,152,381] Rudick and colleagues[542] reported that free kappa light chains in the CSF may be a marker for a poor prognosis. Myelin antibody in the CSF may also help to distinguish clinical forms of MS.[645,646] Glial fibrillary acidic protein in CSF may be a marker for clinical progressive impairment and probably reflects the speed and extent of gliosis.[538] Cytokine networks in MS were recently reviewed (Hohfeld and Lucas 1995).[241b]

SPECIFIC THERAPIES DIRECTED AT THE PATHOGENESIS OF MULTIPLE SCLEROSIS

Table 12–13 lists a number of specific therapies tried in the past and discarded. A number of excellent recent reviews of therapy in MS are available.* *Therapeutic Claims in MS*[568] also examines proposed therapies, many of them proprietary. Table 12–14 lists treatments that may make MS worse.

This chapter focuses on therapies currently considered for use that may have some efficacy in the treatment of either acute exacerbations or the chronic progressive phase of MS. Most therapies for changing the clinical course of MS have focused on the immunopathogenesis theory. The topic has been the subject of several recent symposia, and some controversies surrounding such trials in MS were recently highlighted by a survey conducted by Noseworthy and associates.[458] Cytokines such as tumor necrosis factor-alpha have been implicated in the pathogenesis of MS and EAE.[225a,351b,437a,691a] Blocking TNF holds great promise as a potent anti-inflammatory therapy. Bone marrow transplant has also been suggested as a possible therapy in MS,[84a] and linomide has been found to inhibit EAE[279b] and to benefit MS in a preliminary trial[279a] (see Table 12–33).

Compston[111,112] proposed that future strategies for therapy should include the suppression of inflammatory mediators in the CNS, manipulation of the oligodendrocyte membrane, inhibition of macrophage activity, enhancement of oligodendrocyte regeneration, and reconstitution of defective cell populations in critically placed lesions. The recent interest in the phenomenon of axonal loss in MS (see Chapter 9) has revealed that little is known about the time course and cause of axonal loss. If, as some believe, axonal loss in MS is the only really permanent cause of loss of function, then more should be known concerning its evolution and its cause. If endogenous toxins are found to be important factors in the

---

*References 31a, 111, 428, 457, 506, 580.

Table 12–13. **THERAPIES SHOWN NOT TO BE EFFECTIVE**

Anticoagulants:	Coumadin
	Heparin
Antihistamines:	Diphenhydramine
Anti-infectives:	Adenine arabinoside
	Cytosine arabinoside
	Isoniazid
	Immunoglobulins
	Hyperimmune cow colostrum
	Nystatin
	Vaccines: typhoid, viruses
	Transfusion
Anti-inflammatories:	Aspirin
	Chloroquine
	Penicillamine
	Nonsteroidal anti-inflammatory drugs
	Snake venom
Diets—restricted:	Allergen-free diet
	Gluten-free diet
	Sucrose-tobacco–free diet
	Raw food diet
	Low-fat diet
Diets—supplemented:	Minerals
	Fish oils
	Aloe vera
	Cerebrosides
	Lecithin
	Vitamins
	Cambridge Diet
Metabolic inhibitors or stimulants:	Adenosine-5-monophosphate
	Cytochrome C
	Fever therapy
	Piromen
	Digestive enzymes
	Epsilon aminocaproic acid
	Vitamins, including megavitamins, nicotinic acid, ascorbic acid
	Antidiabetics: tolbutamide

Continued on following page

axonal loss, then the strategies of long-term therapy should turn toward neuroprotection as well as immunomodulation and glial cell repair. Panitch[474a] and Ebers[155] have recently reviewed investigational drug therapies in MS.

Adrenocorticotrophic Hormone and Corticosteroids

Fog in 1951[172] and Glaser and Merritt in 1952[190] were the first to report the use of adrenocorticotrophic hormone (ACTH) in the treatment of relapses of MS (Table 12–15). Subsequently, Miller and Gibbons,[404] Alexander and colleagues,[7] Kelly and Jellinek,[291] and Miller and associates[406] reported successes in the treatment of acute exacerbations with either ACTH or corticosteroids. The definitive study of the use of ACTH in the treatment of acute relapses was that of Rose and colleagues in 1970.[533] This report was a cooperative double blind placebo-controlled study of the use of ACTH in 197 patients with acute relapses. The patients treated with ACTH improved more rapidly than did control subjects, with the most marked improve-

Table 12–13.—*continued*

Immunosuppressants:	Methotrexate: to be tried again (see text) Chlorambucil 5-Fluorouracil
Immune modulators:	Thymus hormones Alpha-fetoprotein Thymectomy Intrathecal tuberculin Dimethyl sulfoxide Various allergens Allergen-free diet
Free radical scavengers:	Superoxide dismutase
Vasoactive drugs:	Histamine Alcohol Papaverine Hydergine Aminophylline Nifedipine Verapamil
Miscellaneous:	Procaine hydrochloride Cells, cell extract, and brain injection or implantation Chelation Blood transfusion
Physical measures:	Acupuncture Hysterectomy Spinal cord stimulation Thymectomy Hyperbaric oxygen Cranial artery surgery Magneto therapy Replacement of mercury amalgam fillings

Source: Adapted from Sibley W.[568]

ment during the first few weeks of therapy. Follow-up at 6 months showed that the improvement curves of the treated and control groups approached each other, suggesting that ACTH accelerated improvement. This trial has been widely quoted as evidence for the effectiveness of ACTH (and by implication, corticosteroids) in the short-term therapy of exacerbations in MS. However, the authors were muted in their enthusiasm about ACTH therapy. In addition, patients were admitted to the study if they had had a significant acute worsening of their MS within 8 weeks. But to be effective, anti-inflammatory therapy probably should be started before or at the height of the inflammatory response. Eight weeks may be too long to wait before initiating anti-inflammatory therapy. However, previous studies had found it very difficult to recruit patients into such a study within the 2 or 3 weeks that most would consider optimal timing. Beck and associates achieved a

Table 12–14. TREATMENTS THAT MAY MAKE MULTIPLE SCLEROSIS WORSE

Intrathecal Depo-Medrol[439]

Intrathecal tuberculin[407]

Levamisole[129]

Interferon gamma[476]

Indomethacin[444]

Isoprinosine[116]

Cyclophosphamide[460]

Table 12–15. SOME RECENT THERAPEUTIC TRIALS OF ACTH AND CORTICOSTEROIDS IN MULTIPLE SCLEROSIS

Year	Senior Author	No. of Patients	Patient Type	Active Agent/ Control Agent	Duration of Therapy or Follow-up	Randomized	Controlled	Blinded	Comments
1970	Rose[533]	197	Relapsing	ACTH/placebo	2 wk/4 wk	+	+	+	Sixty-nine percent of placebo group recovered. ACTH group improved more (p=<0.05) at 6 mo. there was no difference.
1972	Kibler[301]	7	RR	High-dose prednisone/placebo	6 mo	+	+	+	Alternate-day prednisone was randomly withdrawn. Most exacerbations occurred while patients received placebo.
1973	Nelson[439]	23	Relapsing and CP	Intrathecal MP	Mixed	—	—	—	MP was ineffective.
1975	Cendrowski[96]	21	CDMS	Oral steroids/AZA	<14 mo	—	+	—	Steroids reduced relapse severity but had no long-term effect.
1980	Tourtellotte[624]	28	CDMS	ACTH plus steroids	Short	—	—	—	ACTH and steroids reduce intrathecal IgG synthesis.
1980	Dowling[144]	7	Relapsing	IVMP, 500 mg/day, followed by oral prednisone	MP—3 days Prednisone —10–18 wk	—	—	—	Drug improved acute relapse if treatment started early in course of illness.
1980	Trotter[630]	12	CDMS	IVMP 1 g/day	3 days	—	—	—	Improvements occurred in ADL and vision. *Continued on following page*

Table 12–15.—*continued*

Year	Senior Author	Active Agent/ Control Agent	No. of Patients	Patient Type	Duration of Therapy or Follow-up	Randomized	Controlled	Blinded	Comments
1982	Buckley[83]	IVMP 0.25–1 g/day	6	Relapsing	2–5 days	—	—	—	Patients rapidly improved from severe exacerbations, including reversal of weakness, ataxia, and sensory disturbances. This effect is probably due to reduction of inflammation and edema and relief of conduction block.
1983	Goas[191]	IVMP 1 g/day	13	Relapsing	5 days	—	—	—	Drug produced rapid improvement in ten days.
1983	Abbruzzese[1]	IVMP 1 g bolus	30	Two groups	Bolus	+	—	—	IVMP offered no long-term benefit.
1985	Barnes[34]	IVMP 1 g/day/ ACTH	25	Relapsing	7 days	+	+	+	MP was more effective than ACTH but offered no long-term benefit.
1986	Durelli[151]	IVMP 1 g/day with taper/ placebo	23	Relapsing	15 days	+	+	+	Placebo patients received IV steroids after 15 days; all received oral tapering prednisone (120 days). MP associated with: • Decreased IgG synthesis rate • Earlier improvement.
1986	Warren[648]	IVMP,1 60 mg/day or 2 g/day	40	Relapsing	10 days	—	—	—	Clinical improvement was variable. MP reduced IgG synthesis, free antibody to MBP, and MBP levels, especially in acute relapse. *Continued on following page*

467

Table 12–15.—continued

Year	Senior Author	No. of Patients	Patient Type	Active Agent/ Control Agent	Duration of Therapy or Follow-up	Randomized	Controlled	Blinded	Comments
1987	Milligan[408]	50	RR (22) and CP (28)	IVMP 0.5 g/day IV/placebo	4 wk	+	+	+	Patients treated with MP improved ($P<.001$). CP patients improved mostly in spasticity.
1989	Thompson[615]	61	RR (51) CP (10)	IVMP/ACTH	MP—3 days/ ACTH—14 days	+	+	+	No difference occurred in rate of recovery or final outcome between MP and ACTH groups. MP had fewer side effects.
1989	Milanese[389]	30	Relapsing	IVMP (low dose) or IVDM or IVACTH	14 days Tapering dose in all groups	+	+	+	DM was better than MP, MP better than ACTH in this small trial.
1989	Kesselring[293]	50	Relapsing	IVMP 0.5 g/day; MRI studies before and 15 days after treatment	15 days	N/A	N/A	N/A	There was no correlation between MRI changes and clinical observations. Steroids did not change the standard T_2 MRI lesions at 15 days.
1989	Ellison[161]	98	CP	MP vs AZA/ placebo/ both	MP—36 wk AZA—3 yr	+	+	+	No clear therapeutic benefits were obtained. Visual evoked potentials did not change in MP-treated and AZA-treated patients, but did change in controls.

Continued on following page

Table 12–15.—*continued*

Year	Senior Author	Active Agent/Control Agent	No. of Patients	Patient Type	Duration of Therapy or Follow-up	Randomized	Controlled	Blinded	Comments
1990	Whitham[676]	monthly IVMP	33	Mixed	monthly	—	—	—	Patients may be at greater risk for osteoporosis.
1991	Burnham[84]	IVMP 1 g/day	7	Mixed	4–8 days	—	—	—	MP decreased enlarging lesions on MRI.
1991	Barkhof[33]	IVMP 1 g/day	12	MS	10 days	—	—	—	MP decreased enhancement on MRI.
1992	Beck[51]	1. IVMP 250 mg ×4 ×3 days; prednisone tapered over 11 days 2. Prednisone po 1 mg/kg ×14 days 3. Placebo po ×14 days	457	ON with or without MS	<3 wk	+	+	+	MP improved vision faster than other treatments. Low dose prednisone was associated with increased risk of recurrent ON.
1993	Beck[52]	Follow-up on Beck 1992	389	ON only		+	+	+	IVMP treatment was followed by delay in conversion to MS within 2 years.
1994	La Mantia[334a]	High-dose vs low-dose IVMP vs IVDM	31	Relapsing	1-yr follow-up	+	+	+	IVDM was as effective as high-dose MP. Low-dose MP was associated with early reactivation.

ACTH = adrenocorticotropic hormone; AZA = azathioprine; CDMS = clinically definite MS; CP = chronic progressive; DM = dexamethasone; IVMP = intravenous methylprednisolone; MRI = magnetic resonance imaging; MP = methylprednisolone; ON = optic neuritis; RR = relapsing-remitting.
+ = yes; — = no.

one week delay in treatment in the Optic Neuritis Treatment Trial (ONTT)[51] showing that rapid accrual of patients is possible in an acute attack study.

Some of the early studies found ACTH to be effective, but not corticosteroids. More recent experience has suggested that corticosteroids are at least as effective as ACTH, but a long-term effect has yet to be shown.[182] Corticosteroids may be given orally, which makes it easier to administer them on an outpatient basis and easier to achieve large pharmacological doses. More recent approaches advocate IV therapy (pulses) with soluble steroids. A recent treatment trial with ON has suggested that oral prednisone therapy may be associated with a higher than normal risk for early recurrent ON.[51] ACTH and corticosteroids have been used to suppress the inflammatory response in the CNS and also to suppress the immune system. Steroids have many biologic effects aside from their known action on inflammatory and immunologic features. The effectiveness of ACTH and corticosteroids in the treatment and suppression of EAE has supported their widespread use in the treatment of exacerbations in MS. Table 12–15 lists a number of studies of the use of ACTH and corticosteroids.

Other studies examined the effects of long-term ACTH and corticosteroids on chronic progression. In 1954, Meritt and colleagues[383] showed that significant toxicity was seen in all the patients who were treated with corticosteroids for many months, and that a number of patients went on to have exacerbations despite chronic steroid therapy. In 1961, Miller and colleagues[405] randomized patients into treatment groups that received prednisolone, aspirin, chlorquine, gamma globulin, or placebo. Follow-up over 18 months failed to show any difference between the groups treated with placebo, aspirin, or prednisolone. Another study by Millar in 1967[392] showed that ACTH administered daily over 18 months also did not produce any difference in outcome between treated and control patients. The power to detect treatment effects was low in these two studies. In addition, chronic ACTH therapy produced a 25 percent incidence of serious complications such as psychosis, peptic ulcer, septicemia, pathological fracture, and adrenal failure.

The high rate of complications from therapy in these chronic studies points out the potential dangers of long-term corticosteroid use.[356] Current practice dictates that use of ACTH and corticosteroids be limited to the short-term treatment of disabling acute attacks. However, some reports still indicate that ACTH is no better than bedrest in the treatment of acute relapses.[246] The exquisite sensitivity to (and sometimes dependence on) corticosteroids seen in occasional patients may require careful consideration of the benefit-risk ratio. Some patients not only improve with corticosteroid therapy after an acute attack but subsequently deteriorate when the corticosteroids are withdrawn. In our experience, when such deterioration occurs, it is at a dosage level of 20 to 40 mg of prednisone per day has been administered. When withdrawal deterioration occurs, most patients can be withdrawn successfully after a boost in dose to 60 to 80 mg per day followed by slower tapering. Increasing the dose temporarily usually helps to recover the ground lost by the initial taper. Withdrawal of steroids probably does not worsen the disease, but in a double-blind controlled study of a small group of patients, Kibler and his colleagues[301] found that relapses tended to occur after steroids were withdrawn. This finding was in contrast to that of Millar and colleagues,[393] who did not find any effect of withdrawal of corticotropin over a period of 1 year.

Kirk and Compston[309] reported that dexamethasone therapy caused increased response to mitogens. Frequin and colleagues[181] found that IV methylprednisolone caused a reduction in CSF MBP and IgM levels. They also found a correlation between the MBP level and the EDSS in a follow-up study.

Kibler[300] was the first to advocate high doses of oral steroids (200 mg/day of prednisone) in the treatment of acute relapses. This dose was determined by the amount of steroid necessary to reverse paralysis in acute EAE in the rabbit.

PULSED STEROIDS

One recent development in the use of corticosteroids has been the method of pulsed therapy reviewed by Compston.[110] The mechanism of action is unknown but may relate in some way to transient immunomodulation with reduction in cytokine release.[124a] This method of therapy uses very high doses of soluble corticosteroids such as methylprednisolone given intravenously. Several trials of high-dose methylprednisolone in MS have shown significant short-term improvements. In 1980, Dowling and associates[144] gave IV methylprednisolone (300 mg) followed by 150 mg every 6 hours for 2.5 days, which in turn was followed by administration of oral prednisone, 100 mg every other day with gradual tapering doses over 3 months. They contended that if treatment was initiated early in the course of the relapse, the methylprednisolone regimen could be effective in temporarily reversing neurological deficits. Buckley and colleagues[83] and Newman and colleagues[442] also found that patients improved rapidly from severe exacerbations, including reversal of weakness, ataxia, and sensory disturbances, with methylprednisolone. They postulated that the therapeutic effect was due to reduction of inflammation and edema, which in turn relieved conduction block. Goas and associates[191] saw rapid improvement after 5 days of pulsed therapy, but they believed that longer follow-up was required to judge real effectiveness.

Using a complicated regimen, Durelli and his colleagues[147,152] found that clinical improvement occurred earlier in patients who were treated with methylprednisolone than in patients treated with placebo. At the end of the trial, they treated all patients in the study with IV steroids. The placebo-treated patients received a pulsed methylprednisolone after a 15-day course of placebo. Thompson and his colleagues[615] reported no difference in the rate of recovery or the final outcome between patients treated with IV methylprednisolone and IV ACTH. However, they did find that IV methylprednisolone had fewer side effects than did ACTH and therefore was preferable. Milanese[389] treated patients in acute relapse for 14 days with low-dose ACTH, dexamethasone, or methylprednisolone. The response to therapy was best in the dexamethasone treatment group, with a more rapid recovery and higher index of recovery, followed by those in the ACTH and methylprednisolone groups, respectively. In addition, Milligan and colleagues[408] also reported significant short-term improvement in some patients with chronic progressive disease using IV methylprednisolone ($P<0.01$). Our experience confirms these findings; some patients with CPMS improve after pulsed steroid therapy. Most of the chronic progressive patients' improvement is due to reduction in spasticity, but some patients recover strength as well. The dosage of methylprednisolone for pulsed therapy has been 500 to 1000 mg per day intravenously over 3 to 7 days. Alam and colleagues[6] and La Mantia and associates[334a] compared oral methylprednisolone with IV methylprednisolone at equivalent doses and found similar effects. However, low doses of steroids had a negative effect with early clinical reactivation. These results suggest that oral pulsed treatment may be as effective as IV dosage. If so, oral therapy could be much easier for the patient and less expensive.

Some controversy surrounds the use of ACTH versus corticosteroids. ACTH receptors have been found in human lymphocytes, which also can produce ACTH-like substances. Perhaps a well-designed prospective study should compare ACTH with corticosteroids in the therapy of disabling acute relapses.

Some investigators have begun to use pulsed steroids on a monthly basis in an attempt to maintain the initial improvement seen in some chronically active patients.[675] The outcome of these studies is eagerly awaited. At present, the most effective use of steroids for disabling relapses would seem to be intravenous methylprednisolone daily for 3 to 5 days, sometimes followed by an oral tapering dose of prednisone. The tapering dose may not be necessary.

Beck and his colleagues[51] showed that IV methylprednisolone shortened the duration of visual loss in ON. However, oral low-dose prednisone seemed to be associated with an increased risk for recurrent ON. This study suggests a negative effect of low-dose steroids. Although visual function improved over the short term, at the end of 1 year, no differences in visual function could be found between treatment and placebo groups. The most recent publication from Beck and colleagues[52] reported that the methylprednisolone-treated group had a significant effect. It delayed the timing of the second relapse and therefore delayed the onset of clinically definite MS. The reason for such a prolonged protective effect from IV steroids is unknown, but this phenomenon should be studied further in future therapeutic trials.

Beck[49] and Kupersmith and colleagues[325] wrote thoughtful editorials on the IV steroid issue. They propose that IV steroids should be used to treat ON if the MRI shows definite MS-like abnormalities.

Kesselring and his colleagues[293] evaluated the gadolinium-enhanced MRI scan before and after IV methylprednisolone therapy. They found that enhancement diminished after treatment in seven cases, but no other detectable change was found on the MRI scans in 36 of 50 patients. In nine patients, new MRI lesions appeared during the time of therapy, showing that methylprednisolone does not suppress the development of new MRI-detected activity. Subsequent studies from the same group showed that enhancement in MS lesions was dramatically reduced by methylprednisolone therapy, but that the lesions seen on T_2-weighted images did not change. Other studies[33,84,402] have also shown that IV steroid therapy can reduce the duration and degree of enhancement without affecting the lesions seen on the T_2-weighted image. Steroids can also reduce IgG synthesis in the CSF.[46] A recent study of methylprednisolone in SPMS has claimed that a modest benefit might accrue from monthly IV dosing with methylprednisolone.[204a]

COMPLICATIONS OF STEROIDS

Even though short courses of IV or oral corticosteroids seem safe, complications from corticosteroids have been seen, particularly in patients who have additional complicating factors such as urinary tract infection. Aseptic necrosis (osteonecrosis) of the femoral head[363] can be rarely seen after only a few days of therapy. The humeral head is less commonly involved, and avascular necrosis of the capitate has been reported.[288] In our experience, aseptic necrosis of the hip has occurred in only two instances (both in alcoholics) out of more than 2000 short-term courses of oral prednisone. Osteoporosis, another complication of prolonged steroid use, can lead to an increased risk of fractures.[628] One report[676] has recently found that patients with MS in general are at risk for osteoporosis, probably due to inactivity. Patients with MS have reduced bone mass,[443] and therefore only short-term steroids should be used. Several reports of sudden death have also been associated with IV corticosteroid therapy in patients with rheumatological disorders. These deaths were probably due to sudden arrhythmias that occurred after very rapid infusion of large doses (1 or 2 g of methylprednisolone). Sudden death has not been reported in instances where the same dose has been infused over a period of hours. For that reason, we recommend that for pulsed therapy, 1 g of methylprednisolone be placed in 500 mL of normal saline to be infused over a 1- to 2-hour period. Although steroid therapy may result in susceptibility to opportunistic infections, such as varicella and mycobacterial infections including reactivation of tuberculosis, these are rare occurrences in our experience. Other problems include a metallic taste, moon face, electrolyte imbalance, hyperglycemia, hypertension, weight gain, peptic ulcers, manic behavior, depression, insomnia, and seizures, as well as infection.[356] Memory impairment also occurs.[289a] A transient worsening may be seen occasionally. Table 12–16 lists a number of complications of the use of steroids. Herishanu and colleagues[235] reported that patients with ON treated with methylprednisolone converted to MS more readily than did patients who were untreated or treated with prednisone alone. However, the study was small and retrospective in nature, and selection factors were not analyzed.

To summarize, steroids must be administered carefully in MS. The therapeutic effect is short, with its major benefit over the

Table 12–16. COMPLICATIONS OF CORTICOSTEROIDS IN MULTIPLE SCLEROSIS

Short Term
Psychosis
Weight gain
Fluid retention
Increased susceptibility to infection
Peptic ulceration with and without bleeding
Hirsutism
Aseptic necrosis very rarely seen early

Medium and Long Term
Cushingoid features
Aseptic necrosis of the hip and capitate
Osteoporosis
Pathological fracture
Easy bruising
Abdominal striae
Thinning of the skin
Hypertension
Diabetes
Memory loss

first 6 months. Long-term beneficial effects may occur, but this possibility needs to be studied. One problem is that a small but significant number of patients become steroid dependent and may demand continued medication. The therapeutic ratio has not been adequately studied in MS for steroid doses (e.g., alternate day) commonly used in asthma, Crohn's disease, and other diseases. Patients on long-term steroids are particularly prone to serious complications such as osteoporosis, aseptic necrosis of the hip, infections, ulcers, diabetes, hypertension, and opportunistic infections. Death due to sepsis has been seen in two patients who demanded steroids be continued against medical advice (D.W. Paty, unpublished observations, 1990).

One new strategy in the use of steroid analogues has been the use of U740006F in EAE.[279] U740006F is a 21-aminosteroid, derived from the cortisone molecule, that has antioxidant properties.

One form of steroid therapy that can be discarded is intrathecal methylprednisolone (Solu-Medrol). In the 1960s and 1970s, several published papers[55,438,439] suggested improvement, but the complication rate, especially for arachnoiditis, was high. In addition, the reported improvement was probably due to reduction in spasticity rather than to reduction in the severity of the MS process.[137] One recent report of a trial of intrathecal methylprednisolone from Germany demonstrated inconsistent results.[529]

A pharmacological effect of steroids in MS that is not well understood is reduction in spasticity. However, even though very effective against spasticity, the complication rate of long-term steroid use precludes their use in the treatment of spasticity, except in the short term to temporarily reduce severe spasticity in preparation for more permanent therapy.

General Immunosuppression

Many attempts at immunosuppressive or immunomodulating therapy in MS have been made.[441] The rationale for this form of therapy is based on the concept that MS is an autoimmune disease (see Chapters 8 and 11). Patients with MS have a number of nonspecific immunologic changes suggesting an autoimmune disorder. These abnormalities include lowered nonspecific suppressor cell activity,[18,515,519] immunoglobulins in the CSF,[625] inflammatory cells in the CSF,[8] and abnormal natural killer cell numbers and function.[518] In addition, MS has been associated with specific histocompatibility antigens (DR2)[157] and perhaps increased IgG production from peripheral B cells,[19] as well as increased levels of viral antibodies in both the blood and the CSF. The pathology of the acute MS lesion is highly inflammatory, suggesting an immune pathogenesis.[510]

Although the basis of immunosuppression is to dampen autoreactive immune mechanisms, it may have other, perhaps unexpected, effects. For example, Rodriguez and Lindsley[528] showed that immunosuppression can enhance CNS remyelination in a viral model of demyelination. While there is no ideal animal model for MS, the best known of the experimental models (murine EAE) entails a specific autoimmune attack against myelin proteins. Nevertheless, in spite of 50 years of investigation into autoimmune experimental models, no specific target antigen has been identified for MS. No T cells have been found that have antigen specificities unique to MS. The question may be asked, Have we been using immunosuppression too aggressively in MS? Noseworthy and his colleagues[459] found that patients with MS were extraordinarily compliant with potentially toxic therapies. The experience with cyclophosphamide cited later should be considered in that light. The best time to treat patients with immunosuppressives may not be during the chronic progressive stage of the disease but rather during the early stage of the disease to impede the start of the chronic and disabling phase. However, to treat early, it would help to have reliable prognostic markers so that only patients with a poor prognosis are randomized into a treatment protocol. Many studies of prognostic markers are under way, and perhaps in the next few years, we will be able to conduct such a trial (see Chapter 6).

A few immunosuppressive therapeutic trials in MS before 1984 are reviewed here. Full details can be found in two articles.[429,457]

AZATHIOPRINE

Frick and colleagues[183] and Cendrowski[94] gave azathioprine to patients with MS and found a possible beneficial effect (see Tables 12–16 and 12–17). Ring[524] gave azathioprine (AZA) and corticosteroids along with ALG in an uncontrolled trial with 20 patients who had not responded to steroids or AZA alone. The condition of 11 of 20 patients seemed to improve or stabilize, and the condition of 7 was made worse. AZA was subsequently studied by Lhermitte and his colleagues[344,346] in a small group of patients. No difference was seen between steroids alone and a combination of AZA, steroids, and ALG. Subsequent studies have continued to examine the effects of AZA, but most have been unable to show any sustained beneficial effects. Rosen[535] reported on 85 chronic progressive patients that he had treated with AZA over 6 to 14 years, comparing them with historical controls. Only 10 percent of the treated patients progressed to wheelchair status, whereas 65 percent of the historical controls required a wheelchair after the same number of years. Such a study could be considered encouraging, but unless the patients were randomized into treatment and control groups, selection factors could easily produce an erroneous result.

A number of other studies have failed to show a beneficial effect from AZA. Ellison and colleagues[161] randomized patients into AZA, AZA plus methylprednisolone, and double-placebo groups. Based on their endpoint, no clinical benefit from the use of AZA with or without methylprednisolone was demonstrated, although some differences did occur in EPs. A large collaborative study by the British and Dutch[78] suggested a beneficial effect, with a lower relapse rate and a lower progression rate in AZA-treated patients. However, the authors did not recommend AZA as a standard therapy for MS. Some investigators have been sufficiently convinced of its effectiveness that they find it difficult to do placebo-controlled studies.[274] In their eyes, all patients should be on AZA. In a retrospective long-term uncontrolled follow-up of 43 matched pairs of AZA-treated and untreated patients, Kappos and colleagues[274] found that after 10 years, the number of wheelchair-bound, bedridden, or deceased patients was higher by twofold in the untreated group as compared with the treated group. Goodkin and colleagues[201] reported a positive therapeutic effect in a clinical trial of patients with relapsing-remitting disease. His findings were encouraging, but the follow-up lasted only 2 years.

Since several studies had suggested that AZA reduced the relapse rate in the second year of therapy, Yudkin and associates[688] performed a retrospective meta-analysis of the results of all previously published blinded, randomized, controlled trials of AZA in MS. Seven hundred ninety-three patients were evaluated in seven studies. AZA produced some minor benefits, but the authors questioned whether the slight clinical benefits could outweigh side effects. AZA can have significant long-term toxicity, possibly increasing the risk of cancer[242,345] and infections.[242] Mion and colleagues[416] reported on a patient with MS with hepatotoxicity due to AZA. In summary, AZA may have some modest beneficial effect in re-

Table 12–17. **SOME RECENT THERAPEUTIC TRIALS OF AZATHIOPRINE ALONE IN MULTIPLE SCLEROSIS**

Year	Senior Author	Active Agent/ Control Agent	No. of Patients	Patient Type	Duration of Therapy	Randomized	Controlled	Blinded	Comments
1971	Frick[184]	AZA	35	RR	1 yr	−	−	−	AZA decreased relapse rate. Chronic course is not affected.
1971	Cendrowski[94]	AZA/ placebo	30	Mixed	9–14 wk	+	+	+	No significant beneficial effect was seen.
1973	Silberberg[573]	AZA	15	RR (6) CP (6)	78 mo	−	−	−	No significant beneficial effect was seen.
1973	Swinburn[606]	AZA/ vitamin C	19	Mixed All men	2 yr	Balanced pairs	+	+	No significant beneficial effect was seen.
1975	Cendrowski[96]	AZA/ steroids	21/21	Mixed	<14 mo	−	+	+	Steroids reduced relapse severity but had no long-term effect.
1978	Patzold[494]	AZA/ levamisole/ placebo	23/23/22	Mixed	138–314 days	−	+	−	No statistically significant difference was found.
1979	Rosen[535]	AZA/nothing	42	CP	3–6 years	+	+	−	Nine percent of AZA group was in W/C, 65% of the control group was in W/C.
1980	Patzold[496]	AZA/nothing	107	Mixed	732 days	−	+	−	AZA reduced disease severity in patients with least duration.
1980	Frick[183]	AZA	64 24	RR CP	28 mo 34 mo	−	−	−	AZA decreased relapse rate. A possible effect was found in CP group.

Continued on following page

Table 12–17.—*continued*

Year	Senior Author	Active Agent/ Control Agent	No. of Patients	Patient Type	Duration of Therapy	Randomized	Controlled	Blinded	Comments
1980	Dommasch[141]	AZA	8 8 7	RR RP CP	3.5–8 yr >3 yr >3 yr				AZA decreased relapse rate. No effect was found. No effect was found.
1982	Madigand[359]	AZA	261	Mixed	6 yr	—	—	—	AZA decreased relapse rate HLA influenced rate of progression.
1982	Patzold[495]	AZA/nothing	115	Mixed	2 yr	+	+	—	AZA offered benefit in RP group.
1982	Tindall[622]	AZA and PP/ AZA alone	20	CP	12 mo	+	+	+	Combination was better than AZA alone.
1982	Oger[464]	AZA	60	Stable (11) Active (1) Untreated (48)	?	—	+	—	AZA therapy decreased IgG secretion. Untreated controls had increased IgG secretion.
1983	Aimard[4]	AZA	128 47	RR CP	5 yr	—	—	—	AZA delayed the onset of the progressive phase, slowed disability, and delayed occurrence of new attacks.
1984	Lhermitte[346]	AZA treatment	131	Mixed	>1 yr, mean	—	—	—	Ten nonlymphoproliferative cancers were seen.
1984	Sabouraud[544]	AZA	67	CP	5–10 years	—	—	—	Patients had fewer attacks while receiving treatment. AZA had no effect on CP course.

Continued on following page

Table 12–17.—continued

Year	Senior Author	Active Agent/ Control Agent	No. of Patients	Patient Type	Duration of Therapy	Randomized	Controlled	Blinded	Comments
1986	Zeeberg[690]	AZA/placebo	36	Mixed	1 yr	+	+	+	No beneficial effect was seen.
1987	Nuwer[462]	Same trial as Ellison (1989)	101	CP phase	3 yr	+	+	+	EPs remained stable in treated patients.
1988	British-Dutch[78]	AZA/placebo	354	Mixed	3 yr	+	+	+	Only small differences were found between groups. There was a 27% reduction in the number of relapses.
1988	Minderhoud[415]	AZA/placebo	54	Mixed	3 yr	+	+	+	This trial was part of the British-Dutch study. No sign of therapeutic effect was evident.
1989	Ellison[161]	AZA/AZA and MP/placebo	98	CP phase	3 yr	+	+	+	AZA and MP together may have a beneficial effect.
1988	Kappos[275]	AZA/control agents	42 pairs	Mixed	10 yr	−	−	−	This study was retrospectively controlled. AZA-treated patients did better than untreated patients.
1991	Goodkin[201]	AZA/placebo	43	Mixed	2 yr	+	+	+	Results suggest benefit from AZA with a reduced relapse rate in the second year (62%).
1991	Yudkin[688]	Meta-analysis	793	Mixed	Variable	+	+	+	Freedom from relapse was greatest in the AZA-treated groups.

ducing exacerbations and in limiting progression of disability in MS, but the evidence is not strong (see Tables 12–17 and 12–18). The potential influence of publication bias on meta-analysis cannot be ignored. A full scale study of AZA versus interferon beta and placebo is warranted.

CLADRIBINE

A recent report detailed the beneficial effects of cladribine, a highly specific antilymphocyte, antimonocyte immunosuppressive agent, in CPMS.[576,576a] The investigators gave monthly infusions in a controlled double blind fashion to 49 patients and reported a significant reduction in progression of severity on clinical and MRI measures over a 12-month period. A phase III multicenter trial is underway. However, the unusually severe outcome in the control group is troublesome. This finding has not been a harbinger of reproducibility in previous trials.

CYCLOPHOSPHAMIDE

In the 1960s, cyclophosphamide was reported to reduce the severity of or to prevent EAE. Those results led to a number of studies in MS. In 1973, Cendrowski[95] reported on a study of cyclophosphamide used in conjunction with steroids (Table 12–19). He compared this combined treatment to steroids alone. Historical control subjects were used in this study. No significant change in neurological status could be ascribed to the cyclophosphamide, but the follow-up was short. Uncontrolled studies were done in 216 patients.[194,197,198,243,244,614] Two studies claimed stabilization or slowed deterioration in the cyclophosphamide-treated patients.[198,244] One study concluded[614] that cyclophosphamide treatment made no difference to the clinical course.

Subsequently, Hauser and associates[227] reported a study that was neither observer blinded nor placebo controlled in 58 patients with CPMS followed for 12 months. They studied three patient groups, comparing high-dose IV cyclophosphamide plus ACTH, low-dose oral cyclophosphamide plus plasma exchange, and ACTH alone. They claimed a significant stabilization and improvement rate in the 11 cyclophosphamide-treated patients with few treatment failures. The ACTH treatment group did badly, with an aggressive rate of deterioration that exceeded the clinical deterioration rate in all other recently published trials. The cyclophosphamide-treated group, even though it did better than the ACTH-treated group, actually did no better than did the placebo groups in other recent trials. In addition, the definition of CPMS as showing a deterioration of only 0.5 EDSS points in the previous year raises doubt about the true progressive nature of their patients. This entry criterion would admit a relatively high percentage of all patients with MS, some of whom may differ 0.5 to 1 EDSS points between morning and evening of the same day. Furthermore, the control subjects consisted of ACTH failures who were told that they were to receive the same therapy to which they had not responded previously. In our opinion, this scenario could produce a negative "placebo" effect in the ACTH-treated patients. The same team of investigators subsequently reported in uncontrolled trials that stabilization after cyclophosphamide lasts 1 to 2 years, which is then followed by further chronic progressive deterioration.[656] They suggested that intermittent pulsed therapy with cyclophosphamide is "an important method for treatment of progressive MS." This self-assessment seems optimistic. (See Chapter 11 for a more detailed critique of the use of cyclophosphamide in MS.)

Likosky and associates[348] compared IV cyclophosphamide alone with placebo in a randomized, blinded study of 42 patients with CPMS. They found no difference between treated and control groups. Even though the use of cyclophosphamide in MS increased over several years, its therapeutic effectiveness has not been demonstrated in a placebo-controlled trial. Finally, a multicenter double-blinded, randomized, placebo-controlled trial carried out in Canada[449] conclusively showed that there were no statistically significant differences among three treatment groups: (1) high-dose intravenous cyclophosphamide and prednisone, (2) oral cyclophosphamide, oral prednisone, and plasma exchange, and (3) oral double placebo and sham plasma exchange (the control group). By the end of the trial, the cyclophosphamide group had a trend towards a worse outcome than

Table 12–18. **SOME RECENT THERAPEUTIC TRIALS OF AZATHIOPRINE PLUS OTHER DRUGS IN MULTIPLE SCLEROSIS**

Year	Senior Author	Active Agent/ Control Agent	No. of Patients	Patient Type	Duration of Therapy or Follow-up	Randomized	Controlled	Blinded	Comments
1974	Ring[524]	AZA plus ALG plus TDD or steroids	20	Mixed	1 yr	—	—	—	Eleven patients with short-duration disease received benefit.
1975	Lance[336]	AZA plus steroids plus ALG	14	Mixed	1 yr	—	—	—	Nine patients improved. Relapse rate was reduced.
1980	Mertin[384]	AZA plus steroids plus ALG/placebo	30	Mixed	15 mo	+	+	+	Fewer relapses and less progression occurred in treated female patients ($P=.06$).
1987	Nuwer[462]	Same trial as Ellison	101	CP	3 yr	+	+	+	EP measurements were stable with AZA and MP treatment. EP measurements worsened in control group.
1989	Ellison[161]	AZA, MP/ AZA/placebo	98	CP	3 yr	+	+	+	No sustained clinical benefit was achieved. No change occurred after patients stopped treatment.

ALG = antilymphocyte globulin; AZA = azathioprine; CP = chronic progressive; MP = methylprednisolone; TDD = thoracic duct drainage.

Table 12–19. SOME RECENT THERAPEUTIC TRIALS OF CYCLOPHOSPHAMIDE PLUS OTHER DRUGS IN MULTIPLE SCLEROSIS

Year	Senior Author	Active Agent/ Control Agent	No. of Patients	Patient Type	Duration of Therapy or Follow-up	Randomized	Controlled	Blinded	Comments
1973	Cendrowski[95]	Cphos plus steroids/cytosine arabinoside plus steroids	23	Mixed	16–35 days	—	—	—	No significant long-term benefit was observed.
1975	Hommes[244]	Cphos plus prednisone	32	CP	20 days	—	—	—	Seventy-five percent of treated patients improved.
1975	Drachman[145]	Cphos	6	Relapsing	5 days	—	Sequential	—	No benefit was observed.
1977	Gonsette[197]	IV Cphos	110	Mixed	10 days, >2 yr follow-up	—	—	—	Sixty-two percent had stabilization for 2–4 years.
1980	Gonsette[198]	IV Cphos follow-up of 1977 study	201	Mixed	3–5 wk with 2–10 yr follow-up	—	—	—	Intravenous Cphos decreased relapse rate. Sixty percent had long-term benefit.
1980	Hommes[243]	IV Cphos follow-up	39	CP	3 wk, 1–5 yr follow-up	—	—	—	Younger patients with short-duration aggressive disease responded best.
1981	Theys[614]	IV Cphos/ control	21 21	CP CP	1 wk, 2 yr follow-up	—	+	—	In this retrospectively matched analysis, no benefit was seen.
1983	Hauser[227]	Cphos	14	Mixed	Monthly dose × 6 mo	—	—	—	Thirteen of 14 patients improved.
1983	Hauser[227]	ACTH/ACTH plus IV Cphos/ ACTH plus oral Cphos plus PP	58	CP	1 yr	+	+	—	Cphos plus ACTH resulted in stabilization.

Continued on following page

Table 12–19.—continued

Year	Senior Author	Active Agent/ Control Agent	No. of Patients	Patient Type	Duration of Therapy or Follow-up	Randomized	Controlled	Blinded	Comments
1984	Brinkman[77]	Cphos plus pred/ Cphos	17	CP	20 days	—	—	—	Suppressor cell numbers returned to normal after treatment.
1984	Khatri[297]	Oral Cphos plus pred and PP	45	CP (severe)	Variable	—	—	—	Twenty-eight patients improved significantly.
1985	Khatri[298]	Oral Cphos plus pred plus PP/ Cphos plus pred plus sham PP	54	CP (follow-up on Khatri, 1984)	20 wk	+	+	+	Significant improvement was achieved, in PP-treated patients.
1986 1988	Carter[91,92]	IV Cphos	188	CP (follow-up on Hauser, 1983)	2 wk	—	—	—	In this 5-year follow-up study, patients who responded to Cphos began to get worse after 2 years.
1987	Martínez-Maza[367]	Cphos	12	CP	Repeated pulses	—	—	—	Cphos therapy increased numbers of IgG secreting PBL.
1987	Goodkin[205]	IV Cphos	27	CP	Alternate month therapy or no therapy	—	+	—	In this 2-year follow-up, treated patients were more stable.
1987	Myers[433]	IV Cphos	Review	—	Monthly pulses	—	—	—	A dose of 1200 mg/m² was necessary to suppress B cells or CD4 cells. Some patients improved, but drug was too toxic to use this way.

Continued on following page

Table 12–19.—*continued*

Year	Senior Author	Active Agent/Control Agent	No. of Patients	Patient Type	Duration of Therapy or Follow-up	Randomized	Controlled	Blinded	Comments
1988	Killian[304]	IV Cphos/placebo	14	RR	1 yr of monthly treatments	+	+	—	Treatment group showed significant decrease in relapses.
1989	Mauch[374]	IV Cphos/ACTH or cortisone	42	CP	To decrease lymphocyte cell count	—	—	—	Nonrandom controls (self-selected) were used in this study. Cphos was beneficial.
1989	Weiner[652]	ACTH plus oral Cphos ± PP	116	Relapsing	8 wk treatment	+	+	+	Significant improvement was due to PP. No clear long-term benefits were observed.
1991	Noseworthy[449]	IV Cphos plus pred/PP plus oral Cphos plus pred/placebo plus sham PP	168	CP	30 mo	+	+	+	No therapeutic effect was observed. Trend toward improvement in PP-treated. IV Cphos-treated patients did slightly worse than placebo-control group.
1991	Likosky[348]	IV Cphos/placebo	42	CP	2 yr	+	+	+	No therapeutic benefit was achieved.
1993	Weiner[656]	Cphos/ACTH pulse	256	CP	2 yr	+	+	+	A slight benefit was claimed in patients 40 years or younger.

CP = chronic progressive; Cphos = cyclophosphamide; PBL = peripheral blood lymphocytes; PP = plasmapheresis; Pred = prednisone; RR = relapsing-remitting.

the placebo group. Myers and colleagues[433] studied the effects of cyclophosphamide on immunologic monitoring and found that doses high enough to cause decreased numbers of B cells or CD4 cells were too toxic for long-term treatment. The authors concluded that there was no justification for the use of cyclophosphamide therapy in MS.[450] The National MS Society's report[468] on the use of cyclophosphamide points out that its therapeutic effect is not established and that its use should be discouraged.

CYCLOSPORINE

Cyclosporine is an immunosuppressive drug that, when combined with prednisone and AZA, is effective in suppressing transplant rejection. Not only has it been shown to significantly prolong the survival after organ transplants, but it has been reported to delay insulin dependence in juvenile diabetes.[599] Cyclosporine also inhibits and has been successful in the treatment of EAE. The binding of endogenous immunophilins (receptors) appears to mediate its immunosuppressive effect.[558] Included among its effects are suppression of IL-2 production by T cells and selective inhibition of T-cell activation.[572] Preliminary experience (G.C. Ebers and T. Feasby, unpublished data, 1984) showed that all five patients with highly active disease treated in a pilot trial of cyclosporine worsened after a follow-up of less than 1 year (Table 12–20). Several controlled studies have subsequently been reported showing modest or no therapeutic effect. Rudge and associates[539] reported on a 2-year trial comparing cyclosporine A (5 mg/kg per day) with placebo in 196 patients. Based on a number of clinical scoring techniques, a slight difference in outcome was found in the two groups of patients. For patients receiving a high dose (7.2 mg/kg per day), the relapse rate and clinical progression rate were lowered. However, side effects of renal insufficiency, hypertension, and anemia were so severe as to "preclude its [cyclosporine A] use in high enough doses to alter the course of the disease." Many other adverse side effects, including paresthesia and tremor, which were especially common, occurred in at least one arm of the study.

Another study by Kappos and colleagues[275,277] failed to show any therapeutic effect for patients treated with cyclosporine as compared with a control group treated with AZA. This important study was the first to report the use of MRI as an adjunct monitor for extent of disease. A visual assessment scale was used to measure the extent of disease by MRI scan. Patients were scanned 6 months before and at the end of the trial; no baseline scan was obtained, however. No clinical or MRI evidence for a therapeutic effect from cyclosporine was found in this study.

A placebo-controlled study of cyclosporine in patients with CPMS has also been reported.[426] This study was also monitored by MRI, with quantitatively analyzed scans at entry, midpoint, and exit from the study. Although 500 patients were enrolled in the study, 44 percent dropped out of the cyclosporine group and 35 percent dropped out of the placebo group. A subgroup (and secondary) analysis showed a modest effect of the drug in prolonging the time to wheelchair status, but an overall beneficial effect could not be claimed. Furthermore, no difference in MRI features was found comparing cyclosporine with placebo in the study noted above.[321,426] In assessing the reason for the high dropout rate, the authors of this study made the extraordinary claim that it was possible to identify a single cause for dropout in every case. This finding is contrary to our own experience where patients with minor side effects may persist with therapy if they are sensing benefit. If they are worsening, the same side effects may influence them to withdraw. Such side effects are usually a less important factor than lack of benefit.

Nephrotoxicity and hypertension are significant adverse effects of cyclosporine therapy. In addition, there are reports of cyclosporine-induced encephalopathy and white matter lesions in organ and bone marrow transplant patients.[133] Such reports raise serious questions about the safety of cyclosporine use in a white matter disease such as MS, but no proof exists that MS was made worse in any of these studies. Nevertheless, in our opinion, the evidence does not support the use of cyclosporine as a therapy for MS.

It is disappointing that one of the most effective immunosuppressants available, cyclo-

Table 12–20. **SOME RECENT THERAPEUTIC TRIALS OF CYCLOSPORINE**

Year	Senior Author	Active Agent/ Control Agent	No. of Patients	Patient Type	Duration of Therapy	Randomized	Controlled	Blinded	Comments
1980	Rudge[539]	CS/ placebo	196	Mixed	2 yr	+	+	+	No benefit was achieved at nontoxic doses. Toxicity limits CS use.
1981	Ebers and Feasby*	CS	5	CP	6 mo	—	—	—	All patients had continued clinical or scan evidence of activity. One severe relapse occurred while the patient was on CS.
1988	Kappos[275]	CS/AZA	194	Mixed	24–32 mo	+	+	+	No clinical or MRI benefit was observed.
1990	MS Study Group[426]	CS/ placebo	547	CP	2 yr	+	+	+	Very mild benefit was observed on secondary analysis, showing shortened time to W/C in CS-treated patients. Nephrotoxicity was significant.

*Unpublished data, 1980.
AZA = azathioprine; CP = chronic progressive; CS = cyclosporine; W/C = wheelchair.

sporine, does not have a therapeutic benefit in MS. Perhaps the next trial should be done with patients in the early stages of the disease. However, to use a potentially toxic therapy early in MS, investigators must be able to select for therapy only those patients with a poor prognosis. For this reason, reliable prognostic markers are needed for the early stages of the disease. The availability of such markers would allow only those patients with a high probability of a poor prognosis to be randomized into clinical trials.

METHOTREXATE

Currier and colleagues[128] reported a positive effect with low-dose methotrexate (MTX) in a pilot trial of 45 patients in the relapsing phase of the disease but no effect on patients in the chronic progressive phase of the disease. Goodkin and colleagues[206,206a] also reported a clinical and MRI beneficial effect in a 2-year controlled study of weekly (7.5 mg orally) MTX in 60 chronic progressive patients. However, the only effect reaching significance was a reduction of 6+ seconds in the 9-hole peg test, a benefit of uncertain clinical significance. Perhaps more relevant is that at the end of the study neither the patients, the study nurses, nor the physicians found any difference between the treated and placebo groups in the proportion of patients who were thought to have worsened. Fischer and colleagues[171] reported a therapeutic benefit of MTX on cognitive function ($P<0.05$) as well. An improvement in the speed of processing information and two other measures was found in MTX-treated patients with no improvement in placebo-controlled patients. MTX may become an accepted therapy for MS. Additional multicenter studies are needed, especially because of the potential benefit on cognitive function. The doses used to date in MS are far lower than were safe and effective in Crohn's disease[163b] and it is possible that a higher dosage would be more effective.

OTHER IMMUNOSUPPRESSANTS

FK-506,[618] a new immunosuppressant similar to cyclosporine and rapamycin,[423] has been introduced in the transplant set-

ting. It may be ten times more potent than cyclosporine and can inhibit EAE in the same way as does cyclosporine. Unfortunately, FK-506 also may have significant renal toxicity. However, it has been found to have a remarkable steroid-sparing effect in transplant patients, which offers some rationale for its study in MS. Mitoxantrone[40,158a,196,273,323a,452] has been tried in MS. Mitoxantrone has a therapeutic effect on both clinical and MRI monitoring.[158a] Its cardiac toxicity will limit its use, even though it produced a significant treatment effect.

Other immunosuppressants under study include deoxyspergualine.[276] The preliminary analyses of deoxyspergualine are not encouraging, but larger trials are definitely needed.

BIOLOGIC SERA AND COMBINATIONS OF OTHER MODALITIES

A number of biologic agents have been used as immunosuppressives in MS. Gamma globulin was first tried by Miller and colleagues.[403] Other agents include ALG, antithymocyte globulin (ATG), and antilymphocyte serum (ALS) (Table 12–21). Most of these agents have been used in conjunction with other immunosuppressive drugs such as cyclophosphamide and AZA. Ring and associates[523] used ALG in conjunction with AZA in 20 patients of mixed clinical categories. After several years of uncontrolled therapy they reported an apparent reduction in the number of relapses in some of these patients. Lhermitte and colleagues[343] used ALG in conjunction with AZA and corticosteroids in a study that was controlled but not blinded. Serum sickness caused discontinuation of therapy in 12 percent of cases. Even though there was an attempt to control the study, patients were not well matched. The modest improvement reported for some patients must be taken as a suggestive result at best.

MacFadyen and associates[357] treated four patients with chronic progressive disease with ALG plus corticosteroids. All four became worse. In a randomized controlled study, Seland and colleagues[560] compared ATG plus ACTH with ACTH alone in the treatment of acute relapses in 21 patients.

Table 12–21. SOME RECENT THERAPEUTIC TRIALS OF BIOLOGIC PRODUCTS AND COMBINATIONS OF OTHER MODALITIES

Year	Senior Author	Active Agent/ Control Agent	No. of Patients	Patient Type	Duration of Therapy or Follow-up	Randomized	Controlled	Blinded	Comments
1971	Frick[184]	AZA plus ALG/AZA	35	Mixed	1 yr FU	—	—	—	ALG and AZA reduced the relapse rate.
1972	Marteau[366]	ALG plus steroids			1 yr FU	—	—	—	Patients improved transiently or stabilized.
1973	MacFadyen[357]	ALG 7–14 days	4	CP	297–580 days FU	—	—	—	ALG caused serious side effects. No improvement was observed.
1974	Seland[560]	ATG plus ACTH/ ACTH	21	Relapsing	8 mo FU	+	+	—	Patients treated with ACTH plus ATG did better for 7 mo.
1974	Ring[524]	TTD/ALG plus AZA	20	Mixed— AZA and steroid resistant	1 year FU	—	—	—	Eleven patients improved.
1975	Lance[336]	ALG, AZA and prednisone	14	Mixed	1 yr FU	—	—	—	Most patients improved. Relapse rate decreased.
1976	Ring[523]	ALG, TTD, or both plus AZA and ACTH	20	Same as above	1–5 yr FU	—	—	—	Twelve patients improved; others stabilized temporarily.
1976	Walker[644]	ALG plus steroids	23	CP	6 mo FU	—	—	—	Six patients improved. Adverse reactions were frequent.
1978	Kastrukoff[283]	Follow-up of Seland (1974)	21	R	5 yr FU	—	—	+	No long-term benefits were observed.

Continued on following page

Table 12–21.—*continued*

Year	Senior Author	Active Agent/Control Agent	No. of Patients	Patient Type	Duration of Therapy or Follow-up	Randomized	Controlled	Blinded	Comments
1980	Mertin[384]	ALG plus steroids plus AZA/placebo	30	RR	15 mo FU 14 mo FU	+	+	+	Marginal benefit on relapse rate, clinical progression, and EP was found in females.
1986	Weiner[654]	Monoclonal antibodies (anti T-cell)	4	CP	Pilot	–	–	–	No adverse effects occurred. Immune suppression occurred.
1991	Weinshenker[658]	Monoclonal antibodies (OKT3)	15	RR (2) CP (13)	Pilot	–	–	–	This is a very toxic therapy. Rate of progression may be slower.
1991	Myers[432]	Chlorambucil plus prednisone	6	CP	Pilot	–	–	–	No hint of efficacy was observed.
1992	Cook[122]	IV gamma globulin plus IVMP	14	RP	Monthly pulses ×7.8 mo	–	–	–	Agents used were not effective in preventing relapses.
1994	Noseworthy[455]	IV Ig	10	RR	Pulse every 2 weeks ×6	–	–	–	Dosage was well tolerated in this pilot study.
1994	Naida[434]	IV Ig	315	Mixed	Pulse every 3 weeks	–	–	–	Dosage was well tolerated. Patients had decreased relapse rate and disability score while on treatment.
1994	Moreau[420,421]	Antilymphocyte monoclonal (CAMPATH-1)	14	Mixed	12 mo FU	–	–	–	Marked cytokine release, prolonged lymphopenia, MRI effect but no controls.
1996	Rumbach[543a]	Anti CD-4	21	Mixed	1 yr FU	–	–	–	No clearcut clinical or MRI treatment effect was seen.

ALG = antilymphocyte globulin; ATG = antithymocyte globulin; AZA = azathiaprine; CP = chronic progressive; EP = evoked potential; FU = follow-up; IV Ig = IV immunoglobulins; RP = relapsing progressive; RR = relapsing-remitting; TTD = thoracic duct drainage.

Patients were treated for 14 to 28 days after an acute relapse. Both groups improved, but the patients treated with ATG plus ACTH appeared to maintain remission better than the group treated with ACTH alone. Kastrukoff and associates[283] did a blinded 5-year follow-up on the 18 surviving patients from Seland's study (three had died, two from the ACTH group and one from the ATG plus ACTH group) and found no lasting effect that could distinguish the ATG plus ACTH group from the ACTH only group.

Mertin and associates[385] reported on a study of 41 patients treated with intensive immunosuppression, including ALG, AZA, and steroids. This group was compared with a placebo group in a double blind format. The follow-up was a short 15 months. The investigators concluded that the treatment group did marginally better than the placebo group, but it was not an impressive result. Most of the benefit was seen in the HLA-A3-positive patients.

After the report by Rodriguez and colleagues[526,527,528a] that immunoglobulins improved experimental remyelination in the CNS, Van Engelen and colleagues[638] reported that vision loss improved in five patients with visual loss due to stable ON. However, Cross and Hart[125] and others have urged caution in interpreting the results of uncontrolled and small studies.

Naida and Schwaighofer[434] treated 315 patients with long-term immunoglobulins. The mean duration of therapy was 773 days, and the dosage 200 mg/kg every 3 weeks. The investigators found a reduction in the relapse rate from 2.05 relapses per patient per year to 0.47 relapses per patient per year. Sixty-seven percent of the patients had no relapses during therapy. Two patients had mild allergic reactions.

Nos and colleagues[447] compared the effects of IV immunoglobulin versus IV methylprednisone on the blood-brain barrier using MRI methods in 10 patients. They found a profound effect with IV methylprednisolone but no effect with IV immunoglobulin. One patient who received IV immunoglobulin showed worsening of the enhancement after treatment. In a pilot study using IV immunoglobulins, Noseworthy and colleagues[455]

found patients tolerated it well but efficacy is not known at this time.

Tenser and colleagues[612] used IV IgG to treat six patients with secondary progressive MS. They found an immunosuppressive effect after 5 weeks but no clinical effect. They suggested further trials. Cook and colleagues[122] also reported that IV IgG in the treatment of progressive MS did not prevent exacerbation. Francis and associates[178] also studied IV IgG in nine patients with MS with active disease followed up with MRI and clinical measures. They found no beneficial effect. Until recently, studies of IVIG, mostly in Europe, have either been uncontrolled or have not shown benefit. The pre- and post-treatment studies all suffer from the time factor of regression to the mean. An effect on both disability and relapse rate is suggested by a recent well designed study,[163a] but needs to be confirmed.

MONOCLONAL ANTIBODIES

Weinshenker and colleagues[658] reported a pilot study of mouse anti-CD3 monoclonal antibodies. Most of the patients developed a severe serum sickness–like illness. However, only 4 of 16 patients worsened during the follow-up period. Interestingly, enormous elevations in serum γ interferons and TNF-2 were not associated with acute exacerbation. Anti-CD3 monoclonal antibodies can also cause a reversible encephalopathy.[107] Because of this severe side effect, the use of mouse monoclonal antibody therapy has been limited. This type of therapy will be reinstated when human hybrid monoclonal antibodies become available. A chimeric anti-CD4 has been tried in a phase I study[22,350] with variable results.[543a]

Moreau and colleagues[420] treated seven patients with MS with a humanized monoclonal antibody CAMPATH-1, an anti-CDW5 pan-lymphocyte antigen that produces rapid and sustained lymphopenia. The first infusion was accompanied by exacerbation of pre-existing symptoms lasting 4 hours and accompanied by a pulse of systemic cytokine release (TNF-α and interferon gamma peaked at 2 hours with interleukin-6 peaking somewhat later). Pretreatment with 500 mg of IV methylprednisolone blocked the symptoms and the cytokine release. MRI analysis[421] showed a tendency to a decreased active lesion rate after therapy that a "meta-analysis" found to be significant ($P = 0.001$). Thymectomy has also been tried without success.[631] A recent report of two patients treated with a monoclonal antibody to TNF suggested caution because of apparent immune activation.[639a] In addition, a study of soluble TNF receptor therapy not only showed no therapeutic effect, but may have aggravated the disease for both outcome measures of relapse rate and MRI activity. (Personal observations, D.W. Paty and G.C. Ebers, March 1997).

In summary, the results of trials of immunosuppressive drugs and biologic agents show some modest therapeutic effect, but these drugs are not without harmful effects. The possible effects must be balanced against the natural history of the disease. The clinician does not want to harm patients with a relatively benign prognosis by treating them with toxic drugs that may have only marginal benefits.

Immunomodulation

LEVAMISOLE

Several clinical trials have been conducted involving levamisole (Table 12–22). Some of these trials involved uncontrolled observations in mixed-category patients. One study[129] reported that five of seven treated patients deteriorated significantly during the short term, one patient improved, and one patient remained stable. Myers and associates[430] reported a mixed picture in four patients, with modest improvement in one and stabilization in another. Cendrowski and Czlonkowska[98] reported no clear benefit from levamisole in 19 patients. Gonsette and associates[199] compared levamisole with placebo in a randomized, controlled, double blind trial involving 54 patients followed up for more than 9 months. Although the treatment group's condition tended to stabilize, the difference between groups was not statistically

significant. Massaro and colleagues[370] have published a 4-year controlled study that found relapses to be much less common in levamisole-treated patients. Levamisole has also been implicated in a causal role in three patients with adenocarcinoma of the colon, who developed a multifocal inflammatory CNS disease which, by MRI and biopsy, looked just like MS, after receiving both levamisole and 5-fluorouracil.[248] At this time, no clear consensus exists concerning the use of levamisole. Some data suggest that it may have a weak effect in exacerbating MS. However, the results of one study[370] suggest that the drug should be reassessed.

LINOMIDE

Linomide is an immunomodulator which inhibits EAE. It also has a beneficial effect on relapsing and remitting[280] and secondary progressive MS. The most dramatic effect has been on the MRI monitoring.[17a] However, the rate of side effects, particularly serositis including pericarditis and pleuritis, is high and may limit its use even if effective. In fact, two large phase 3 studies were cancelled as of April 9, 1997, due to an increased risk of myocardial infarction and other side effects.[380a]

TRANSFER FACTOR

At least nine studies have been conducted to evaluate the effect of transfer factor (TF) (Table 12–23). In 1976, Behan and his colleagues[54] reported on a double blind study of TF versus placebo in 29 patients. No significant difference was found between treated and control groups. Others[38,108,174,335,639] subsequently reported on controlled trials suggesting either no therapeutic effect or a modest trend toward stabilization in the TF-treated patients. One study[335] monitored the results using evoked potentials and CT scans, as well as clinical evaluations. Basten[38] initially reported a modest benefit from TF therapy in mildly affected patients in the early stage of their disease when followed up for greater than 18 months. A longer follow-up based on the same study has been completed[27] showing

Table 12–22. SOME RECENT THERAPEUTIC TRIALS OF LEVAMISOLE

Year	Senior Author	Active Agent/ Control Agent	No. of Patients	Patient Type	Duration of Therapy	Randomized	Controlled	Blinded	Comments
1976	Dau[129]	Lev	7	Mixed	12 wk	—	—	—	Five of 7 patients got worse.
1977	Myers[430]	Lev	4	CP	6 mo	—	—	—	Variable effect was seen.
1978	Cendrowski[98]	Lev	35	Mixed	1 mo	—	—	—	No effect was seen.
1978	Patzold[494]	Lev/ AZA/ fatty acids	24 23 22	Mixed	10 mo	—	—	—	Lev had no effect. AZA slowed deterioration.
1982	Gonsette[199]	Lev/ placebo	54	Mixed	2 yr	+	+	+	Twenty-eight patients discontinued therapy. No significant therapeutic effect was observed. There was a trend for benefit from Lev.
1990	Massaro[370]	Lev/ placebo	41	Stable	4 yr	+	+	+	Lev group had significantly fewer relapses than placebo group.

AZA = azathioprine; CP = chronic progressive; Lev = levamisole.

Table 12–23. SOME RECENT THERAPEUTIC TRIALS OF TRANSFER FACTOR IN MULTIPLE SCLEROSIS

Year	Senior Author	Active Agent/ Control Agent	No. of Patients	Patient Type	Duration of Therapy	Randomized	Controlled	Blinded	Comments
1976	Behan[54]	TF/placebo	30	Mixed	3 mo	+	+	+	No therapeutic effect was observed.
1978	Fog[174]	TF/placebo	32	CP	13 mo	+	+	+	No therapeutic effect was observed.
1978	Colins[108]	TF/placebo	56	Mixed	1 yr	+	+	+	No therapeutic effect was observed.
1980	Basten[38]	TF/placebo	58	Mixed	2 yr	+	+	+	TF retarded progression after 18 months in less severe patients.
1981	Lamoureux[335]	TF/placebo	27	RR	3 mo	+	+	+	No therapeutic effect was observed.
1986	Van Haver[639]	TF relatives/ TF random/ placebo	105	Mixed	18 mo	+	+	+	TF had no effect on ADL, disability, or EP.
1986	Frith[185]	1. Follow-up on Basten (1980) 2. Open study	45 209	Mixed Mixed	18 mo 3 yr	− −	− −	− −	TF slowed progression (tentative conclusion) in both follow-up and open studies.
1986	Nordenbo[445]	Follow-up on Fog (1978)	32	CP	8 yr follow-up after original study	+	+	+	No therapeutic effect was observed.
1989	AUSTIMS[27]	TF/alpha IFN/placebo	153	Mixed	2 yr	+	+	+	No therapeutic effect was observed. TF-treated patients possibly worse. IFN groups had more withdrawals and more side effects.

ADL = activities of daily living; CP = chronic progressive; EP = evoked potentials; IFN = interferon; RR = relapsing-remitting; TF = transfer factor.

Table 12–24. **SOME RECENT THERAPEUTIC TRIALS OF MYELIN BASIC PROTEIN IN MULTIPLE SCLEROSIS**

Year	Senior Author	Active Agent/ Control Agent	No. of Patients	Patient Type	Duration of Therapy	Randomized	Controlled	Blinded	Comments
1973	Campbell[87]	Human MBP/ placebo	64	Mixed	1 yr	+	+	+	Evaluation was conducted by questionnaire. No therapeutic or adverse effect was found.
1977	Gonsette[195]	Human and bovine MBP	35	RR	3–11 mo	—	—	—	No change in relapse rate occurred.
1979	Romine[531]	Porcine MBP	9	Mixed	10 mo	—	—	—	MBP caused no adverse effects. No therapeutic effect was observed.
1993	Weiner[655]	Oral bovine	30	RR	1 yr	—	+	+	Possible benefit (see text).
1995	Warren[646a]	MBP peptides IT	14	CP	10 weeks	—	—	—	No neurological worsening was seen.

CP = chronic progressive; IT = intrathecal; MBP = myelin basic protein; RR = relapsing and remitting.

no therapeutic benefit after continued and prolonged use of either TF or interferon alpha. (The TF-treated group actually did somewhat worse than the placebo-controlled group.) Most TF studies have shown some effect on immune function, however.

MYELIN BASIC PROTEIN

As previously discussed, MBP has been considered a prime candidate for the specific myelin antigen that may be under attack in MS (see Chapter 11). Therefore, the use of MBP as an analogue to modulate the immune response has had strong support.[11] Several pilot trials have examined the effect of MBP in the treatment of MS (Table 12–24). Campbell and colleagues[87] reported on a double blind study of 64 patients who were given subcutaneous human MBP (5 mg/week) or placebo over 1 year. After 52 weeks, placebo-controlled patients were also given MBP and the results were evaluated by questionnaire. Unfortunately, no neurological examination data were given. MBP-treated patients reported some subjective improvement, but almost one-half withdrew from the study. The report is difficult to interpret, but most observers consider this trial to be a treatment failure for MBP.

In an open trial, Gonsette and his colleagues[195] gave either human or bovine MBP (5 mg/week) over 3 to 11 months to 35 relapsing patients. Even though the study was uncontrolled, the authors concluded that because there was no decrease in the relapse rate subsequent to MBP administration, there was no therapeutic effect. Romine and Salk[531] reported on a trial of porcine MBP in a single blind, randomized, controlled study in nine patients followed up for up to 1 year. One MBP-treated patient had a fulminating and severe clinical course. Overall, the authors found no detectable improvement related to the administration of MBP.

Weiner and colleagues[655] have reported on a pilot trial of oral bovine MBP in an attempt to produce oral tolerance. A multicenter trial has been completed and was negative. This approach seems fundamentally flawed. The consequences of oral tolerance to ingested pathogens causing pulmonary disease would at least theoretically preclude this as a viable mechanism for turning off a secondary autoimmue response. Another study of combined oral MBP and interferon beta therapy showed that interferon beta enhanced the production of oral tolerance in rodents with EAE.[9] Warren and Catz[646a] used myelin basic protein peptides intrathecally and saw no adverse effects.

COPOLYMER I

In an attempt to develop a nonencephalitogenic yet immunologically active analogue of MBP, Arnon and associates[25] and Teitelbaum and Sela[610,611] developed a copolymer made by the mixture of four amino acids called copolymer I (COP I). COP I was shown to suppress EAE. A pilot study by Abramsky and colleagues[3] in terminal patients with MS showed no obvious toxic effects. COP I was subsequently used by Bornstein and colleagues[69] (Table 12–25). Bornstein and his colleagues reported their experience with 12 patients with CPMS and four patients with relapsing disease in an open trial. During a mean follow-up of 2 years, the authors found that three of the patients with chronic progressive disease improved and two of the patients with relapsing disease improved. On the basis of these initial impressions, they moved on to stage two, a single-center, randomized, placebo-controlled pilot trial using 50 patients with relapsing disease. The side effects from the administration of COP I were minimal, but most COP I–treated patients developed a local skin reaction. The presence of this local skin reaction may have made blinding of the study difficult. The lack of blinding, shown by the results of a questionnaire given to both neurologists and patients, could have influenced the results. Bornstein and colleagues reported that the relapse rate in the COP I–treated patients was significantly less than in the placebo-treated patients. The patients had a high prestudy relapse rate, and that rate would be expected to fall with time. Of the COP I group, 56 percent had no relapses as compared with 26 percent of the placebo group.

COP I has been subjected to a multicenter, double blind, controlled therapeutic

Table 12–25. **SOME RECENT THERAPEUTIC TRIALS OF COPOLYMER I**

Year	Senior Author	Active Agent/ Control Agent	No. of Patients	Patient Type	Duration of Therapy	Randomized	Controlled	Blinded	Comments
1977	Abramsky[3]	COP I	4	Terminal	2–5 mo	—	—	—	COP I caused no side effects.
1982	Bornstein[69]	COP I	12	Mixed	2 yr	—	—	—	COP I caused no undesirable effect. Five patients got better.
1987	Bornstein[67]	COP I/ placebo	50	RR	2 yr	+	+	+	COP I–treated patients had a lower exacerbation rate. Overall, COP I did not significantly affect progression.
1989	Miller[395]	COP I/ placebo	106	CP	2 yr	+	+	+	No clear-cut effect was observed.
1995	Johnson[267b,269]	COP I/ placebo	251	RR	24 yr	+	+	+	COP I produced a 29 percent reduction in relapse rate.

CP = chronic progressive; COP I = copolymer I; RR = relapsing-remitting.

trial in patients with relapsing disease.[267b] A 23 percent reduction in relapse rate was reported[269] with a trend towards improvement in EDSS. The MRI data[105a,362a] also suggested some therapeutic effect. It is encouraging that a therapeutic modality with so few side effects might have a major effect on relapse. However, in future trials, blinding should be stringently carried out and the evaluation done as objectively as possible, using serial MRI in the full cohort in addition to clinical evaluations.[399,485] Additional follow-up studies will help place these promising short-term results in context.

COP I has also been investigated in patients with CPMS.[68,395] Some trends were observed in COP I–treated patients, but the study concluded that no significant therapeutic benefits were found. A most unusual center effect was noted, which is difficult to understand because much difference occurred between the two participating centers.

T-CELL VACCINATION

Anti-T-cell vaccination is currently being evaluated in a pilot study.[641,641a] There were some immune function changes and no adverse clinical effects. However, the rationale for such a study in part depends on the concept of restricted T-cell-receptor gene usage in MS, which is yet to be proven.

INTERFERONS

Interferon gamma augments immune responses[60] and appears to increase the relapse rate in MS, but does not affect suppressor activity.[446] It may also potentiate antibody-mediated demyelination in vivo.[642] Interferon gamma also can be localized in nerve roots during the active inflammation stage of experimental autoimmune neuritis,[557] in addition to augmenting the disease.[223] Type I interferon (alpha and beta) can also suppress EAE.[79]

Interferon beta has been reported as decreasing mitogen driven IL-2 expression, perhaps reducing T-cell activation.[540] Interferon gamma also changes the behavior of human brain endothelial cells in culture, allowing greater leakages through tight junctions.[253,397] However, both interferon alpha and interferon beta seem to augment

suppression in MS.[446] Interferon beta also blocks the immune activation effects of interferon gamma.[253] Therefore, the antagonism to interferon gamma effects could be considered as a scientific rationale for the clinical studies with interferon alpha and interferon beta. Johnson and Panitch,[268] Panitch,[474] and Weinstock-Gutmann and colleagues[664] have reviewed the use of interferons in MS. Oral interferons may also be effective.[80]

Interferon Alpha. Interferon alpha has significant biologic activity, showing both immunomodulation and antiviral properties. It is effective against non-A, non-B hepatitis but can exacerbate autoimmune hepatitis.[481] It may be effective against the common cold.[143,230] It may also be modestly effective against subacute sclerosing panencephalitis.[683] However, because of the selective effects of the interferons in viral and autoimmune diseases, the clinician must be very careful with its use in putative autoimmune diseases such as MS. Knobler and his colleagues[312] undertook a study of interferon alpha in 24 patients with relapsing disease using a double blind, randomized, placebo-controlled crossover design (Table 12–26). Patients were treated for 6 months, allowed a 6-month washout period, and then crossed over to the other treatment arm for a second 6-month treatment period. In that trial, there was a high frequency of symptomatic side effects such as fever, fatigue, and malaise. Knobler reported a tendency for the interferon-treated patients to have less in the way of clinical relapses, but the crossover design prohibited the analysis of the long-term effects of their short (6 months) course of therapy. Pavol and colleagues[496a] reported cognitive deficits associated with interferon alpha therapy in a controlled study. Few investigators are convinced that the interferon alpha was effective in either suppressing relapses or in altering the outcome of MS. Panitch and colleagues[473,475] reported an 18 months' or longer follow-up on the Knobler study, which did not clarify the situation, mostly because of the crossover design.

Camenga and his colleagues[86] studied interferon alpha-2 (recombinant) by randomizing 98 patients with relapsing or

Table 12–26. SOME RECENT THERAPEUTIC TRIALS OF INTERFERON ALPHA

Year	Senior Author	Active Agent/ Control Agent	No. of Patients	Patient Type	Duration of Therapy or Follow-up	Randomized	Controlled	Blinded	Comments
1984	Knobler[312]	IFN alpha/ placebo	24	RR	18 mo	+	+	+	This study used a crossover design. Relapse rate was reduced in both placebo and IFN groups, with greatest reduction in IFN. Outcome was not influenced.
1986	Camenga[86]	Recombinant IFN alpha-2/ placebo	98	RR	1 yr	+	+	+	All patients had reduced relapse rate. No therapeutic benefit was observed (see text).
1987	Panitch[473]	Follow-up on Knobler (1984)	24	RR	2.3 yr FU	—	—	—	Reduced relapse rate was observed over time.
1989	AUSTIMS[27]	IFN alpha /TF/ placebo	153	Mixed	2 yr	+	+	+	No therapeutic effect was observed. Side effects were significant in the IFN group.
1990	Kastrukoff[285]	IFN alpha/ placebo	100	CP	6 months' treatment, 2-year FU	+	+	+	No therapeutic effect was observed by clinical or MRI measures.
1993	Koopmans[319]	IFN alpha* same trial as Kastrukoff (1990)	63	CP	6 mo	+	+	+	No therapeutic effect was observed on MRI.
1994	Durelli[148,149]	Recombinant IFN alpha-2a/ placebo	20	RR	6 mo	+	+	+	A treatment effect was seen on relapses and MRI monitoring for active lesions.
1994	Massaro[371]	Recombinant IFN alpha-2a	14	RR	4 yr	+	+	+	Patients had reduced relapse rate and reduced disability change while on treatment.
1996	Durelli[149a]	Follow-up on 1994 study	20	RR	12 mo	—	—	—	Drug effects were restricted to time of therapy.

CP = chronic progressive; FU = follow-up; IFN = interferon; IT = intrathecal; RR = relapsing-remitting.
*Lymphoblastoid IFN.

CPMS into treatment and placebo groups. Treated patients received 2 million interferon alpha units subcutaneously three times a week for 12 months. A dramatic fall in the relapse rate occurred in both experimental and control groups. This fall probably represents the known tendency for high rates of activity to regress toward the mean over time. There was no difference between the two treatment groups. In addition, the interferon-treated patients converted to a progressive stage of the disease after treatment more frequently than did controls.

Massaro and colleagues[371] reported a 4 year follow-up of recombinant interferon alpha-2a in 14 patients. Some tendency to improvement in the first 2 years was lost if the treatment was stopped. Four years of therapy seemed to be safe, and the patients treated for 4 years (N = 7) had only one relapse in the group and no increase in EDSS. A large Australian multicenter study[27] also found no treatment effect from interferon alpha.

A subsequent interferon alpha (lymphoblastoid) study has been reported by Kastrukoff and associates.[284–286] In this randomized, controlled, double blind study, 100 patients with CPMS were treated with either subcutaneous interferon alpha (5 million units per day) or placebo. Treatment continued for 6 months, but observation, using MRI as well as clinical endpoints, continued for 2 years. There was no significant difference between treatment and control groups at 2 years. At 6 months, nine interferon-treated patients had done better than expected. However, the number of patients was not large enough to make an overall difference in the statistics. The quantitative MRI studies also showed a trend toward less extent of disease at 6 months in the treated patients as compared with control subjects.[319] However, at 2 years, there was no difference between the two groups in the MRI-detected extent of disease. The immune function studies showed that interferon alpha therapy increased CD5+ and CD4+ cells significantly, whereas the CD8+ cells decreased slowly during the therapy. The inconclusive result of the study probably reflects the short duration of the treatment phase (6 months). In future studies, patients selected because of

poor prognostic markers early in their course may need to be treated for 3 years or possibly 5 years to see a decisive clinical result. Six months or even 2 years of therapy is a very short time in a disease that evolves over 35 years.

Cavello and colleagues[93] and Durelli and colleagues[149,149a] repeated a controlled pilot study of recombinant interferon alpha and found a reduction in relapse rate and MRI activity over a 4-month period. However, after patients stopped the therapy, all signs of disease activity returned to baseline levels.[149] Follow-up of their patients revealed that interferon alpha-2a therapy reduced mononuclear cell production of TNF-α and IFN gamma.[150] Tumor growth factor (TGF-β) synthesis was increased. After therapy was stopped, cytokine production also returned to baseline levels.

In an uncontrolled study, Kinnunen and colleagues[307] found that 3 million units of interferon alpha-2b (recombinant) was associated with an increase in the intrathecal IgG synthesis rate and may have augmented the disease progression. They contended that the mean progression index was higher after treatment than it had been before treatment. This finding is intriguing but cannot be considered conclusive because the sample consisted of only six patients and, furthermore, the study was not placebo controlled. Kinkel and colleagues[305] reported a rapid neurological decline in a patient treated with a combination of systemic IL-2 and interferon alpha-2b. IFN alpha may also be effective in HTLV-1 myelopathy.[258a] In addition, interferon alpha may have some persistent neurotoxicity.[387,481]

Interferon Beta. As noted previously, interferon beta blocks some of the immune activation effects of interferon gamma. However, since interferons turn on what may be hundreds of genes, any proposals concerning mechanism of action in MS are speculative. Intrathecal interferon beta therapy has been reported in several studies (Table 12–27). The goal of the trials was to measure the relapse rate in patients with active relapsing disease. Jacobs and his colleagues[262,264] first reported that 10 patients with high relapse rates had dramatically lowered relapse rates after starting intrathe-

Table 12–27. **SOME RECENT THERAPEUTIC TRIALS OF INTERFERON BETA**

Year	Senior Author	Active Agent/ Control Agent	No. of Patients	Patient Type	Duration of Therapy or Follow-up	Randomized	Controlled	Blinded	Comments
1981	Jacobs[262]	IT IFN beta (Natural)	20	Mixed	6-mo Rx, 1.5-yr FU	+	+	+	Relapse rate was reduced in comparison to pre-study relapse rate (not observed).
1982	Jacobs[264]	IT IFN beta follow-up on Jacobs (1981)	20	Mixed	1.7-yr FU	—	—	—	IFN beta reduced relapse rate.
1985	Jacobs[263]	IT IFN beta follow-up on Jacobs (1981)	20	Mixed	4-yr FU	—	—	—	This study used a crossover design. IFN beta reduced relapse rate.
1986,87	Jacobs[261]	IT IFN beta/ placebo	69	RR	6 mo, 2-yr FU	+	+	+	IFN beta–treated patients had a lower relapse rate.
1988	Huber[249]	IV IFN beta	9	Mixed	5-mo Rx, 1.2-yr FU	—	—	—	One severe exacerbation occurred in a treated patient. No treatment effect was seen.
1990	Milanese[390]	IT IFN beta	16	Mixed	6-mo Rx, 22-mo FU	+	+	+	An increased relapse rate occurred during treatment. No overall benefit was seen.
1993	Knobler[311]	Systemic (SC) recombinant IFN beta-1b/ placebo	30	RR	3-yr, pilot study	+	+	+	The trend was towards treatment efficacy.

Continued on following page

Table 12–27.—continued

Year	Senior Author	Active Agent/ Control Agent	No. of Patients	Patient Type	Duration of Therapy or Follow-up	Randomized	Controlled	Blinded	Comments
1993	IFNB Study Group[254,492]	Systemic (SC) recombinant IFN beta-1b/ placebo	372	RR	3 yr	+	+	+	1. The high dose of IFN beta-1b had a 34 percent effect in reducing the relapse rate. 2. MRI effects were more dramatic than the clinical effect, with median 70 percent reduction in MRI activity.
1995	IFNB Study Group[256] final report	Systemic (SC) recombinant IFN beta-1b/ placebo	217	RR	4 or 5 yr	+	+	+	Those patients completing 4 and 5 yr of treatment had a sustained reduction in relapse rate and in MRI BOD measure (see text).
1996	Jacobs[260]	Systemic (IM) IFN beta-1a/ placebo	301	RR	2 yr Rx (see text)	+	+	+	1. Progression of disability 33% in placebo vs. 21% in Rx group. 2. The drug decreased exacerbation frequencies by 18% overall. 3. It also reduced the number of gadolinium-enhancing lesions on MRI.
1996	Pozzilli[507a]	Systemic (SC) IFNβ-1a	68	RR	6 mo crossover	+	—	—	Treatment reduced MRI and clinical activity.

BOD = burden of disease; CP = chronic progressive; FU = follow-up; IFN = interferon; IM = intramuscular; IT = intrathecal; IV = intravenous; RR = relapsing-remitting; Rx = treatment; SC = subcutaneous.

cal interferon. A historical control group did not have such a high relapse rate. All patients were eventually treated with interferon and the authors claim that treated patients continued to show a low relapse rate when compared with the patients' own pretreatment (historical) relapse rate. All patients treated with intrathecal interferon beta had a chemical meningitis with increased cells and protein in the CSF.[266]

Jacobs and colleagues[261,263,265,266] subsequently completed a randomized, controlled, double blind, stratified 2-year study of intrathecal interferon beta in 69 high–relapse-rate patients. Treatment was given for 6 months. Control patients had sham lumbar punctures following the same schedule as used for the interferon-treated patients. Evaluation was done by a neurologist who was unaware of the treatment schedule or treatment modality. Indomethacin was given to mask the systemic side effects of the interferon.[419] Seventy-nine percent of the interferon recipients and 64 percent of the control subjects believed that they were getting the true interferon beta.

The relapse rate fell in both treatment and control groups, but more so (P<0.04) in the interferon group. The authors argued that the relapse rate would not be expected to fall on its own; therefore, they attributed the fall to the therapy and a placebo effect. However, the principle of regression to the mean would predict that patients selected for a high pretrial relapse rate would naturally regress towards the mean rate. See the alpha interferon study by Camenga.[86] CSF pleocytosis and elevated protein again occurred. Milanese and colleagues[391] also reported an intrathecal interferon beta study without any beneficial effects. Huber et al[249] reported a trial monitored by MRI that was inconclusive.

Interferon Beta-1b. Interferon Beta-1b (IFNB-1b) is a recombinant interferon made in E-coli. It is non-glycosylated and has two amino acids different from natural IFNB. Three hundred seventy-two patients with relapsing disease from across North America were entered into a three-arm trial with recombinant interferon beta-1b in two doses plus placebo.[254] The effectiveness of inteferon beta in reducing the relapse rate

was strongly suggested by the results of the pilot study.[312] Entry criteria included an EDSS score of 0 to 5.5 and at least two relapses in the previous 2 years. Patients were randomized into three groups of high-dose [8 million international units (MIU)] and low-dose [1.6 MIU] interferon beta and placebo subcutaneously. Primary endpoints were the differences in relapse rates and the proportion of patients who were relapse-free. At two years, the mean annual relapse rate was 1.27 for the placebo group, 1.17 for the low-dose group, and 0.83 for the high-dose group. These differences were highly significant statistically (P = 0.0001) and represented a 34 percent reduction in the relapse rate in the high dose group. Although a positive result was seen in relapse rate, unfortunately there was no significant impact on clinical neurological impairment and disability.

The most striking results were seen on MRI monitoring.[492] Over a 2-year period the treated group at one site with frequent scanning had a median reduction of 83 percent in the number of active lesions and a 50 percent reduction in the rate of active scans.[492] The quantitative increase in disease burden on MRI monitoring of the entire cohort was 20 percent in the placebo group contrasted to a 0.1 percent reduction in the high-dose interferon beta group. IFNB-1b may also have a benefit on cognitive aspects of MS.[502,502a] The study was designed for 2 years and was twice extended, so some patients went past 4 and 5 years on the drug. Many patients chose to discontinue the drug after the first extension without knowing the results.

Over the 5 years of follow-up in this trial,[256] using a double blind protocol, individual patients remained in the trial for 3.5 to 5 years with a median study time of 4 years. There were 155 dropouts, but the dropout rate did not seem to affect outcome. Dropouts from the placebo arm tended to have a higher exacerbation rate, a greater increase in mean EDSS[256,322] and a greater increase in the MRI changes than did the non-dropouts.

Major long-term side effects from the drug were not found. The most common side effect was the flulike symptoms, which decreased from 100 to 10 percent, usually by

2 months into the study. NSAIDs such as ibuprofen decreased this initial problem. A gradual increase in the dosage of interferon beta also helped to decrease side effects. Injection site reactions were common in IFNB treated patients. However, blinding was preserved by having two doses of drug and the clinical examination of the patients by a neurologist blinded to side effects. Early leukopenia and mild liver enzyme abnormalities disappeared by 3 to 4 months. While the reduction in exacerbation rate continued, prevention of disease progression was again not noted; however, further studies in patients with progressive disease are being carried out. (Neilley and colleagues[437b] have reported on the side effects on 72 patients treated in an open label trial.)

The MRI component of the study showed three significant findings.[492] For one, interferon beta in both high and low doses led to a 50 percent reduction in the formation of new lesions. The second observation was a decrease in enlargement of periventricular lesions (BOD), which may have some relevance to disease progression. The third observation was the confirmation of the drug effect into the 5th year. Even though the numbers of active lesions were low on the yearly scans, the results of therapy were still highly significant.[256,322] McDonald and colleagues[378] provide a thoughtful discussion of the MRI results; they urge caution in interpretation until the clinical implications of MRI activity are fully understood.

Letters to the editor related to this trial appear in the January 1994 issue of *Neurology*.* Sibley and colleagues[571] reviewed the data and considered and commented on the following issues:

1. Why the primary outcome was exacerbation rate and not EDSS.
2. Lack of effect on EDSS.
3. Was the study a true intent to treat? How were the dropouts handled?
4. How was blinding maintained in the face of skin reactions?
5. How was the determination of MRI changes + or − 10% derived? Was it a prospective set?
6. Was there MRI stratification?

7. What was the availability of the raw data to the investigators?
8. What is the cost effectiveness of the drug?
9. How does one explain the suicide attempts?

Goodkin and Kanoti[204] wrote a thoughtful essay on the ethics of continued placebo-controlled trials subsequent to the availability of interferon beta-1b. They make a distinction between *efficacy* (effect of a drug in a controlled setting such as a controlled clinical trial) and *effectiveness* (clinical benefit outside the controlled trial). Their conclusion was that placebo-controlled trials are still possible with the following stipulations:

1. Proper informed consent that details the loss of benefit related to exclusion from interferon beta treatment
2. An external monitoring process to ensure appropriate sample size

Our interpretation of this study is that interferon beta-1b has made a significant impact on the MS disease process. The relapse rate was reduced and the patients who were treated went longer during the study before their first, second, and subsequent relapses. Relapses were less severe in the treated group. The clinical effects were modest but clear cut. However, the MRI results suggest that interferon beta treatment has a profound impact on the pathology of the disease as detected by MRI. The expected increase in burden of disease and the rate of formation of new lesions was reduced. All clinical and MRI data were internally consistent, whatever the endpoint. The disappointing feature is that even with longer than 4 years' participation, the chronic impairment as measured by the EDSS was not slowed enough to reach statistical significance. The reason for such a profound effect on the inflammatory nature of the disease on MRI scan and a relative lack of clinical impact may be that the long-term clinical impairment in MS is due not to the primary inflammatory factors but to secondary or even independent features such as axonal loss and gliosis. It is very encouraging, however, that the total BOD increase was retarded along with the suppression of the inflammatory activity. The use of IFNB-1b has been reviewed.[502b]

---

*References 81, 135, 310, 351, 353, 365, 375, 386, 472.

Interferon beta-1b has been released for use in the United States, Canada, Australia, and Europe.[231] A consensus conference has made suggestions on management.[353a] It should be used only in early relapsing patients because of its demonstrated ability to reduce the relapse rate and to prolong the time between relapses. The American Academy of Neurology has released a practice advisory on selection of patients with MS for treatment with interferon beta-1b (Betaseron).[10]

The final data from the double blind follow-up (4 to 5 years)[255] showed that the high dose had a persistent effect on exacerbation rate and was relatively free of long-term side effects. Of 372 patients, 217 completed the 4 years. No systematic bias identified the dropouts except that they were generally those patients who had the highest relapse rates, the greatest change on EDSS, and the greatest change in MRI BOD measure. The MRI BOD measure continued to show a significant therapeutic benefit in the high-dose group until the end ($P = 0.001$). There was a statistically significant percent change per year also (baseline to year 1, year 1 to year 2, year 2 to year 3, year 3 to year 4) at each interval in the 72 placebo patients who had yearly scans through to year 4 or 5. The correlations between outcome measures were strengthened (see Table 12–12).

Neutralizing antibodies (NAB) were found in 35 percent of patients on the high dose.[256a] The presence of NAB was associated with a reduction in therapeutic efficacy so that the NAB-positive patients' relapse rate resembled that of the placebo group. In contrast, the removal of the NAB-positive patients from the treatment group revealed that the NAB-negative patients had a superior therapeutic effect. Guidelines for the use of NAB data have also been published.[488a] In fact, there is reason to believe that the patients who form NAB have more active diseases (J. Petkan, personal communication, March 1997) and can be predicted by their baseline IgG secretion rates.[465a]

Interferon beta-1b has not yet been shown to be effective in the chronic phase of the disease. Studies focusing on the chronic progressive phase are under way,

and we can hope that this drug and others will have a long-term impact on the disease process. Interferon beta-1b does not have direct glial toxic effects.[686] In fact, it blocks the IFN gamma astrocyte proliferating effect.[550a] In addition, COP I and interferon beta had additive, and sometimes synergistic, suppressive effects on in vitro responses to MBP,[409] increasing hopes that combination therapies will be effective towards stronger and more enduring control of at least the inflammatory aspects of the disease. Additional studies will be necessary to determine whether disease outcome (disability) can be improved.

Stone and colleagues[602] reported that starting patients with relapsing-remitting disease on interferon beta-1b produced a remarkable reduction in enhancing lesions on serial MRI evaluations. However, the response was not homogenous.[178a] These investigators had a number of patients in a natural history study using MRI. They observed the change in MRI activity after the patients were started on interferon beta-1b. Although the number of enhancing lesions appeared to be dropping even prior to initiation of therapy.

Panitch and colleagues[478] monitored viral infections during the trial and found no reduction in upper respiratory tract infections (URIs) due to interferon beta. Clinical attacks followed 34 percent of URIs. The same group was able to show detectable levels of IFNB-1b at 8 to 24 hours after injection.[295a]

A recent study by Reder and Lowy[514] showed that the therapeutic effect of interferon beta is not mediated by stimulating cortisol levels. Shakir and colleagues[564] also showed that interferon beta induced interleukin (IL-10) production in mononuclear cells. Because IL-10 suppresses secretion of inflammatory cytokines and inhibits immune responses, that mechanism may also be important in the interferon beta-1b therapeutic effect. IL-10 alone may also be a reasonable therapeutic agent for MS. Interferon beta also depresses collagenase expressions from T cells.[651] Because T-cell collagenases are important in degrading the collagen in adhesion molecules, this action may also be important in its therapeutic effect. The main mechanism by which interferon beta-1b is effective is probably by blocking the effect of interferon gamma (see following discussion).[253,253a,516a,550a] In addition, preliminary data suggest that some cognitive functions were less affected in the treated patients as compared with controls.[502,502a] Faulds and Benfield[163] have reviewed interferon beta-1b and its basic biology and uses.

Fernandez and colleagues reported on their study using natural interferon beta; their preliminary results suggest a reduction in relapse rate and a reduction in enhancing and T_2 lesions on the MRI scan. We await their full published results.

Interferon Beta-1a. Jacobs and colleagues[260] reported the results of a study of one intramuscular injection of 6 MIU per week of recombinant interferon beta-1a. This product is believed to be identical to the natural human molecule and is genetically engineered in mammalian cells. It is fully glyosylated and contains no amino acid substitution. Three hundred and one patients were randomized into a double blind placebo-controlled multicenter phase II trial. The primary outcome measure was tied to a sustained EDSS progression of at least one point. Due to an excellent rate of compliance, the study was stopped one year prior to the expected end. The early termination of the study resulted in only 61 percent of the placebo and 54 percent of the treated patients being followed for a full 2 years. The authors found a statistically significant treatment effect on EDSS ($P = 0.02$) and relapse rate ($P = 0.04$). There was an extrapolation of the results from the actual follow-up to 2 years for the Kaplan-Meier 2-year analysis.

The MRI analysis was primarily done on yearly gadolinium enhanced scans. The number of active scans (containing at least one enhancing lesion) was 42.3 percent in the placebo group and 30 percent in the treated group ($P = 0.05$).

The number of enhancing lesions (white spots on the post–gadolinium scan) was reduced from a mean of 1.50 to 1.04 ($P = 0.02$) at 1 year and 1.65 to 0.80 at year 2 ($P = 0.05$). The extent of the enhancing lesions and T_2 lesions was determined by measuring the area of involvement on the scan, which was then converted to volume by a conversion

factor calculated by the slice thickness. Even though the T_2 measurements decreased in both groups of patients over the 2 years, there was a significant effect at 1 year ($P = 0.02$). For some reason (probably technical) the authors did not find the expected increase over time usually seen in the extent of T_2 lesions in the placebo group.

Another preparation of IFNB-1a has been used in a pre- and posttreatment randomized design in 68 patients over 1 year.[507a] The treatment (3 and 9 MIU subcutaneously 3 times per week) resulted in a significant ($P = <0.001$) posttreatment reduction (49 and 64 percent for each dose studied) in enhancing lesions. The treatment effect was seen after the first month of the study. The relapse rate was also reduced by 60 percent in the period after treatment ($P = <0.001$).

COMMENT

Interferon beta-1a (IFNB-1a) differs from IFNB-1b in that it is a recombinant product of a mammalian cell line (Chinese hamster ovary cells—CHO). It is glycosylated, and has the amino acid sequence typical of natural human IFN-beta. It is not clear whether glycosylation confers any significant advantage over IFNB-1b. A modest treatment effect was seen in the EDSS measure in the treated arm compared to placebo patients.[260]

The results are not directly comparable to those for IFNB-1b since the molecules are different. The dose and route of administration and the outcome measures also differed. Nevertheless a few inferences seem appropriate. The relapse rate reduction in the overall study was 18 percent for 1a as compared with 30 percent for 1b. The effect on disability is much more problematic. The 1a study involved patients with low disability (EDSS 0 to 3.5), while the 1b study entered patients from EDSS 0 to 5.5. Both studies had a similar definition of disease progression, i.e. a confirmed worsening of one point on the EDSS (6 months in the 1a study and 3 months in the 1b study). In the 1b study, 28 percent of patients in the placebo group had "progressed" at 3 years compared to 20 percent in the high-dose treatment group. For 1a the progression rate was 35 percent in the placebo group compared with 22 percent for the treatment group at 2 years. The 1a study claimed to have demonstrated a significant effect on slowing disability at 2 years (from the extrapolated Kaplan-Meier curves) but looking at all patients at 2 years (completed by only 85 of 158 treated patients) progression did not differ significantly from the placebo group ($P = 0.07$).

The postitive outcome message in the 1a study was equated with disability even though it is clear that worsening of one point on the EDSS scale at the lower levels of the scale is often as trivial as an abnormal reflex and/or a mild sensory loss or change. Since the levels of significance in this study were borderline, the soft nature of outcome at lower disability scale levels may be relevant. A more important issue concerns the question of progression of disability since there is only borderline significance, it is somewhat unsettling that the placebo group in the 1a study did worse than expected compared to natural history data and the data from other trials. Thirty-five percent deterioration at 2 years closely rivals the change seen in secondary-progressive MS trials. Natural history studies show that the time spent at EDSS 1 to 3.5 is longer than spent at EDSS 4 to 5.5, implying that the rate of progression for the mild placebo group in the 1a patients entering at 0 to 3.5 would be expected to be less than was reported. In fact, if one examines the 82 patients from the placebo group from the 1b study[234] who would have satisfied the 1a entry criteria (excluding the 4.0 to 5.5 patients) one finds a progression rate in 2 years of only 17 percent, and at 3 years of only 20 percent (Ebers, unpublished data, 1996). This rate of change is as good as or better than that in the *treated* patients from the 1a study and is consistent with the 20% placebo rate of worsening in a recently reported study of sulfasalazine[461a] in low-disability relapsing-remitting patients.

We recognize the potential hazards in comparing one study to another and that there are often small differences that interfere with such comparisons. However the inability of the result of the IFNB-1a study to stand up to cross-study comparison implies a certain lack of robustness in what

otherwise appears to be a positive result. These observations in which the control group did worse than expected (accounting for the "treatment effect") are reminiscent of the earlier study data[227] in which the poor outcome in the control group was the outlier. Finally, this study uses as an outcome measure a one-point increase in EDSS.

Our conclusion at this point is that neither IFN-1b nor 1a can yet be considered to significantly prevent the unremitting disability that accumulates with time in the great majority of MS patients.

INTERFERON BETA-1A, -1B AND COP I. A rather difficult choice faces neurologists today in the selection of therapy for relapsing-remitting patients. On the surface, it appears that three different therapies have comparable efficacy in relapse reduction and in reducing MRI activity.

It is important to bear in mind that relapse rate reduction, MRI lesion reduction, and even delay in progression on the disability scales are all surrogate markers for what matters most to patients and their families—a reduction in long-term disability. The social and economic costs of this disease are concentrated at the higher end of the disability scale. Unfortunately, however, the duration of clinical trials is limited and few studies can carry a large cohort of patients beyond 3 or 4 years. Even with appropriate intention to treat analyses, evaluation of outcome rapidly becomes constrained by the accumulating number of dropouts. This phenomenon raises the chances of type II (false negative) errors when attempts are made to assess long-term efficacy. There is no convincing evidence for an impact on long-term disability for either IFNB or COP I.

The idea of direct head-to-head comparisons of these drugs to one another and to older immunosuppressive drugs such as azathioprine and methotrexate is most attractive. Until such studies are done there will be considerable variability in the drugs chosen and even more so in the patients for whom therapy can be recommended.

It may be that validating surrogate markers such as MRI will be easier than demonstrating efficacy on long-term clinical outcome measures. In addition, cognitive function, a very important factor in employability, is probably equally as important for clinical trials as is neurological function. Modern trials are just beginning to use cognitive and quality of life measures as outcomes. Every attempt needs to be made to show an impact on the latter if skeptical critics of therapy are to be convinced. This kind of critical approach is appropriate for any proposed new treatment.

NEUTRALIZING ANTIBODIES (NAB)—AND DOSAGE. It has long been known that NAB may form against a variety of injectable biological products. This phenomenon was seen in the early days of insulin therapy and continues to be a problem even for occasional patients injected with the human product. Previously the switch from beef insulin to pork insulin in patients in whom antibodies occurred could modify the reduced efficacy due to NAB. Accordingly it is not a surprise that NAB might develop against recombinant interferon even though the product is a naturally occurring human molecule. Antibodies to the Beta Interferons definitely occur.[256a] However, in interpreting studies, one must be sure that the antibodies measured are actually neutralizing ones. Many patients can be antibody-positive on ELISA but negative for NAB. The phenomenon has attained clinical significance because some 38 percent of patients in the original IFNB-1b study developed NAB, most of these in the first 12 to 18 months. These antibodies appeared to have a marked effect on efficacy outcome measures in terms of both the relapse rate and MRI activity. NAB positive patients were found to revert to placebo levels of exacerbation from the time they developed sustained antibody levels. A reduction in, but not abolition of, MRI efficacy was also seen in the NAB positive group. However, NAB negative patients had an even more marked reduction in exacerbation rate than the whole population of patients; in this subgroup it approached 50 percent.[256a] The NAB question is under active investigation, and there is reason to believe that the effect of NAB on individual patients is not as significant as the grouped data would suggest (J. Petkau, unpublished data, 1996). In the IFNB-1a study the development of antibodies was reported to be 22 percent, but this finding is not directly comparable

to the 1b study because the assay methodology and the cutoff titer were apparently not the same.

Underdosing may be a factor in the 1a study. The treatment effect on exacerbation rate was less than in the 1b study. The MRI results were less impacted, and adverse events were much less frequent. The expected reductions in lymphocyte count and the common findings of liver function abnormalities were also much less than in the 1b trial. For example, the in vivo production of interferon in response to a variety of viral infections in normal subjects is an important mediator of the flu-like symptoms that are seen. Therefore, it seems unlikely that the difference in efficacy and adverse events could be attributed to glycosylation or some other molecular difference in the preparation. However, the specific activity of these two types of interferon preparations needs to be further studied. It is possible that underdosing accounts for both the efficacy and adverse-event differences between the two studies. Further studies of both drugs with larger doses may help resolve this question.

MECHANISM OF ACTION. The mechanism of action of IFNB could be one or more of the following effects:

1. Inhibition of pro-inflammatory cytokine (IFN gamma or TNF) effects[79a,365a,374a, 542a,550a]
2. Increasing anti-inflammatory cytokines (IL-4 or IL-10)[132b,581a]
3. Inhibition of T-cell metalloproteases[340a]
4. Decrease of nitrous oxide production[373b]
5. Increase of IL-6 production[79a]

However, IFNB does not affect IgG secretion of MS B cells.[36a] In addition, transretinoic acid may be synergestic with IFNB in modulating IFN gamma effect in vivo.[132a]

INTERFERON GAMMA. The biology of interferon gamma has been recently reviewed by Farrer and Schreiber.[162] It is produced by T cells in response to specific antigenic challenges and has been shown to activate macrophages and to enhance the generalized Shwartzman reaction.[63] It also augments experimental autoimmune neuritis[223] and causes human brain endothelial cells to express Ia antigen and form a leaky model blood-brain barrier.[253] In addition, interferon gamma enhances intercellular adhesion molecule-1 expression.[396] Therefore, interferon gamma may be involved in the signaling mechanisms seen in inflammatory disorders. One mechanism of action is that it activates a calcium channel in T lymphocytes via protein kinase C.[368] Because interferon gamma can be measured in patients,[219] future studies of this molecule should shed a great deal of light on the problem of MS lesion activity.

Future strategies for therapy in MS include the use of agents that block the effects of interferon gamma. As noted previously, both interferon alpha and interferon beta antagonize the immune effects of interferon gamma. However, the lymphocytes of patients with MS produce very little interferon gamma when stimulated with phytohemagglutinins.[480] Olsson and his colleagues,[469] however, used the CSF and blood lymphocyte secretion of interferon gamma in response to MBP as a measure of autoreactivity in MS.

Panitch and his colleagues[476] reported the use of interferon gamma in a phase I therapeutic study of 18 patients with relapsing disease. They found a striking increase in the relapse rate after interferon gamma therapy (Table 12–28). For this reason, the trial was stopped. Those patients who developed additional relapses, attributed by the authors to the interferon gamma, were subsequently reported to have recovered and have had no permanent ill effects (H.S. Panitch, personal communication, 1990). However, because of potential adverse effects on the MS, interferon gamma has been discarded as a viable therapeutic modality. Noronha and associates[446] studied both interferon alpha and interferon beta in MS and found both to augment sup-

pressor cell function as measured by the ConA-generated suppressor cell assay. Interferon gamma had no effect on suppressor cell function, however.

In contrast to this therapeutic trial, Bever and his colleagues[59] measured the interferon gamma response to the interferon inducer poly ICLC. They found that even though the levels of interferon gamma rose as expected, there was no associated clinical worsening. The observations of Panitch noted previously are important, however, because they are consistent with the autoimmune theory of MS pathogenesis. Cytokine antagonists and soluble adhesion molecules are possibly going to dominate treatment trials in the next several years.[134,186,521,522,626,650] Leukotrienes may also play a role[234] in tissue damage. Therapies designed to moderate their effect seems to be a rational approach.

Compston[112] wrote a thoughtful editorial on the future of MS treatment trials, discussing strategies to limit the spread of damage by immune manipulation and by enhancing axonal regeneration and glial repair.

Other Therapies

ESSENTIAL FATTY ACIDS

Baker and his colleagues[31] reported that hospitalized patients with MS had lower than normal levels of linoleic acid (LA) in the serum. That finding led to several trials of LA supplementation to the diet for the treatment of MS (Table 12–29). In 1972, Millar and colleagues[394] reported on a double blind comparison of LA to oleic acid

Table 12–28. **A PILOT TRIAL OF INTERFERON GAMMA**

Year	Senior Author	Active Agent/ Control Agent	No. of Patients	Patient Type	Duration of Therapy or Follow-up	Comments
1987	Panitch[476]	IFN gamma	18	RR	4 wk	Relapse rate increased.
1987	Panitch[477]	IFN gamma	Same	Same	4 wk	Immune responses were augmented.

IFN = interferon; RR = relapsing-remitting.

Table 12–29. **SOME RECENT THERAPEUTIC TRIALS OF LINOLEIC ACID AND FISH OIL**

Year	Senior Author	Active Agent/ Control Agent	No. of Patients	Patient Type	Duration of Therapy and Follow-up	Randomized	Controlled	Blinded	Comments
1973	Millar[394]	LA/OA	75	Mixed	2 yr	+	+	+	Relapses were less frequent in LA group. No influence on outcome was observed.
1977	Bates[42]	LA, LE, OA	152	CP	2 yr	+	+	+	No therapeutic effect was observed.
1978	Bates[43]	LA, LE, OA	116	RR	2 yr	+	+	+	LA treatment had a marginal effect in reducing relapse severity.
1978	Paty[487]	LA/OA	76	Mixed	2 yr	+	+	+	No therapeutic effect was observed.
1984	Dworkin[153]	Reanalysis of earlier trials	181	Mixed	2 yr	N/A	N/A	N/A	Reanalysis suggested benefit in less disabled patients. An analysis of three controlled trials was carried out.
1989	Bates[41]	Fish oil (n-3)/OA	292	RR	2 yr	+	+	+	No significant difference was observed. Trend was toward therapeutic effect.

CP = chronic progressive; LA = linoleic acid; LE = gamma lenolenic acid; N/A = not applicable; OA = oleic acid (controls); RR = relapsing-remitting.

Table 12–30. **SOME RECENT THERAPEUTIC TRIALS OF PLASMAPHERESIS AND LYMPHOCYTAPHERESIS**

Year	Senior Author	Active Agent/ Control Agent	No. of Patients	Patient Type	Duration of Follow-up	Randomized	Controlled	Blinded	Comments
1978	Schauf[554]	PP alone	3	Mixed	10 days	—	—	—	Two patients improved during treatment.
1980	Dau[130]	PP, AZA, and steroids	8	CP	2–15 mo	—	—	—	Modest improvement occurred in seven.
1980	Weiner[653]	PP, AZA, and steroids	8	CP	3 mo	—	—	—	Moderate temporary improvement occurred in 6 to 8 patients.
1982	Tindall[622]	PP plus AZA/PP	20	CP	1 yr	Matched	+	—	Transient subjective improvement occurred.
1983	Rose[534]	LP alone	7	CP	3–4 wk	—	—	—	Two of 7 patients improved.
1983	Valbonesi[636]	PP alone	6	CP	1 treatment	—	—	—	Four patients had moderate improvement.
1984	Khatri[297]	PP plus Cphos plus steroids	45	CP	1 yr	—	—	—	Twenty-eight of 45 patients improved.
1984	Medaer[380]	LP	9	Mixed	1 yr	—	—	—	Four of 9 patients improved. Relapses were not prevented.
1984	Hauser[229]	LP alone	5	CP	2–6 mo	—	—	—	No clinical effect was observed.
1985	Gordon[211]	PP plus AZA plus steroids/ AZA plus steroids	20	CP	6 mo	+	+	+	No sustained therapeutic benefit was observed.

Continued on following page

Table 12–30. — *continued*

Year	Senior Author	Active Agent/ Control Agent	No. of Patients	Patient Type	Duration of Follow-up	Randomized	Controlled	Blinded	Comments
1985	Khatri[298]	PP plus Cphos plus steroids/ Cphos plus steroids plus sham PP	54	CP	11 mo	+	+	+	Sustained benefit especially in cognitive function was achieved in PP group.
1986	Maida[361]	LP alone	9	RR	1 yr	—	—	—	Severe vein complications occurred in two patients. There was some suggestion of a reduced relapse rate.
1989	Weiner[652]	PP/sham; All patients received oral Cphos plus ACTH	116	Acute attacks	8 wk	+	+	+	PP-treated patients had a shorter recovery period. No long-term benefits were observed.
1991	CDN[449]	Cphos/PP/sham	168	CP	2 yr	+	+	+	PP treated patients had a trend towards improvement.
1996	Sorensen[586a]	PP and AZA	11	SP	6 mo crossover	+	—	+	A modest MRI treatment effect was seen.

AZA = azathioprine; ACTH = adrenocorticotrophic hormone; CDN = Canadian Cooperative MS Study Group; CP = chronic progressive; Cphos = cyclophosphamide; LP = lymphocytapheresis; PP = plasmapheresis; SP = secondary progressive.

(OA) over a treatment period of 2 years in 75 patients. They confirmed that LA levels were low in MS and that LA levels could be raised by dietary supplementation. The LA-treated group had a modest but statistically significant lower rate of relapses than did the OA group. This study and the others cited below, all showed that serum levels of LA could be corrected by oral administration of LA.

Subsequently, Bates and colleagues[43] and Paty and associates[487] tried to replicate Millar's result. Bates and colleagues found a marginal effect in reducing the frequency and severity of relapses, with no effect on the overall outcome. Paty and associates found no treatment effect. Dworkin and colleagues[153] pooled the data and reanalyzed the three therapeutic trials. Their reanalysis suggested that if only the mildly affected patients were considered, (a post-hoc subgroup analysis) the LA-treated patients had less neurological deterioration and a lower relapse rate than the OA-treated patients. The retrospective pooling of subgroup data from separate trials is not statistically sound methodology, even though the trial design had purposefully been similar in all three studies. Bates[41] also reported on a controlled trial of three long-chain polyunsaturated fatty acids versus placebo in 312 patients with relapsing-remitting MS over 2 years. The treatment group tended to benefit, but the difference between the groups was not statistically significant. A recent report of LA[341] in RA showed a significant treatment effect in the acute phases of RA flare-up. If this report can be confirmed, perhaps this agent should be reinvestigated in MS. A pilot study of 13-*cis*-retinoic acid has also been tried.[369]

Many patients take essential fatty acid preparations on their own. In the absence of a clear-cut contraindication to taking such preparations, we have taken the position that we cannot object to or condone such self therapy. It certainly would be helpful to have a clear-cut clinical trial result as a guide. However, one can understand the patient's desire to take a preparation that is not harmful if it might possibly have a beneficial effect.

PLASMAPHERESIS AND LYMPHOCYTAPHERESIS

Plasmapheresis (PP) is a physical method of separating the plasma from the red cell mass with plasma replacement by either fresh or frozen plasma or albumin. One of several hematologic, renal, and neurological indications for PP therapy include myasthenia gravis. In conditions with clear indications for PP therapy, antibodies exist that are considered important pathogenic factors in the production of the disease. No such knowledge or indication exists for MS.

Dau and colleagues[130] were the first to claim a therapeutic effect using PP in MS (Table 12–30). Eleven patients were treated in an uncontrolled fashion with PP, steroids, or AZA alone or in combination. "Neurological examination parameters" improved in seven patients. Later several other groups[525,622,635,653] reported a therapeutic effect in uncontrolled trials. Khatri and his colleagues[296–299] reported a controlled study using 55 patients with CPMS. They claimed improvement after 10 exchanges, with some startling figures for improvement in several very ill patients. Many critics have interpreted their results as being too good to be true, suggesting that the marked improvement must have occurred in some patients that were recovering from unrecorded or unrecognized acute attacks. Gordon and his colleagues[211] studied 20 patients with severely progressive disease and failed to find any beneficial therapeutic effect from PP. The study by Weiner and his colleagues[653] included a group treated with oral cyclophosphamide and plasmapheresis. They claimed a mild benefit for PP over placebo. Sorensen and colleagues[586a] have reported a randomized study of PP and AZA in eight secondary progressive patients followed by MRI during pre- and post-treatment. There were some modest treatment effects but the authors did not feel that the treatment effects were significant.

A trend towards PP effectiveness was also seen in a double blind, three-arm, multi-center randomized controlled clinical trial completed in Canada.[449] However, it is unclear whether this effect can be attributed to the PP alone; to the other simultaneous therapies, which included oral prednisone and oral cyclophosphamide; or to all these therapies in combination. Therefore, plasma exchange therapy cannot be endorsed for standard use until there is more clear-cut evidence of long-term benefit.

TOTAL LYMPHOID IRRADIATION

In 1986, Cook and his colleagues[118] reported a trial of total lymphoid irradiation (TLI) in patients with both relapsing remitting and chronic progressive MS (Table 12–31). They reported the treatment to significantly slow the rate of progression and to be very low in serious side effects. TLI or sham irradiation was given to 40 patients with CPMS in a double-blind, randomized, prospective clinical trial for an average follow-up of 21 months. The patients treated with TLI had a slower rate of functional decline than did the controls ($P<0.01$). The controls did somewhat worse than expected and patient blinding probably was not successful since 90 percent of the females developed amenorrhea and two-thirds of patients loss pubic/axillary hair. Although this report is interesting, the data require independent confirmation. Several aspects of trial design were suboptimal, including the use of a new, unvalidated impairment scale and reliance on a secondary ad hoc analysis. In contrast, preliminary results of a trial from Italy showed no therapeutic benefit.[89] In addition, follow-up of the TLI-treated patients from Cook and colleagues' report showed that five died, mostly from infectious complications.[121] The study was therefore put on hold for a time but has recently been restarted,[117a] combined with low-dose prednisone. The investigators also found that patients with the lowest lymphocyte counts seemed to respond the best.[119,120] The long-term effects of TLI must be clearly documented in a controlled and blinded trial done in an independent institution before it can be endorsed as beneficial. Wiles and colleagues[680] have reported on a trial using clinical and MRI monitoring where TLI treatment failed to confer a therapeutic benefit. In addition, brain irradiation may have an adverse effect on MS lesions.[500]

HYPERBARIC OXYGEN

In the 1970s, some practitioners began to use hyperbaric oxygen (HBO) ad hoc for the treatment of MS. The rationale for such therapy was unclear. Perhaps the practitioners had a treatment available and were looking for a disease to treat. More probable, however, because of the well-known tendency for patients with MS to remit spontaneously, some centers were claiming a therapeutic benefit in uncontrolled trials. In 1983, Fischer and his colleagues[170] reported on a highly controversial clinical trial in 37 patients with chronic stable MS (Table 12–32). Oxygen was compared with room air, both at two atmospheres of pressure in a double blind, randomized, controlled trial. Fischer and his colleagues reported a temporary (less than 1 year) modest improvement in several areas of neurological function, especially bladder control. Minor fluctuations were considered significant. Several subsequent controlled trials[35,115,220,347,382,679] have failed to show any therapeutic benefit from HBO, although some studies have reported some subjective improvement (some of the patients reported feeling better). In several of the studies, bladder function was marginally better in the treated patients. However, in one study the reverse was found.

OTHER AGENTS

A number of trials using other agents (Table 12–33) have demonstrated no sustained benefit. A recent trial of sulfasalazine has found that a modest early effect on relapse rate was more than offset later in the trial. By a higher rate of progression in disability in the treated group compared to controls. Sulfasalazine is currently in trial. However, one patient has been described in the literature[192] and we have personal experience with three patients who developed MS while on sulfasalazine therapy. It also fails to influence experimental autoimmune encephalomyelitis (EAE).[633] Colchicine has been tried in EAE[355] and has been tried in humans. Poly ICLC has been tried with indeterminate results.[58,59,61] Antioxidants have also been tried and found to be safe.[360]

Table 12–31. **SOME RECENT THERAPEUTIC TRIALS OF TOTAL LYMPHOID IRRADIATION**

Year	Senior Author	Active Agent/ Control Agent	No. of Patients	Patient Type	Duration of Follow-up	Randomized	Controlled	Blinded	Comments
1984	Hafstein[217]	TLI/sham	19	CP	6 mo	+	+	+	Trend was toward treatment effectiveness.
1986	Cook[118]	TLI/sham [extension of Hafstein (1984)]	40	CP	21 mo	+	+	+	A slower decline occurred in TLI-treated patients.
1987	Cook[121]	TLI/sham [extension of Cook (1986)]	45	CP	2 yr	+	+	+	Response was seen in patients with low lymphocyte count (secondary outcome measure).
1989	Cook[123]	TLI	Follow-up on earlier studies	CP	Over 2 yr	N/A	N/A	N/A	Five deaths occurred in TLI-treated patients.
1990	Cook[119]	TLI	24	CP	1 yr	+	+	+	A therapeutic effect was observed. Slower progression also occurred.
1990	Cook[119]	TLI	19	CP	1 yr	—	—	—	Response was better if lymphocyte count was low.
1992	Capra[89]	TLI	6	CP	4 yr	—	—	—	No reduction of worsening of disability was observed. One patient died of pneumonia.
1994	Wiles[680]	TLI	27	CP	2 yr	+	+	+	No clinical benefit was seen. MRI monitoring showed a reduction in lesion scores in TLI-treated patients. TLI was not recommended.

CP = chronic progressive; FU = follow-up; N/A = not applicable; TLI = total lymphoid irradiation.

Table 12–32. SOME RECENT THERAPEUTIC TRIALS OF HYPERBARIC OXYGEN

Year	Senior Author	Active Agent/ Control Agent	No. of Patients	Patient Type	Duration of Therapy or Follow-up	Randomized	Controlled	Blinded	Comments
1980	Neubauer[440]	HBO/air	250	CP	20 treatments	—	—	—	Improvement occurred in some patients.
1983	Fischer[170]	HBO/air	40	CP	1-yr follow-up	+	+	+	Transient subjective bladder improvement occurred.
1985	Barnes[35]	HBO/air	120	CP	4 wk	+	+	+	Transient subjective bladder improvement occurred in 12/51 HBO-treated patients. No sustained benefit.
1985	Rosen[536]	HBO/air	12	CP	2 mo	—	—	—	No therapeutic benefit was observed. Some transient subjective bladder improvement occurred.
1986	Harpur[220]	HBO/air	82	Chronic stable	7 mo	+	+	+	No therapeutic benefit was observed on clinical, EP, or MRI.
1986	Lhermitte[347]	HBO/air	49	Stable or progressive	6 mo	+	+	+	No clinical benefit was observed.
1987	Barnes[36]	Follow-up on Barnes (1985)	120	Chronic	18 treatments with 1-yr follow-up	+	+	+	No significant overall benefit was observed
1990	Meneghetti[382]		15	Progressive	2 yr	—	—	—	Subjective improvement in bladder function occurred.

CP = chronic progressive; EP = evoked potentials; HBO = hyperbaric oxygen; MRI = magnetic resonance imaging.

Table 12–33. **SOME RECENT MISCELLANEOUS THERAPEUTIC TRIALS**

Year	Senior Author	Active Agent/Control Agent	No. of Patients	Patient Type	Duration of Therapy or Follow-up	Randomized	Controlled	Blinded	Comments
1972	Neumann[441]	6-MP or methotrexate vs. placebo*	27	Mixed	10–23 mo	+	+	+	Significant clinical improvement was not evident
1979	Gore[212]	IT Cytarabine	4	Mixed	20 days	−	−	−	Meningeal reaction stopped treatment.
1980	Tourellotte[624]	Cytarabine IV or IT	10	Mixed	2 wk	−	−	−	No improvements or adverse effects were observed.
1980	Brage[74]	Thymectomy	166	Mixed	N/A	−	−	−	No complications occurred. Some patients did better.
1980	Cendrowski[97]	Thymus factor (TF)	13	Mixed	1–14 mo	−	−	−	TF does not abolish relapses.
1980	Ellison[160]	Amantadine/placebo	14	Mixed	40 wk	−	+	+	No therapeutic benefit was observed in this matched pair design.
1985	Stefoski[590]	Mannitol/ACTH/NaHCO$_3$/placebo	34	Relapsing	1 hr to 10 days	+	+	+	Temporary benefit was derived from mannitol, NaHCO$_3$, and ACTH.
1985	Trotter[629]	Thymectomy ± AZA	34	Mixed	3 yr	−	−	−	No therapeutic benefit was observed.
1987	Plaut[501]	Amantadine/placebo	53	Mixed	3–4 yr	+	+	+	Relapse rate was reduced. No effect on neurological deterioration.
1990	Kappos[273]	Mitoxantrone	14	SP	3 mo	−	−	−	Eight patients remained stable or did better in 6 mo. MRI monitoring showed benefit.

Continued on following page

Table 12–33.—*continued*

Year	Senior Author	Active Agent/ Control Agent	No. of Patients	Patient Type	Duration of Follow-up	Randomized	Controlled	Blinded	Comments
1991, 1993	Noseworthy[452,453]	IV mitoxantrone	13	CP	Up to 18 mo	–	–	–	Potentially helpful.
1994	Milligan[407a]	Isoprinosine	52	Mixed	2 yr	+	+	+	No treatment effect was observed.
1995	Calabresi[85a]	TGF-β_2	18	CP	—	–	–	–	This study was open label.
1995	Karussis[279c,280a]	Linomide	30	SP	Up to 1 yr	+	+	+	Linomide reduced EDSS change and reduced number of enhancing lesions on MRI.
1995	Krapf[323a]	Mixtoxantrone	10	Rapid	2 yr	–	–	–	MRI activity (gadolinium enhancement) decreased from baseline.
1996	Edan[158a]	Mitoxantrone/ placebo. All patients received IVMP monthly.*	42	Active	6 mo	+	+	+	A marked decrease in enhancing lesions on MRI scan, a decrease in relapse rate, and a decrease in EDSS change were seen in mitoxantrone treated patients.
1995–96	Goodkin[206,206a]	Methotrexate	56	CP	6 mo	+	+	+	Clinical and MRI treatment effects were seen.
1996	Anderson[17a]	Linomide	31	RR	6 mo to 2 yr	+	+	+	MRI activity was reduced.
1996	Vandenbark[641a]	T-cell receptor vaccination	23	CP	1 yr	–	–	–	Treatment was safe.

ACTH = adrenocorticotrophic hormone; AZA = Azathioprine; CP = chronic progressive; Cytarabine = cytosine arabinoside; EDDS = Extended Disability Status Scale; 6-MP = 6-mercaptopurine; MRI = magnetic resonance imaging; NaHCO$_3$ = sodium bicarbonate; SP = secondary progressive; TF = thymus factor; TGF = tumor growth factor; IT = intrathecal.

*The drugs were alternated every 3 months, placebo patients remained on placebo.

Table 12–34. SOME THERAPEUTIC TRIALS CURRENTLY UNDER WAY

2-Chlorodewxyadenosine (2-CDA) (Cladribine)	Deprenyl (selegiline HCl)
3-4-Diaminopyridine (3-4-DAP)	Extracorporeal irradiation of blood
4-Aminopyridine (4-AP)	Fatty acids
15-Deoxyspanqualin	FK-506
Adhesion molecules (soluble)	Fluoxetine
Anergix (antigen/MHC complex binder)	Gallium nitrate
Antidepressants	Glial growth factor
Amitriptyline	Gluthemide
Azathioprine (Imuran)	Gold sodium thiomalate
Bee venom (purified)	Human gamma globulins
Botulinum A exotoxin	Hydrolases
Bromocriptine	Hydroxyzine HCl
CD2 receptor	Immunoglobulin G
CD4 analogue	Immunosuppressants
Chlorambucil and prednisone	Interferons—various
Colchicine	Interleukin-2 bound toxin
Copolymer I (COP I)	Interleukin-10 (IL-10)
Cyclophosphamide (Cytoxan)	Interleukin-6 (IL-6)
Cytokines (interferons, TGF-β_2, interleukin-10)	Irradiation—extracorporeal
Cytokine blocker (Anti-interleukin-2, Anti-tumor necrosis factor)	Isoprinisine
	L-Thrionine
Cytosine arabinoside	Leuprolide acetate
Desferrioxamine B	Linomide
Digitalis	Methotrexate
Deoxyspergualin	

Continued on following page

During that trial, the glutathone peroxidase activity was found to be low in the patients with MS. In addition, Stefoski and colleagues[590] reported that mannitol, ACTH, and sodium bicarbonate each produced temporary benefit in patients during an acute relapse. The short-lived benefits of these agents may be due to osmotic or electrolyte effects on conduction in demyelinated axons. Table 12–34 lists some of the substances currently under study around the world.[435]

Summary of Specific Therapies

We can say at this time that MS has changed from an untreatable disease to a partially treatable one, but no known treatment for MS significantly alters the long-term outcome of the disease. Recovery from acute exacerbations is hastened by corticosteroids, but corticosteroid therapy, either short-term or long-term, does not appear to affect long-term outcome. Furthermore, there is no clear-cut evidence that intermittent corticosteroid therapy for relapses alters the long-term outcome. Several therapeutic approaches appear to modestly influence the rate of progression in the short term for patients with CPMS. Most of these therapies use some form of immunosuppression. Several agents have also been reported to reduce the relapse rate. Most of these agents are under continued study. The high level of therapeutic trial activity with encouraging reports suggests that a rational strategy for treating malignantly active MS may soon be available[435,436] (see Table 12–34).

New approaches such as TNF-α receptor blockade, soluble adhesion molecule blockade, monoclonal antibody therapy, and T-cell vaccination add to the diversity of

Table 12–34.—*continued*

Methylprednisolone	Steroids and ACTH
Micophenolate mofetil	Sulfasalazine
Misoprostol (Cytotek)	T-cell vaccination
Mitoxantrone	T-cell receptor peptides
Monoclonal antibodies	Terbutaline
Antiadhesion molecules	Thalidomide
Antilymphocyte (Campath-1H)	Tizanidine (Sirdulad)
Anti–interferon gamma	Total lymphoid irradiation
Anti–T-cell receptor (TcR)	Transfer factor
Anti–tumor necrosis factor (TNF)	Transforming growth factor (TGF)-β (Betakine)
Chimeric anti-CD4	Tumor necrosis factor blockers—antibodies, soluble receptors
Anti-TAC:33B31, Anti-CD52	Vaccination studies
OKT3	T-cell receptors
Anti-integrin receptor	T-cell receptor peptides
Mycophenolate mofetil	Potential therapies being considered (effective in EAE):
Myelin plus myelin basic protein (MBP) (oral)	Monoclonal antibodies—anti-MHC (OX6)
Peptide—immunizations (various)	Omega 3 fatty acids—anti-CD11
Pentoxyfylline (Trental)	Metaloproteinases
Plasmapheresis	Antioxidants (MK801)
Platelet activation factor antagonists	Polyamine blockade
Poly ICLC	Cytokine IL-12 blockade (P40 Homo Dymer)
Prednisone	Verapamil
Psoralen UV-A irradiation (PUVA)	TMI—block metalloproteinases (BB 3644)
Rapamycin	
13-*cis*-Retinoic acid and azathioprine	

Source: National Multiple Sclerosis Society,[436] whole publication, with permission.
ACTH = adrenocorticotrophic hormone; EAE = experimental allergic encephalomyelitis.

therapeutic strategies that, when fully evaluated, may achieve a more profound clinical effect. Clearly, objective measurements of disease activity are sorely needed during this most important time in the history of MS therapeutic trials. MRI seems to offer such an objective method of assessment. The results of several trials show that MRI monitoring is not only an objective outcome measure, but is more sensitive to treatment effects than are other currently used clinical methods. In addition, if an analogy to cancer chemotherapy is appropriate, perhaps the next step after the demonstration of a modest therapeutic effect of single agents should be to combine the best of the single agents into regimens using multiple agents, with each agent being used in its most effective form.

When an accurate index for prognosis is determined (see Chapter 6), patients with a predetermined level of poor prognostic indicators could be randomized and stratified into treatment and control groups early in the course of their disease. A long-term (5 years or so) controlled study using these patients could then be conducted using an aggressive regimen as suggested previously avoiding dropouts will always be problematic. Without such a prognostic scale, few investigators would be willing to undertake a long-term study using toxic drugs in patients with early disease and perhaps benign prognosis. One should be fearful of making the treatment worse than the disease in those patients who would otherwise follow a benign clinical course. In the meantime, the interferons, which are mostly nontoxic, should be studied intensely to find the optimum dose, most appropriate treatment group, and persistence of effect.

RECOMMENDED REGIMEN FOR LONG-TERM MANAGEMENT OF RELAPSING MULTIPLE SCLEROSIS*

Early Multiple Sclerosis

1. Establish the diagnosis with maximum certainty.
2. Take time to educate the patient and family about MS.
3. Be encouraging concerning the outlook for new therapies being effective.
4. See the patient in follow-up frequently enough to continue the dialogue.
5. Interferon beta seems appropriate (if available) for patients with early RRMS, particularly for those with frequent disabling relapses.

Relapses

1. Treat only relapses that interfere significantly with function and that do not spontaneously improve after a week or so of follow-up.
2. Treat the relapses with oral prednisone, ACTH, bedrest, or IV corticosteroids. Bedrest alone can be effective in some severe relapses. Severe relapses warrant IV methylprednisolone, 1 g/day for 3 to 5 days, possibly followed by a tapering dose of oral prednisone.
3. Interferon beta, COP I, and AZA reduce the rate of relapses, but direct comparison between AZA and interferon preparations would help put these therapies in context.

TREATMENT OF THE CHRONIC PROGRESSIVE PHASE OF MS

There is no specific therapy that has been proven to make a significant impact on the chronic progressive phase of MS. Azathioprine, cladribine, linomide, methotrexate, mitoxantrone, and other immunosuppressant agents may have a modest impact and are under further study. The IFN Betas have not been shown to be effective and are being studied as this section is being written. Intermittent pulses of methylprednisone or dexamethasone may have a place. Plasma exchange is used in some centers for very rapidly advancing MS, especially in those patients with cognitive problems.

Most of the management of the chronic progressive phase is by the use of symptomatic drug treatment, rehabilitation strategies, and other supportive therapies seeking to improve quality of life. We therefore recommend the following approach when it is apparent that the chronic progressive phase of MS has begun:

1. Optimize a supportive program with OT, PT, and social work. A maintenance program of supportive therapy is very important.
2. By titrating the dose, develop a drug strategy designed to reduce spasticity and control bladder problems. Anticipate and treat bladder infections aggressively. Remember that intermittent self-catheterization can have a very beneficial effect in patients with a high chronic residual urinary volume.
3. Give at least one course of IV methylprednisolone 3 to 5 days at 1 gram per day. Some patients with chronic active MS respond to IV steroids. Such therapy can be given easily in an outpatient setting. Some patients may require a tapering dose of oral prednisone. If patients respond to IVMP, booster injections every 3 months may help sustain mobility. Some neurologists are using 1 day of pulse therapy per month for maintenance but efficacy is not established.
4. Monitor the patients carefully for osteoporosis by bone density measurements. Also give calcium supplements, estrogen as needed, and a bone metabolism regulator (for example, etidronate disodium or alendronate sodium), especially to women.

---

*The authors refer the reader to the section of management in Sibley[568]: *Therapeutic Claims in MS*, and other books by R. Schapiro[552] and L. Scheinberg.[555]

5. If patients are relentlessly progressing, we will sometimes use azathioprine or methotrexate in addition to intermittent IV steroids.

The only aspects of this management strategy that are definitely going to improve patients' function and quality of life are the rehabilitation measures and symptomatic drug management. We anticipate more definitive direction will come from the many ongoing studies presently underway.

Long-Term Management

MS is a disease that impairs the quality of life, and symptomatic management can be highly effective in improving quality of life.

1. Respond to the patient's questions and take time to know both the patient and the family.
2. Monitor the patient for complications such as infection, depression, mania, decubiti, and so forth.
3. Do not hesitate to use knowledgeable consultants such as social workers, psychologists, psychiatrists, ophthalmologists, urologists, sexual medicine specialists, and physical and occupational therapists.
4. Use drugs for symptomatic control sparingly. Remember that control of urinary incontinence is important for social and medical reasons. Anticholinergic drugs and intermittent self-catheterization can be effective measures in improving bladder function. Antispasticity drugs can be useful in both ambulation and nursing care. Attention to diet and fluid intake are important for bowel management. In addition, sleep is important to overall well-being. Improvement in sleep can be obtained by providing appropriate therapy for conditions that may interrupt sleep, such as nocturia, spasms, and depression, and by the use of low doses of benzodiazepines.
5. Interferon beta should be given to actively relapsing patients early in the course of their disease to suppress relapses and, it is hoped, to prolong the time to significant disability. It is not yet indicated for patients with progressive impairment.

Long-Term Home Care

1. Patients should be kept at home as long as possible. However, the needs of caregivers must be identified and met; otherwise, patients will go into institutional care earlier than they otherwise would.
2. Local agencies, including the MS Society, social services, and coalitions for the disabled can help to identify support services for both patients and families.
3. Regular home visits by nurses, therapists, and physicians can help the patient and the family caregivers to continue with home management.
4. Respite care, with intermittent institutionalization, is an invaluable alternative to home care for families requiring a break from the demands of caregiving. Many centers provide such services; if they are not available, pressure should be applied to develop respite care beds in the local area.

Longer-Term Institutional Care

Some patients require nursing care that cannot be provided at home. Those patients are best maintained in an institution that has experience with patients with MS. Specific wards that cater to the younger disabled are preferable to those that mix patients with MS and elderly, likely demented, patients. The International Federation of MS Societies and individual country MS societies are currently looking at this very important issue.[127] Pressure must be applied to convince medical care providers that a coordinated approach to long-term care for the younger disabled patient is not only urgently needed, but economically feasible, particularly when linked to the concept of widely accessible respite and day-care facilities.

REFERENCES

1. Abbruzzese G, Gandolfo C, and Loeb C: "Bolus" methylprednisolone versus ACTH in the treatment of multiple sclerosis. Ital J Neurol Sci 4: 169–172, 1983.

2. Abramowicz M (ed): Drugs that cause sexual dysfunction. Med Lett Drugs Ther 25:73–76, 1983.

3. Abramsky O, Teitelbaum D, and Arnon R: Effect of a synthetic polypeptide (cop 1) on patients with multiple sclerosis and with acute disseminated encephalomyelitis. J Neurol Sci 31:433–438, 1977.

3a. Adler CH, Zimmerman RA, Savino PJ, Bernardi B, Bosley TM and Sergott RC: Hemifacial spasm: Evaluation by magnetic resonance imaging and magnetic resonance tomographic angiography. Ann Neurol 32:502–506, 1992.

4. Aimard G, Confavreux C, Trouillas P, and Devic M: L'azathioprine dans les traitement de la sclérose en plaques. Une expérience de 10 ans à propos de 77 malades. Rev Neurol (Paris) 134:215–222, 1978.

5. Aisen ML, Holzer M, Rosen M, Dietz M, and McDowell F: Glutethimide treatment of disabling action tremor in patients with multiple sclerosis and traumatic brain injury. Arch Neurol 48:513–515, 1991.

6. Alam SM, Kyriakides T, Lawden M, and Newman PK: Methylprednisolone in multiple sclerosis: A comparison of oral with intravenous therapy at equivalent high dose. J Neurol Neurosurg Psychiatry 56:1219–1220, 1993.

7. Alexander L, Berkeley AW, and Alexander AM: Multiple Sclerosis: Prognosis and Treatment. Thomas, Springfield, IL, 1961.

8. Allen JC, Sheremata W, Cosgrove JBR, Osterland K, and Shea M: Cerebrospinal fluid T and B lymphocyte kinetics related to exacerbations of multiple sclerosis. Neurology 26:579–583, 1976.

9. Al-Sabbagh A, Nelson P, and Weiner HL: Beta interferon enhances oral tolerance to MBP and PLP in experimental autoimmune encephalomyelitis. Neurology 44(suppl 2):A242, 1994.

10. Alter M, Byrne TN, Daube JR, Franklin G, and Goldstein ML: Quality Standards Subcommittee: Practice advisory on selection of patients with multiple sclerosis for treatment with Betaseron. Neurology 44:1537–1540, 1994.

11. Alvord EC Jr, Shaw CM, Hruby S, and Kies MW: Has myelin basic protein received a fair trial in the treatment of multiple sclerosis? Ann Neurol 6:461–468, 1979.

12. Amato MP, Fratiglioni L, Groppi C, Siracusa G, and Amaducci L: Interrater reliability in assessing functional systems and disability on the Kurtzke Scale in multiple sclerosis. Arch Neurol 45:746, 1988.

13. Amato MP, Groppi C, Siracusa GF, and Fratiglioni L: Inter and intra-observer reliability in Kurtzke scoring systems in multiple sclerosis. Ital J Neurol Sci 6:129–132, 1987.

14. Amato MP, Ponziani G, Pracucci G, Siracusa G, and Amaducci L: Validation of self-administered version of the minimal record of disability for multiple sclerosis. Neurology 44(suppl 2):A392, 1994.

15. Aminoff MJ: The use of somatosensory evoked potentials in the evaluation of the central nervous system (review). Neurol Clin 6:809–823, 1988.

16. Aminoff MJ, Davis SL, and Panitch HS: Serial evoked potential studies in patients with definite multiple sclerosis. Arch Neurol 41:1197–1202, 1984.

17. Anderson DC, Slater GE, Sherman R, and Ettinger MG: Evoked potentials to test a treatment of chronic multiple sclerosis. Arch Neurol 44:1232–1236, 1987.

17a. Andersen O, Lycke J, Tollesson PO, et al: Linomide reduces the rate of active lesions in relapsing-remitting multiple sclerosis. Neurology 47:895–900, 1996.

18. Antel JP, Arnason BGW, and Medof ME: Suppressor cell function in multiple sclerosis: Correlation with clinical disease activity. Ann Neurol 5:338–342, 1979.

19. Antel JP, Rosenkoetter M, Reder AT, Oger J-F, and Arnason BGW: Multiple sclerosis: Relation of in vitro IgG secretion to T suppressor cell number and function. Neurology 34:1155–1160, 1984.

20. Anzola GP, Bevilacqua L, Cappa SF, et al: Neuropsychological assessment in patients with relapsing-remitting multiple sclerosis and mild functional impairment: correlation with magnetic resonance imaging. J Neurol Neurosurg Psychiatry 53:142–145, 1990.

21. Aring CD: Observations on multiple sclerosis and conversion hysteria. Brain 88:663, 1965.

22. Armspach JP, Rumbach L, Namer IJ, et al: Evaluation of anti-CD4 monoclonal antibody treatment in multiple sclerosis. 10th Congress of the European Committee for Treatment and Research in Multiple Sclerosis, Book of Abstracts. Athens, Greece, 1994, p 30.

23. Arnold DL, De Stefano N, Collins DL, et al: Imaging of axonal damage in multiple sclerosis. Neurology 44(suppl 2):A340, 1994.

24. Arnold DL, Riess GT, Mathews PM, et al: Use of proton magnetic resonance spectroscopy for monitoring disease progression in multiple sclerosis. Ann Neurol 36:76–82, 1994.

25. Arnon R, Teitelbaum D, and Sela M: Suppression of experimental allergic encephalomyelitis by COP1: Relevance to multiple sclerosis. Isr J Med Sci 25:686–689, 1989.

26. Atlas SW, Grossman RI, Goldberg HI, Hackney DB, Bilaniuk LT, and Zimmerman RA: MR diagnosis of acute disseminated encephalomyelitis. J Comput Assist Tomogr 10:798–801, 1986.

27. AUSTIMS Research Group: Interferon-α and transfer factor in the treatment of multiple sclerosis: a double-blind, placebo-controlled trial. J Neurol Neurosurg Psychiatry 52:566–574, 1989.

28. Azouvi P, Roby-Brami A, Biraben A, Theibaut JB, Thurel C, and Bussel B: Effect of intrathecal baclofen on the monosynaptic reflex in humans: Evidence for a postsynaptic action. J Neurol Neurosurg Psychiatry 56:515–519, 1993.

29. Bach MA, Martin C, Cesaro P, Eizenbaum JF, and Degos JD: T cell subsets in multiple sclerosis: A longitudinal study of exacerbating-remitting cases. J Neuroimmunol 7:331–343, 1985.

30. Bach MA, Tournier E, Phan-Dinh-Tuy F, Chatenovo L, and Bach JF: Deficient of suppressor T cells in active multiple sclerosis. The Lancet 2:1221–1224, 1980.

31. Baker RW, Thompson RH, and Zilkha KJ: Changes in the amounts of linoleic acid in the serum of patients with multiple sclerosis. J Neurol Neurosurg Psychiatry 29:95–98, 1966.

31a. Bansil S, Cook SD, and Rohowsky-Kochan C: Multiple sclerosis: Immune mechanism and update on current therapies. Ann Neurol 37(suppl 1): S87–S101, 1995.

32. Barkhof F, Frequin ST, Hommes OR, et al: A correlative triad of gadolinium-DTPA MRI, EDSS, and CSF-MBP in relapsing multiple sclerosis patients treated with high-dose intravenous methylprednisolone. Neurology 42:63, 1992.

33. Barkhof F, Hommes OR, Scheltens P, and Valk J: Quantitative MRI changes in gadolinium-DTPA enhancement after high-dose intravenous methylprednisolone in multiple sclerosis. Neurology 41:1219–1222, 1991.

34. Barnes MP, Bateman DE, Cleland PG, et al: Intravenous methylprednisolone for multiple sclerosis in relapse. J Neurol Neurosurg Psychiatry 48:157–159, 1985.

35. Barnes MP, Bates D, Cartlidge NEF, French JM, and Shaw DA: Hyperbaric oxygen and multiple sclerosis: Short-term results of a placebo-controlled, double-blind trial. The Lancet 1:297–300, 1985.

36. Barnes MP, Bates D, Cartlidge NEF, French JM, and Shaw DA: Hyperbaric oxygen and multiple sclerosis: Final results of a placebo-controlled, double-blind trial. J Neurol Neurosurg Psychiatry 50:1402–1406, 1987.

36a. Barrett KA, Guthikonda P, Goodman A and Mattson D: The effect of in vitro and in vivo interferon-β1b on immunoglobulin G synthesis by peripheral blood lymphocytes. Neurology 46: 136–137, 1996.

37. Bass B, Weinshenker B, Rice GPA, et al: Tizanidine versus baclofen in the treatment of spasticity in patients with multiple sclerosis. Can J Neurol Sci 15:15–19, 1988.

37a. Basso MR, Beason-Hazen S, Lynn J, Rammohan K and Bornstein RA: Screening for cognitive dysfunction in multiple sclerosis. Arch Neurol 53:980–984, 1996.

38. Basten A, Pollard JD, Stewart GJ, et al: Transfer factor in treatment of multiple sclerosis. The Lancet 2:931–934, 1980.

39. Bastianello S, Pozzilli C, Bernardi S, et al: Serial study of gadolinium-DTPA MRI enhancement in multiple sclerosis. Neurology 40:591–595, 1990.

40. Bastianello S, Pozzilli C, D'Andrea F, et al: A controlled trial of mitoxantrone in multiple sclerosis: Serial MRI evaluation at one year. Can J Neurol Sci 21:266–270, 1994.

40a. Bastianello S, Pozzilli C, Gasperini C, et al: Surrogate markers of disease activity in multiple sclerosis: Monthly enhanced imaging versus 6-month T2 assessment. Neurology 46:A367, 1996.

41. Bates D, Cartlidge NEF, French JM, et al: A double-blind controlled trial of long chain n-3 polyunsaturated fatty acids in the treatment of multiple sclerosis. J Neurol Neurosurg Psychiatry 52:18–22, 1989.

42. Bates D, Fawcett PRW, Shaw DA, and Weightman D: Trial of polyunsaturated fatty acids in non-relapsing multiple sclerosis. BMJ 2:932–933, 1977.

43. Bates D, Fawcett PRW, Shaw DA, and Weightman D: Polyunsaturated fatty acids in treatment of acute remitting multiple sclerosis. BMJ 2:1390–1391, 1978.

44. Baumhefner RW, Syndulko K, Ke D, Paty DW, Ellison GW, and Tourtellotte WW: Relationship between total MRI lesion area above the spinal cord and clinical and neuroperformance outcome assessments in chronic progressive multiple sclerosis. Neurology 44(suppl 2):1994.

45. Baumhefner RW, Tourtellotte WW, Paty DW, Mertin J, Merrill J, and Lisak RP: Peripheral, cerebrospinal fluid and CNS immune cell subset and functional alterations in multiple sclerosis. In Hommes OR, Mertin J, and Tourtellotte WW (eds): Immunotherapies in MS. S Phillips Publications, Sutton, England, 1986, pp 1–36.

46. Baumhefner RW, Tourtellotte WW, Syndulko K, Staugaittis A, and Shapshak P: Multiple sclerosis intra-blood-brain-barrier IgG synthesis: Effect of pulse intravenous and intrathecal corticosteroids. Italian Journal of Neurological Sciences 10:19–32, 1989.

47. Baumhefner RW, Tourtellotte WW, Syndulko K, et al: Quantitative multiple sclerosis plaque assessment with magnetic resonance imaging: Its correlation with clinical parameters, evoked potentials, and intra-blood-brain barrier IgG analysis. Arch Neurol 47:19, 1990.

48. Beatty WW, and Scott JG: Issues and developments in the neuropsychological assessment of patients with multiple sclerosis. Journal of Neurologic Rehabilitation 7(3–4):87, 1993.

49. Beck RW: Corticosteroid treatment of optic neuritis: A need to change treatment practices—The Optic Neuritis Study Group (editorial). Neurology 42:1133–1135, 1992.

50. Beck RW, Arrington J, Murtagh FR, Cleary PA, Kaufman DI, and the Optic Neuritis Study Group. Brain Magnetic Imaging in Acute Optic Neuritis: Experience of the Optic Neuritis Study Group. Arch Neurol 50:841–846, 1993.

51. Beck RW, Cleary PA, Anderson MM, et al: A randomized, controlled trial of corticosteroids in the treatment of acute optic neuritis. New Engl J Med 326:581–588, 1992.

52. Beck RW, Cleary PA, Trobe JD, et al: The effect of corticosteroids for acute optic neuritis on the subsequent development of multiple sclerosis: The Optic Neuritis Study Group. New Engl J Med 329:1764–1769, 1993.

52a. Becker WJ, Harris CJ, Long ML, Ablett DP, Klein GM, and DeForge DA: Long term intrathecal baclofen therapy in patients with intractable spasticity. Can J Neurol Sci 22:208–217, 1995.

53. Becker WJ, and Richards IM: Serial pattern shift visual evoked potentials in multiple sclerosis. Can J Neurol Sci 11:53–59, 1984.

54. Behan PO, Durward WF, Behan WMH, Melville ID, and McGeorge AP: Transfer-factor therapy in multiple sclerosis. The Lancet 988–990, 1976.

55. Bernat JL, Sadowsky CH, Vincent FM, Nordgren RE, and Margolis G: Sclerosing spinal pachy-

meningitis: A complication of intrathecal administration of Depo-Medrol for multiple sclerosis. J Neurol Neurosurg Psychiatry 39:1124–1128, 1976.

56. Betts CD, D'Mellow MT, and Fowler CJ: Urinary symptoms and the neurological features of bladder dysfunction in multiple sclerosis. J Neurol Neurosurg Psychiatry 56:245–250, 1993.

56a. Bever CT, Anderson PA, Leslie J, Treatment with oral 3,4 diaminopyridine improves leg strength in multiple sclerosis patients: Results of a randomized, double-blind, placebo-controlled, crossover trial. Neurology 47:1457–1462, 1996.

57. Bever CT Jr, Leslie J, Camenga DL, Panitch HS, and Johnson KP: Preliminary trial of 3,4-diaminopyridine in patients with multiple sclerosis. Ann Neurol 27:421–427, 1990.

58. Bever CT Jr, McFarland HF, Levy HB, and McFarlin DE: Cortisol induction by poly ICLC: Implications for clinical trials of interferon. Ann Neurol 23:196–199, 1988.

59. Bever CT Jr, McFarlin DE, and Levy HB: A comparison of interferon responses to poly ICLC in males and females. J Interferon Res Spec No:85–90, 1992.

60. Bever CT Jr, Panitch HS, Levy HB, McFarlin DE, and Johnson KP: Gamma-interferon induction in patients with chronic progressive MS. Neurology 41:1124–1127, 1991.

61. Bever CT Jr, Salazar AM, Neely E, et al: Preliminary trial of poly ICLC in chronic progressive multiple sclerosis. Neurology 36:494–498, 1986.

62. Bever CT Jr, Young D, Anderson PA, et al: The effects of 4-aminopyridine in multiple sclerosis patients: Results of a randomized, placebo-controlled, double-blind, concentration-controlled, crossover trial. Neurology 44:1054–1059, 1994.

63. Billiau A: Gamma-interferon: The match that lights the fire? Immunol Today 9:37–40, 1988.

64. Blaivas JG: Management of bladder dysfunction in multiple sclerosis. Neurology 30:12–18, 1980.

65. Bogousslavsky J, Fox AJ, Carey LS, et al: Correlates of brain-stem oculomotor disorders in multiple sclerosis (magnetic resonance imaging). Arch Neurol 43:460–463, 1986.

66. Boller F, and Frank E: Sexual Dysfunction in Neurological Disorders: Diagnosis, Management, and Rehabilitation. Raven Press, New York, 1982.

67. Bornstein MB, Miller A, Slagle S, et al: A pilot trial of cop 1 in exacerbating-remitting multiple sclerosis. N Engl J Med 317:408–414, 1987.

68. Bornstein MB, Miller AI, Slagle S, et al: A placebo-controlled, double-blind, randomized, two-center, pilot trial of Cop 1 in chronic progressive multiple sclerosis. Neurology 41:533–539, 1991.

69. Bornstein MB, Miller AI, Teitelbaum D, Arnon R, and Sela M: Multiple sclerosis: Trial of a synthetic polypeptide. Ann Neurol 11:317–319, 1982.

70. Bourdette D, Prochazka AV, Mitchell W, Burks J, and Licari P: Evidence that a multidisciplinary team care clinic is more effective than standard medical care in treating veterans with multiple sclerosis. Neurology 41:353, 1991.

70a. Bourgouin PM, Lapierre Y, Wolfson C, Duquette P, Duong HD and Trudel GC: Spinal cord multiple sclerosis: A study of disease activity with gadolinium-enhanced MRI. Neurology 46:A368, 1996.

71. Boyle EA, Clark CM, Klonoff H, Paty DW, and Oger JJF: Empirical support for psychological profiles observed in multiple sclerosis. Arch Neurol 48:1150–1154, 1991.

72. Bozek CB, Kastrukoff LF, Wright JM, Perry TL, and Larsen TA: A controlled trial of isoniazid therapy for action tremor in multiple sclerosis. Neurology 234:36–39, 1987.

73. Bradbury K, Aparicio SR, Sumner DW, MacFie A, and Bird CC: In vitro toxicity of MS sera correlates with new clinical signs. Acta Neurol Scand 70:456–459, 1984.

74. Brage D: Observations in 166 patients with multiple sclerosis after thymectomy. In Bauer HJ, Poser S, and Ritter G (eds): Progress in Multiple Sclerosis Research. Springer-Verlag, New York, 1980, pp 451–454.

75. Brar SP, Smith MB, Nelson LM, Franklin GM, and Cobble ND: Evaluation of treatment protocols on minimal to moderate spasticity in multiple sclerosis. Arch Phys Med Rehabil 72:186–189, 1991.

76. Brett DC, Ferguson GG, and Paty DW: Percutaneous trigeminal rhizotomy: Treatment of trigeminal neuralgia secondary to multiple sclerosis. Arch Neurol 39:219–221, 1982.

77. Brinkman CJJ, Nillesen WM, and Hommes OR: The effect of cyclophosphamide on T lymphocytes and T lymphocyte subsets in patients with chronic progressive multiple sclerosis. Acta Neurol Scand 69:90–96, 1984.

78. British and Dutch Multiple Sclerosis Azathioprine Trial Group: Double-masked trial of azathioprine in multiple sclerosis. The Lancet 2:179–183, 1988.

79. Brod SA, and Burns DK: Suppression of relapsing experimental autoimmune encephalomyelitis in the SJL/J mouse by oral administration of type I interferons. Neurology 44:1144–1148, 1994.

79a. Brod SA, Marshall GD, Henninger EM, Sriram S, Khan M, and Wolinsky JS: Interferon-β_{1b} treatment decreases tumor necrosis factor-α and increases interleukin-6 production in multiple sclerosis. Neurology 46:1633–1638, 1996.

80. Brod SA, and Khan M: Oral administration of human or murine type I interferons prevents relapses and adoptive transfer in experimental allergic encephalitis. Paper presented at the 119th Annual Meeting of the American Neurological Association, San Francisco, October 1994. Ann Neurol 36:92, 1994.

81. Broderick JP, and Samaha FJ: Interferon beta treatment of multiple sclerosis (letter). Neurology 44:186, 1994.

82. Brown JR, Beebe GW, Kurtzke JF, Loewenso RB, Silberberg DH, and Tourtellotte WW: The design of clinical studies to assess therapeutic efficacy in multiple sclerosis. Neurology 29:3–23, 1979.

82a. Brunet DG, Hopman WM, Singer MA, Edgar CM, and MacKenzie TA: Measurement of health-related quality of life in multiple sclerosis patients. Can J. Neurol. Sci. 23:99–103, 1996.

83. Buckley C, Kennard C, and Swash M: Treatment of acute exacerbations of multiple sclerosis with intravenous methylprednisolone. J Neurol Neurosurg Psychiatry 45:179–186, 1982.

84. Burnham JA, Wright RR, Driesbach J, and Murray RS: The effect of high-dose steroids on MRI gadolinium enhancement in acute demyelinating lesions. Neurology 41:1349–1354, 1991.

84a. Burt RK, Burns W, and Hess A: Bone marrow transplantation for multiple sclerosis. Bone Marrow Transplant 16:1–6, 1995.

85. Butterworth FM, Ristow GE, and Collarini E: Fluctuation of plasma cortisol levels in multiple sclerosis. Can J Neurol Sci 6:59–63, 1979.

85a. Calabresi PA, Hanham A, Carlino J, et al: Report of an ongoing phase 1 trial of recombinant transforming growth factor-Beta 2 (TGF-β2) in chronic progressive multiple sclerosis. Neurology 45(suppl 4)417:1995.

86. Camenga DL, Johnson KP, Alter M, et al: Systemic recombinant alpha-2 interferon therapy in relapsing multiple sclerosis. Arch Neurol 43:1239–1246, 1986.

87. Campbell B, Vogel PJ, Fisher E, and Lorenz R: Myelin basic protein administration in multiple sclerosis. Arch Neurol 29:10–15, 1973.

88. Canadian MS Research Group: A randomized controlled trial of amantadine in fatigue associated with multiple sclerosis. Can J Neurol Sci 14:273–278, 1987.

89. Capra R, Marcianó N, Mattioli F, et al: Total lymphoid irradiation in chronic progressive multiple sclerosis. Ital J Neurol Sci 13:131–134, 1992.

90. Caroscio JT, Kochwa S, Sacks H, Makuku S, Cohen JA, and Yahr MD: Quantitative cerebrospinal fluid IgG measurements as a marker of disease activity in multiple sclerosis. Arch Neurol 43:1129–1131, 1986.

91. Carter JL, Dawson DM, Hafler DA, et al: Five-year experience with intensive immunosuppression in progressive multiple sclerosis using high-dose IV cyclophosphamide plus ACTH. Neurology 36(suppl 1):284, 1986.

92. Carter JL, Hafler DA, Dawson DM, Orav J, and Weiner HL: Immunosuppression with high-dose IV cyclophosphamide and ACTH in progressive multiple sclerosis: Cumulative 6-year experience in 164 patients. Neurology 38(suppl 2):9–14, 1988.

93. Cavallo R, Durelli L, Ferri R, et al: Chronic high-dose systemic recombinant-alpha-2a-interferon (r-alpha-2a-IFN) in relapsing/remitting (R/R) MS: Clinical and MRI evaluation. Neurology 43:A164, 1993.

93a. Cella DF, Dineen K, Arnason B, et al: Validation of the functional assessment of multiple sclerosis quality of life instrument. Neurology 47:129–139, 1996.

94. Cendrowski WS: Therapeutic trial of imuran (azathioprine) in multiple sclerosis. Acta Neurol Scand 47:254–260, 1971.

95. Cendrowski WS: Combined therapeutic trial in multiple sclerosis: Hydrocortisone hemisuccinate with cyclophosphamide or cytosine arabinoside. Acta Neurol Belg 73:209–219, 1973.

96. Cendrowski WS: Pilot-study on large-dose alternate-day steroid therapy in multiple sclerosis: Comparison of oral corticosteroids verus azathioprine. Schweiz Arch Neurol Neurochir Psychiatr 117:197–203, 1975.

97. Cendrowski WS: Clinical impressions on the treatment of multiple sclerosis with thymus factor. Schweiz Arch Neurology Neurochir Psychiatr 127:199–203, 1980.

98. Cendrowski WS, and Czlonkowska A: Levamisole in multiple sclerosis, with special reference to immunological parameters: A pilot study. Acta Neurol Scand 57:354–359, 1978.

99. Chancellor MB, and Blaivas JG: Diagnostic evaluation of incontinence in patients with neurological disorders. Compr Ther 17:37–43, 1991.

100. Chang YY, Wu HS, Tsai TC, and Liu JS: Intractable hiccup due to multiple sclerosis: MR Imaging of medullary plaque. Can J Neurol Sci 21:271–272, 1994.

101. Chao R, and Clowers DE: Experience with intra-cavernosal tri-mixture for the management of neurogenic erectile dysfunction. Arch Phys Med Rehabil 75:276–278, 1994.

102. Chao R, Mayo ME, Bejany DE, and Bavendam T: Bladder neck closure with continent augmentation of suprapubic catheter in patients with multiple sclerosis. Journal of the American Paraplegia Society 16:18–22, 1993.

103. Chrousos GP, Wilder RL, and Gold PW: The stress response and the regulation of inflammatory disease. Ann Intern Med 117:854–866, 1992.

104. Clark CM, James G, Li DKB, Oger JJF, Paty DW, and Klonoff H: Ventricular size, cognitive function and depression in patients with multiple sclerosis. Can J Neurol Sci 19:352–356, 1992.

105. Clifford DB, and Trotter JL: Pain in multiple sclerosis. Arch Neurol 41:1270–1272, 1984.

105a. Cohen JA, Grossman RI, Udupa JK, et al: Assessment of the efficacy of Copolymer-1 in the treatment of multiple sclerosis by quantitative MRI. Neurology 45 (suppl 4):A418, 1995.

106. Cohen RA, and Fisher M: Amantadine treatment of fatigue associated with multiple sclerosis. Arch Neurol 46:676–678, 1989.

107. Coleman AE, and Norman DJ: OKT3 Encephalopathy. Ann Neurol 28:837–838, 1990.

108. Colins RC, Espinoza LR, Plank CR, Ebers GC, Rosenberg RA, and Zabriskie JB: A double-blind trial of transfer factor vs placebo in multiple sclerosis patients. Clin Exp Immunol 33:1–11, 1978.

108a. Comi G, Filippi M, Martinelli V, et al: Brain MRI correlates of cognitive impairment in primary and secondary progressive multiple sclerosis. J Neurol Sci 132:222–227, 1995.

109. Compston DAS: Lymphocyte subpopulations in patients with multiple sclerosis. J Neurol Neurosurg Psychiatry 46:105–114, 1983.

110. Compston D: Methylprednisolone and multiple sclerosis. Arch Neurol 45:669–670, 1988.

111. Compston DAS: The management of multiple sclerosis. QJM 70:93–101, 1989.

112. Compston DAS: Limiting and repairing the damage in multiple sclerosis. J Neurol Neurosurg Psychiatry 54:945–948, 1991.

113. Compston DAS, Emre M, and UK Tizanidine Study Group: Safety and efficacy of tizanidine in

therapy of spasticity secondary to multiple sclerosis (MS). Neurology 44(suppl 2):A375, 1994.

114. Confavreux C, Compston DAS, Hommes OR, McDonald WI, and Thompson AJ: EDMUS, a European database for multiple sclerosis. J Neurol Neurosurg Psychiatry 55:671–676, 1992.

115. Confavreux C, Mathieu C, Chacornac R, Aimard G, and Devic M: Inefficacité de l'oxygénothérapie hyperbare dans la sclérose en plaques. Essai randomisé contrôlé par placebo en double aveugle. Presse Méd. 15:1319–1322, 1986.

116. Confavreux C, Thivolet C, Ventre JJ, Aimard G, and Devic M: Isoprinosine treatment of multiple sclerosis: 52 cases (letter). Presse Med 15: 2256–2257, 1986.

117. Constantino A, Black SE, and Carr T: Dorsal midbrain syndrome in multiple sclerosis with magnetic resonance imaging correlation. Can J Neurol Sci 13:62–65, 1986.

117a. Cook SD, Bansil S, Boos J, et al: Total lymphoid irradiation (TLI) and low-dose prednisone (LDP) in progressive multiple sclerosis (PMS). Neurology 45 (suppl 4):A417, 1995.

117b. Constantinescu CS, Kamoun M, Dotti M, Farber RE, Galetta SL, and Rostami A: A longitudinal study of the T cell activation marker CD26 in chronic progressive multiple sclerosis. J Neurol Sciences 130:178–182, 1995.

118. Cook SD, Devereux C, Troiano R, et al: Effect of total lymphoid irradiation in chronic progressive multiple sclerosis. The Lancet 1:1405–1409, 1986.

119. Cook SD, Devereux C, Troiano R, et al: The treatment of patients with chronic progressive multiple sclerosis with total lymphoid irradiation. In Cook SD (ed): Handbook of Multiple Sclerosis. Marcel Dekker, New York, 1990, p 403.

120. Cook SD, Devereux C, Troiano R, Rohowsky-Kochan C, Zito G, and Dowling PC: Effect of lymphoid irradiation on clinical course, lymphocyte count, and T-cell subsets in chronic progressive multiple sclerosis. Ann NY Acad Sci 540:533–534, 1988.

121. Cook SD, Devereux C, Troiano R, et al: Total lymphoid irradiation in multiple sclerosis: Blood lymphocytes and clinical course. Ann Neurol 22:634–638, 1987.

122. Cook SD, Troiano R, Rohowsky-Kochin C, et al: Intravenous gamma globulin in progressive MS. Acta Neurol Scand 86:171–175, 1992.

123. Cook SD, Troinano R, Zito G, Rohowsky-Kochan R, Sheffit C, Dowling PC, and Devereux CK: Deaths after total lymphoid irradiation for multiple sclerosis (letter). The Lancet 2:277–278, 1989.

124. Cooper IS: Neurosurgical alleviation of intention tremor of multiple sclerosis and cerebellar disease. N Engl J Med 263:441–444, 1960.

124a. Crockard AD, Treacy MT, Droogan AG, McNeill TA, and Hawkins SA: Transient immunomodulation by intravenous methylprednisolone treatment of multiple sclerosis. Multiple Sclerosis 1:20–24, 1995.

125. Cross AH, and Hart WM Jr: Caveat regarding immunoglobulin therapy in multiple sclerosis (letter and comment). Ann Neurol 33:660, 1993.

126. Curé JK, Cromwell LD, and Case JL: Auditory dysfunction caused by multiple sclerosis: Detection with MR imaging. AJNR 11:817–820, 1990.

127. Currey J, Barton PB, and Dansie O: Danesbury: Changing patterns in the care of the younger disabled over three decades. International Disability Studies 9:41–44, 1987.

128. Currier RD, Haerer AF, and Meydrech EF: Low dose oral methotrexate treatment of multiple sclerosis: A pilot study. J Neurol Neurosurg Psychiatry 56:1217–1218, 1993.

129. Dau PC, Johnson KP, and Spitler LE: The effect of levamisole on cellular multiple sclerosis. Clin Exp Immunol 26:302–309, 1976.

130. Dau PC, Petajan JH, Johnson KP, Panitch HS, and Bornstein MB: Plasmapheresis in multiple sclerosis: Preliminary findings. Neurology 30: 1023–1028, 1980.

130a. Davie CA, Barker GJ, Webb S, et al: Persistent functional deficit in multiple sclerosis and autosomal dominant cerebellar ataxia is associated with axon loss. Brain 118:1583–1592, 1995.

131. Davie CA, Miller DH, Barker GJ, Webb S, Thompson AJ, and McDonald WI: Use of magnetic resonance spectroscopy to investigate disability in multiple sclerosis. Paper presented at the 119th Annual Meeting of the American Neurological Association, San Francisco, October 1994. Ann Neurol 36:301, 1994.

132. Davis FA, Stefoski D, and Rush J: Orally administered 4-aminopyridine improves clinical signs in multiple sclerosis. Ann Neurol 27:186–192, 1990.

132a. Dayal A, Qu ZX, Jensen M, and Arnason BGW: Transretinoic acid reverses induction of interferon-γ-secreting cells by interferon β-1B. Neurology A165, 1996.

132b. Dayal AS, Jensen MA, and Arnason BGW: Changes induced in interferon-γ-secreting cell number and production by class I interferons. Ann Neurol 40:520–521, 1996.

133. De Groen PC, Aksamit AJ, Rakela J, Forbes GS, and Krom RAF: Central nervous system toxicity after liver transplantation: The role of cyclosporine and cholesterol. N Engl J Med 317: 861–866, 1987.

133a. De Stefano N, Matthews PM, Phil D, et al: Chemical pathology of acute demyelinating lesions and its correlation with disability. Ann Neurol 38:901–909, 1995.

134. Debets R, and Savelkoul HFJ: Cytokine antagonists and their potential therapeutic use. Immunol Today 15:455–458, 1994.

135. Deming QB: Interferon beta treatment of multiple sclerosis (letter). Neurology 44:186, 1994.

136. Detels R, Myers LW, Ellison GW, et al: Changes in immune response during relapses in MS patients. Neurology 31:492–495, 1981.

136a. Devinsky O: Outcome research in neurology: Incorporating health-related quality of life. Ann Neurol 37:141–142, 1995.

137. Dewey RB, and Nelson MD: Dangers from methylprednisolone acetate therapy by intraspinal injection. Arch Neurol 45:804, 1988.

138. Dewis M, and Thorton NG: Sexual dysfunction in multiple sclerosis. J Neurosci Nurs 21:175–179, 1989.

139. Dimitriadis G, Ioannidis E, Hatzichristou D, Yannakoyorgos K, and Kalinderis A: Bladder Neuropathy in MS patients: 10 Year follow up. 10th Congress of the European Committee for Treatment and Research in Multiple Sclerosis, Book of Abstracts. Athens, Greece, 1994, p 74.

140. Dohrn M: Pharmakolgie Einiger Pyridinderivate. Arch Exp Pathol Pharmakol 105:10–11, 1924.

141. Dommasch D, Lurati M, Albert E, and Mertens HG: Long-term azathioprine therapy in multiple sclerosis. In Bauer HJ, Poser S, and Ritter G (eds): Progress in Multiple Sclerosis. Springer-Verlag, New York, 1980, pp 381–387.

142. Dore-Duffy P, Donaldson JO, Koff T, Longo M, and Perry W: Prostaglandin release in multiple sclerosis: Correlation with disease activity. Neurology 36:1587–1590, 1986.

143. Douglas RM, Moore BW, and Miles HB: Prophylactic efficacy of intra-nasal alpha2-interferon against rhinovirus infections in the family setting. N Engl J Med 314:65–70, 1986.

144. Dowling PC, Bosch VV, and Cook SD: Possible beneficial effect of high-dose intravenous steroid therapy in acute demyelinating disease and transverse myelitis. Neurology 30:33–36, 1980.

145. Drachman DA, Paterson PY, Schmidt RT, and Spehlmann RF: Cyclophosphamide in exacerbations of multiple sclerosis: Therapeutic trial and a strategy for pilot drug studies. J Neurol Neurosurg Psychiatry 38:592–597, 1975.

146. Duquette P, Pleines J, and du Souich P: Isoniazid for tremor in multiple sclerosis: A controlled trial. Neurology 35:1772–1775, 1985.

146a. Duquette P, Bourgouin PM, Wolfson C, Lapierre Y, Duong HD, and Trudel GC: Spinal cord multiple sclerosis: Detection of lesions with MRI and correlation with neurologic examination. Neurology 46:A368, 1996.

147. Durelli L, Baggio GF, Bergamasco B, et al: Early immunosuppressive effect of parenteral methylprednisolone in the treatment of multiple sclerosis. Acta Neurol (Napoli) 7:338–344, 1985.

148. Durelli L, Bongioanni MR, Cavallo R, et al: Chronic systemic high-dose recombinant interferon alfa-2a reduces exacerbation rate, MRI signs of disease activity, and lymphocyte interferon gamma production in relapsing-remitting multiple sclerosis. Neurology 44:406–413, 1994.

149. Durelli L, Bongioanni MR, Ferrero B, Geuna M, Ferri R, and Aimo G: Chronic effects of high-dose recombinant-alpha-2a-interferon in MS: Cytokine profile and clinical-MRI results during and after treatment. 10th Congress of the European Committee for Treatment and Research in Multiple Sclerosis, Book of Abstracts. 1994, p 25.

149a. Durelli L, Bongioanni MR, Ferrero B, et al: Interferon alpha-2a treatment of relapsing-remitting multiple sclerosis: Disease activity resumes after stopping treatment. Neurology 47:123–129, 1996.

150. Durelli L, Bongioanni MR, Ferri R, et al: Interferon (IFN)-Alpha2A treatment of relapsing/remitting (R\R) multiple sclerosis (MS): Disease activity resumes after stopping treatment. Neurology 44 (suppl 2):A358, 1994.

151. Durelli L, Cocito D, Riccio A, et al: High-dose intravenous methylprednisolone in the treatment of multiple sclerosis: clinical-immunologic correlations. Neurology 36:238–243, 1986.

152. Durelli L, Poccardi G, and Cavallo R: CD8+ high CD11b+ low T cells (T suppressor-effectors) in multiple sclerosis cerebrospinal fluid are increased during high dose corticosteroid treatment. J Neuroimmunol 31:221–228, 1991.

153. Dworkin RH, Bates D, Millar JHD, and Paty DW: Linoleic acid and multiple sclerosis: A reanalysis of three double-blind trials. Neurology 34:1441–1445, 1984.

154. Ebers GC: Multiple sclerosis and other demyelinating diseases. In Asbury A, McKhann G, and McDonald I (eds): Diseases of the Nervous System. WB Saunders, Philadelphia, 1986, pp 1268–1281.

155. Ebers GC: Treatment of multiple sclerosis (review). Lancet 343:275–279, 1994.

156. Ebers GC, Bulman DE, Sadovnick AD, et al: A population-based twin study in multiple sclerosis. N Engl J Med 315:1638–1642, 1986.

157. Ebers GC, and Paty DW: The major histocompatibility complex, the immune system and multiple sclerosis. Clin Neurol Neurosurg 81:69, 1979.

158. Ebers GC, Vinuela FV, Feasby TE, and Bass B: Multifocal CT enhancement in MS. Neurology 34:341–346, 1984.

158a. Edan G, Miller D, Clanet M, et al: Therapeutic effect of mitoxantrone combined with methylprednisolone in multiple sclerosis: A randomised multi-centre study of active disease using MRI and clinical criteria. (in press). J Neurol Neurosurg Psychiatry 62:1997.

159. Edwards MK, Farlow MR, and Stevens JC: Multiple sclerosis: MRI and clinical correlation. AJR 147:571–574, 1986.

160. Ellison GW, Mickey MR, Myers LW, and Rose AS: A pilot study of amantadine treatment of multiple sclerosis. In Bauer HF, Poser S, and Ritter G (eds): Progress in Multiple Sclerosis Research. Springer-Verlag, Berlin, 1980, pp 407–408.

161. Ellison GW, Myers LW, Mickey MR, et al: A placebo-controlled, randomized, double-masked, variable dosage, clinical trial of azathioprine with and without methylprednisolone in multiple sclerosis. Neurology 39:1018–1026, 1989.

162. Farrar M, and Schreiber RD: The molecular cell biology of interferon-γ and its receptor. Annu Rev Immunol 11:571–611, 1993.

163. Faulds D, and Benfield P: Inteferon beta-1b in multiple sclerosis: an initial review of its rationale for use and therapeutic potential. Clinical Immunotherapy 1:79–87, 1994.

163a. Fazekas F, Deisenhammer F, Strasser-Fuchs S, Nahlker G, Mamoli B, The Austrian Immunoglobulin in Multiple Sclerosis Study Group. The Lancet 349:589–593, 1997.

163b. Flagan BG, Rochon J, Fedorak RN, et al: Methotrexate for the treatment of Crohn's Disease N Eng J Med 332:292–297, 1995.

164. Feinstein A, Kartsounis LD, and Miller DH: Clinical isolated lesions of the type seen in multiple sclerosis: A cognitive, psychiatric and MRI

follow-up study. J Neurol Neurosurg Psychiatry 55:869–876, 1992.

165. Fernández O, Antiquédad A, Arbizu T, et al: Treatment of relapsing-remitting multiple sclerosis with natural interferon beta: A multicenter, randomized clinical trial. Multiple Sclerosis 1:67–69, 1995.

166. ffrench-Constant C: Pathogenesis of multiple sclerosis. Lancet 343:271–275, 1994.

166a. Filippi M, Campi A, Martinelli V, et al: A brain MRI study of different types of chronic-progressive multiple sclerosis. Acta Neurol Scand 91:231–233, 1995.

167. Filippi M, Horsfield MA, Bressi S, et al: Intra- and inter-observer agreement of brain MRI lesion volume measurements in multiple sclerosis: A comparison of techniques. 10th Congress of the European Committee for Treatment and Research in Multiple Sclerosis, Book of Abstracts. Athens, Greece, 1994, p 10.

168. Filippi M, Horsfield MA, Morrissey SP, et al: Quantitative brain MRI lesion load predicts the course of clinically isolated syndromes suggestive of multiple sclerosis. Neurology 44:635–641, 1994.

169. Filippi M, Miller DH, Paty DW, et al: Correlations between changes in disability and MRI activity in multiple sclerosis: A two-year follow-up study. Neurology 44 (suppl 2):A339, 1994.

170. Fischer BH, Marks M, and Reich T: Hyperbaric-oxygen treatment of multiple sclerosis: A randomized, placebo-controlled, double-blind study. N Engl J Med 308:181–186, 1983.

171. Fischer JS, Goodkin DE, Rudick RA, et al: Low-dose (7.5 mg) oral methotrexate improves neuropsychological function in patients with chronic progressive multiple sclerosis. 119th Annual Meeting of the American Neurological Association. Ann Neurol 36:54, 1994.

172. Fog T: ACTH therapy of multiple sclerosis. Nord Med 46:1742–1748, 1951.

173. Fog T, and Linnemann F: The course of multiple sclerosis in 73 cases with computer-designed curves. Acta Neurol Scand (suppl) 46:1–175, 1970.

174. Fog T, Raun NE, Mellerup E, Pedersen L, and Kam-Hansen S: Long-term transfer-factor treatment for multiple sclerosis. The Lancet 851–853, 1978.

175. Foley FW: Comprehensive evaluation of outcome of care in multiple sclerosis (special focus issue). Journal of Neurologic Rehabilitation 7:85–182, 1993.

176. Fowler CJ, van Kerrebroeck PE, Nordenbo A, and Van Poppel H: Treatment of lower urinary tract dysfunction in patients with multiple sclerosis. Committee of the European Study Group of SUDIMS (Sexual and Urological Disorders in Multiple Sclerosis). J Neurol Neurosurg Psychiatry 55:986–989, 1992.

177. Francis DA, Bain P, Swan AV, and Hughes RA: An assessment of disability rating scales used in multiple sclerosis. Arch Neurol 48:299–301, 1991.

178. Francis GS, Arnaoutelis R, and Antel JP: Lack of efficiency of IVIG in multiple sclerosis. Neurology 44 (suppl 2):A357, 1994.

178a. Frank JA, Stone LA, Calebresi P, Bash CN, Maloni H, and McFarland HF: Heterogeneous response of MRI characteristics in patients treated with beta interferon 1b. Neurology 46:A480–A481, 1996.

179. Franklin GM, Heaton RK, Nelson LM, Filley CM, and Seibert C: Correlation of neuropsychological and MRI findings in chronic/progressive multiple sclerosis. Neurology 38:1826–1829, 1988.

180. Fredrikson S, Link H, and Eneroth P: CSF neopterin as marker of disease activity in multiple sclerosis. Acta Neurol Scand 75:352–355, 1987.

181. Frequin STF, Barkhof F, Lamers KJB, Hommes OR, and Borm GF: CSF myelin basic protein, IgG and IgM levels in 101 MS patients before and after treatment with high-dose intravenous methylprednisolone. Acta Neurol Scand 86:291, 1992.

182. Frequin STF, Lamers KJB, Barkhof F, Borm GF, and Hommes OR: Follow-up study of MS patients treated with high-dose intravenous methylprednisolone. Acta Neurol Scand 90:105–110, 1994.

183. Frick E, Angstwurm H, Blomer R, and Strauss G: Long-term treatment of multiple sclerosis with azathioprine. In Bauer HJ, Poser S, and Ritter G (eds): Progress in Multiple Sclerosis Research. Springer-Verlag, Berlin, 1980, pp 377–380.

184. Frick E, Angstwurm H und Späth G: Immunosuppressive therapie der multiplen sklerose 1. Vorläufige mitteilung der behandlungsergebnisse mit azathioprin und antilymphozytenglobulin. Münch Med Wochenschir 113:221–231, 1971.

185. Frith JA, McLeod JG, Basten A, et al: Transfer factor as a therapy for multiple sclerosis: A follow-up study. Clinical and Experimental Neurology 22:149–154, 1986.

186. Gallo P, Sivieri S, Rinaldi R, et al: Intrathecal synthesis of interleukin-10 (IL-10) in viral and inflammatory diseases of the central nervous system. J Neurol Sci 126:49–53, 1994.

187. Garabedian-Ruffalo SM, and Ruffalo RL: Adverse effects secondary to baclofen withdrawal. Drug Intelligence and Clinical Pharmacy 19:304–306, 1985.

187a. Gawne-Cain ML, O'Riordan JI, and Miller DH: Could fast FLAIR replace conventional dual spin echo in the MR arm of MS treatment trials: A preliminary sequence comparison. Multiple Sclerosis 2:27–28, 1996.

188. Geny C, Ricolfi F, Degos JD, Cesaro P, and Nguyen JP: Chronic thalamic stimulation for treatment of tremor in multiple sclerosis. Neurology 44(suppl 2):A393, 1994.

189. Giesser B: Evoked potentials as outcome measures in multiple sclerosis. Journal of Neurolic Rehabilitation 7(3–4):99, 1993.

189a. Giovannoni G, Lai M, Thorpe J, et al: Intercellular adhesion molecule-1 correlates with gadolinium enhancement serial magnetic resonance imaging in multiple sclerosis. Neurology 46:A367, 1996.

190. Glaser GH, and Merritt HH: Effects of corticotrophin (ACTH) and cortisone on disorders of the nervous system. JAMA 148:898, 1952.

191. Goas JY, Marion JL, and Missoum A: High dose intravenous methyl prednisolone in acute exacerbations of multiple sclerosis (letter). J Neurol Neurosurg Psychiatry 46:99, 1983.

192. Gold R, Kappos L, and Becker T: Development of multiple sclerosis in patient on long-term sulfasalazine. Lancet 335:409, 1990.

193. Goldberger RF: Bridging the gap between patient and physician: Reflections of a scientist-patient on outcomes in MS. Journal of Neurologic Rehabilitation 7 (3–4):105, 1993.

194. Gonsette RE, Defalque A, and Demonty L: Effects of immunosuppressive agents and particularly of cyclophosphamide on lymphocytes subsets in treated multiple sclerosis patients. Rivista Di Neurologia 57:181–184, 1987.

195. Gonsette RE, Delmotte P, and Demonty L: Failure of basic protein therapy for multiple sclerosis. J Neurol 216:27–31, 1977.

196. Gonsette RE, and Demonty L: Immunosuppression with mitoxantrone in multiple sclerosis: A pilot study for 2 years in 22 patients (abstract). Neurology 40:261, 1990.

197. Gonsette RE, Demonty L, and Delmotte P: Intensive immunosuppression with cyclophosphamide in multiple sclerosis: Follow up of 110 patients for 2–6 years. J Neurol 214:173–181, 1977.

198. Gonsette RE, Demonty L, and Delmotte P: Intensive immunosuppression with cyclophosphamide in remittent forms of multiple sclerosis. A follow-up of 134 patients for 2–10 years. In Bauer HJ, Poser S, and Ritter G (eds): Progress in MS Research. Springer Verlag, New York, 1980, pp 401–406.

199. Gonsette RE, Demonty L, Delmotte P, Decree J, de Cock W, Verhaeghen H, and Symoens J: Modulation of immunity in multiple sclerosis: A double-blind levamisole-placebo controlled study in 85 patients. J Neurol 228:65–72, 1982.

200. Gonzalez CF, Vinitski S, Seshagiri S, Lublin FD, and Knobler RL: Volumetric regional analysis of MS lesions of the brain using 3D segmentation. Neurology 44 (suppl 2):A339, 1994.

201. Goodkin DE, Bailly RC, Teetzen ML, Hertsgaard D, and Beatty WW: The efficacy of azathioprine in relapsing-remitting multiple sclerosis. Neurology 41:20–25, 1991.

202. Goodkin DE, Cookfair D, Wende K, et al: Inter-and intrarater variability for grades 1.0–3.5 of the Kurtzke expanded disability status scale (EDSS). Neurology 41:145, 1992.

203. Goodkin DE, Hertsgaard D, and Seminary J: Upper extremity function in multiple sclerosis: Improving assessment sensitivity with box-and-block and nine-hole peg tests. Arch Phys Med Rehabil 69:850–854, 1988.

204. Goodkin DE, and Kanoti GA: Ethical considerations raised by the approval of interferon beta-1b for the treatment of multiple sclerosis. Neurology 44:166–170, 1994.

204a. Goodkin DE, Kinkel RP, Weinstock-Guttman B, et al: A randomized, double-masked, dose-comparison, Phase II study of bimonthly intravenous methylprednisolone (IVMP) to modify progression of disability in patients with sec-ondary progressive multiple sclerosis (SPMS). Neurology 48:A339, March 1997.

205. Goodkin DE, Plencner S, Palmer-Saxerud J, Teetzen M, and Hertsgaard D: Cyclophosphamide in chronic progressive multiple sclerosis. Maintenance vs non-maintenance therapy. Arch Neurol 44:823–827, 1987.

206. Goodkin DE, Rudick A, VanderBrug-Medendorp S, et al: Low-dose (7.5 mg) oral methotrexate reduces the rate of progression in chronic progressive multiple sclerosis. Ann Neurol 37:30–40, 1995.

206a. Goodkin DE, Rudick RA, Mededorp SVB, Daughtry MM, and Van Dyke C: Low-dose oral methotrexate in chronic progressive multiple sclerosis: Analyses of serial MRIs. Neurology 47:1153–1157, 1996.

207. Goodkin DE, Rudick RA, and Ross JS: The use of brain magnetic resonance imaging in multiple sclerosis. Arch Neurol 51:505–516, 1994.

208. Goodkin DE, Vanderburg-Medendorp S, and Ross J: The effect of repositioning error on serial magnetic resonance imaging scans (letter). Arch Neurol 50:569–571, 1993.

209. Goodman SJ, and Berlin JA: The use of predicted confidence intervals when planning experiments and the misuse of power when interpreting results. Ann Intern Med 121:200–206, 1994.

210. Goodman SJ, and Young RF: Dorsal column stimulation in the treatment of multiple sclerosis. Surgical Forum 29:507–509, 1978.

211. Gordon PA, Carroll DJ, Etches WS, et al: A double-blind controlled pilot study of plasma exchange versus sham apheresis in chronic progressive multiple sclerosis. Can J Neurol Sci 12:39–44, 1985.

212. Gore M, Buckman R, and Stern G: Intrathecal cytarabine in multiple sclerosis. The Lancet 2:204, 1979.

213. Gorman E, Rudd A, and Ebers GC: Giving the diagnosis of multiple sclerosis. In Poser CM (ed): The Diagnosis of Multiple Sclerosis. Thieme-Stratton, N.Y., 1984, pp 216–222.

214. Goust JM, Hogan EL, and Arnaud P: Abnormal regulation of IgG production in multiple sclerosis. Neurology (New York) 32:228–234, 1982.

215. Grant I, McDonald WI, Patterson TL, and Trimble MR: Multiple sclerosis. In Brown GW, and Harris T (eds): Life Events and Illness: Studies of Psychiatric and Physical Disorders. Guilford Press, New York, 1989, pp 295–311.

216. Grossman RI, Lenkinski RE, Ramer KN, Gonzalez-Scarano F, and Cohen JA: MR proton spectroscopy in multiple sclerosis. AJNR 13:1535–1543, 1992.

217. Hafstein MP, Devereux C, Troiano R, et al: Total lymphoid irradiation in chronic progressive multiple sclerosis: A preliminary report. Ann NY Acad Sci 397–409, 1984.

218. Hallett M, Lindsey W, Adelstein BD, and Riley PO: Controlled trial of isoniazid therapy for severe postural cerebellar tremor in multiple sclerosis. Neurology 35:1374–1377, 1985.

219. Hammann KP, and Hopf HC: Determination of interferon-gamma in the peripheral blood of

multiple sclerosis patients in remission, using a chemiluminescence technique. J Neuroimmunol 13:9–18, 1986.

220. Harpur GD, Suke R, Bass BH, et al: Hyperbaric oxygen therapy in chronic stable multiple sclerosis: Double-blind study. Neurology 36:988–991, 1986.

221. Harris JO, Frank JA, Patronas N, McFarlin DE, and McFarland HF: Serial gadolinium-enhanced magnetic resonance imaging scans in patients with early, relapsing-remitting multiple sclerosis: Implications for clinical trials and natural history. Ann Neurol 29:548–555, 1991.

222. Harrison SA, and Wood CA Jr: Hallucinations after preoperative baclofen discontinuation in spinal cord injury patients. Drug Intelligence and Clinical Pharmacy 19:747–749, 1985.

222a. Hartung HP, Reiners K, Archelos JJ, et al: Circulating adhesion molecules and tumor necrosis factor receptor in multiple sclerosis: Correlation with magnetic resonance imaging. Ann Neurol 38:186–193, 1995.

223. Hartung HP, Schafer B, van der Meide PH, Fierz W, Heininger K, and Toyka KV: The role of interferon-gamma in the pathogenesis of experimental autoimmune disease of the peripheral nervous system. Ann Neurol 27:247–257, 1990.

224. Hashmat AI, Abrahams J, Fani K, and Nostrand I: A lethal complication of papaverine-induced priapism. J Urol 145:146–147, 1991.

225. Hatzichristou DG, Basile G, Payton T, Kalinderis A, and Goldstein I: Multiple sclerosis and spinal cord injury patients in pharmacological erection program(PEP): Efficacy and patient satisfaction. 10th Congress of the European Committee for Treatment and Research in Multiple Sclerosis, Book of Abstracts. Athens, Greece, 1994, p 41.

225a. Hauser SL: Tumor necrosis factor: Immunogenetics and disease (editorial). Annals of Neurology. Vol. 38, pg 702–703, 1995.

226. Hauser SL, Bresnan MJ, Reinherz EL, and Weiner HL: Childhood multiple sclerosis: Clinical features and demonstration of changes in T cell subsets with disease activity. Ann Neurol 11:463–468, 1982.

227. Hauser SL, Dawson DM, Lehrich JR, et al: Intensive immunosuppression in progressive multiple sclerosis. A randomized, three-arm study of high-dose intravenous cyclophosphamide, plasma exchange, and ACTH. N Engl J Med 308:173–180, 1983.

228. Hauser SL, Doolittle TH, Lopez-Bresnahan M, et al: An antispasticity effect of threonine in multiple sclerosis. Arch Neurol 49:923–926, 1992.

229. Hauser SL, Fosburg M, Kevy SV, and Weiner HL: Lymphocytapheresis in chronic progressive multiple sclerosis: Immunologic and clinical effects. Neurology 34:922–926, 1984.

230. Hayden FG, Albrecht JK, Kaiser DL, and Gwaltney JM Jr: Prevention of natural colds by contact prophylaxis with intranasal alpha-interferon. N Engl J Med 314:71–75, 1986.

231. Health and Human Services News. US Dept of Health and Human Services, Washington, DC, 1983, publication P-93–31.

232. Heller L, Keren O, Aloni R, and Davidoff G: An open trial of vacuum penile tumescence: Constriction therapy for neurological impotence. Paraplegia 30:550–553, 1992.

233. Henderson JS: Intermittent clean self-catheterization in clients with neurogenic bladder resulting from multiple sclerosis. J Neurosci Nurs 21:160–164, 1989.

234. Henderson WR Jr: The role of leukotrienes in inflammation. Ann Intern Med 121:684–697, 1994.

235. Herishanu YO, Badarna S, Sarov B, Abarbanel JM, Segal S, and Bearman JE: A possible harmful late effect of methylprednisolone therapy on a time cluster of optic neuritis. Acta Neurol Scand 80:569–574, 1989.

236. Herndon RM, and Murray TJ: Multiple Sclerosis: Proceedings of the International Conference on Therapeutic Trials in Multiple Sclerosis-Grand Island, NY. Arch Neurol 40(special issue):663–710, 1992.

237. Herroelen L, de Keyser J, and Ebinger G: Central-nervous-system demyelination after immunization with recombinant hepatitis B vaccine. Lancet 338:1174–1175, 1991.

238. Hilton P, Hertogs K, and Stanton SL: The use of desmopressin (DDAVP) for nocturia in women with multiple sclerosis. J Neurol Neurosurg Psychiatry 46:854–855, 1983.

239. Hinds JP, and Wald A: Colonic and anorectal dysfunction associated with multiple sclerosis (review). Am J Gastroenterol 84:587–595, 1989.

240. Hirsch RL, Johnson KP, and Camenga DL: The placebo effect during a double blind trial of recombinant alpha2 interferon in multiple sclerosis patients: Immunological and clinical findings. Int J Neurosci 39:189–196, 1988.

241. Ho SY, Catalanotto FA, Lisak RP, and Dore-Duffy P: Zinc in multiple sclerosis. II. Correlation with disease activity and elevated plasma membrane-bound zinc in erythrocytes from patients with multiple sclerosis. Ann Neurol 20:712–715, 1986.

241a. Hohol MJ, Orav EJ, and Weiner HL: Disease steps in multiple sclerosis: A simple approach to evaluate disease progression. Neurology 45: 251–255, 1995.

241b. Hohlfeld R, and Lucas K: Cytokine networks in multiple sclerosis. Neurology 45 (suppl 6):S1–S55, 1995.

242. Hohlfeld R, Michels M, Heininger K, Besinger U, and Toyka KV: Azathioprine toxicity during long-term immunosuppression of generalized myasthenia gravis. Neurology 38:258–261, 1988.

243. Hommes OR, Lamers KJB, and Reekers P: Effect of intensive immunosuppression on the course of chronic progressive multiple sclerosis. J Neurol 223:177–190, 1980.

244. Hommes OR, Prick JJG, and Lamers KJB: Treatment of the chronic progressive form of multiple sclerosis with a combination of cyclophosphamide and prednisone. Clin Neurol Neurosurg 78:59–72, 1975.

245. Honer WG, Hurwitz T, Li DK, Palmer M, and Paty DW: Temporal lobe involvement in multiple sclerosis patients with psychiatric disorders. Arch Neurol 44:187–190, 1987.

246. Hoogstraten MC, Cats A, and Minderhoud JM: Bed rest and ACTH in the treatment of exacerbations in multiple sclerosis patients. Acta Neurol Scand 76:346–350, 1987.

247. Hoogstraten MC, van der Ploeg RJ, v.d. Burg W, Vreeling A, Van MS, and Minderhoud JM: Tizanidine versus baclofen in the treatment of spasticity in multiple sclerosis patients. Acta Neurol Scand 77:224–230, 1988.

248. Hook CC, Kimmel DW, Kvols LK, et al: Multifocal inflammatory leukoencephalopathy with 5-fluorouracil and levamisole. Ann Neurol 31:262–267, 1992.

249. Huber M, Bamborschke S, Assheuer J, and Heib WD: Intravenous natural beta interferon treatment of chronic exacerbating-remitting multiple sclerosis: Clinical response and MRI/CSF findings. J Neurol 235:171–173, 1988.

250. Huddlestone JR, and Oldstone MBA: T suppressor (Tg) lymphocytes fluctuate in parallel with changes in the clinical course of patients with multiple sclerosis. J Immunol 123:4, 1979.

251. Hugenholtz H, Nelson RF, and Dehoux E: Intrathecal baclofen: The importance of catheter position. Can J Neurol Sci 20:165–167, 1993.

252. Hugenholtz H, Nelson RF, Dehoux E, and Bickerton R: Intrathecal baclofen for intractable spinal spasticity: Double-blind cross-over comparison with placebo in 6 patients. Can J Neurol Sci 19:188–195, 1992.

252a. Hutchinson J, and Hutchinson M: The functional limitations profile may be a valid, reliable and sensitive measure of disability in multiple sclerosis. J Neurol 242:650–657, 1995.

253. Huynh HK, and Dorovini-Zis KA: Effects of interferon-γ on primary cultures of human brain microvessel endothelial cells. Am J Pathol 142:1265–1278, 1993.

253a. Huynh HK, Oger J, and Dorovini-Zis K: Interferon-β downregulates interferon-γ-induced class II MHC molecule expression and morphological changes in primary cultures of human brain microvessel endothelial cells. Journal of Neuroimmunology 60:63–73, 1995.

254. IFNB Multiple Sclerosis Study Group: Interferon beta-1b is effective in relapsing-remitting multiple sclerosis. I. Clinical results of a multicenter, randomized, double-blind, placebo-controlled trial. Neurology 43:655–661, 1993.

255. IFNB Multiple Sclerosis Study Group: Treatment of MS with interferon beta-1b—final clinical results of the betaseron trial. IVth International Congress of Neuroimmunology, the Netherlands, October 1994. J Immunol 54:178, 1994.

256. The IFNB Multiple Sclerosis Study Group and the University of British Columbia MS/MRI Analysis Group: Interferon beta-1b in the treatment of multiple sclerosis: Final outcome of the randomized controlled trial. Neurology 45:1277–1285, 1995.

256a. The IFNB Multiple Sclerosis Study Group and the University of British Columbia MS/MRI Analysis Group: Neutralizing antibodies during treatment of multiple sclerosis with interferon beta-1b: Experience during the first three years. Neurology 47:889–894, 1996.

257. Isaac C, Li DKB, Genton M, et al: Multiple sclerosis: A serial study using MRI in relapsing patients. Neurology 38:1511–1515, 1988.

258. Izquierdo G, Campoy F Jr, Mir J: Memory and learning disturbances in multiple sclerosis. MRI lesions and neuropsychological correlation. Eur J Radiol 13:220–224, 1991.

258a. Izumo S, Goto I, Itoyama Y, et al: Interferon-alpha is effective in HTLV-I-associated myelopathy: A multicenter, randomized, double-blind, controlled trial. Neurology 46:1016–1021, 1996.

259. Jackson EF, Narayana PA, Wolinsky JS, and Doyle TJ: Accuracy and reproducibility in volumetric analysis of multiple sclerosis lesions. J Comput Assist Tomogr 17:200–205, 1993.

260. Jacobs LD, Cookfair DL, Rudick RA, et al: Intramuscular interferon beta-1a for disease progression in relapsing multiple sclerosis. Ann Neurol 39:285–294, 1996.

261. Jacobs L, Herndon R, Freeman A, et al: Multicentre double-blind study of effect of intrathecally administered natural human fibroblast interferon on exacerbations of multiple sclerosis. The Lancet 2(8521–8522):1411–1413, 1986.

262. Jacobs L, O'Malley J, Freeman A, and Ekes R: Intrathecal interferon reduces exacerbations of multiple sclerosis. Science 214:1026–1028, 1981.

263. Jacobs L, O'Malley JA, Freeman A, Ekes R, and Reese PA: Intrathecal interferon in the treatment of multiple sclerosis: Patient follow-up. Arch Neurol 42:841–847, 1985.

264. Jacobs L, O'Malley J, Freeman A, Murawski J, and Ekes R: Intrathecal interferon in multiple sclerosis. Arch Neurol 39:609–615, 1982.

265. Jacobs L, O'alley JA, Freeman A, and Reese PA: Intrathecal interferon as treatment of multiple sclerosis: A planned multicenter study. Arch Neurol 40:683–686, 1983.

266. Jacobs L, Salazar AM, Herndon R, et al: Intrathecally administered natural human fibroblast interferon reduces exacerbations of multiple sclerosis: Results of a multicenter, double-blinded study. Arch Neurol 44:589–595, 1987.

267. Jacobson S, and McFarland HF: Measles virus persistence in human lymphocytes: A role for virus-induced interferon. J Gen Virol 63:351–357, 1982.

267a. Jansen HML, Willemsen ATM, Sinnige LGF, et al: Cobalt-55 positron emission tomography in relapsing-progressive multiple sclerosis. J Neurol Sci 132:139–145, 1995.

267b. Johnson KP, Brooks BR, Cohen JA, et al: Copolymer 1 reduces relapse rate and improves disability in relapsing-remitting multiple sclerosis: Results of a phase III multicenter, double-blind, placebo-controlled trial. Neurology 45:1268–1276, 1995.

268. Johnson KP, and Panitch HS: Interferon therapy for multiple sclerosis. Md Med J 41:601–603, 1992.

269. Johnson KP, and the Copolymer I Multiple Sclerosis Treatment Group: Copolymer I: Positive results from a phase III trial in relapsing-remitting multiple sclerosis. 119th Annual Meeting of

the American Neurological Association, San Francisco, 1994. Ann Neurol 36:23, 1994.

270. Kaji R, Happel L, and Sumner AJ: Effect of digitalis on clinical symptoms and conduction variables in patients with multiple sclerosis. Ann Neurol 28:582–584, 1990.

271. Kalb RC, La Rocca NG, and Kaplan SR: Sexuality. In Scheinberg LC, and Holland NJ (eds): A Guide for Patients and Their Families. Raven Press, New York, 1987.

272. Kapoor R, Brown P, Thompson PD, and Miller DH: Propriospinal myoclonus in multiple sclerosis. J Neurol Neurosurg Psychiatry 55:1086–1088, 1992.

273. Kappos L, Gold R, and Künstler E, et al: Mitoxantrone (Mx) in the treatment of rapidly progressive MS: A pilot study with serial gadolinium (Gd)-enhanced MRI (abstract). Neurology 40(supp 1):261, 1990.

274. Kappos L, Heun R, and Mertens HG: A 10-year matched-pairs study comparing azathioprine and no immunosuppression in multiple sclerosis. Eur Arch Psychiatry Neurol Sci 240:34–38, 1990.

275. Kappos L, Patzold U, Dommasch D, et al: Cyclosporine versus azathioprine in the long-term treatment of multiple sclerosis: Results of the German multicenter study. Ann Neurol 23:56–63, 1988.

276. Kappos L, Radü EW, Haas J, Hartard CH, and Hartung HP: European multicenter trial deoxyspergualine (DSG) versus placebo: Results of the first interim analysis. J Neurol 241(suppl 1):S27, 1994.

277. Kappos L, Städt D, Keil W, Ratzka M, Heitzer T, and Schneiderbanger-Grygier S: An attempt to quantify magnetic resonance imaging in multiple sclerosis: Correlation with clinical parameters. Neurosurg Rev 10:133–135, 1987.

278. Kappos L, Städt D, Ratzka M, Keil W, et al: Magnetic resonance imaging in the evaluation of treatment in multiple sclerosis. Neuroradiology 30:299–302, 1988.

279. Karlik SJ, Noseworthy J, Gilbert JJ, St. Louis J, and Strejan G: Nuclear magnetic resonance (NMR) spectroscopy studies in experimental allergic encephalomyelitis (EAE). Proceedings of the Society of Magnetic Resonance in Medicine, Scientific Program Third Annual Meeting. Academic Press, San Diego, 1984, p 399.

279a. Karussis DM, Lehmann D, Slavin S, et al: Inhibition of acute, experimental autoimmune encephalomyelitis by the synthetic immunomodulator linomide. Ann Neurol 34:654–660, 1993.

279b. Karussis DM, Lehmann D, Slavin S, et al: Immunomodulation of autoimmunity by linomide. Israel J Med Sci 31:38–41, 1995.

279c. Karussis D, Meiner Z, Lehmann, et al: Treatment of secondary progressive multiple sclerosis with the immunomodulator linomide: results of a double-blind placebo-controlled study with monthly MRI evaluation. Neurology 45(suppl 4):A417, April 1995.

280. Karussis D, Meiner Z, Lehmann D, et al: A novel therapeutic approach for multiple sclerosis, through immunomodulation with linomide: Preliminary results of the Israeli linomide, double-blind placebo controlled study in secondary progressive MS with monthly MRI evaluation. 10th Congress of the European Committee for Treatment and Research in Multiple Sclerosis, Book of Abstracts. Athens, Greece, 1994, p 27.

280a. Karussis DM, Meiner Z, Lehmann D, et al: Treatment of secondary progressive multiple sclerosis with the immunomodulator linomide: A double-blind, placebo-controlled pilot study with monthly magnetic resonance imaging evaluation. Neurology 47:341–346, 1996.

281. Kassirer JP: Clinical trials and meta-analysis. N Engl J Med 327:273–274, 1992.

282. Kastrukoff LF, Hashimoto SA, Oger JJF, et al: A study of namalwa interferon in patients with chronic progressive multiple sclerosis: Clinical and magnetic resonance imaging results. Ann Neurol 22:154, 1987.

283. Kastrukoff LF, McLean DR, and McPherson TA: Multiple sclerosis treated with antithymocyte globulin: A five year follow-up. Can J Neurol Sci 5:175–178, 1978.

284. Kastrukoff LF, Morgan NG, Aziz TM, Zecchini D, Berkowitz J, and Paty DW: Natural killer (NK) cells in chronic progressive multiple sclerosis patients treated with lymphoblastoid interferon. J Neuroimmunol 20:15–23, 1988.

285. Kastrukoff LF, Oger JJ, Hashimoto SA, et al: Systemic lymphoblastoid interferon therapy in chronic progressive multiple sclerosis. I. Clinical and MRI evaluation. Neurology 40:479–486, 1990.

286. Kastrukoff LF, Oger JJF, Tourtellotte WW, Sacks SL, Berkowitz J, and Paty DW: Systemic lymphoblastoid interferon therapy in chronic progressive multiple sclerosis. II. Immunologic evaluation. Neurology 41:1936–1941, 1991.

287. Kastrukoff LF, and Paty DW: A serial study of peripheral blood T lymphocyte subsets in relapsing-remitting multiple sclerosis. Ann Neurol 15:250–256, 1984.

288. Kato H, Ogino T, and Minami A: Steroid-induced avascular necrosis of the capitate: A case report. Handchir Mikrochir Plast Chir 23:15–17, 1991.

289. Katz D, Taubenberger JK, Cannella B, McFarlin DE, Raine CS, and McFarland HF: Correlation between magnetic resonance imaging findings and lesion development in chronic, active multiple sclerosis. Ann Neurol 34:661–669, 1993.

289a. Keenan PA, Jacobson MW, Soleymani RM, Mayes MD, Stress ME, and Yaldoo DT: The effect on memory of chronic prednisone treatment in patients with systemic disease. Neurology 47:1396–1402, 1996.

290. Kelly RE, Ellison GW, Myers LW, Goymerac V, Larrick SB, and Kelley CC: Abnormal regulation of in vitro IgG production in multiple sclerosis. Ann Neurol 9:267–272, 1981.

291. Kelly RE, and Jellinek EH: Treatment of multiple sclerosis with corticotrophin. Lancet 2:1258, 1961.

292. Kermode AG, Tofts PS, Thompson AJ, et al: Heterogeneity of blood-brain barrier changes in

multiple sclerosis: An MRI study with gadolinium-DTPA enhancement. Neurology 40:229–235, 1990.

293. Kesselring J, Miller DH, MacManus DG, et al: Quantitative magnetic resonance imaging in multiple sclerosis: The effect of high dose intravenous methylprednisolone. J Neurol Neurosurg Psychiatry 52:14–17, 1989.

294. Ketelaer P, and Battaglia MA: Rehabilitation in Multiple Sclerosis (RIMS). Proceedings of the 1st European Workshop, Associazione Italiana Sclerosi Multipla, Milano, 1991.

295. Khan OA: Treatment of paroxysmal symptoms in multiple sclerosis with Ibuprofen. Neurology 44:571–572, 1994.

295a. Khan OA, Xia Q, Bever Jr. CT, Johnson KP, Panitch HS, and Dhib-Jalbut SS: Interferon beta-1b serum levels in multiple sclerosis patients following subcutaneous administration. Neurology 46:1639–1643, 1996.

296. Khatri BO: Experience with use of plasmapheresis in chronic progressive multiple sclerosis: The pros. Neurology 38:50–52, 1988.

297. Khatri BO, Koethe SM, and McQuillen MP: Plasmapheresis with immunosuppressive drug therapy in progressive multiple sclerosis: A pilot study. Arch Neurol 41:734–738, 1984.

298. Khatri BO, McQuillen MP, Harrington GJ, Schmoll D, and Hoffmann RG: Chronic progressive multiple sclerosis: Double-blind controlled study of plasmapheresis in patients taking immunosuppressive drugs. Neurology 35:312–319, 1985.

299. Khatri BO, McQuillen MP, Hoffmann RG, Harrington GJ, and Schmoll D: Plasma exchange in chronic progressive multiple sclerosis: A long-term study. Neurology 41:409–414, 1991.

299a. Khoury SJ, Guttmann CRG, Orav EJ, et al: Longitudinal MRI in multiple sclerosis: Correlation between disability and lesion burden. Neurology 44:2120–2124, 1994.

299b. Khoury SJ, Guttmann CRG, Orav EJ, et al: Correlation between changes in lymphocyte populations and disease activity in multiple sclerosis. Neurology 46:A367–A368, 1996.

300. Kibler RF: Large dose corticosteroid therapy of experimental and human demyelinating diseases. NY Acad Sci 122:469–479, 1965.

301. Kibler RF, Paty DW, Re PK, McPhedran AM, and Karp HR: Effect of large doses of adrenocorticosteroids on the course of EAE and multiple sclerosis. In Wolfgram F, Ellison GW, Stevens JG, and Andrews DM (eds): Multiple Sclerosis. Immunology, Virology and Ultra Structure. Academic Press, New York, pp 511–529, 1972.

302. Kidd D, Thompson AJ, Kendall BE, Miller DH, and McDonald WI: Benign form of multiple sclerosis: MRI evidence for less frequent and less inflammatory disease activity. J Neurol Neurosurg Psychiatry 57:1070–1072, 1994.

302a. Kidd D, Thorpe JW, Kendall BE, et al: MRI dynamics of brain and spinal cord in progressive multiple sclerosis. J Neurol Neurosurg Psychiatry 60:15–19, 1996.

303. Kidd D, Thorpe JW, Thompson AJ, et al: Spinal cord MRI using multi-array coils and fast spin echo. II. Findings in multiple sclerosis. Neurology 43:2632–2637, 1993.

304. Killian JM, Bressler RB, Armstrong RM, and Huston DP: Controlled pilot trial of monthly intravenous cyclophosphamide in multiple sclerosis. Arch Neurol 45:27–30, 1988.

305. Kinkel RP, and Rudick RA: Rapid neurologic decline in an MS patient treated with systemic interleukin 2 (IL-2) and interferon alpha (INF-alpha 2b). Neurology 44 (suppl 2):A392, 1994.

306. Kinn AC, and Larsson PO: Desmopressin: A new principle for symptomatic treatment of urgency and incontinence in patients with multiple sclerosis. Scand J Urol Nephrol 24:109–112, 1990.

307. Kinnunen E, Timonen TP, Pirttilä T, et al: Effects of recombinant α-2b-interferon therapy in patients with progressive MS. Acta Neurologica Scandinavica 87:457–460, 1993.

308. Kinnunen E, and Wikstrom J: Prevalence and prognosis of epilepsy in patients with multiple sclerosis. Epilepsia 27:729–733, 1986.

309. Kirk P, and Compston DAS: The effect of methylprednisolone on lymphocyte phenotype and function in patients with multiple sclerosis. J Neuroimmunol 26:1–8, 1990.

310. Klapper JA: Interferon beta treatment in multiple sclerosis (letter). Neurology 44:188, 1994.

311. Knobler RL, Greenstein JI, Johnson KP, et al: Systemic recombinant human interferon-beta treatment of relapsing-remitting multiple sclerosis: Pilot study analysis and six-year follow-up. Journal of Interferon Research 13:333–340, 1993.

312. Knobler RL, Panitch HS, Braheny SL, et al: Systemic alpha-interferon therapy of multiple sclerosis. Neurology 34:1273–1279, 1984.

313. Kocsis JD, Bowe CM, and Waxman SG: Different effects of 4-aminopyridine on sensory and motor fibers: Pathogenesis of paresthesias. Neurology 36:117–120, 1986.

314. Kofler M, and Leis AA: Prolonged seizure activity after baclofen withdrawal. Neurology 42:697–698, 1991.

315. Kondziolka D, Lunsford DL, and Bissonette DJ: Long-term results after glycerol rhizotomy for multiple sclerosis-related trigeminal neuralgia. Can J Neurol Sci 21:137–140, 1994.

316. Koopmans RA, Li DKB, Oger JJF, et al: Chronic progressive multiple sclerosis: Serial magnetic resonance brain imaging over six months. Ann Neurol 26:248–256, 1989.

317. Koopmans RA, Li DKB, Grochowski E, Cutler PJ, and Paty DW: Benign versus chronic progressive multiple sclerosis: Magnetic resonance imaging features. Ann Neurol 25:74–81, 1989.

318. Koopmans RA, Li DKB, Oger JJF, Mayo J, and Paty DW: The lesion of multiple sclerosis: Imaging of acute and chronic stages. Neurology 39:959–963, 1989.

319. Koopmans RA, Li DKB, Redekop WK, et al: The use of magnetic resonance imaging in monitoring interferon therapy of multiple sclerosis. American Society of Neuroimaging 3:163–168, 1993.

320. Koopmans RA, Li DKB, Zhao GJ, Allen PS, Penn A, and Paty DW: Magnetic resonance spec-

troscopy of multiple sclerosis: In-vivo detection of myelin breakdown products (letter). The Lancet 341:631–632, 1993.

321. Koopmans RA, Li DKB, Zhao GJ, Redekop WK, and Paty DW: MRI assessment of cyclosporine therapy of MS in a multi-center trial. Neurology 42(suppl 3):210, 1992.

322. Koopmans RA, Zhao GJ, Paty DW, and Li DKB: Lesion activity assessment by yearly serial MRI in monitoring a therapeutic trial interferon beta in the treatment of relapsing and remitting MS. Neurology 44(suppl 2):A392, 1994.

323. Kornhuber HH, and Schütz A: Efficient treatment of neurogenic bladder disorders in multiple sclerosis with initial intermittent catheterization and ultrasound-controlled training. Eur Neurol 30:260–267, 1990.

323a. Krapf H, Mauch E, Fetzer U, Laufen H, and Kornhuber HH: Serial gadolinium-enhanced magnetic resonance imaging in patients with multiple sclerosis treated with mitoxantrone. Neuroradiology 37:113–119, 1995.

324. Kroin JS, Bianchi GD, and Penn RD: Intrathecal baclofen down-regulates GABAb receptors in the rat substantia gelatinosa. J Neurosurg 79:544–549, 1993.

324a. Krupp LB, Coyle PK, Doscher C, et al: Fatigue therapy in multiple sclerosis: Results of a double-blind, randomized, parallel trial of amantadine, pemoline, and placebo. Neurology 45:1956–1961, 1995.

325. Kupersmith MJ, Kaufman DO, Paty DW, et al: Megadose corticosteroids in multiple sclerosis. Neurology 44:1–4, 1994.

326. Kurtzke JF: A new scale for evaluating disability in multiple sclerosis. Neurology 5:580–583, 1955.

327. Kurtzke JF: On the evaluation of disability in multiple sclerosis. Neurology 11:686–694, 1961.

328. Kurtzke JF: Neurologic impairment in multiple sclerosis and the disability status scale. Acta Neurol Scand 46:493–512, 1970.

329. Kurtzke JF: Rating neurologic impairment in multiple sclerosis: An expanded disability status scale (EDSS). Neurology 33:1444–1452, 1983.

330. Kurtzke JF: Neuroepidemiology. II: Assessment of Therapeutic Trials. Ann Neurol 19:311–319, 1986.

331. Kurtzke JF: The Disability Status Scale for multiple sclerosis: Apologia pro DSS sua. Neurology 39:291–302, 1989.

332. Kurtzke JF: Clinical definition for multiple sclerosis treatment trials. Ann Neurol 36 (suppl):373–379, 1994.

333. Kurtzke JF, Beebe GW, Nagler B, Nefzger MD, Auth TL, and Kurland LT: Studies on the natural history of multiple sclerosis. V. Long-term survival in young men. Arch Neurol 22:215–225, 1970.

334. Kuzma JW, Namerow NS, Tourtellotte WW, et al: An assessment of the reliability of three methods used in evaluating the status of multiple sclerosis patients. Journal of Chronic Diseases 21:803–814, 1969.

334a. La Mantia L, Eoli M, Milanese C, Salmaggi A, Dufour A, and Torri V: Double-blind trial of dexamethasone versus methylprednisolone in

multiple sclerosis acute relapses (abstract). Eur Neurol 34:199–203, 1994.

335. Lamoureux G, Cosgrove J, Duquette P, Lapierre Y, Jolicoeur R, and Vanderland F: A clinical and immunological study of the effects of transfer factor on multiple sclerosis patients. Clin Exp Immunol 43:557–564, 1981.

336. Lance EM, Kremer M, Abbosh J, Jones VE, Knight S, and Medawar PB: Intensive immunosuppression in patients with disseminated sclerosis. I. Clinical response. Clin Exp Immunol 21:1–12, 1975.

336a. Langdon D, and Thompson AJ: Predicting outcome of neuro-rehabilitation in multiple sclerosis. Multiple Sclerosis 2:33, 1996.

337. Lapides J, Diokno AC, Lowe BS, and Kalish MD: Follow up on unsterile, intermittent self-catheterization. J Urol 3:184–187, 1974.

338. Lapides J, Diokno AC, Silber SJ, and Lowe BS: Clean, intermittent self-catheterization in the treatment of urinary tract disease. J Urol 107:458–461, 1972.

339. LaRocca NG, Kalb RC, Foley FW, and Caruso LS: Assessment of psychosocial outcomes in multiple sclerosis. Journal of Neurologic Rehabilitation 7(3–4):109, 1993.

340. LaRocca NG, Scheinberg LC, Slater RJ, et al: Field testing of a minimal record of disability in multiple sclerosis: The United States and Canada. Acta Neurologica Scandinavica Supplementum 101:126–138, 1984.

340a. Leppert D, Waubant E, Oksenberg J, and Hauser SL: Interferon-β inhibits gelatinase production and basement membrane transmigration of human T cells. Neurology 46:A165–A166, 1996.

341. Leventhal LJ, Boyce EG, and Zurier RB: Treatment of rheumatoid arthritis with gammalinolenic acid. Ann Intern Med 119:867–874, 1993.

342. Levine RA, Gardner JC, Fullerton BC, Stufflebeam SM, Furst M, and Rosen BR: Multiple sclerosis lesions of the auditory pons are not silent. Brain 117:1127–1141, 1994.

343. Lhermitte F, Marteau R, and de Saxe H: Traitement des formes graves de sclerose en plaques par le serum antilymphocytaire: Resultats d'une etude pilote de 50 malades suivis 4 ans. Rev Neurol (Paris) 135:389–400, 1979.

344. Lhermitte F, Marteau R, and de Saxe H: Treatment of progressive and severe forms of multiple sclerosis using a combination of antilymphocyte serum, azathioprine and prednisone: Clinical and biological results–Comparison with a control group treated with azathioprine and prednisone only. 4-year follow-up. Rev Neurol (Paris) 143:98–107, 1987.

345. Lhermitte F, Marteau R, and Roullet E: Not so benign long-term immunosuppression in multiple sclerosis (letter)? Lancet 1:276–277, 1984.

346. Lhermitte F, Marteau R, Roullet E, de Saxcé H, and Loridan M: [Prolonged treatment of multiple sclerosis with average doses of azathioprine. An evaluation of 15 years' experience]. Rev Neurol (Paris) 140:553–558, 1984.

347. Lhermitte F, Roullet E, Lyon-Caen, O, et al: Double-blind treatment of 49 cases of chronic multiple sclerosis using hyperbaric oxygen. Rev Neurol (Paris) 142:201–206, 1986.

348. Likosky WH, Fireman B, Elmore R, et al: Intense immunosuppression in chronic progressive multiple sclerosis: The Kaiser study. J Neurol Neurosurg Psychiatry 54:1055–1060, 1991.

349. Likosky WH, Starr-Schneidkraut NJ, and Wilson S: Coping with MS effectively: A proactive psychosocial intervention for patients with multiple sclerosis. Neurology 44 (suppl 2):A393, 1994.

350. Lindsey JW, Hodgkinson S, Mehta R, et al: Phase 1 clinical trial of chimeric monoclonal anti-CD4 antibody in multiple sclerosis. Neurology 44: 413–419, 1994.

351. Longstreth WT, and Franklin GM: Interferon beta treatment of multiple sclerosis (letter). Neurology 44:186–187, 1994.

351a. Loseff NA, Kingsley DPE, McDonald WI, Miller DH, and Thompson AJ: Clinical and magnetic resonance imaging predictors of disability in primary and secondary progressive multiple sclerosis. Multiple Sclerosis 1:218–222, 1996.

351b. Losseff NA, Wang L, Lai M, et al: A serial MRI study of cerebral atrophy in multiple sclerosis. Multiple Sclerosis 2:29, 1996.

351c. Losseff NA, McDonald WI, Miller DH, and Thompson AJ: Spinal cord atrophy in multiple sclerosis: A new reproducible and sensitive MRI technique to monitor disease progression. Multiple Sclerosis 2:28–29, 1996.

352. Lubetzki C, Thuillier Y, Galli A, Lyon-Caen O, Lhermitte F, and Zalc B: Galactosylceramide: A reliable serum index of demyelination in multiple sclerosis. Ann Neurol 26:407–409, 1989.

353. Lubic LG: Interferon beta treatment of multiple sclerosis (letter). Neurology 44(1):186, 1994.

353a. Lublin FD, Whitaker JN, Eidelman BH, Miller AE, Arnason BGW, and Burks JS: Management of patients receiving interferon beta-1b for multiple sclerosis: Report of a consensus conference. Neurology 45:12–18, 1996.

354. Lundberg PO: Sexual dysfunction in female patients with multiple sclerosis. International Rehabilitation Medicine 3:32–34, 1984.

355. Lyons MJ, Amador R, Petito C, Nagashima K, Weinreb H, and Zabriskie JB: Inhibition of acute experimental allergic encephalomyelitis in mice by colchincine. J Exp Med 164:1803, 1986.

356. Lyons PR, Newman PK, and Saunders M: Methylprednisolone therapy in multiple sclerosis: A profile of adverse effects. J Neurol Neurosurg Psychiatry 51:285–287, 1988.

357. MacFadyen DJ, Reeve CE, Bratty PJA, and Thomas JW: Failure of antilymphocytic globulin therapy in chronic progressive multiple sclerosis. Neurology 23:592–598, 1973.

358. MacKay AL, Whittall KP, Cover KS, Li DK, and Paty DW: In vivo T2 relaxation measurements of brain may provide myelin concentration. Society of Magnetic Resonance in Medicine, 10th Annual Meeting, Vol I. San Francisco, Book of Abstracts. August 1991, p 917.

359. Madigand M, Oger J-F, Fauchet R, Sabouraud O, and Genetet B: HLA profiles in multiple sclerosis suggest two forms of disease and the existence of protective haplotypes. J Neurol Sci 53:519–529, 1982.

360. Mai J, Sorensen PS, and Hansen JC: High dose antioxidant supplementation to MS patients. Effects on glutathione peroxidase, clinical safety, and absorption of selenium. Biological Trace Element Research 24:109–117, 1990.

361. Maida E, Hocker P, and Mann E: Long-term lymphocytapheresis therapy in multiple sclerosis: Preliminary observations. Eur Neurol 25:225–232, 1986.

362. Mammi S, Filippi M, Campi A, et al: A quantitative brain MRI study in different types of chronic-progressive multiple sclerosis patients. Neurology 44(suppl 2):A391, 1994.

362a. Mancardi GL, Sardanelli F, Parodi RC, et al: The effect of copolymer 1 on serial gadolinium-enhanced magnetic resonance scans in relapsing multiple sclerosis. Ann Neurol 40:521, 1996.

363. Mankin HJ: Nontraumatic necrosis of bone (osteonecrosis). N Engl J Med 326:1473–1479, 1992.

364. Mann U, Staedt D, Kappos L, Wense AV, and Haubitz I: Correlation of MRI findings and neuropsychological results in patients with multiple sclerosis. Psychiatry Res 29:293–294, 1989.

365. Markovitz D: Interferon beta treatment of multiple sclerosis (letter). Neurology 44:1994.

365a. Marshall GD, Henninger E, Khan M, Wolinsky J, and Brod S: Interferon-β-1b treatment of relapsing-remitting multiple sclerosis decreases CD3-mediated tumor necrosis factors-α and increases CD3-mediated interleukin-6 production ex vivo. Neurology 46:A136, 1996.

366. Marteau R: Treatment of multiple sclerosis (recent concepts) [in French]. Rev Méd Liège 27:543–546, 1972.

367. Martinez-Maza O, Moody DJ, Rezai AR, et al: Increased spontaneous immunoglobulin secretion associated with cyclophosphamide-induced immune suppression. J Clin Immunol 7:107–113, 1987.

368. Martino G, Clementi E, Brambilla E, et al: A new γ-interferon-activated Ca²+ channel in T-lymphocytes from patients with multiple sclerosis. Neurology 44(suppl 2):A146, 1994.

369. Massacesi L, Siracusa G, Gran B, Raimondi L, Pirisino A, and Amaducci L: Safety of 13-cis retinoic acid in the treatment of chronic progressive multiple sclerosis: Pilot clinical study. 10th Congress of the European Committee for Treatment and Research in Multiple Sclerosis, Book of Abstracts. Athens, Greece, 1994, p 28.

370. Massaro AR, Cioffi RP, Laudisio A, Schiavino D, and Mariani M: Four year double-blind controlled study of levamisole in multiple sclerosis. Ital J Neurol Sci 11:595–599, 1990.

371. Massaro AR, Scivoletto G, Rumi C, Laudisio A, and Tonali P: Four year follow-up of multiple sclerosis (MS) patients treated with alpha-2A interferon. 10th Congress of the European Committee for Treatment and Research in Multiple

Sclerosis, Book of Abstracts. Athens, Greece, 1994, p 24.

372. Massey EW, and Pleet AB: Penile prosthesis for impotence in multiple sclerosis. Ann Neurol 6:451–453, 1979.

373. Matias-Guiu J, Sanz M, Gili J, Molins A, and Bonaventura ICA: Correlation of MRI with the clinical status of patients with multiple sclerosis (letter). Neurology 36:1626, 1986.

373a. Mattson D, Petrie M, Srivastava DK, McDermott M: Multiple sclerosis: Sexual dysfunction and its response to medications. Arch Neurol 52:862–868, 1995.

373b. Mattson D, and Guthikonda P: Interferon-β-1b decreases induced nitric oxide production by a human astrocytoma cell line. Ann Neurol 40:515, 1996.

374. Mauch E, Kornhuber HH, Pfrommer U, Hähnel A, Laufen H, and Krapf H: Effective treatment of chronically progressive multiple sclerosis with low-dose cyclophosphamide with minor side-effects. European Archives of Psychiatry and Neurological Sciences 238:115–117, 1989.

374a. McLaurin J, Antel JP, and Yong VW: Immune and non-immune actions of interferon-β-1b on primary human neural cells. Multiple Sclerosis 1:10–19, 1995.

375. McDonald MA, and McDonald CM: Interferon beta treatment of multiple sclerosis (letter). Neurology 44:187, 1994.

376. McDonald WI, and Barnes D: Lessons from magnetic resonance imaging in multiple sclerosis. Trends Neurosci 12:376–379, 1989.

377. McDonald WI, Miller DH, and Barnes D: The pathological evolution of multiple sclerosis. Neuropathol Appl Neurobiol 18:319–334, 1992.

378. McDonald WI, Miller DH, and Thompson AJ: Are magnetic resonance findings predictive of clinical outcome in therapeutic trials in multiple sclerosis? The dilemma of interferon-β. Ann Neurol 36:14–18, 1994.

379. Meador KJ, Loring DW, Hugh K, Gallagher BB, and King DW: Comparative cognitive effects of anticonvulsants. Neurology 40:391–394, 1990.

380. Medaer R, Eeckhout C, Gautama K, and Vermijlen C: Lymphocytapheresis therapy in multiple sclerosis: A preliminary study. Acta Neurol Scand 69:111–115, 1984.

380a. Medical memo dated April 10, 1997, MS Society of Canada.

381. Mehta PD, Kulczycki J, Patrick BA, Sobczyk W, and Wisniewski HM: Effect of treatment on oligoclonal IgG bands and intrathecal IgG synthesis in sequential cerebrospinal fluid and serum from patients with subacute sclerosing panencephalitis. J Neurol Sci 109:64–68, 1992.

382. Meneghetti G, Spartà S, Rusca F, Facco E, Martini A, Comacchio F, and Schiraldi C: Hyperbaric oxygen therapy in the treatment of multiple sclerosis. A clinical and electrophysiological study in a 2 year follow-up. Rivista Di Neurologia 60:67–71, 1990.

383. Meritt HH, Glaser GH, and Herrmann C: A study of the short and long-term effects of

384. Mertin J, Knight SC, Rudge P, Thompson EJ, and Healy MJR: Double-blind, controlled trial of immunosuppression in treatment of multiple sclerosis. The Lancet 2:949–951, 1980.

385. Mertin J, Rudge P, Kremer M, et al: Double-blind controlled trial of immunosuppression in the treatment of multiple sclerosis: Final report. Lancet 2:351–354, 1982.

386. Metz L, Bell R, and Zochodne D: Interferon beta treatment of multiple sclerosis (letter). Neurology 44:187–188, 1994.

387. Meyers CA, Scheibel RS, and Forman AD: Persistent neurotoxicity of systemically administered interferon-alpha. Neurology 41:672–676, 1991.

388. Mickey MR, Ellison GW, and Myers LW: An illness severity score for multiple sclerosis. Neurology 34:1343–1347, 1984.

389. Milanese C, La Mantia L, Salmaggi A, et al: Double-blind randomized trial of ACTH versus dexamethasone versus methylprednisolone in multiple sclerosis bouts: Clinical, cerebrospinal fluid and neurophysiological results. European Neurology 29:10–14, 1989.

390. Milanese C, Salmaggi A, La Mantia L, et al: Double blind study of intrathecal beta-interferon in multiple sclerosis: Clinical and laboratory results. J Neurol Neurosurg Psychiatry 53:554–557, 1990.

391. Milanese C, Salmaggi A, La Mantia L, Corridore F, and Nespolo A: Intrathecal beta-interferon in multiple sclerosis (letter). Lancet 2:563–564, 1988.

392. Millar JHD, Noronha MJ, Liversedge LA, and Rawson MD: Long-term treatment of multiple sclerosis with corticotrophin. Lancet 2:429–431, 1967.

393. Millar JHD, Rahman R, Vas CJ, Noronha MJ, Liversedge LA, and Swinburn WR: Effect of withdrawal of corticotrophin in patients on long-term treatment for multiple sclerosis. Lancet 700–701, 1970.

394. Millar JHD, Zilkha KJ, Langman MJS, Wright HP, Smith AD, Belin J, and Thompson RHS: Double-blind trial of linoleate supplementation of the diet in multiple sclerosis. BMJ 1:765–768, 1973.

395. Miller A, Borenstein M, Slagle S, et al: Clinical trial of Cop 1 in chronic progressive multiple sclerosis. Neurology 39(suppl 1):356, 1989.

396. Miller A, Lanir N, Revel M, Honigman S, Kinarty A, and Lahat N: Diverse modulation of HLA and ICAM-1 expression on human microvessel endothelial cells by IFN-β ad interacting cytokines, implications for multiple sclerosis. 10th Congress of the European Committee for Treatment and Research in Multiple Sclerosis, Book of Abstracts. Athens, Greece, 1994, p 31.

397. Miller A, Lanir N, Revel M, Honigmann S, Kinarty A, and Lahat N: Immunoregulatory effects of recombinant human interferon-β on human microvessel endothelial cells: Interactions with IFN-γ. Paper presented at the 119th Annual Meeting of the American Neurological Associa-

tion, San Francisco, October 1994. Ann Neurol 36:290, 1994.

398. Miller DH: Magnetic resonance in monitoring the treatment of multiple sclerosis. Ann Neurol 36(suppl):S91–S94, 1994.

398a. Miller DH, Albert PS, Barkhof F, et al: Guidelines for the use of magnetic resonance techniques in monitoring the treatment of multiple sclerosis. Ann Neurol 39:6–16, 1996.

399. Miller DH, Barkhof F, Berry I, Kappos L, Scotti G, and Thompson AJ: Magnetic resonance imaging in monitoring the treatment of multiple sclerosis: Concerted action guidelines. J Neurol Neurosurg Psychiatry 54:683–688, 1991.

400. Miller DH, Gass A, Thompson AJ, and McDonald WI: Correlation of clinical disability with magnetization transfer ratio (MTR) imaging in multiple sclerosis. Neurology 44 (suppl 2):A339, 1994.

400a. Miller DH, Lai HM, Moseley IF, et al: A comparison and methods for measuring MRI disease activity in multiple sclerosis. Neurology 46:A366, 1996.

401. Miller DH, Rudge P, Johnson G, et al: Serial gadolinium enhanced magnetic resonance imaging in multiple sclerosis. Brain 111:927–939, 1988.

402. Miller DH, Thompson AJ, Morrissey SP, et al: High dose steroids in acute relapses of multiple sclerosis: MRI evidence for a possible mechanism of therapeutic effect. J Neurol Neurosurg Psychiatry 55:450–453, 1992.

403. Miller HG, Forester JB, Newell DJ, Barwick DD, and Brewis RAL: Multiple sclerosis: therapeutic trials of chloroquine, soluble aspirin and gamma globulin. BMJ 5370:1436–1439, 1963.

404. Miller HG, and Gibbons JL: Acute disseminated encephalomyelitis and acute disseminated sclerosis: Results of treatment with ACTH. BMJ 2:1345–1349, 1953.

405. Miller HG, Newell DJ, and Ridley A: Multiple sclerosis. Trials of maintenance treatment with prednisolone and soluble aspirin. Lancet 1:127–129, 1961(b).

406. Miller HG, Newell DJ, and Ridley A: Treatment of multiple sclerosis with corticotrophin (ACTH). Lancet 2:1361–1362, 1961.

407. Miller HG, Newell DJ, Ridley A, and Schapira K: Therapeutic trials in multiple sclerosis: Preliminary report on effects of intrathecal injection of tuberculin (P.P.D.). J Neurol Neurosurg Psychiatry 24:118–120, 1961.

407a. Milligan NM, Miller DH, and Compston DAS: A placebo-controlled trial of isoprinosine in patients with multiple sclerosis. J Neurol Neurosurg Psychiatry 57:164–168, 1994.

408. Milligan NM, Newcombe R, and Compston DAS: A double-blind controlled trial of high dose methylprednisolone in patients with multiple sclerosis. I. Clinical effects. J Neurol Neurosurg Psychiatry 50:511–516, 1987.

409. Milo R, and Panitch H: Additive effects of COP-1 and IFN-Beta on immune responses to myelin basic protein. Neurology 44 (suppl 2):A212, 1994.

410. Minden SL: Psychotherapy for people with multiple sclerosis. J Neuropsychiatry Clin Neurosci 4:198–213, 1992.

411. Minden SL, Orav J, and Reich P: Depression in multiple sclerosis. Gen Hosp Psychiatry 9:426–434, 1987.

412. Minden SL, Orav J, and Schildkraut JJ: Hypomanic reactions to ACTH and prednisone treatment for multiple sclerosis. Neurology 38:1631–1634, 1988.

413. Minderhoud JM, Leemkius JG, Kremer J, Laban E, and Smits PML: Sexual disturbances arising from multiple sclerosis. Acta Neurol Scand 70:299–306, 1984.

414. Minderhoud JM, Mooyaart EL, Kamman RL, et al: In vivo phosphorus magnetic resonance spectroscopy in multiple sclerosis. Arch Neurol 49:161–165, 1992.

415. Minderhoud JM, Prange AJA, and Luyckx GJ: A long-term double-blind controlled study on the effect of azathioprine in the treatment of multiple sclerosis. Clin Neurol Neurosurg 90:25–28, 1988.

416. Mion F, Napoleon B, Berger F, Chevallier M, Bonvoisin S, and Descos L: Azathioprine induced liver disease: nodular regenerative hyperplasia of the liver and perivenous fibrosis in a patient treated for multiple sclerosis. Gut 32:715–717, 1991.

417. Mochizuki A, Hamanouchi H, and Murata M: Medullary lesion revealed by MRI in a case of MS with respiratory arrest. Neuroradiology 30:574–576, 1988.

418. Montalban J, Fernandez AL, Duran I, Tintor M, Galan I, and Acarin N: Antiganglioside antibodies in sera of MS patients (abstract). J Neurol 241(suppl 1):S73, 1994.

419. Mora JS, Munsat TL, and Kao KP: Intrathecal administration of natural human interferon alpha in amyotrophic lateral sclerosis. Neurology 36:1986.

419a. Moreau T, Coles A, Wing M, et al: Transient increase in symptoms associated with cytokine release in patients with multiple sclerosis. Brain 119:225–237, 1996.

420. Moreau T, Thorpe J, Miller D, et al: Preliminary evidence from magnetic resonance imaging for reduction in disease activity after lymphocyte depletion in multiple sclerosis. 10th Congress of the European Committee for Treatment and Research in Multiple Sclerosis, Book of Abstracts. Athens, Greece, 1994, p 45.

421. Moreau T, Wing M, Waldmann H, and Compston A: Cytokine release increases symptoms in patients with multiple sclerosis. 10th Congress of the European Committee for Treatment and Research in Multiple Sclerosis, Book of Abstracts. Athens, Greece, 1994, p. 26.

422. Morimoto C, Hafler DA, Weiner HL, et al: Selective loss of the suppressor-inducer T-cell subset in progressive multiple sclerosis: Analysis with anti-2H4 monoclonal antibody. N Engl J Med 316:67–72, 1987.

423. Morris RE: Rapamycin: FK506's fraternal twin or distant cousin? Immunol Today 12:137–140, 1991.

424. Morrissey SP, Miller DH, Kendall BE, et al: The significance of brain magnetic resonance imaging abnormalities at presentation with clinically isolated syndromes suggestive of multiple sclerosis: A 5-year follow-up study. Brain 116(pt 1):135–146, 1993.

425. Moulin DE: Pain in multiple sclerosis. Neurol Clin 7:321–331, 1989.

426. Multiple Sclerosis Study Group: Efficacy and toxicity of cyclosporine in chronic progressive multiple sclerosis: A randomized, double-blinded, placebo-controlled clinical trial. Ann Neurol 27:591–605, 1990.

427. Murray TJ: Amantadine therapy for fatigue in multiple sclerosis. Can J Neurol Sci 12:251–254, 1985.

428. Myers LW: Therapy of multiple sclerosis. Current Opinion in Neurology and Neurosurgery 3:208–212, 1990.

429. Myers LW, and Ellison GW: The peculiar difficulties of therapeutic trials for multiple sclerosis. Neurologic Clinics 8:119–141, 1990.

430. Myers LW, Ellison GW, Levy J, Holevoet MI, MA BI, and Tourtellotte WW: Evaluation of levamisole as a treatment for multiple sclerosis (abstract). Neurology 4(suppl 1)27:363, 1977.

431. Myers LW, Ellison GW, Lucia M, Novom S, Holevoet MI, and Madden D: Swine influenza virus vaccination in patients with multiple sclerosis. J Infect Dis 136(suppl):546–554, 1977.

432. Myers LW, Ellison GW, Nuwer MR, Packwood JW, Craig SL, and Leake BD: A preliminary clinical trial of chlorambucil and prednisone in multiple sclerosis (abstract). Ann Neurol 30: 271, 1991.

433. Myers LW, Fahey JL, Moody DJ, Mickey MR, Frane MV, and Ellison GW: Cyclophosphamide 'pulses' in chronic progressive multiple sclerosis: A preliminary clinical trial. Arch Neurol 44:828–832, 1987.

434. Naida E, and Schwaighofer B: Long-term therapy with high-dose IV immunoglobulins in MS clinical and MRI observations. 10th Congress of the European Committee for Treatment and Research in Multiple Sclerosis, Book of Abstracts. Athens, Greece, 1994.

434a. Nance P, Schryvers O, Schmidt B, Dubo H, Loveridge B, and Fewer D: Intrathecal baclofen therapy for adults with spinal spasticity: Therapeutic efficacy and effect on hospital admissions. Can J Neurol. Sci. 22:22–29, 1995.

435. National Multiple Sclerosis Society: Clinical Trials of New Agents in MS: Planned, in Progress, Recently Completed. Research and Medical Program Department, NMSS, New York, 1994.

436. National Multiple Sclerosis Society: Experimental drugs hold promise. Research Highlights (newsletter). NMSS, New York, 1994.

437. Nauta JJ, Thompson AJ, Barkhof F, and Miller DH: Magnetic resonance imaging in monitoring the treatment of multiple sclerosis patients: Statistical power of parallel-groups and cross-over designs. J Neurol Sci 122:6–14, 1994.

437a. Navikas V, He B, Linkn J, et al: Augmented expression of tumour necrosis factor-a and lymphotoxin in mononuclear cells in multiple sclerosis and optic neuritis. Brain 119:213–223, 1995.

437b. Neilley LK, Goodin DS, Goodkin DE, and Hauser SL: Side effect profile of interferon beta-1b in MS: Results of an open label trial. Neurology 46:552–554, 1996.

438. Nelson DA: Dangers from methylprednisolone acetate therapy by interspinal injection. Arch Neurol 45:804, 1988.

439. Nelson DA, Vates TS Jr, and Thomas RB Jr: Complications from intrathecal steroid therapy in patients with multiple sclerosis. Acta Neurol Scand 49:176–188, 1973.

440. Neubauer RA: Exposure of multiple sclerosis patients to hyperbaric oxygen at 1.5–2 ATA: A preliminary report. J Fla Med Assoc 67:498, 1980.

441. Neumann JW, and Ziegler DK: Therapeutic trial of immunosuppressive agents in multiple sclerosis. Neurology 22:1268–1271, 1972.

442. Newman PK, Saunders M, and Tilley PJB: Methylprednisolone therapy in multiple sclerosis. J Neurol Neurosurg Psychiatry 45:941, 1982.

443. Nieves J, Cosman F, Herbert J, Shen V, and Lindsay R: High prevalence of vitamin D deficiency and reduced bone mass in multiple sclerosis. Neurology 44:1994.

444. Niewodniczy A, and Pózniak-Patewicz E: Negative results following use of indomethacin in treatment of multiple sclerosis. Neurol Neurochir Pol 7:291, 1973.

445. Nordenbo AM, and Zeeberg I: An 8 years follow-up study of transfer factor treatment on the course of multiple sclerosis. In Hommes OR (ed): Multiple Sclerosis Research in Europe. MTP Press, Lancaster, 1986, pp 81–83.

446. Noronha A, Toscas A, and Jensen MA: Contrasting effects of alpha, beta and gamma interferons on nonspecific suppressor function in multiple sclerosis. Ann Neurol 31:103–106, 1992.

447. Nos C, Montalban X, Rovira A, Tintore M, Rio J, and Codina A: Blood brain barrier changes after IVIG treatment. 10th Congress of the European Committee for Treatment and Research in Multiple Sclerosis, Book of Abstracts. Athens, Greece, 1994, p 39.

448. Noseworthy JH: Concordance between examining neurologists on multiple sclerosis disability scales in a blinded, prospective clinical trial. Neurology 38:195, 1988.

449. Noseworthy JH: The Canadian cooperative trial of cyclophosphamide and plasma exchange in progressive multiple sclerosis. The Lancet 337: 441–446, 1991.

450. Noseworthy JH, Ebers GC, and Roberts R: Cyclophosphamide and MS (letter). Neurology 44:579–581, 1994.

451. Noseworthy JH, Ebers GC, Vandervoort MK, Farquhar RE, Yetisir E, and Roberts R: The impact of blinding on the results of a randomized, placebo-controlled multiple sclerosis clinical trial. Neurology 44:16–20, 1994.

452. Noseworthy JH, Hopkins MB, Vandervoort MK, et al: An open-trial evaluation of mitoxantrone in the treatment of progressive MS. Neurology 43:1401–1406, 1993.

453. Noseworthy JH, Lee D, Penman M, et al: A phase II evaluation of mitoxantrone HCI in the treatment of progressive multiple sclerosis. Neurology 41:146, 1991.

454. Noseworthy JH, O'Brien PC, Naessens JM, and the Mayo Clinic-Canadian Cooperative MS Study Group: Outcome measures in randomized, placebo-controlled, double-blind multiple sclerosis clinical trial. Neurology 44 (suppl 2):A392, 1994.

455. Noseworthy JH, Rodriguez M, An KN, et al: IVIg treatment in multiple sclerosis: Pilot study results and design of a placebo-controlled, double-blind clinical trial. Paper presented at the 119th Annual Meeting of the American Neurological Association, San Francisco, October 1994. Ann Neurol 36:325, 1994.

456. Noseworthy JH, Rodriguez M, Weinshenker BG, et al: The assessment of muscle strength in an MS clinical trial. 10th Congress of the European Committee for Treatment and Research in Multiple Sclerosis, Book of Abstracts. Athens, Greece, 1994.

457. Noseworthy JH, Seland TP, and Ebers GC: Therapeutic trials in multiple sclerosis. Can J Neurol Sci 11:355–362, 1984.

458. Noseworthy JH, Vandervoort MK, Ebers GC, and the Canadian Cooperative Multiple Sclerosis Study Group: Acceptance of placebo-controlled trial design by progressive multiple sclerosis patients. Neurology 39:606–607, 1989.

459. Noseworthy JH, Vandervoort MK, Hopkins M, and Ebers GC: A referendum on clinical trial research in multiple sclerosis: The opinion of the participants at the Jekyll Island Workshop. Neurology 39:977–981, 1989.

460. Noseworthy JH, Vandervoort MK, Penman M, et al: Cyclophosphamide and plasma exchange in multiple sclerosis (letters to the editor). The Lancet 337:1540–1541, 1991.

461. Noseworthy JH, Vandervoort MK, Wong CJ, and Ebers GC: Interrater variability with the Expanded Disability Status Scale (EDSS) and Functional Systems (FS) in a multiple sclerosis clinical trial: The Canadian Cooperation MS Study Group. Neurology 40:971–975, 1990.

461a. Noseworthy JH, O'Brien PC, and the Mayo Clinic-Canadian Cooperative MS Study Group: The Mayo Clinic-Canadian Cooperative Study of Sulfasalazine (Salazopyrin EN) in active multiple sclerosis: Preliminary report. Neurology 48:A340, March 1997.

462. Nuwer MR, Packwood JW, Myers LW, and Ellison GW: Evoked potentials predict the clinical changes in a multiple sclerosis drug study. Neurology 37:1754–1761, 1987.

463. Ochs G, Struppler A, Meyerson BA, et al: Intrathecal baclofen for long-term treatment of spasticity: A multicenter study. J Neurol Neurosurg Psychiatry 52:933–939, 1989.

464. Oger J-F, Antel JP, Han Hwa Kuo BS, and Arnason BGW: Influence of azathioprine (Imuran) on in vitro immune function in multiple sclerosis. Ann Neurol 11:177–181, 1982.

465. Oger J, Willoughby E, and Paty D: Serial studies of relapsing multiple sclerosis: Reduced IgG secretion in vitro and reduced suppressor cell function correlate with disease activity as recognized by magnetic resonance imaging. Ann Neurol 22:152, 1987.

465a. Oger JJF, Vorobeychick G, Al-Fahim A, Aziz T, Edan G and Paty D: Neutralizing antibodies in Betaseron-treated MS patients and in vitro immune function before treatment. Neurology 48: A80, March 1997.

466. Okada S, Kinoshita M, Fujioka T, and Yoshimura M: Two cases of multiple sclerosis with painful tonic seizures and dysesthesia ameliorated by the administration of mexiletine. Jpn J Med 30:373–375, 1991.

467. O'Keeffe F, Stanton H, Woods R, and Kirrane S: T helper/suppressor ratio and acute attacks in multiple sclerosis. Ir Med J 77:39–41, 1984.

468. O'Looney PA, and Reingold SC: Report on the use of the immunosuppressive drug cyclophosphamide (Cytoxan) for progressive multiple sclerosis. Research and Medical Programs Department News, National Multiple Sclerosis Society, New York, 1993.

469. Olsson T, Wei Zhi W, Hojeberg B, Yu-Ping J, Anderson G, Ekre HP, and Link H: Autoreactive T lymphocytes in multiple sclerosis determined by antigen-induced secretion of interferon-γ. J Clin Invest 86:981–985, 1990.

470. O'Riordan JI, Doherty C, Javed M, Brophy D, Hutchinson M, and Quinlan D: Indoramin for lower urinary tract dysfunction in multiple sclerosis. 10th Congress of the European Committee for Treatment and Research in Multiple Sclerosis, Book of Abstracts. Athens, Greece, 1994, p 73.

470a. O'Riordan JI, McDonald WI, and Miller DH: The predictive value of MRI in clinically isolated syndromes suggestive of demyelination. Multiple Sclerosis 2:29, 1996.

471. Ormerod IE, Miller DH, McDonald WI, et al: The role of NMR imaging in the assessment of multiple sclerosis and isolated neurological lesions. Brain 110:1579–1616, 1987.

472. Pachner AR: Interferon beta treatment of multiple sclerosis (letter). Neurology 44(1):188, 1994.

473. Panitch HS: Systemic alpha-interferon in multiple sclerosis: Long-term patient follow-up. Arch Neurol 44:61–63, 1987.

474. Panitch HS: Interferons in multiple sclerosis. A review of the evidence. Drugs 44:946–962, 1992.

474a. Panitch HS: Investigational drug therapies for treatment of multiple sclerosis. Multiple Sclerosis 2:66–77, 1996.

475. Panitch HS, Francis GS, Hooper CJ, Merigan TC, and Johnson KP: Serial immunological studies in multiple sclerosis patients treated systemically with human alpha interferon. Ann Neurol 18:434–438, 1985(b).

476. Panitch HS, Haley AS, Hirsch RL, and Johnson KP: Exacerbations of multiple sclerosis in patients treated with gamma interferon. The Lancet 893–894, 1987.

477. Panitch HS, Hirsch RL, Schindler J, and Johnson KP: Treatment of multiple sclerosis with

gamma interferon: Exacerbations associated with activation of the immune system. Neurology 37:1097–1102, 1987.

478. Panitch HS, Katz E, and Johnson KP: Effects of beta interferon treatment on viral infections and relapses of multiple sclerosis. Neurology 44 (suppl 2):A358, 1994.

479. Panzer VP, Smith ME, Martin R, et al: Functional evaluation of clinical status in multiple sclerosis. Annals of Neurology. Seattle, Washington, Vol 30, 1991, p 271.

480. Papiha SS, Boddy J, Roberts D, and Bates D: PHA-induced interferon in multiple sclerosis: association between gamma interferon and clinical and genetical variables. Acta Neurol Scand 80:145–150, 1989.

481. Papo T, Marcellin P, Bernuau J, Durand F, Poynard T, and Benhamou JP: Autoimmune chronic hepatitis exacerbated by alpha-interferon. Ann Intern Med 116:51–53, 1992.

482. Paschalidou M, Tsounis S, Barba V, Heliopoulos I, Milonas I, and Constas C: Effect of clonazepam on ataxia and tremor in multiple sclerosis. 10th Congress of the European Committee for Treatment and Research in Multiple Sclerosis, Book of Abstracts. Athens, Greece, 1994, p 87.

483. Paty DW: Multiple sclerosis: Assessment of disease progression and effects of treatment. Can J Neurol Sci 14:518–520, 1987.

484. Paty DW: Magnetic resonance imaging in the assessment of disease activity in multiple sclerosis. Can J Neurol Sci 15:266–272, 1988.

485. Paty DW: Trial measures in multiple sclerosis: The use of magnetic resonance imaging in the evaluation of clinical trials. Neurology 38:82–83, 1988.

486. Paty DW, Bergstrom J, Palmer M, MacFadyen J, and Li DKB: A quantitative magnetic resonance image of the multiple sclerosis brain. Neurology 35(suppl 1):137, 1985.

487. Paty DW, Cousin HK, Read S, and Adlakha K: Linoleic acid in multiple sclerosis: Failure to show any therapeutic benefit. Acta Neurol Scand 58:53–58, 1978.

488. Paty DW, Ebers GC, and Wonnacott TH: Prognostic markers in multiple sclerosis. 12th World Congress of Neurology, International Congress Series, Vol 548. Excerpta Medica. Hamburg, Germany, 1981, p 56.

488a. Paty DW, Goodkin D, Thompson A, and Rice G: Guidelines for physicians with patients on IFNβ-1b: The use of an assay for neutralizing antibodies (NAB). Neurology 47:865–866, 1996.

489. Paty DW, and Kastrukoff LF: Suppressor T Cells in MS: Do changes in numbers vary with clinical activity? Ann NY Acad Sci 436:227–266, 1984.

490. Paty DW, Kastrukoff L, Morgan N, and Hiob L: Suppressor T-lymphocytes in multiple sclerosis: Analysis of patients with acute relapsing and chronic progressive disease. Ann Neurol 14:445–449, 1983.

491. Paty DW, Koopmans RA, Li DKB, and Oger JJF: Magnetic resonance imaging (MRI) as an outcome measure in multiple sclerosis. Journal of Neurologic Rehabilitation 7(3–4):117, 1993.

491a. Paty DW, Koopmans RA, Redekop WK, Oger JJF, Kastrukoff LF, and Li DKB: Does the MRI activ-

ity rate predict the clinical course of MS? Neurology 42 (suppl 3):427, 1992.

492. Paty DW, and Li DKB, UBC MS/MRI Study Group, and the IFNB Multiple Sclerosis Study Group: Interferon beta-1b is effective in relapsing-remitting multiple sclerosis. II. MRI analysis results of a multicenter, randomized, double-blind, placebo-controlled trial. Neurology 43: 662–667, 1993.

493. Paty DW, Li DKB, and Koopmans RA: Matters arising: MRI in monitoring the treatment of multiple sclerosis: Concerted action guidelines. J Neurol Neurosurg Psychiatry 55:978, 1992.

494. Patzold U, Haller P, Haas J, Pocklington P, and Deicher H: Therapie der multiplen sklerose mit Levamisol und Azathioprin. Nervenarzt 49:285–294, 1978.

495. Patzold U, Hecker H, and Pocklington P: Azathioprine in treatment of multiple sclerosis. J Neurol Sci 54:377–394, 1982.

496. Patzold U, and Pocklington P: Azathioprine in multiple sclerosis: A 3-year controlled study of its effectiveness. J Neurol 223:97–117, 1980.

496a. Pavol MA, Meyers CA, Rexer JL, Valentine AD, Mattis PJ, and Talpaz M: Pattern of neurobehavioral deficits associated with interferon alpha therapy for leukemia. Neurology 45:947–950, 1995.

497. Penn RD: Intrathecal baclofen for spasticity of spinal origin: Seven years of experience. J Neurosurg 77:236–240, 1992.

498. Penn RD, and Kroin JS: Long-term intrathecal baclofen infusion for treatment of spasticity. J Neurosurg 66:181–185, 1987.

499. Penn RD, Savoy M, Corcos D, et al: Intrathecal baclofen for severe spinal spasticity. N Engl J Med 320:1517–1521, 1989.

499a. Petajan JH, Gappmaier E, White AT, Spencer MK, Mino L, and Hicks RW: Impact of aerobic training on fitness and quality of life in multiple sclerosis. Ann Neurol 39:432–441, 1996.

500. Peterson K, Rosenblum MK, Powers JM, Alvord E, Walker RW, and Posner JB: Effect of brain irradiation on demyelinating lesions. Neurology 43:2105–2112, 1993.

501. Plaut GS: Effectiveness of amantadine in reducing relapses in multiple sclerosis. J R Soc Med 80:91, 1987.

502. Pliskin NH, Towle VL, Hamer DP, et al: The effects of interferon-beta on cognitive function in multiple sclerosis. Ann Neurol 36:326, 1994.

502a. Pliskin NH, Hamer DP, Goldstein DS, et al: Improved delayed visual reproduction test performance in MS patients receiving interferon β-1b. Neurology 47:1463–1468, 1996.

502b. Polman CH: Interferon beta-1b in multiple sclerosis — a seminar-in-print. Clinical Immunotherapeutics 5 (suppl 1): 1–58, 1996.

503. Polman CH, Bertelsmann FW, van Loenen AC, and Koetsier JC: 4-aminopyridine in the treatment of patients with multiple sclerosis: Long-term efficacy and safety. Arch Neurol 51:292–296, 1994.

504. Polman CH, Smits R, Bertelsmann F, van Loenen A, Emmen H, and Kulig B: The effects of 4-aminopyridine on cognitive function of MS patients. Neurology 44 (suppl 2):A374, 1994.

505. Polman CH, van Diemen HA, van Dongen MM, Koetsier JC, van Loenen AC, and van Walbeek HK: 4-Aminopyridine in multiple sclerosis (letter and comment). Ann Neurol 28:589, 1990.

506. Poser S: Management of patients with multiple sclerosis. In Koetsier JC (ed): Handbook of Clinical Neurology. Demyelinating Diseases. Vol. 47. Elsevier, 1985, p 147.

507. Potvin AR, Tourtellotte WW, Syndulko K, and Potvin J: Quantitative methods in assessment of neurologic function. Critical Reviews in Bioengineering 6:177–224, 1981.

507a. Pozzilli C, Bastianello S, Koudriavtseva T, et al: Magnetic resonance imaging changes with recombinant human interferon-β-1a: a short term study in relapsing-remitting multiple sclerosis. J Neurol Neurosurg Psychiatry 61:251–258, 1996.

508. Pozzilli C, Fieschi C, Perani D, et al: Relationship between corpus callosum atrophy and cerebral metabolic asymmetries in multiple sclerosis. J Neurol Sci 112:51–57, 1992.

509. Pozzilli C, Passafiume D, Bernardi S, et al: SPECT, MRI and cognitive functions in multiple sclerosis. J Neurol Neurosurg Psychiatry 54:110–115, 1991.

510. Prineas JW: The neuropathology of multiple sclerosis. In Koetsier JC (ed): Handbook of Clinical Neurology. Vol. 45. Elsevier, Amsterdam, 1985, pp 213–257.

511. Rao SM: Neuropsychology of multiple sclerosis: A critical review. J Clin Exp Neuropsychol 8:503–542, 1986.

512. Redekop WK: Prognosis in Multiple Sclerosis: The predictors and prediction of specified functional impairments. Dissertation. University of British Columbia, Vancouver, 1995.

513. Redekop WK, Studney DR, Farquhar RE, and Paty DW: Achieving standardization to support data pooling. In Lun KC, Degoulet P, Piemme TE, Rienhoff O (eds): MEDINFO 92. Amsterdam: Elsevier Science Publishers, 860–865, 1992.

514. Reder AT, and Lowy MT: Interferon-beta treatment does not elevate cortisol in multiple sclerosis. Journal of Interferon Research 12:195–198, 1992.

515. Reinherz EL, Weiner HL, Hauser SL, Cohen JA, Distaso JA, and Schlossman SF: Loss of suppressor T cells in active multiple sclerosis. Analysis with monoclonal antibodies. N Engl J Med 303:125–129, 1980.

516. Reischies FM, Baum K, Bräu H, Hedde JP, and Schwindt G: Cerebral magnetic resonance imaging findings in multiple sclerosis. Arch Neurol 45:1114–1116, 1988.

516a. Revel M, Chebath J, Mangelus M, Harroch S, and Moviglia GA: Antagonism of interferon beta on interferon gamma: inhibition of signal transduction in vitro and reduction of serum levels in multiple sclerosis patients. Multiple Sclerosis 1:S5–S11, 1995.

517. Revesz T, Kidd D, Thomspon AJ, Barnard RO, and McDonald WI: A comparison of the pathology of primary and secondary progressive multiple sclerosis. Brain 117:759–765, 1994.

518. Rice GPA, Casali P, Merigan TC, and Oldstone MBA: Natural killer cell activity in patients with multiple sclerosis given alpha interferon. Ann Neurol 14:333–338, 1983.

519. Rice GPA, Finney D, Braheny SL, Knobler RL, Sipe JC, and Oldstone MBA: Disease activity markers in multiple sclerosis: Another look at suppressor cells defined by monoclonal antibodies OKT4, OKT5 and OKT8. J Neuroimmunmol 6:75–84, 1984.

520. Richards TL: Proton MR spectroscopy in Multiple Sclerosis: Value in establishing diagnosis, monitoring progression, and evaluating therapy. AJR 157:1073–1078, 1991.

521. Rieckmann P, Martin S, Albrecht M, Michel U, and MS Research Group *Department of Neurology: Soluble adhesion molecules in MS: Indicator for relapse and new therapeutic perspectives. 10th Congress of the European Committee for Treatment and Research in Multiple Sclerosis, Book of Abstracts. Athens, Greece, 1994, p 33.

522. Rieckmann P, Martin S, Weichselbraun I, et al: Serial analysis of circulating adhesion molecules and TNF receptor in serum from patients with multiple sclerosis: ICAM-1 is an indicator for relapse. Neurology 44:2367–2372, 1994.

523. Ring J, Angstwurm H, Mertin J, Backmund H, Brendel W, Seifert J, Frick E, Brass B, and Lob G: Pilot study with antilymphocyte globulin in the treatment of multiple sclerosis. Postgrad Med J 52(suppl 5):123–128, 1976.

524. Ring J, Lob G, Angstwurm H, et al: Intensive immunosuppression in the treatment of multiple sclerosis. The Lancet 7889:1093–1096, 1974.

525. Rodriguez M, Karnes WE, Bartleson JD, and Peneda AA: Plasmapheresis in acute episodes of fulminant CNS inflammatory demyelination. Neurology 43:1100–1104, 1993.

526. Rodriguez M, Lennon VA, Benveniste EN, and Merrill JE: Remyelination by oligodendrocytes stimulated by antiserum to spinal cord. J Neuropathol Exp Neurol 46:84–95, 1987.

527. Rodriguez M, and Lennon VA: Immunoglobulins promote remyelination in the central nervous system. Ann Neurol 27:12–17, 1990.

528. Rodriguez M, and Lindsley MD: Immunosuppression promotes CNS remyelination in chronic virus-induced demyelinating disease. Neurology 42:348–358, 1992.

528a. Rodriquez M, Miller DJ, Lennon VA: Immunoglobulins reactive with mylelin basic protein promote CNS remyelination. Neurology 46:538–545, 1996.

529. Rohrbach E, Kappos L, Stadt D, Kaiser D, Hennes A, Domasch D, and Mertens HG: Intrathecal versus oral corticosteroid therapy of spinal symptoms in multiple sclerosis: A double-blind controlled trial. Neurology 38:256, 1988.

530. Romijn JA, van Lieshout JJ, and Velis DN: Reversible coma due to intrathecal baclofen. Lancet 2:696, 1986.

531. Romine JS, Salk J, Wiederholt WC, Westall FC, and Jablecki CK: Preliminary phase studies of myelin basic protein in multiple sclerosis: II Clinical observations. Neurology 29:572, 1979.

532. Ron M, and Feinstein A: Multiple sclerosis and the mind. J Neurol Neurosurg Psychiatry 55:1–3, 1992.

533. Rose AS, Kuzuma JW, Kurtzke JF, Namerow NS, Sibley WA, and Tourtellotte WW: Cooperative study in the evaluation of therapy in multiple sclerosis: ACTH vs. placebo. Final Report. 20:1–59, 1970.

534. Rose J, Klein H, Greenstein J, McFarlin D, Gerber L, and McFarland H: Lymphocytapheresis in chronic progressive multiple sclerosis: Results of a preliminary trial. Ann Neurol 14:593–594, 1983.

535. Rosen JA: Prolonged azathioprine treatment of non-remitting multiple sclerosis. J Neurol Neurosurg Psychiatry 42:338–344, 1979.

536. Rosen JA: Hyperbaric oxygenation does not improve chronic progressive multiple sclerosis. Ann Neurol 17:615, 1985.

537. Rosenberg GA, and Appenzeller O: Amantadine, fatigue, and multiple sclerosis. Arch Neurol 45:1104–1106, 1988.

538. Rosengren LE, Lycke J, and Andersen O: Glial fibrillary acidic protein in CSF of multiple sclerosis patients: Relation to neurological deficit. J Neurol Sci 133:61–65, 1995.

539. Rudge P, Koetsier JC, Mertin J, et al: Randomized double blind controlled trial of cyclosporin in multiple sclerosis. J Neurol Neurosurg Psychiatry 52:559–565, 1989.

540. Rudick RA, Carpenter CS, Cookfair DL, Tuohy VK, and Ransohoff RM: In vitro and in vivo inhibition of mitogen-driven T-cell activation by recombinant interferon beta. Neurology 43:2080, 1993.

540a. Rudick R, Antel J, Confavreux C, Cutter G, Ellison G, Fischer J, Lublin F, et al: Clinical outcomes assessment in multiple sclerosis. Ann Neurol 49:469–479, 1996.

541. Rudick RA, and Goodkin DE: Treatment of Multiple Sclerosis: Trial Design, Results, and Future Perspectives. Springer-Verlag, London, 1992.

542. Rudick RA, Medendorp S, Namey M, Boyle S, and Fischer J: CSF free kappa light chains predict subsequent physical deterioration in prospectively followed multiple sclerosis (MS) patients. Neurology 44(suppl 2):A393, 1994.

542a. Rudick RA, Ransohoff RM, Peppler R, Mendendorp SV, Lehmann P, and Alam J: Interferon beta induces interleukin-10 expression: relevance to multiple sclerosis. Ann Neurol 40:618–627, 1996.

543. Rudick RA, Shasin CA, and VanderBrug-Mendendorp S: Clinical significance of upper extremity impairment in multiple sclerosis patients. Paper presented at the 119th Annual Meeting of the American Neurological Association, San Francisco, October 1994. Ann Neurol 36:290, 1994.

543a. Rumbach L, Racadot E, Armspach JP, et al: Biological assessment and MRI monitoring of the therapeutic efficacy of a monoclonal anti-T CD4 antibody in multiple sclerosis patients. Multiple Sclerosis 1:207–212, 1996.

543b. Ryan L, Clark CM, Klonoff H, Li D, and Paty D: Patterns of cognitive impairment in relapsing-remitting multiple sclerosis and their relationship to neuropathology on magnetic resonance images. Neuropsychology 10:176–193, 1996.

544. Sabouraud O, Oger G, Darcel F, Madigand M, and Merienne M: Long-term immunosuppression in multiple sclerosis: Evaluation of treatments begun before 1972. Rev Neurol (Paris) 140:125–130, 1984.

545. Sabra AF, Hallett M, Sudarsky L, and Mullally W: Treatment of action tremor in multiple sclerosis with isoniazid. Neurology 32:912–913, 1982.

546. Sacks HS, Berrier J, Reitman D, Ancona-Berk VA, and Chalmers TC: Meta-analyses of randomized controlled trials. N Engl J Med 1987.

547. Sadovnick AD, and Baird PA: The familial nature of multiple sclerosis: Age-corrected empiric recurrence risks of children and siblings of patients. Neurology 38:990–991, 1988.

548. Sadovnick AD, Ebers GC, Eisen KA, and Paty DW: Cause of death in patients attending multiple sclerosis clinics. Neurology 41:1193–1196, 1991.

549. Sadovnick AD, Eisen KA, Hashimoto SA, et al: Multiple sclerosis and pregnancy: A prospective study. Arch Neurol 51:1120–1124, 1994.

550. Sadovnick AD, and Macleod PM: The familial incidence of multiple sclerosis: Empiric recurrence risks for first, second and third degree relatives of patients. Neurology 31:1039–1041, 1981.

550a. Satoh J, Paty DWP, and Kim SU: Counteracting effect of IFN-β on IFN-γ-induced proliferation of human astrocytes in culture. Multiple Sclerosis 1:279–287, 1996.

551. Schapira K, Poskanzer DC, Newell DJ, and Miller H: Marriage, pregnancy and multiple sclerosis. Brain 89:419–428, 1966.

552. Schapiro RT: Management and MS: A Rehabilitation Approach. Demos Publication, New York, 1991.

553. Schapiro RT, and Langer SL: Symptomatic therapy of multiple sclerosis. Curr Opin Neurol 7:229–233, 1994.

554. Schauf CL, and Davis FA: The occurrence, specificity, and role of neuroelectric blocking factors in multiple sclerosis. Neurology 28(pt 2):34–39, 1978.

555. Scheinberg LC: Multiple Sclerosis: A Guide for Patients and Their Families (ed 2). Raven Press, New York, 1987.

556. Schiffer RB, Herndon RM, and Rudick RA: Treatment of pathologic laughing and weeping with amitriptyline. N Engl J Med 312:1480–1482, 1985.

557. Schmidt B, Stoll G, van Der Meide P, Jung S, and Hartung HP: Transient cellular expression of γ-interferon in myelin-induced and γ-cell line-mediated experimental autoimmune neuritis. Brain 115:1633—1646, 1992.

558. Schreiber SL, and Crabtree GR: The mechanism of action of cyclosporin A and FK506. Immunol Today 13:136–142, 1992.

559. Sechi GP, Zuddas M, Piredda M, et al: Treatment of cerebellar tremors with carbamazepine: A controlled trial with long-term follow-up. Neurology 39:1113–1115, 1989.

560. Seland TP, McPherson TA, Grace M, Lamoureux G, and Blain JG: Evaluation of antithymocyte globulin in acute relapses of multiple sclerosis. Neurology 24:34–40, 1974.

561. Selmaj K, Alam R, Perkin GD, and Rose FC: T lymphocyte-derived demyelinating activity in multiple sclerosis patients in relapse. J Neurol Neurosurg Psychiatry 50:532–537, 1987.

562. Semmlow JL, and Lubowsky J: Sexual instrumentation. IEEE Trans Biomed Eng 30:309–319, 1983.

563. Shafey H: The effect of fluoxetine in depression associated with multiple sclerosis (letters). Clinical Journal Psychiatry 37:2:147–148, 1990.

564. Shakir S, Byskosh PV, and Reder AT: Interferon-β induces interleukin-10 MRNA in mononuclear cells (MNC). Neurology 44(suppl 2):A211, 1994.

565. Sharief MK, Phil M, and Hentges R: Association between tumor necrosis factor-α and disease progression in patients with multiple sclerosis. N Engl J Med 325:467–472, 1991.

566. Sharief MK, Phil M, and Thompson EJ: Correlation of interleukin-2 and soluble interleukin-2 receptor with clinical activity of multiple sclerosis. J Neurol Neurosurg Psychiatry 56:169–174, 1993.

566a. Sharrack B, and Hughes RAC: Clinical scales for multiple sclerosis. (Review article). J Neurological Sciences 135:1–9, 1996.

567. Sibley WA: Drug treatment of multiple sclerosis. Handbook of Clinical Neurology. Vol. 45. Amsterdam Demyelinating Disease. 1985, p 383.

568. Sibley WA: International Federation of Multiple Sclerosis Societies: Therapeutic claims in multiple sclerosis. Demos Publications, New York, 1993.

569. Sibley WA, Bamford CR, and Clark K: Clinical viral infections and multiple sclerosis. Lancet 1313–1315, 1985.

570. Sibley WA, Bamford CR, Clark K, Smith MS, and Laguna JF: A prospective study of physical trauma and multiple sclerosis. J Neurol Neurosurg Psychiatry 54:584–589, 1991.

571. Sibley WA, Ebers GC, Panitch HS, and Reder AT: Interferon beta treatment of multiple sclerosis (reply from the authors). Neurology 44:188–190, 1994.

572. Sigal NH, and Dumont FJ: Cyclosporin A, FK-506, and Rapamycin: pharmacologic probes of lymphocyte signal transduction. Annu Rev Immunol 10:519–560, 1992.

573. Silberberg D, Lisak R, and Zweiman B: Multiple sclerosis unaffected by azathioprine in pilot study. Arch Neurol 28:210–212, 1973.

574. Simon LT, Hsu B, and Adornato BT: Carbamazepine-induced aseptic meningitis. Ann Intern Med 112:627–628, 1990.

575. Sipe JC, Knobler RL, Braheny SL, Rice GPA, Panitch HS, and Oldstone MBA: A neurologic rating scale (NRS) for use in multiple sclerosis. Neurology 34:1368–1372, 1984.

576. Sipe JC, Romine J, Zyroff J, Koziol J, McMillan R, and Beutler E: Cladribine favorably alters the clinical course of progressive multiple sclerosis (MS). Neurology 44(suppl 2):A357, 1994.

576a. Sipe JC, Romine JS, Koziol JA, McMillan R, Zyroff J, and Beutler E: Cladribine in treatment of chronic progressive multiple sclerosis. The Lancet 344:9–13, 1994.

577. Slater RJ: Criteria and uses of the minimal record of disability in multiple sclerosis. Acta Neurol Scand Suppl 101:16–20, 1984.

578. Smith C, Birnbaum G, Carter JL, Greenstein J, Lublin FD, and the US Tizanidine Study Group: Tizanidine treatment of spasticity caused by multiple sclerosis: Results of a double-blind, placebo-controlled trial. Neurology 44 (suppl 9):S34-S43, 1994.

579. Smith CR: Encephalomyelopathy as an idiosyncratic reaction to carbamazepine: A case report. Neurology 41:760–761, 1991.

580. Smith CR, Aisen ML, and Scheinberg LC: Symptomatic management of multiple sclerosis. Multiple Sclerosis. Butterworth's International Medical Reviews. 1986, Ch 10.

581. Smith CR, LaRocca NG, Giesser BS, and Scheinberg LC: High-dose oral baclofen: Experience in patients with multiple sclerosis. Neurology 41:1829–1831, 1991.

581a. Smith DR, Balachov K, Halfer DA, Khoury SJ, and Weiner HL: Beta-interferon increases anti-CD3-induced IL-4 production in multiple sclerosis patients. Neurology 46:A164–A165, 1996.

582. Smith ME, Martin R, Frank JA, Harris JO, Patronas N, and McFarlin DE/HF: Gadolinium-enhanced magnetic resonance imaging and its correlation with expanded disability status score in multiple sclerosis. Ann Neurol 30:270, 1991.

583. Smith ME, Stone LA, Albert PS, et al: Clinical worsening in multiple sclerosis is associated with increased frequency and area of gadopentetate dimeglumine-enhancing magnetic resonance imaging lesions. Ann Neurol 33:480–489, 1993.

584. Smith T, Zeeberg I, and Sjo O: Evoked potentials in multiple sclerosis before and after high-dose methylprednisolone infusion. Eur Neurol 25:67, 1986.

585. Smits RCF, Emmen HH, Bertelsmann FW, Kulig BM, van Loenen AC, and Polman CH: The effects of 4-aminopyridine on cognitive function in patients with multiple sclerosis: A pilot study. Neurology 44:1701–1705, 1994.

586. Snow BJ, Tsui JK, Bhatt MH, Varelas M, Hashimoto SA, and Calne DB: Treatment of spasticity with botulinum toxin: a double-blind study. Ann Neurol 28:512–515, 1990.

586a. Sorensen PS, Wanscher B, Szpirt W, et al: Plasma exchange combined with azathioprine in multiple sclerosis using serial gadolinium-enhanced MRI to monitor disease activity: A randomized single-masked cross-over pilot study. Neurology 46:1620–1625, 1996.

587. Spackman AJ, Doulton DC, Roberts MHW, Martin JP, and McLellan DL: Caring at night for people with multiple sclerosis. BMJ 299:1433, 1989.

588. Stamm WE, and Hooton TM: Managment of urinary tract infections in adults. N Engl J Med 1328–1334, 1993.

588a. Starr NJ, Likosky WH, Wilson SR, and Hayes BW: Improved quality of life outcomes in multiple sclerosis (MS) patients after participation in the "Coping with MS effectively" program. Neurology 46:A427, 1996.

589. Stefoski D, Davis FA, Fitzsimmons WE, Luskin SS, Rush J, and Parkhurst GW: 4-Aminopyridine in multiple sclerosis: Prolonged administration. Neurology 41:1344–1348, 1991.

590. Stefoski D, Davis FA, and Schauf CL: Acute improvement in exacerbating multiple sclerosis produced by intravenous administration of mannitol. Ann Neurol 18:443–450, 1985.

591. Stenager E, Stenager EN, and Jensen K: Sexual aspects of multiple sclerosis. Semin Neurol 12:120–124, 1992.

592. Stenager E, Stenager EN, and Jensen K: Sexual function in multiple sclerosis: A 5-year follow-up study. 10th Congress of the European Committee for Treatment and Research in Multiple Sclerosis, Book of Abstracts. Athens, Greece, 1994, p 18.

593. Stewart WA: Proton Spin Relaxation as a Means of Characterizing the Pathology of multiple sclerosis. Dissertation. University of British Columbia, Vancouver, British Columbia, Canada, 1989.

594. Stewart WA: Spin-spin relaxation in experimental allergic encephalomyelitis: Analysis of CPMG data using a non-linear least squares method and linear inverse theory. Magn Reson Med 29:767–775, 1993.

595. Stewart WA, Alvord EC, Hruby S, Hall LD, and Paty DW: Early detection of experimental allergic encephalomyelitis by magnetic resonance imaging. Lancet 2:898, 1985.

596. Stewart WA, Alvord EC Jr: Magnetic resonance imaging of experimental allergic encephalomyelitis in primates. Brain 114:1069–1096, 1991.

597. Stewart WA, Hall LD, Berry K, and Paty DW: Correlation between NMR scan and brain slice: Data in multiple sclerosis. Lancet 2:412, 1984.

598. Stewart WA, Whittall KP, and Paty DW: Analysis of CPMG data from CNS tissue: A potential method for detecting demyelination in multiple sclerosis. Society of Magnetic Resonance in Medicine, 10th Annual Meeting, Washington, D.C., Book of Abstracts. Vol 1. 1989, p 85.

599. Stiller CR, Dupre J, and Gent M: Effects of cyclosporine immunosuppression in insulin-dependent diabetes mellitus of recent onset. Science 223:1362–1367, 1984.

600. Stommel EW: Carbamazepine encephalopathy (letter). Neurology 42:705, 1992.

601. Stone LA, DeCarli C, Smith ME, Albert PS, Frank J, and McFarland HF: Quantitation of white matter hyperintensity on magnetic resonance imaging in multiple sclerosis over two years. Paper presented at the 119th Annual Meeting of the American Neurological Association, San Francisco, October 1994. Ann Neurol 36:292, 1994.

602. Stone LA, Frank JA, Albert PS, et al: The effect of interferon-b on blood brain barrier disruptions demonstrated by contrast enhanced magnetic resonance imaging in relapsing-remitting multiple sclerosis. Ann Neurol 37:611–619, 1995.

602a. Stone LA, Smith ME, Albert PS, et al: Blood-brain barrier disruption on contrast-enhanced MRI in patients with mild relapsing-remitting multiple sclerosis: Relationship to course, gender, and age. Neurology 45:1122–1126, 1995.

603. Stone LA, Smith ME, Frank JA, et al: Incidence of contrast enhancement on MRI over time in MS patients. Neurology 44(suppl 2):A391, 1994.

604. Studney DR, Lublin F, Marcucci L, et al: MS COSTAR: A computerized record for use in clinical research in multiple sclerosis. Journal of Neurologic Rehabilitation 7:145–152, 1993.

605. Swank RL, and Dugan BB: Effect of low saturated fat diet in early and late cases of multiple sclerosis. Lancet 336:37–39, 1990.

606. Swinburn WR, and Liversedge LA: Long-term treatment of multiple sclerosis with azathioprine. J Neurol Neurosurg Psychiatry 36:124–126, 1973.

607. Swirsky-Sacchetti T, Mitchell DR, et al: Neuropsychological and structural brain lesions in multiple sclerosis: A regional analysis. Neurology 42:1291–1295, 1992.

608. Syndulko K, Tourtellotte WW, Baumhefner RW, et al: Neuroperformance evaluation of multiple sclerosis disease progression in a clinical trial: Implications for neurological outcome measurement. Journal of Neurologic Rehabilitation 7(3–4):153, 1993.

608a. Syndulko K, Ke D, Ellison GW, et al: Comparative evaluations of neuroperformance and clinical outcome assessments in chronic progressive multiple sclerosis: I. Reliability, validity and sensitivity to disease progression. Multiple Sclerosis 2:142–156, 1996.

609. Szasz G, Paty DW, and Maurice WL: Sexual dysfunctions in multiple sclerosis. Ann NY Acad Sci 436:443–452, 1984.

610. Teitelbaum D, Meshorer A, Hirshfeld T, Arnon R, and Sela M: Suppression of experimental allergic encephalomyelitis by a synthetic polypeptide. Eur J Immunol 1:242, 1971.

611. Teitelbaum D, Webb C, Meshorer A, Arnon R, and Sela M: Suppression by several synthetic polypeptides of experimental allergic encephaloymyelitis induced in guinea pigs and rabbits with bovine and human basic encephalitogen. Eur J Immunol 3:273–279, 1973.

612. Tenser RB, Hay KA, and Aberg JA: Immunoglobulin G immunosuppression of multiple sclerosis: Suppression of all three major lymphocyte subsets. Arch Neurol 50:417–420, 1993.

612a. Therapeutics and Technology Assessment Subcommittee: Assessment: Neurological evaluation of male sexual dysfunction. Neurology 45:2287–2292, 1995.

613. Theriot KO, and Brar S: Rehabilitation and physical therapy outcomes in multiple sclerosis. Journal of Neurologic Rehabilitation 7(3–4):139, 1993.

614. Theys P, Gosseye-Lissoir F, Ketelaer P, and Carton H: Short-term intensive cyclophosphamide treatment in multiple sclerosis: A retrospective controlled study. J Neurol 225:119–133, 1981.

615. Thompson AJ, Kennard C, Swash M, et al: Relative efficacy of intravenous methylprednisolone and ACTH in the treatment of acute relapse in MS. Neurology 39:969–971, 1989.
616. Thompson AJ, Kermode AG, MacManus DG, et al: Patterns of disease activity in multiple sclerosis: Clinical and magnetic resonance imaging study. BMJ 300:631–634, 1990.
617. Thompson AJ, Kermode AG, Wicks D, et al: Major differences in the dynamics of primary and secondary progressive multiple sclerosis. Ann Neurol 29:53–62, 1991.
618. Thomson AW: FK-506 enters the clinic. Immunol Today 11:35–36, 1990.
618a. Thorpe JW, Barker GJ, Jones SJ, et al: Magnetization transfer ratios and tranverse magnetization decay curves in optic neuritis: Correlation with clinical findings and electrophysiology. J Neurol Neurosurg Psychiatry 59:487–492, 1995.
619. Thorpe JW, Halpin SF, Barker GJ, et al: A comparison of fast spin echo and conventional spin echo in multiple sclerosis. Proceedings of the Society of Magnetic Resonance in Medicine, New York, 1993, p 325.
620. Thorpe JW, Kidd D, Kendall BE, et al: Spinal cord MRI using multi-array coils and fast spin echo. I. Technical aspects and findings in healthy adults. Neurology 43:2625–2631, 1993.
620a. Thorpe JW, Kidd D, Moseley IF, et al: Serial gadolinium-enhanced MRI of the brain and spinal cord in early relapsing-remitting multiple sclerosis. Neurology 46:373–378, 1996.
621. Tienari PJ, Salonen O, Wikström J, Valanne L, and Palo J: Familial multiple sclerosis: MRI findings in clinically affected and unaffected siblings. J Neurol Neurosurg Psychiatry 55:883–886, 1992.
622. Tindall RSA, Walker JE, Ehle AL, Near L, Rollins J, and Becker D: Plasmapheresis in multiple sclerosis: Prospective trial of pheresis and immunosuppression versus immunosuppression alone. Neurology 32:739–743, 1982.
623. Tofts PS, Wicks DAG, and Barker GJ: The MRI measurement of NMR and physiological parameters in tissue to study disease process. Prog Clin Biol Res 363:313–325, 1991.
624. Tourtellotte WW, Baumhefner RW, Potvin AR, et al: Multiple sclerosis de novo CNS IgG synthesis: Effect of ACTH and corticosteroids. Neurology 30:1155–1162, 1980.
625. Tourtellotte WW, Walsh MJ, Baumhefner RW, Staugaitis SM, and Shapshak P: The current status of multiple sclerosis intra-blood-brain IgG synthesis. Ann NY Acad Sci 436:52–67, 1984.
626. Trinchieri G, and Scott P: The role of interleukin 12 in the immune response, disease and therapy. Immunology Today 15:460–463, 1994.
627. Troiano RA, Hafstein M, Ruderman M, Dowling PC, and Cook SD: Effect of high-dose intravenous steroid administration on contrast-enhancing computed tomographic scan lesions in multiple sclerosis. Ann Neurol 15:257–263, 1984.
628. Troiano RA, Jotkowitz A, Cook SD, Bansil S, and Zito G: Rate and types of fractures in corticosteroid-treated multiple sclerosis patients. Neurology 42:1389–1391, 1992.

629. Trotter JL, Clifford DB, Montgomery EB, and Ferguson TB: Thymectomy in multiple sclerosis: A 3-year follow up. Neurology 35:1049–1051, 1985.
630. Trotter JL, and Garvey WF: Prolonged effects of large dose methylprednisolone infusion in multiple sclerosis. Neurology (Minneapolis) 30:702–708, 1980.
631. Trotter JL, Gebel HM, Ferguson TB, Garvey WF, and Rodey GE: Thymectomy-induced decrease in T gamma cells and OKT8+ cells in multiple sclerosis. Ann Neurol 14:656–661, 1983.
632. Truyen L, Gheuens J, Van de Vyver FL, Parizel PM, Peersman GB, and Martin JJ: Improved correlation of magnetic resonance imaging (MRI) with clinical status in multiple sclerosis (MS) by use of an extensive standardized imaging-protocol. J Neurol Sci 96:173–182, 1990.
632a. Truyen L, van Waesberghe JHTM, van Walderveen MAA, et al: Accumulation of hypointense lesions ("black holes") on T_1 spin-echo MRI correlates with disease progression in multiple sclerosis. Neurology 47:1469–1476, 1996.
633. Uitdehaag BM, Polman CH, de Groot CJ, Huitinga I, and Dijkstra CD: Failure of sulfasalazine to influence experimental autoimmune encephalomyelitis (letter). Acta Neurol Scand 84:173–174, 1991.
634. United Kingdom Tizanidine Trial Group: A double-blind, placebo-controlled trial of tizanidine in the treatment of spasticity caused by multiple sclerosis. Neurology 44(suppl 9):S70–S78, 1994.
635. Valbonesi M, and Garelli S: Plasma exchange in neurological diseases. A critical approach. Vox Sang (review) 44:65–80, 1983.
636. Valbonesi M, Garelli S, Montani F, et al: Plasma-exchange in neurological diseases. Ricerca in Clinica e in Laboratorio 13:75–84, 1983.
636a. Valiquette G, Herbert J, and Meade-D'Alisera P: Desmopressin in the management of nocturia in patients with multiple sclerosis. Arch Neurol 53:1270–1275, 1996.
637. Van Diemen HA, van Dongen MM, Dammers JW, and Polman CH: Increased visual impairment after exercise (Uhthoff's phenomenon) in multiple sclerosis: Therapeutic possibilities. Eur Neurol 32:231–234, 1992.
638. Van Engelen BGM, Hommes OR, Pinckers A, Cruysberg JRM, Barkhof F, and Rodriguez M: Improved vision after intravenous immunoglobulin in stable demyelinating optic neuritis. Ann Neurol 32:834–835, 1992.
639. Van Haver H, Lissoir F, Droissart C, et al: Transfer factor therapy in multiple sclerosis: A three-year prospective double-blind clinical trial. Neurology 36:1399–1402, 1986.
639a. van Oosten BW, Barkhof F, Truyen L, et al: Increased MRI activity and immune activation in two multiple sclerosis patients treated with the monoclonal anti-tumor necrosis factor antibody cA2. Neurology 47:1531–1534, 1996.
640. Van Walderveen MMA, Barkhof F, Hommes OR, et al: Correlating MRI and clinical disease activity in multiple sclerosis: Relevance of hypointense lesions on short-TR/short-TE (T_1

weighted) spin-echo images. Neurology 45: 1684–1690, 1995.

641. Vandenbark AA, Chou YK, Bourdette DN, Whitham R, Hashim GA, and Offner H: T cell receptor peptide therapy for autoimmune disease. J Autoimmun 5(suppl A):83–92, 1992.

641a. Vandenbark AA, Chou YK, Whitham R, et al: Treatment of multiple sclerosis with T-cell receptor peptides: results of a double-blind pilot trial. Nature Medicine 2:1109–1115, 1996.

642. Vass K, Heininger K, Schafer B, Linington C, and Lassmann H: Interferon-γ potentiates antibody-mediated demyelination in vivo. Ann Neurol 32:198–206, 1992.

642a. Vercoulen JHMM, Hommes OR, Swanink CMA, et al: The measurement of fatigue in patients with multiple sclerosis: a multidimensional comparison with patients with chronic fatigue syndrome and healthy subjects. Arch Neurol 53: 642–649, 1996.

643. Verdier-Taillefer MH, Zuber M, Lyon-Caen O, et al: Observer disagreement in rating neurologic impairment in multiple sclerosis: facts and consequences. Eur Neurol 31:117–119, 1991.

644. Walker JE, Hoehn MM, and Kashiwagi N: A trial of antilymphocyte globulin in the treatment of chronic progressive multiple sclerosis. J Neurol Sci 29:303–309, 1976.

645. Warren KG, and Catz I: Myelin antigen-specific forms of multiple sclerosis. Neurology 44 (suppl 2):A300, 1994(a).

646. Warren KG, and Catz I: Relative frequency of autoantibodies to myelin basic protein and proteolipid protein in optic neuritis and multiple sclerosis cerebrospinal fluid. J Neurol Sci 121:66–73, 1994(b).

646a. Warren KG, and Catz I: Administration of myelin basic protein synthetic peptides to multiple sclerosis patients. Journal of the Neurological Sciences 133:85–94, 1995.

647. Warren KG, and Catz I: A correlation between cerebrospinal fluid myelin basic protein and anti-myelin basic protein in multiple sclerosis patients. Ann Neurol 21:183–189, 1987.

648. Warren KG, Catz I, Jeffrey VM, and Carroll DJ: Effect of methylprednisolone on CSF IgG parameters, myelin basic protein and anti-myelin basic protein in multiple sclerosis exacerbations. Can J Neurol Sci 13:25–30, 1986.

649. Warren SA, Warren KG, Greenhill S, and Paterson M: How multiple sclerosis is related to animal illness, stress and diabetes? Can Med Assoc J 126:377–385, 1982.

650. Washington R, Burton J, Todd R III, Newman W, Dragovic L, and Dore-Duffy P: Expression of immunologically relevant endothelial cell activation antigens on isolated central nervous system microvessels from patients with multiple sclerosis. Ann Neurol 35:89–97, 1994.

651. Waubant E, Leppert D, and Hauser SL: Inhibition of T lymphocyte migration through subendothelial basement membrane by inhibiting two collangenases secreted by these lymphocytes (abstract). J Neurol 241(suppl 1):S28, 1994.

651a. Weiner HL: Correlation of magnetic resonance imaging with immune and clinical measures in 45 MS patients receiving 20–24 MRI scans each over a one year period. Works in Progress for Expedited Presentation, WIP 1. Washington, D.C. National Institute of Health, 1995, NIH publication N01-NS-0–2397.

652. Weiner HL, Dau PC, and Kharti BO, et al: Double-blind study of true vs. sham plasma exchange in patients treated with immunosuppression for acute attacks of multiple sclerosis. Neurology 39:1143–1149, 1989.

653. Weiner HL, and Dawson DM: Plasmapheresis in multiple sclerosis: Preliminary study. Neurology 30:1029–1033, 1980.

654. Weiner HL, Fallis RJ, Aoun M, and Hafler DA: Immunologic effects in progressive MS patients treated with anti-T11 and anti-T4 monoclonal antibodies. Neurology 36(suppl 1):284, 1986.

655. Weiner HL, Mackin GA, Matsui M, et al: Double-blind pilot trial of oral tolerization with myelin antigens in multiple sclerosis. Science 259: 1321–1324, 1993.

656. Weiner HL, Mackin GA, Orav EJ, et al: Intermittent cyslophosphamide pulse therapy in progressive multiple sclerosis: Final report of the Northeast Cooperative Multiple Sclerosis Treatment Group. Neurology 43: 910–918, 1993.

657. Weiner HL, and Paty DW: Diagnostic and therapeutic trials in multiple sclerosis: A new look: Summary of Jekyll Island Workshop. Neurology 39:972–976, 1989.

658. Weinshenker BG, Bass B, Karlik S, Ebers GC, and Rice GPA: An open trial of OKT3 in patients with multiple sclerosis. Neurology 41: 1047–1052, 1991.

659. Weinshenker BG, Bass B, Rice GPA, et al: The natural history of multiple sclerosis: A geographically based study. I. Clinical course and disability. Brain 112:133–146, 1989.

660. Weinshenker BG, Carriere W, Baskerville J, and Ebers GC: The natural history of multiple sclerosis: A geographically based study. IV. Applications to planning and interpretation of clinical therapeutic trials. Brain 114:1057–1060, 1991.

661. Weinshenker BG, and Ebers GC: The natural history of multiple sclerosis. Can J Neurol Sci 14:255–261, 1987.

661a. Weinshenker BG, Issa M, and Baskerville J: Meta-analysis of the placebo-treated groups in clinical trials of progressive MS. Neurology 46:1613–1619, 1996.

661b. Weinshenker BG, Issa M, and Baskerville J: Long-term and short-term outcome of multiple sclerosis. A 3-year follow-up study. Arch Neurol 53:353–358, 1996.

662. Weinshenker BG, Penman M, Bass B, Ebers GC, and Rice GPA: A double-blind, randomized, crossover trial of pemoline in fatigue associated with multiple sclerosis. Neurology 42:1468–1471, 1992.

663. Weinshenker BG, and Sibley WA: Natural history and treatment of multiple sclerosis. Current Opinion in Neurology and Neurosurgery 5:203–211, 1992.

664. Weinstock-Gutmann B, Ransohoff RM, Philip-Kinkel R, and Rudick RA: The Interferons: Biological effects, mechanisms of action, and use in

multiple sclerosis. Ann Neurol 37:7–15, 1995.

665. Weiss W, and Stadlan EM: Design and statistical issues related to testing experimental therapy in multiple sclerosis. In Rudick RA, and Goodkin DE (eds): Treatment of Multiple Sclerosis: Trial Design, Results, and Future Perspectives. Springer-Verlag, New York, 1992, pp 91–122.

666. Whitaker JN: Indicators of disease activity in multiple sclerosis: Studies of myelin basic protein-like materials. Ann NY Acad Sci 436:140–150, 1984.

667. Whitaker JN: Expanded clinical trials of treatments for multiple sclerosis: The Advisory Committee Clinical Trials of New Agents in Multiple Sclerosis of the National MS Society. Ann Neurol 34:755–756, 1993.

668. Whitaker JN: Rationale for immunotherapy in multiple sclerosis (review). Ann Neurol 36 (suppl):S103-S107, 1994.

669. Whitaker JN, Kachelhofu RD, Bradley EL, Burgard S, et al: Urinary myelin basic protein-like material as a correlate of the progressive phase of multiple sclerosis. Ann Neurol 38:625–632, 1995.

670. Whitaker JN, Layton BA, Herman P, Burgard S, and Bartolucci AA: The level of cerebrospinal fluid myelin basic protein-like material in patients with multiple sclerosis as a predictor of the response to glucocorticoids. Ann Neurol 30:304, 1991.

671. Whitaker JN, McFarland HF, Rudge P, and Reingold SC: Outcomes assessment in multiple sclerosis clinical trials: A critical analysis. Multiple Sclerosis 1995.

672. Whitaker JN, and Mitchell GW: Experimental allergic encephalomyelitis as a guide to the understanding and treatment of multiple sclerosis (editorial). Ann Neurol 34:636–637, 1993.

673. Whitaker JN, Mitchell GW, and Cutter GR: Clinical outcomes and documentation of partial beneficial effects of immunotherapy for multiple sclerosis. Ann Neurol 37:5–6, 1995.

674. Whitaker JN, Williams PH, Layton BA, et al: Correlation of clinical features and findings on cranial magnetic resonance imaging with urinary myelin basic protein-like material in patients with multiple sclerosis. Ann Neurol 35:577–585, 1994.

675. Whitham RH, and Bourdette DN: Treatment of multiple sclerosis with high-dose methylprednisolone pulse therapy. Neurology (suppl 1) 39:357, 1989.

676. Whitham RH, Schaumann BA, McClung M, Perry B, Gehling AM, and Bourdette D: Premature osteoporosis in multiple sclerosis: implications for corticosteroid therapy. Neurology (suppl 1) 40:284, 1990.

677. Wicks DAG, Tofts PS, Miller DH, et al: Volume measurement of multiple sclerosis lesions with magnetic resonance images: A preliminary study. Neuroradiology 34:475–479, 1992.

678. Wiebe S, Lee DH, Karlik SJ, et al: Serial cranial and spinal cord magnetic resonance imaging in multiple sclerosis. Ann Neurology 32:643–650, 1992.

679. Wiles CM, Clarke CR, Irwin HP, Edgar EF, and Swan AV: Hyperbaric oxygen in multiple sclerosis: a double blind trial. BMJ 292:367–371, 1986.

680. Wiles CM, Omar L, Swan AV, et al: Total lymphoid irradiation in multiple sclerosis. J Neurol Neurosurg Psychiatry 57:154–163, 1994.

681. Willoughby EW, Grochowski E, Li DKB, Oger J, Kastrukoff LF, and Paty DW: Serial magnetic resonance scanning in multiple sclerosis: A second prospective study in relapsing patients. Ann Neurol 25:43–49, 1989.

682. Willoughby EW, and Paty DW: Scales for rating impairment in multiple sclerosis: A critique. Neurology 38:1793–1798, 1988.

683. Yalaz K, Anlar B, Oktem F, et al: Intraventricular interferon and oral inosiplex in the treatment of subacute sclerosing panencephalitis. Neurology 42(3 pt 1):488, 1992.

684. Yetkin FZ, Haughton VM, Papke RA, Fischer ME, and Rao SM: Multiple sclerosis: Specificity of MR for diagnosis. Radiology 178:447–51, 1991.

685. Yokota T, Matsunaga T, Okiyama R, et al: Sympathetic skin response in patients with multiple sclerosis compared with patients with spinal cord transection and normal controls. Brain 114(pt 3):1381–1394, 1991.

686. Yong VW, Antel JP, and Williams K: In vitro effects of β-interferon on human CNS cells. Neurology 44(suppl 2):A212, 1994.

687. Youl BD, Turano G, Miller DH, et al: The pathophysiology of acute optic neuritis: An association of gadolinium leakage with clinical and electrophysiological deficits. Brain 114:2437–2450, 1991.

688. Yudkin PL, Ellison GW, Ghezzi A, et al: Overview of azathioprine treatment in multiple sclerosis. The Lancet 338:1051–1055, 1991.

689. Zabriskie JB, Mayer L, Fu SM, Yeadon C, Cam V, and Plank C: T-cell subsets in multiple sclerosis: Lack of correlation between helper and suppressor T cells and the clinical state. J Clin Immunol 5:7–12, 1985.

689a. Zajicek J, and Compston A: Mechanisms of damage and repair in multiple sclerosis: A review. Multiple Sclerosis 1:61–72, 1995.

690. Zeeberg IE: Azathioprine assessment in progressive multiple sclerosis. Clinical aspects. In Hommes OR (ed): MS Research in Europe. MTP Press, Lancaster, 1986, pp 61–70. 1986.

690a. Zhao GJ, Koopmans RA, Li DIB, et al: Corticospinal tract lesions in multiple sclerosis: Relationship between MRI activity and clinical course. Neurology 43:A246, 1993.

691. Zimmerman GA, Martin SB, and Tracey KJ: The neuroimmunology of tumour necrosis factor-a. Clin Immunother 1:67–78, 1994.

691a. Zipp F, Weber F, Huber S, et al: Genetic control of multiple sclerosis: increased production of lymphotoxin and tumor necrosis-factor-a by HLA-DR2⁺ T cells. Ann Neurol 38:723–730, 1995.

692. Zoukos Y, Kidd D, Woodroofe MN, Kendall BE, Thompson AJ, and Cuzner ML: Increased expression of high affinity IL-2 receptors and beta-adrenoceptors on peripheral blood mononuclear cells is associated with clinical and MRI activity in multiple sclerosis. Brain 117 (pt 2): 307–315, 1994.

INDEX

ISBN 0-8036-6784-1

90000 >

EAN

9 780803 667846